# Improving Outcomes in
# Colon and Rectal Surgery

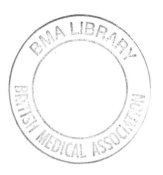

# Improving Outcomes in Colon and Rectal Surgery

Edited by

**Brian R. Kann,** MD, FACS, FASCRS
**David E. Beck,** MD, FACS, FASCRS
**David A. Margolin,** MD, FACS, FASCRS
**H. David Vargas,** MD, FACS, FASCRS
**Charles B. Whitlow,** MD, FACS, FASCRS
Department of Colon and Rectal Surgery
Ochsner Clinic Foundation
New Orleans, Louisiana

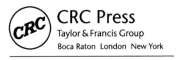

CRC Press
Taylor & Francis Group
Boca Raton  London  New York

CRC Press is an imprint of the
Taylor & Francis Group, an **informa** business

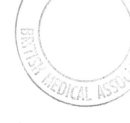

CRC Press
Taylor & Francis Group
6000 Broken Sound Parkway NW, Suite 300
Boca Raton, FL 33487-2742

© 2019 by Taylor & Francis Group, LLC
CRC Press is an imprint of Taylor & Francis Group, an Informa business

No claim to original U.S. Government works

Printed on acid-free paper

International Standard Book Number-13: 978-1-138-62683-6 (Pack- Hardback and eBook)

---

**Library of Congress Cataloging-in-Publication Data**

---

Names: Kann, Brian R., editor. | Beck, David E., editor. | Margolin, David A., editor. | Vargas, H. David., editor. | Whitlow, Charles B., editor.
Title: Improving outcomes in colon and rectal surgery / edited by Brian R. Kann, David E. Beck, David A. Margolin, H. David Vargas, Charles B. Whitlow.
Description: Boca Raton : CRC Press, [2018] | Includes bibliographical references and index.
Identifiers: LCCN 2018011083| ISBN 9781138626836 (pack - book and e-book : alk. paper) | ISBN 9781351816786 (e-book)
Subjects: | MESH: Colonic Diseases--surgery | Rectal Diseases--surgery | Treatment Outcome | Colon--surgery | Rectum--surgery | Colorectal Surgery--methods
Classification: LCC RD543.C57 | NLM WI 650 | DDC 617.5/547--dc23
LC record available at https://lccn.loc.gov/2018011083

---

**Visit the Taylor & Francis Web site at**
**http://www.taylorandfrancis.com**

**and the CRC Press Web site at**
**http://www.crcpress.com**

# Contents

# Preface

Quality measures and outcomes are receiving greater attention by the lay and medical communities. The occurrence or mismanagement of complications often results in poor outcomes, increased cost, and significant morbidity. Answering the call for transparency and improvement requires action by all involved in the care of patients. Collection of objective data and quality measures allows documentation of optimal care and desired outcomes while identifying areas for improvement.

The goal of this book is to present the current knowledge of outcomes, as well as the techniques for minimizing and managing complications from the common diseases and procedures of this specialty. This information will aid providers in optimizing care and encourage research in outcome and quality measurement.

*Improving Outcomes of Colon and Rectal Surgery* represents the collaborative efforts of many individuals. The contributing authors were selected for their knowledge of colorectal surgery and ability to present their surgical judgment and experience in written form. They represent a spectrum of experienced providers who have made significant contributions to younger individuals who will shape the future of their specialty. In addition to reviewing the available literature, they have described their personal approach to complications in colorectal surgery. Numerous technical descriptions and highlights from multiple discussions held in surgical locker rooms, morbidity and mortality conferences, and the hallways of conferences and symposiums have been included. Using this approach, we hope this book will provide initial guidance to the less-experienced provider and stimulate additional thought and research to the more-experienced provider.

The editors gratefully acknowledge the efforts of the many individuals who made this book possible. This book carries on the vision of previous editors and contributors to the first two editions of *Complications in Colon and Rectal Surgery* and *Improved Outcomes in Colon and Rectal Surgery*.

**Brian R. Kann, MD, FACS, FASCRS**
**David E. Beck, MD, FACS, FASCRS**
**David A. Margolin, MD, FACS, FASCRS**
**H. David Vargas, MD, FACS, FASCRS**
**Charles B. Whitlow, MD, FACS, FASCRS**

# Editors

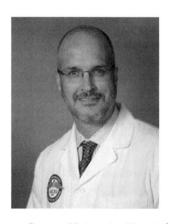 **Brian R. Kann, MD, FACS, FASCRS** earned his undergraduate degree from Old Dominion University in Norfolk, VA in 1993, followed by his medical degree from Hahnemann University in Philadelphia, PA in 1997. He completed his internship and residency in general surgery, including a one-year research fellowship focusing on transplant immunology, at Cooper University Hospital, University of Medicine and Dentistry of New Jersey (UMDNJ)/Robert Wood Johnson Medical School in Camden, New Jersey in 2003, then went on to complete a residency in colon and rectal surgery at the Ochsner Clinic in New Orleans, Louisiana in 2004. He has previously held academic appointments at Cooper University Hospital, UMDNJ/Robert Wood Johnson Medical School, where he was assistant professor of surgery and program director of the General Surgery Residency from 2004 to 2010, and at the University of Pennsylvania Perelman School of Medicine, where he was assistant professor of clinical surgery and program director of the Colon and Rectal Surgery Residency from 2010 to 2014. In 2015, he returned to the Ochsner Clinic in New Orleans, where he currently serves as a senior staff surgeon and associate program director of the Colon and Rectal Surgery Residency.

Dr. Kann is certified by both the American Board of Surgery and the American Board of Colon and Rectal Surgery. He is an active member of the American College of Surgeons, the American Society of Colon and Rectal Surgeons (ASCRS), the Association of Program Directors in Colon and Rectal Surgery, and the Society for Surgery of the Alimentary Tract. He has served on numerous committees within these organizations and has been selected as program chair for 2019 ASCRS national meeting. He has published numerous original scientific manuscripts, reviews, and book chapters in the field of colon and rectal surgery. While his practice spans the field of colon and rectal surgery, he has particular clinical interest in the surgical management of inflammatory bowel disease.

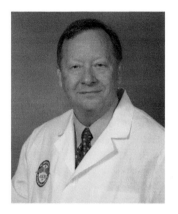 **David E. Beck, MD, FACS, FASCRS** was a distinguished graduate of the United States Air Force (USAF) Academy and attended medical school at the University of Miami. He completed his residency in general surgery at Wilford Hall USAF Medical School, Lackland AFB, Texas and completed a fellowship in colorectal surgery at the Cleveland Clinic Foundation, Cleveland, Ohio. He is board certified in general and colon and rectal surgery and is a fellow of the American College of Surgeons and the American Society of Colon and Rectal Surgeons. After retiring from the Air Force, where he was chairman and residency program director of the Department of General Surgery at Wilford Hall USAF Medical Center and the military consultant to the air force surgeon general in colon and rectal surgery, Dr. Beck joined Ochsner in 1993, served as chairman of the Colon and Rectal Surgery Department from 1995 to 2014, and is now chairman emeritus.

Dr. Beck conducts research on colorectal diseases, has authored and edited nine medical textbooks, and written over 300 scientific publications. He was the president of the American Society of Colon and Rectal Surgeons (ASCRS) from 2010 to 2011 and is a member of many other medical associations. He served as a member of the Board of Governors of the Ochsner Clinic Foundation from 2005 to 2012 and currently serves on the American Board of Colon and Rectal Surgery. Dr. Beck is on the editorial board of several prestigious medical journals. In addition to his clinical and administrative duties, he is a professor of surgery at the University of Queensland, Australia and is on the clinical faculty at the Louisiana State University and Uniformed Services University Schools of Medicine. Dr. Beck is listed in Who's Who, Best Doctors in America, Good Housekeeping's Top Cancer Doctors for Women, and Best Surgeons in New Orleans. Dr. Beck is a nationally recognized expert in inflammatory bowel disease, anal, rectal and colon cancer, stomas, adhesions, bowel preparation, sphincter saving surgery for cancer, laparoscopic surgery, and postoperative pain management.

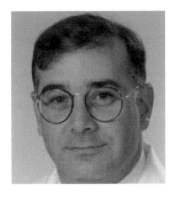

**David A. Margolin, MD, FACS, FASCRS** earned his medical degree from the Medical College of Ohio in Toledo and completed his internship and residency at Case Western Reserve University in Cleveland, Ohio. He completed his fellowship in colon and rectal surgery at Ochsner. Dr. Margolin is board certified in general surgery and colon and rectal surgery and has been on staff at Ochsner since the beginning of 2003. Dr. Margolin is te current President of the American Society of Colon and Rectal Surgeons and is listed in Best Doctors in America. He serves as Director of Colon and Rectal Surgery Research. His professional interests include laparoscopic colon and rectal surgery, inflammatory bowel disease, complex anorectal conditions and incontinence.

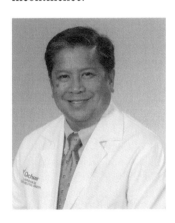

**H. David Vargas, MD, FACS, FASCRS** graduated with distinction with a major in Religious Studies from the University of Virginia in Charlottesville, Virginia. He stayed at the University of Virginia and graduated from the School of Medicine. He completed a residency in General Surgery and served as Chief Surgical Resident at the Lehigh Valley Hospital in Allentown Pennsylvania. Dr. Vargas then pursued additional training here in New Orleans performing a fellowship at the Ochsner Clinic in the specialty of Colon Rectal Surgery. He became board certified (and has been re-certified) by the American Board of Surgery and the American Board of Colon Rectal Surgery. Of note, Dr. Vargas distinguished himself by attaining the highest score on the written examination administered by the American Board of Colon and Rectal Surgery.

After leaving fellowship training in New Orleans, Dr. Vargas gained extensive clinical experience in both private practice and academic surgery all the while remaining involved in medical education and postgraduate surgery resident training. He has been active in local, regional, and national professional organizations and has held positions of leadership. He has authored multiple book chapters as well as scientific articles published in peer-reviewed surgical journals.

While Dr. Vargas' clinical practice encompasses the breadth of Colon Rectal Surgery, in particular he has gained recognition for minimally invasive or laparoscopic colorectal surgery which led to his recruitment in 2007 to the University of Kentucky College of Medicine as Chief of Colon Rectal Surgery.

After five years in Kentucky, he returned to New Orleans in 2012 and joined the Department of Colon and Rectal Surgery of the Ochsner Clinic where he now serves as Staff Surgeon and Program Director of the Colon Rectal Surgery Fellowship. In addition, he is a Assistant Medical Director of Endoscopy Services at Ochsner Medical Center.

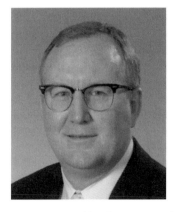

**Charles B. Whitlow, MD, FACS, FASCRS** earned his medical degree from the University of Arkansas and completed his internship and residency at William Beaumont Army Medical Center in El Paso, Texas. He completed his colon and rectal surgery fellowship at Ochsner. Dr. Whitlow is board certified in general surgery and colon and rectal surgery and has been on staff at Ochsner since the Summer of 2002. Dr. Whitlow is the chairman of the Department of Colon and Rectal Surgeins. He is listed in Best Doctors in America and is a Past President of the American Board of Colon and Rectal Surgery. His particular areas of professional interest include transanal excision of large benign rectal tumors, sphincter-preserving surgery for rectal cancer, surgical treatment of inflammatory bowel disease, laparoscopic and robotic colon and rectal surgery, surgery for rectal prolapse, and treatment of anorectal fistulas.

# Contributors

**Cary B. Aarons** MD, FACS, FASCRS
Department of Surgery
University of Pennsylvania
Philadelphia, Pennsylvania

**Joseph C. Adongay** MD
Section of Colon and Rectal Surgery
Grant Medical Center
Columbus, Ohio

**Alison Althans** BA
Case Western Reserve University School of Medicine
Cleveland, Ohio

**Lara McKean Basté** MD
Department of Colon and Rectal Surgery
Ochsner Clinic Foundation
New Orleans, Louisiana

**Jennifer S. Beaty** MD, FACS, FASCRS
Department of Colon and Rectal Surgery, Inc.
Omaha, Nebraska

**David E. Beck** MD, FACS, FASCRS
Department of Colon and Rectal Surgery
Ochsner Clinic Foundation
New Orleans, Louisiana

**Joshua I. S. Bleier** MD, FACS, FASCRS
Department of Surgery
University of Pennsylvania
Philadelphia, Pennsylvania

**Kristina K. Booth** MD, FACS, FASCRS
Division of Colon and Rectal Surgery
University of Oklahoma Health Science Center
Oklahoma City, Oklahoma

**Scott A. Brill** MD
Department of Colon and Rectal Surgery
OhioHealth Colon and Rectal Surgeons
Columbus, Ohio

**Shaun R. Brown** MD, FACS, FASCRS
Department of Colon and Rectal Surgery
Womack Army Medical Center
Fort Bragg, North Carolina

**Huisar Dao Campi** MD
Department of Surgery
University of Texas Health Science Center
San Antonio, Texas

**Thomas E. Cataldo** MD, FACS, FASCRS
Department of Colon and Rectal Surgery
Brown University
Providence, Rhode Island

**Heidi K. Chua** MD, FACS, FASCRS
Department of Colon and Rectal Surgery
Mayo Clinic
Rochester, Minnesota

**Bradley R. Davis** MD, FACS, FASCRS
Department of Colon and Rectal Surgery
Carolinas Medical Center
Charlotte, North Carolina

**Kurt G. Davis** MD, FACS, FASCRS
Department of Colon and Rectal Surgery
Louisiana State University
New Orleans, Louisiana

**Scott E. Delacroix, Jr.** MD
Department of Urology
Louisiana State University School of Medicine
New Orleans, Louisiana

**J. Marcus Downs** MD, FACS, FASCRS
Department of Colon and Rectal Surgery
UT Southwestern Medical School
Dallas, Texas

**Laura Melina Fernandez** MD
Angelita & Joaquim Gama Institute
São Paulo, Brazil

**James Fleshman, Jr.** MD, FACS, FASCRS
Department of Surgery
Baylor University
Dallas, Texas

**Jesus Flores** MD
Texas Colon and Rectal Surgeons
Dallas, Texas

**Luanne M. Force** MD
Department of colorectal Surgery
University of Miami
Miami, Florida

**Molly M. Ford** MD, FACS, FASCRS
Department of Colon and Rectal Surgery
Vanderbilt University
Nashville, Louisiana

**Sharon G. Gregorcyk** MD, FACS, FASCRS
Texas Colon and Rectal Surgeons
Dallas, Texas

**Leander M. Grimm, Jr.** MD, FACS, FASCRS
Division of Colon and Rectal Surgery
Department of Surgery
University of South Alabama
Mobile, Alabama

**Jason F. Hall** MD, FACS, FASCRS
Department of Colon and Rectal Surgery
Boston Medical Center
Boston, Massachusetts

**Alexander T. Hawkins** MD, MPH
Division of General Surgery
Department of Colon and Rectal Surgery
Vanderbilt University Medical Center
Nashville, Tennessee

**Roland Hawkins** MD
Radiation Oncology
Ochsner Cancer Institute
New Orleans, Louisiana

**Traci L. Hedrick** MD, MS, FACS, FASCRS
Department of Surgery
University of Virginia Health System
Charlottesville, Virginia

**Terry C. Hicks** MD, FACS, FASCRS
Department of Colon and Rectal Surgery
Ochsner Clinic Foundation
New Orleans, Louisiana

**M. Benjamin Hopkins** MD, FACS, FASCRS
Division of General Surgery
Department of Colon and Rectal Surgery
Vanderbilt University Medical Center
Nashville, Tennessee

**Steven R. Hunt** MD, FACS, FASCRS
Department of Colon and Rectal Surgery
Washington University
St. Louis, Missouri

**John D. Hunter** MD
Division of Colon and Rectal Surgery
Department of Surgery
University of South Alabama
Mobile, Alabama

**Syed G. Husain** MD, FACS, FASCRS
Department of Colon and Rectal Surgery
Brown University
Providence, Rhode Island

**Mohammed Iyoob Mohammed Ilyas** MBBS, MS, MRCS
Division of Colon and Rectal Surgery
Department of Surgery
Henry Ford Hospital
Detroit, Michigan

**Arjun N. Jeganathan** MD
Department of Surgery
University of Pennsylvania
Philadelphia, Pennsylvania

**Michelle C. Julien** MD, FACS, FASCRS
Division of Colon and Rectal Surgery
Lehigh Valley Hospital
Allentown, Pennsylvania

**Brian R. Kann** MD, FACS, FASCRS
Department of Colon and Rectal Surgery
Ochsner Clinic Foundation
New Orleans, Louisiana

**Kevin R. Kasten** MD, FACS, FASCRS
Department of Colon and Rectal Surgery
Carolinas Medical Center
Charlotte, North Carolina

**Aaron L. Klinger** MD
Department of Colon and Rectal Surgery
Ochsner Clinic Foundation
New Orleans, Louisiana

**Jonathan Lu** MD
Department of Hematology and Oncology
Ochsner Clinic Foundation
New Orleans, Louisiana

**Farouq Manji** MD
Department of Colon and Rectal Surgery
Ferguson Clinic Spectrum Health Medical Group
Michigan State University
Grand Rapids, Michigan

**David A. Margolin** MD, FACS, FASCRS
Department of Colon and Rectal Surgery
Ochsner Clinic Foundation
New Orleans, Louisiana

**David J. Maron** MD, MBA, FACS, FASCRS
Department of Colorectal Surgery
Cleveland Clinic Florida
Weston, Florida

**Marc R. Matrana** MD, MS
Department of Hematology and Oncology
Ochsner Clinic Foundation
New Orleans, Louisiana

**Nijjia N. Mahmoud** MD, FACS, FASCRS
Department of Colon and Rectal Surgery
University of Pennsylvania
Philadelphia, Pennsylvania

**Andrew C. Matthews** MD
Department of Radiology
Ochsner Clinic Foundation
New Orleans, Louisiana

**Charles C. Matthews** MD, FACR
Department of Radiology
Ochsner Clinic Foundation
New Orleans, Louisiana

**Shannon McChesney** MD
Department of General Surgery
Tulane University School of Medicine
New Orleans, Louisiana

**Allison B. McCoy** PhD
Tulane University School of Public Health
and Tropical Medicine
New Orleans, Louisiana

**Jacob A. McCoy** MD
Department of Urology
Ochsner Clinic Foundation
New Orleans, Louisiana

**Genevieve B. Melton-Meaux** MD, PhD, FACS, FASCRS
Division of Colon and Rectal Surgery
University of Minnesota
Minneapolis, Minnesota

**Jeffery Mino** MD
Department of Colon and Rectal Surgery
Cleveland Clinic
Cleveland, Ohio

**Mary T. O'Donnell** MD
Department of Surgery
University of Pennsylvania
Philadelphia, Pennsylvania

**Supriya S. Patel** MD, FACS, FASCRS
Kaiser Permanente Department of General Surgery
San Jose, California

**Rodrigo O. Perez** MD
University of São Paulo School of Medicine
São Paulo, Brazil

**W. Brian Perry** MD, FACS, FASCRS
Department of Surgery
University of Texas Health Science Center
San Antonio, Texas

**Danielle Pickham** MD, FACS, FASCRS
Kaiser Permanente Department of General Surgery
San Jose, California

**Craig A. Reickert** MD, FACS, FASCRS
Division of Colon and Rectal Surgery
Henry Ford Hospital
Detroit, Michigan

**Rocco Ricciardi** MD, MPH, FACS, FASCRS
Department of Colon and Rectal Surgery
Massachusetts General Hospital
Boston, Massachusetts

**Daniel E. Sarmiento** MD
Division of Colon and Rectal Surgery
Lehigh Valley Hospital
Allentown, Pennsylvania

**Nicole M. Saur** MD, FACS, FASCRS
Department of Surgery
University of Pennsylvania
Philadelphia, Pennsylvania

**Skandan Shanmugan** MD
Department of Surgery
University of Pennsylvania
Philadelphia, Pennsylvania

**Benjamin D. Shogan** MD
Department of Colon and Rectal Surgery
University of Chicago
Chicago, Illinois

**Robert J. Sinnott** DO, FACS, FASCRS
Division of Colon and Rectal Surgery
Lehigh Valley Hospital
Allentown, Pennsylvania

**Arida Siripong** MD, FACS, FASCRS
Department of Colon and Rectal Surgery
Ferguson Clinic Spectrum Health Medical Group
Michigan State University
Grand Rapids, Michigan

**Scott R. Steele** MD, FACS, FASCRS
Colorectal Surgery
Cleveland Clinic
Cleveland, Ohio

**Sharon L. Stein** MD, FACS, FACRS
University Hospitals Cleveland Medical Center
Case Western Reserve University
Cleveland, Ohio

**Emily Steinhagen** MD
University Hospitals Cleveland Medical Center
Case Western Reserve University
Cleveland, Ohio

**W. David Sumrall, III** MD
Department of Anesthesia
Ochsner Clinic Foundation
New Orleans, Louisiana

**H. David Vargas** MD, FACS, FASCRS
Department of Colon and Rectal Surgery
Ochsner Clinic Foundation
New Orleans, Louisiana

**Charles C. Vining** MD
Department of Colon and Rectal Surgery
University of Pennsylvania
Philadelphia, Pennsylvania

**Katerina O. Wells** MD
Department of Surgery
Baylor University
Dallas, Texas

**Charles B. Whitlow** MD, FACS, FASCRS
Department of Colon and Rectal Surgery
Ochsner Clinic Foundation
New Orleans, Louisiana

**J. Christian Winters** MD
Department of Urology
Louisiana State University School of Medicine
New Orleans, Louisiana

**Moriah E. Wright** MD
Department of Colon and Rectal Surgery, Inc.
Omaha, Nebraska

**Massarat Zutshi** MD, FACS, FASCRS
Department of Colon and Rectal Surgery
Cleveland Clinic
Cleveland, Ohio

# Preexisting conditions

ARIDA SIRIPONG AND FAROUQ MANJI

## CHALLENGING CASE

A 63-year-old woman is referred to your office with a right colon cancer found on screening colonoscopy. Her past medical history is significant for stable coronary artery disease.

## CASE MANAGEMENT

You order a complete blood count (CBC) and basic metabolic profile. A chest x-ray and a computed tomography (CT) scan of the abdomen and pelvis are obtained for staging purposes. No other workup is needed prior to scheduling the patient for surgery.

## INTRODUCTION

A thorough preoperative assessment is essential to identify, treat, and optimize preexisting comorbidities and minimize morbidity and mortality after colorectal surgery. Paying early attention to patient risk factors and recognizing their potential impact on outcomes is the surgeon's responsibility. This will often require a multidisciplinary approach and coordination with other physicians; however, these extra steps and dedicated attention are as critical as the technical aspects of the procedure to ensure maximal benefit for each patient.

This chapter highlights preoperative optimization of the patient undergoing elective colorectal surgery. In the setting of emergent surgery, additional testing or modification of preexisting conditions is a luxury, and the risk of delaying surgery will seldom justify the benefit of additional workup. In these cases, intensive intraoperative and perioperative care is necessary to minimize complications.

## PREOPERATIVE TESTING

For healthy patients undergoing surgery, routine laboratory tests may be unnecessary. In a large study of 2,000 patients undergoing elective surgery, only 0.22% of routine preoperative laboratory results found abnormalities that prompted intervention (1). This testing can unnecessarily delay surgery and lead to an increase in health-care costs without clinical benefit. Therefore, the decision to order preoperative tests in the healthy individual should be guided by the patient's clinical history, physical exam findings, disease pathology, and risk of planned surgery.

Ambulatory anorectal procedures are considered low risk and do not require routine laboratory testing in the asymptomatic patient (2). The remaining colorectal procedures, however, generally involve intraabdominal dissection and are classified as elevated risk. Baseline blood count and type and screen are indicated in these patients undergoing major surgery where significant blood loss is a potentiality and/or is anticipated. Coagulation studies are reserved for patients with a history of bleeding or coagulopathy, on chronic anticoagulation medications, or with comorbidities that may affect normal coagulation (renal disease or liver failure). Creatinine level is warranted in older patients (older than 60 years old), as well as in those with a history of diabetes or baseline renal insufficiency. Patients with recent weight loss, infection, or hospital admission may benefit from albumin assessment to guide recommendations for preoperative nutritional support and discussion regarding the role of stoma creation.

## CARDIAC EVALUATION

Cardiovascular disease (CVD) is the leading cause of death in the industrialized world (3), and 25%–30% of all patients undergoing noncardiac surgery have significant coronary artery disease at the time of operation (4). The goal of preoperative cardiac evaluation is to identify those who will benefit from additional testing and intervention prior to surgery. In general, prophylactic cardiac interventions are not advised, and additional workup should only be recommended if also warranted outside of the surgical setting.

Perioperative risk stratification for noncardiac surgical patients is calculated based on procedure-related risk, cardiac risk indices, and assessment of exercise tolerance based on metabolic equivalents (METs). Currently the American College of Cardiology/American Heart Association (ACC/AHA) categorizes noncardiac surgery into *low risk*, which conveys a risk of myocardial infarction or major adverse cardiac event (MACE) <1%, and *elevated risk*, which conveys risk ≥1% (5). Historically, this risk was stratified into three groups; however, recommendations for those of intermediate and high risk were similar. Therefore, in current guidelines, these groups have been combined and most major colorectal procedures are classified as elevated risk.

Various cardiac risk indices have been described. The Goldman Cardiac Risk Index is a multivariate risk index and precursor to the widely used Lee Revised Cardiac Risk Index (RCRI) (6,7). The RCRI is a simple and validated evaluation tool, based on six predictors of perioperative cardiac risk (high-risk surgery, history of ischemic heart disease, congestive heart failure, cerebrovascular disease, diabetes mellitus requiring insulin treatment, and renal dysfunction with creatinine >2). A patient with none, one, two, or more than three risk factors has a MACE rate of 0.4%, 1.0%, 2.4%, and 5.4%, respectively (6). The American College of Surgeons National Surgical Quality Improvement Program (ACS NSQIP) Myocardial Infarction and Cardiac Arrest (MICA) Risk Calculator is a tool based on multivariate analysis, derived from prospectively collected data from over 500 hospitals and one million operations (8). The advantage of the NSQIP calculator is the greater number of input variables required to generate risk estimations, therefore deriving more accurate results. MICA has been shown to outperform the RCRI in discriminative power among the same group of patients (8). Regardless of which model is chosen, practitioners should be comfortable using one of these risk indices in the preoperative assessment.

The recommended 2014 ACA/AHA algorithm for preoperative cardiac evaluation is shown in Figure 1.1 (5). As previously noted, patients needing emergent surgery require close perioperative monitoring and management but often cannot delay surgery for additional testing. Those with acute coronary symptoms undergoing nonemergent surgery should be treated based on guideline-directed medical therapy (GDMT). Asymptomatic patients with cardiac risk factors are stratified based on surgical and clinical risk. Low-risk procedures do not require additional testing, whereas those undergoing elevated-risk procedures are further categorized based on METs. METs, a measure of exercise tolerance, can be evaluated based on a few simple questions during the initial encounter. Patients unable to walk two blocks on level ground or carry two bags of groceries up one flight of stairs without symptoms of angina or dyspnea have poor exercise tolerance, equivalent

to <4 METs. The role of cardiac stress testing is closely related to METs and functional capacity of the patient. Patients with elevated surgical risk and poor (<4 METs) or unknown functional capacity should undergo exercise or pharmacological stress testing if it will change management. In the setting of elective surgery, findings of severe cardiac ischemia on stress testing should prompt intervention with medical therapy and/or preoperative revascularization. Of note, in those with <4 METs, additional cardiac testing or intervention should not be pursued if it will not impact surgical decision-making (decision to proceed with surgery or palliative measures).

## TESTING AND INTERVENTIONS

As mentioned previously, prophylactic cardiac interventions have no proven benefit in outcomes and should only be considered in patients who would also require it in the nonsurgical setting (5). In those who present with indications for urgent cardiac intervention before noncardiac surgery, the type of cardiac intervention should be guided by the urgency of the noncardiac surgery.

Coronary artery bypass graft (CABG) is indicated in patients with triple vessel disease or myocardial ischemia with concomitant decreased left ventricular function, who require elective noncardiac surgery with a high bleeding risk (9). There is a paucity of data regarding optimal timing of elective noncardiac surgery after CABG, although one compelling study suggests a significant increase in mortality for patients undergoing high-risk vascular surgery within 30 days of CABG (10). Therefore, when possible, noncardiac surgery should be postponed for 30 days after recent CABG and may not be a feasible option for the patient with symptomatic colorectal pathology.

Percutaneous coronary intervention (PCI) with drug-eluting or bare metal stents is indicated in (1) patients with left main disease whose comorbidities preclude bypass surgery without undue risk and (2) patients with unstable coronary artery disease who would be appropriate candidates for emergency or urgent revascularization (11,12). While bare metal stents require uninterrupted antiplatelet therapy for 30 days, this recommendation is extended to 365 days after placement of a drug-eluting stent. These recommendations are based on several studies that show convincing evidence that disruption of dual-antiplatelet therapy within a short time period results in higher adverse cardiac outcomes, and is the leading predictor of coronary thrombosis and restenosis (13,14). In the setting of a recent stent and urgent indications for major abdominal surgery, discussion with the patient's cardiologist regarding the use of bridging antiplatelet agents, such as Integrillin or Tirofiban, may be beneficial (15). When used as a bridging agent for Plavix, these short-acting agents should be started as an infusion therapy 24 hours after the last dose of Plavix (5 days prior to surgery) and continued up to 4 hours prior to surgery. The infusion is then resumed 2 hours postoperatively until Plavix is restarted.

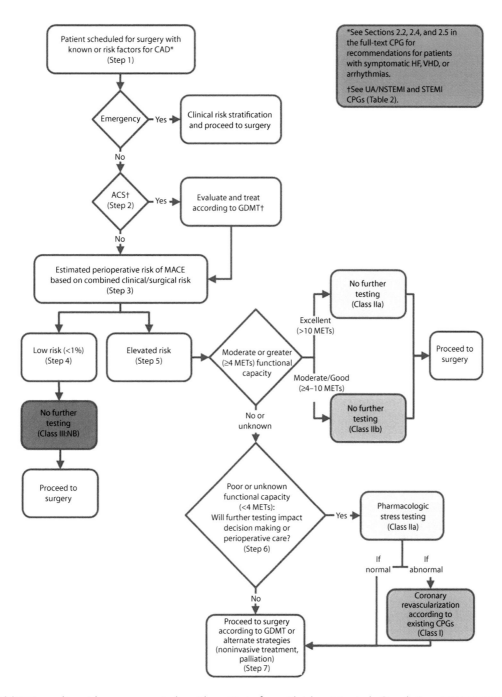

**Figure 1.1** ACC/AHA cardiac risk assessment algorithm. (Data from Fleisher LA et al. *Circulation*. 2014;130(24):2215–45.)

Balloon angioplasty should be considered for those who do not meet criteria for CABG, require time-sensitive noncardiac surgery, and/or are at high risk for bleeding (16). A patient with a new diagnosis of colon cancer with findings of severe cardiac ischemia may fall into this category. The main benefit of balloon angioplasty is the ability to carry out noncardiac surgery immediately without necessitating dual-antiplatelet therapy, although ideally such surgery should be postponed a minimum of 14 days (5). Ultimately, decisions regarding type of PCI and management of perioperative antiplatelet therapy should be coordinated between the surgeon, cardiologist, anesthesiologist, and patient, weighing the relative risk of bleeding versus stent thrombosis.

## PERIOPERATIVE β-BLOCKADE

β-Blockers should be continued in patients who were using them chronically, and postoperative management should be guided by clinical circumstances, such as hypotension, bradycardia, or bleeding (5). In patients at intermediate or high risk of myocardial ischemia, or with three or more RCRI factors, it may be reasonable to start β-blockers in the preoperative setting. Importantly, though, β-blockers should be initiated in advance of surgery to assess safety and titrate dosage appropriately. β-Blockers should not be started on the day of surgery, and this may actually be harmful, as illustrated by results of the POISE (Perioperative Ischemic

Evaluation Study) trial (17). In this study of 9,000 participants, although β-blockade diminished the incidence of myocardial infarction, patients also experienced higher rates of death, stroke, hypotension, and bradycardia.

## PULMONARY ASSESSMENT

Postoperative pulmonary complications (PPCs) are common after noncardiac surgery and play an important role in patient outcomes. Definitions of PPCs vary across studies, and therefore, the true incidence is difficult to describe, with reported rates ranging from 6% to 80% (18). Patient-related factors that increase risk of PPCs include smoking, age older than 60 years, congestive heart failure, chronic obstructive pulmonary disease (COPD), functional dependency, and American Society of Anesthesiologists (ASA) Physical Status Classification of III or above (18–20). Surgery-specific factors include general anesthesia, longer operating room times (more than 2–3 hours), emergency surgery, and site-specific surgery, with the greatest risk among upper abdominal and thoracic procedures, which contribute to splinting and a restrictive pulmonary physiology (21,22). In a recent multicenter prospective study of ASA III patients undergoing prolonged general anesthesia (more than 2 hours), 33.4% of patients experienced at least one PPC. In this study, even mild PPCs, including atelectasis or prolonged oxygen requirement, were predictors of increased mortality, intensive care unit admission, and prolonged length of stay. Furthermore, modifiable factors from this review included colloid administration, higher intraoperative blood loss, prolonged surgery and anesthesia time, and higher intraoperative tidal volumes (18).

COPD is a significant predictor for pulmonary complications, with an observational study based on the NSQIP database describing risk of pneumonia, prolonged ventilation, and reintubation at 6.5%, 8.8%, and 5.5% among COPD patients (23). However, despite the increased risk seen in COPD patients, there is no prohibitive level of pulmonary function that serves as a contraindication to noncardiac surgery. Prior studies demonstrate that COPD severity does not incrementally correlate with risk of PPCs; therefore, routine spirometry is also not recommended in COPD patients without clinical changes in pulmonary function (21).

Smoking is widely accepted as a risk factor for PPC. Rates of respiratory failure, pneumonia, and other related complications are demonstrably higher in active smokers (24–26). These patients are more likely to have prolonged hospital stay, obtain wound infections, and experience venous emboli and cardiac complications (27–29). Thus, patients should be screened for smoking status, previous smoking history, and in specific cases, occupational or secondhand exposure. Prior debate centered on the duration of smoking cessation before intervention and the potential increase in PPC if patients stop smoking shortly before surgery. This

was based on a small study published in 1989, which suggested PPCs could be higher in patients who cease smoking less than 8 weeks before surgery versus those who continue smoking (30). More recent analysis, however, challenges these results. Two recent meta-analyses demonstrate no evidence to suggest an increased risk of PPC when smoking cessation occurs within a few weeks of surgery. Furthermore, there is a time-related decrease in postoperative complications the longer smoking is stopped before surgery (31,32). The current data demonstrate that it is safe to encourage patients to stop smoking any time in the preoperative period, and ideally 6–8 weeks before the procedure.

Obstructive sleep apnea (OSA) is defined by a state of upper airway obstruction leading to apneic episodes. The incidence of OSA has increased with the rise in obesity and is associated with higher risk of postoperative hypoxemia, cardiopulmonary events, intensive care unit admission, and increased hospital length of stay (33). Unfortunately, OSA may be undetected in the preoperative setting, as symptoms may deviate from the traditional description of daytime sleepiness and snoring, and instead manifest as headaches, difficulty concentrating, altered mood, and nocturia. Given the challenges in diagnosing OSA based on symptoms alone, screening tools including the STOP-Bang questionnaire have helped identify patients who may benefit from pulmonary evaluation prior to major abdominal surgery (34). This questionnaire includes four objective patient measures and four additional questions regarding sleeping habits. Preoperative recognition of OSA can minimize anesthetic complications as well as PPC with the anticipated use of continuous positive airway pressure postoperatively.

Guidelines regarding preoperative chest radiography and spirometry emphasize clinical assessment, relying on the history and physical exam (21). Guidelines from the American College of Physicians do not recommend routine preoperative chest radiography for predicting risk of PPC, as it does not alter outcomes (35). Patients who should have chest radiography include those with new or unstable cardiopulmonary signs or symptoms, and patients at increased risk of postoperative pulmonary complication if the results would alter perioperative management (i.e., informed decision-making, timing, and type/technique of surgery). For example, a COPD patient diagnosed with pneumonia on chest x-ray may benefit from delaying elective surgery until the infectious process is treated and pulmonary status is optimized to baseline.

## RENAL DISEASE

Chronic renal failure is present in over 20% of patients over the age of 60, and is reported in 15% of the population overall (36). Renal failure encompasses a wide range of kidney dysfunction, ranging from glomerular filtration rate <60 mL/min to dialysis-dependent renal failure. Regardless of disease severity, it is crucial to prevent additional kidney injury in these patients who are highly susceptible to post-operative acute renal failure. Intraoperatively, significant blood loss and hypovolemia are poorly tolerated and should be minimized. Avoidance of nephrotoxic agents, including nonsteroidal anti-inflammatory agents and IV contrast, and recognizing the impact of decreased renal function on medication clearance, such as nondepolarizing neuromuscular blocking agents, are critical components to periop-erative care.

Chronic kidney disease is associated with a host of comorbidities, but most significantly it increases risk of CVD and is an independent predictor of adverse cardiac events. CVD and kidney disease are closely related, and in the nonsurgical setting, CVD is the leading cause of morbidity and mortality in chronic renal failure patients. Postoperatively, these patients experience a higher rate of cardiovascular complications and noncancer mortality after colorectal cancer surgery; the rate in this population has been reported at 5%–10% after elective and up to 40% after emergency procedures (37). Given this relationship between CVD and chronic kidney disease, there should a high index of suspicion for underlying cardiac disease in all renal failure patients.

In end-stage renal failure, surgery should be timed soon after dialysis to minimize electrolyte and fluid shift changes. Prior to surgery, it is also important to recognize the physiologic changes that accompany underlying chronic kidney disease. Progressive renal disease can lead to hypo-albuminemia, anemia, hyperkalemia, decreased leukocyte and immunologic function, and increased bleeding time due to uremic platelet dysfunction. These changes contrib-ute to higher rates of infectious and wound complications in this population and should be carefully considered and discussed with the patient when consenting for surgery. As coagulopathy is secondary to platelet dysfunction in the uremic patient, in the emergent setting, DDAVP (desmo-pressin acetate) or dialysis may be used to mitigate bleeding complications.

## LIVER DISEASE

Cirrhosis and underlying liver disease represent the most significant predictors of mortality after colorectal surgery, noting a 6.5-fold increased risk (38). Fortunately, it is rare for patients to present with colorectal disease in the set-ting of cirrhosis. For these unique situations, it is critical to consider the natural history of the colorectal pathology, the severity of liver dysfunction, and potential candidacy for liver transplantation. Thorough preoperative counseling facilitates informed decision-making, allowing the surgeon to review goals of care and outline realistic expectations regarding risks of any intervention.

Liver failure is a well-known predictor of mortality after abdominal surgery. Two available metrics, the Child-Turcotte-Pugh (CTP) and Model for End-Stage Liver Disease (MELD) scores, are used to assess surgical risk in liver fail-ure patients. The CTP classification was originally described to assess operative risk in patients undergoing shunt surgery for portal hypertension but has also been utilized in risk assessment for other abdominal surgeries (39). Designed to quantify liver dysfunction, the CTP score uses albumin, bilirubin, prothrombin time (INR), presence of ascites, and encephalopathy to assign points and subsequently classify patients into three categories, A–C (maximal dysfunction). Mortality associated with Child's class A, B, and C has been reported at 10%, 17%, and 63% (40), respectively, in a review of nonhepatic abdominal procedures. In a study of cirrhotic patients undergoing colectomy, in-hospital mortality was 24%, with the highest mortality rates in those with enceph-alopathy, ascites, hypoalbuminemia, and anemia (38). The MELD score is derived from a complex formula based on INR, bilirubin, and creatinine and is calculated using Web-based tools. In general, MELD scores classified as less than 10, 10–15, and greater than 15 correlate to Child's class A, B, and C, respectively. MELD scores greater than 15 have been associated with a higher risk of complications, mortality due to complications, and overall mortality after colorectal surgery (41).

Postoperative morbidity in the cirrhotic patient is largely related to anastomotic, bleeding, and stoma complica-tions (42). Damaged hepatocytes decrease production of clotting factors, with subsequent coagulopathy, and pre-operative anticipation of bleeding risk is critical. Although minimizing the severity of a significant anastomotic leak, stoma creation in the setting of ascites has inherent risks of peristomal leakage and varices as well. Furthermore, ascites can increase infectious complications, wound dehiscence, or evisceration. Meunier evaluated 41 cirrhotic patients who underwent colorectal surgery and identified postopera-tive infection as the most significant risk factor for mortal-ity, increasing it from 11% to 53% (43).

Preoperative findings, such as portal hypertension, vari-ces, and a large amount of ascites, represent decompensated liver failure and may be an indication to consider preopera-tive transjugular intrahepatic portosystemic shunt (TIPS), if colectomy is deemed necessary. One study of severely cirrhotic patients with abdominal malignancies reported outcomes of abdominal surgery 1 month after TIPS was performed, noting decreased portal hypertension, ascites, and venous congestion; less intraoperative blood loss; and decreased need for blood transfusion (44). Nonetheless, TIPS increases the rate and severity of hepatic encepha-lopathy, and 1-year mortality rate after TIPS is estimated at 50%, related to the overwhelming severity of liver fail-ure. Regardless of whether or not TIPS is pursued, medical optimization of ascites with diuretic agents should also be employed throughout the perioperative period to minimize fluid overload.

A rare but significant dilemma arises when a cirrhotic patient presents with colorectal cancer. It is important to remember that a cirrhotic patient will not be a trans-plant candidate until deemed cancer free for 5 years. These cases should be discussed in a multidisciplinary setting, to review overall goals of care, both short and long term. Nonetheless, metastatic colorectal cancer to the liver is low (<10%), with theorized low rates due to poor tissue environment for tumor growth (45). Given the host of physiologic changes that accompany this disease process, patients with liver failure present several perioperative challenges.

## DIABETES

In 2012, it was estimated that 29.1 million people in the United States had diabetes, with approximately 20% (8.1 million) of patients undiagnosed (46). Diabetic patients harbor microvascular and macrovascular pathology that contribute to long-term complications, including nephropathy, CVD, cerebrovascular disease, neuropathy, and retinopathy and have been associated with increased morbidity and mortality after colorectal surgery (47). This increase in complications is likely a manifestation of both hyperglycemia and the associated comorbid conditions, with higher rates of postoperative renal failure and myocardial infarction identified in diabetic patients (48).

Surgery induces a physiologic disruption in glucose homeostasis due to release of stress hormones and insulin resistance. For diabetic patients, who have marginal insulin secretion at baseline, the above factors contribute to a significant catabolic state. The subsequent hyperglycemia is a well-described risk factor for delayed wound healing and infectious complications after colorectal surgery. Hyperglycemia impairs monocyte and neutrophil function, with a resultant increase in surgical site infections (49–51). In a review of 11,633 general surgery patients undergoing colorectal and bariatric surgeries, hyperglycemia (>180 mg/dL) was associated with adverse infectious complications, with effects mitigated in those who received insulin (52). Close glycemic monitoring, however, is critical to prevent and treat not only hyperglycemia but also *hypo*glycemia. Prolonged hypoglycemia can lead to neurologic sequelae, including somnolence, unconsciousness, seizures, and irreversible neurologic damage (53), and play an equally detrimental role in the recovery period.

Hemoglobin A1c serves as an indicator of global long-term glucose control, and studies suggest a relationship between preoperative levels and postoperative morbidity (54). A prospective study of 438 patients undergoing abdominal surgery reported higher rates of major postoperative complications in those with preoperative HbA1c levels >6.5% and perioperative hyperglycemia (54). Similarly, Gustaffson and colleagues reported increased morbidity after colorectal surgery in patients with HbA1c >6 mg/dL (55). Although firm guidelines do not exist regarding optimal preoperative levels, a recent HbA1c level should be obtained prior to surgery to optimize glycemic control leading up to elective procedures.

## OBESITY

Based on the most recent data from the Centers for Disease Control and Prevention, 38% of the adult U.S. population is obese, defined as body mass index (BMI) >30 kg/m$^2$ (56). Furthermore, more than 5% of men and 10% of women are classified as morbidly obese, with BMI >40 kg/m$^2$. The obesity epidemic places a significant socioeconomic burden on our health-care system and predisposes patients to additional comorbidities, including insulin resistance and diabetes, CVD, hypertension, and obstructive sleep apnea (57,58).

Physically, these patients pose specific technical challenges for the colorectal surgeon, and the obese patient significantly benefits from a minimally invasive approach when feasible (59). Despite these technical challenges, obese patients have a decreased mortality rate compared to their nonobese counterparts, referred to as the "obesity paradox" (60). This favorable outcome is thought to be a result of increased nutritional stores and a chronically inflamed state of obesity that may better prepare these patients for the physiological stress of surgery.

Despite this lower mortality rate, obese patients harbor a prothrombotic and pro-inflammatory state and experience increased morbidity after colorectal surgery, with higher rates of venous thromboembolism (VTE) and surgical site infection (SSI). In a study of 7,020 colectomy patients, obese patients had an increased rate of SSI compared with nonobese patients (14.5% versus 9.5%, $p < 0.001$) and overall increased risk of SSI by 60% (61). In addition, obese patients demonstrate a significantly increased risk of pulmonary embolism (2.18; 95% confidence interval [CI], 2.16–2.19) and deep vein thrombosis (relative risk [RR] 2.5; 95% CI, 2.49–2.51), with these results magnified in those under the age of 40 (62). Measures to decrease VTE and infectious complications in the obese population may include patient selection for secondary or delayed primary closure and consideration for extended thromboprophylaxis, in the section "Considerations for Extended Thromboprophylaxis".

## MALNUTRITION

One of the most important yet often underrecognized factors to assess at the initial encounter is nutritional status. Malnutrition is common among colorectal cancer patients, and it is a well-known predictor of postoperative complications (63). Furthermore, obstruction, fistulization, and infection related to inflammatory bowel disease (IBD) or malignancy can prevent adequate nutrient and fluid absorption. Therefore, strategies to optimize nutrition are a critical component of preoperative planning.

Malnutrition is a well-known predictor of adverse postoperative outcomes after colorectal surgery and is traditionally defined by an albumin level 3.5 g/dL, BMI <18.5 kg/m$^2$, or weight loss of >10% of total body weight over a 6-month period. A recent review of the ACS NSQIP database showed a high rate of malnutrition in colorectal cancer patients (27.8%), much higher than all other cancer types (64). In this study, the three listed criteria were used to define malnutrition, but only albumin <3.5 g/dL independently predicted 30-day mortality and postoperative outcomes including sepsis, renal failure, and cardiovascular events, return to operating room, and need for reintubation. In reality, however, several factors can affect fluctuations in albumin level, and it should not be taken as a sole indicator of nutritional status and the implied risks.

When identified, malnutrition should be addressed and treated in the nonemergent setting. In the last two decades, the role of immune-enhancing nutritional supplementation, or immunonutrition (IMN), has been well studied with promising results from several randomized controlled trials. These formulas are composed of specific immune-modulating substances, including arginine, nucleotides, glutamine, and omega-3 fatty acids/fish oil, which have been shown to modify postsurgical stress and immune response, resulting in lower infectious complications and shorter length of stay (65). Arginine is an essential amino acid found at low resting levels in the normal state, but serves as the primary fuel source for T cells. During trauma or surgery, arginine production cannot meet the demands of the body; therefore, IMN can significantly support immune function by supplementing this deficiency.

Even a short course of high arginine-rich protein and nutrient supplements prior to colorectal surgery significantly reduces postoperative morbidity. In a randomized controlled trial of patients undergoing surgery for gastrointestinal malignancies (colorectal, stomach, and pancreas), Braga et al. found significant clinical benefit in those randomized to receive immunonutrition versus a control enteral formula (66). In this study, patients were separated into four groups: (1) preoperative IMN, (2) preoperative and postoperative IMN, (3) preoperative control isoenergetic/isonitrogenous formula, and (4) no supplementation, demonstrating a significant reduction in infection rates in those who received IMN (12% versus 32%, $p < 0.05$). These results have been replicated with subsequent randomized controlled trials, and most recently, Thornblade et al. published results from Surgical Care Outcomes Assessment Program (SCOAP) in a community setting (67). In this prospective cohort study of 3,357 colorectal surgery patients, the authors reported the applicability of these results outside of a clinical trial. In general, patients receiving IMN had a higher ASA class (III–IV) and were more likely to require an ostomy (18% versus 14%, $p = 0.02$). Although results were not statistically significant, those receiving IMN had lower rates of prolonged length of stay (13.8% versus 17.3%, $p = 0.04$) and decreased rates of serious adverse events (6.8% versus 8.3%, $p = 0.25$). In combination with other components of enhanced recovery pathways, including avoidance of nasogastric tubes, early enteral feeding, carbohydrate loading, and close glucose control, IMN has proven to be a critical component of optimizing surgical outcomes.

## IMMUNOSUPPRESSION

Several medications alter the immune response of colorectal surgery patients. In elective surgery, the surgeon may minimize the adverse effects of these medications by careful decision-making regarding surgery timing, technique, and selection for stoma creation.

Steroids are often used to treat IBD in the acute setting and achieve symptomatic control prior to surgical intervention. However, steroids negatively impact all phases of wound healing and are associated with increased rates of venous thromboembolism (68), decreased bone density, and adrenal suppression. Available literature investigating the relationship between steroids and surgical outcomes is largely based on varying definitions of "recent steroid administration" and dosages; however, results are consistent, describing the negative impact of steroids on healing. In a review of NSQIP data, perioperative steroid use was associated with increased rates of superficial SSI (5% versus 2.9%), deep surgical site infections (1.8% versus 0.8%), a two- to threefold higher risk of dehiscence and organ space SSI, and a fourfold increase in mortality in those undergoing abdominal surgery (69). In a study of 250 colorectal patients undergoing left-sided resections with anastomoses, Slieker et al. identified a 7.5% leak rate, with corticosteroid use inferring a sevenfold increased risk of anastomotic leak (70). In particular, the authors emphasized a significantly higher leak rate in those receiving "long-term steroids" (50% leak rate), although duration and dosage of steroids were not described and numbers were small for this subgroup. Similarly, a meta-analysis of 12 studies including 9,565 patients identified an anastomotic leak rate of 6.77% compared to 3.27% in those receiving steroids versus no steroids (71). Despite the variability in defining perioperative steroids regimens, these studies emphasize the increased surgical risk inherent to patients unable to wean or stop long-term or perioperative steroids prior to surgery.

In the last two decades, the treatment of IBD has transformed with the introduction of biologic agents. Biologics are monoclonal antibodies or fusion proteins that bind to strictly defined molecules that play a crucial role in the inflammatory process. Antitumor necrosis factor-alpha (anti-TNF-α) agents, including infliximab and adalimumab, and more recently vedolizumab, are commonly utilized in the treatment of IBD with promising results. Despite these advancements in medical management, up to one-third of patients with Crohn disease will still require surgical resection within 5 years of diagnosis and overall two-thirds of Crohn disease patients will require major abdominal surgery at some point in their lifetime (72,73). Therefore, the impact of biologics on perioperative outcomes remains an area of active interest.

TNF-α increases angiogenesis and collagen production, and therefore it is hypothesized that inhibition of TNF-α delays wound healing, increasing postoperative complications. While this topic has been extensively studied, results are conflicting. In 2008, Appau et al. demonstrated the negative impact of recent infliximab administration (within 3 months) on ileocolic resection for Crohn disease, reporting a significantly higher rate of postoperative sepsis (20% versus 5.8%, $p = 0.021$), anastomotic leak (10% versus 1.4%, $p = 0.045$), and hospital readmission (20% versus 2.9%, $p = 0.007$) among those receiving infliximab. Syed and colleagues similarly published a single-center study of anti-TNF agents in 325 patients undergoing surgery for Crohn disease, highlighting the negative impact of biologics. In this cohort, 150 patients were exposed to anti-TNF therapy within 8 weeks of abdominal surgery, noting no difference in preoperative nutritional status or corticosteroid or immunomodulator use in the two groups. On multivariate analysis, recent anti-TNF therapy was a predictor for overall infectious (odds ratio [OR] 2.43; 95% CI, 1.18–5.03) and surgical site (OR 1.96; 95% CI, 1.02–3.77) complications (74).

More recently, however, emerging studies have challenged these findings and repeatedly demonstrate the safety of continuing biologics in the perioperative period. In a Danish study of 2,293 patients with Crohn disease who underwent intestinal resection, biologic therapy within 12 weeks of surgery did not predict a higher rate of morbidity and mortality. Furthermore, a subanalysis of this data showed no increased risk of postoperative complications when given within 14 days of surgery (75). Waterman et al. similarly looked at a cohort of 195 IBD patients who were exposed to biologic therapy before surgery and found no difference in postoperative infectious rates when exposure was within 14 days, 15–30 days, or 31–180 days before surgery compared with controls (76). Review of the available data highlights the controversial nature of this topic but increasingly supports the practice of continuing biologic therapy. Perhaps more relevant, however, is the overall impact of combined immunosuppressive agents on wound healing. In the study by Waterman et al., while shorter interval between last dose of biologic therapy and surgery did not increase surgical complications, combination therapy with thiopurine and biologics was associated with higher rates of perioperative morbidity. This point underscores the cumulative effect of immunomodulating agents and cautions one to consider temporary stoma creation in the setting of multimodal immunosuppression.

With continuing advancements in medical immunosuppression regimens, transplant recipients are living longer, and it is not uncommon for the colorectal surgeon to encounter these patients in practice. In the emergent setting, particularly after initial transplantation, these patients are often receiving high-dose immunosuppression, with minimal physiologic reserve, and intestinal anastomoses should be avoided when possible. In the elective setting, however, limited data exist to guide the surgeon in preoperative counseling and decision-making. A study of rodent models undergoing intestinal anastomoses and abdominal wall closure showed that tacrolimus was associated with no difference in wound healing or tensile strength in the early postoperative period (77). In this study, however, wound strength was measured out to 7 days only, while in reality anastomotic complications may present up to 2–3 weeks after the index procedure. Although similar studies of human cohorts are unavailable, Dean and colleagues identified a higher incidence of SSIs and incisional hernias in patients randomized to either sirolimus versus tacrolimus after renal transplantation (47% versus 8%, $p < 0.0001$) (78). Given the lack of evidence to support cessation of these drugs in the perioperative period and the critical role they play in preventing transplant rejection, transitioning from sirolimus to tacrolimus 6 weeks leading up to surgery may be reasonable.

Among colorectal cancer patients, 28,000 patients (20%) will present with metastatic disease at the time of diagnosis. Metastatic colorectal cancer requires a patient-specific, multidisciplinary approach due to the variation in disease burden and distribution. Patients who are asymptomatic at initial presentation often benefit from initial chemotherapy, and those with a favorable response may be appropriate surgical candidates in the future. For those patients who present for elective surgery after neoadjuvant chemotherapy, surgery timing is left to the discretion of the surgeon. The cytotoxic effect of chemotherapy leads to induction of cell death in the setting of colorectal cancer, and theoretically also delays wound and anastomotic healing. Bevacizumab, a humanized monoclonal antibody targeting vascular endothelial growth factor (VEGF) receptor, is considered first-line therapy with FOLFOX in the treatment of metastatic colorectal cancer. Bevacizumab prevents tumor growth by inhibiting neoangiogenesis but can also lead to deleterious effects on healthy tissue in the postoperative setting, delaying wound healing and increasing the risk of infectious, ischemic, and bleeding complications. Bevacizumab has been associated with increased rates of early and late anastomotic complications, including fistula formation up to 5 months after surgery (79–81). With a half-life of 20 (11–50) days, this drug should be held at least 28–40 days prior to elective surgery and postoperatively resumed no earlier than 28 days, and ideally 6 weeks after surgery (82). For those who are unable to afford a drug holiday due to clinical deterioration (obstruction and perforation), stoma creation should be strongly considered, and increased bleeding risk should be anticipated prior to arriving to the operating room.

## CHRONIC ANTICOAGULATION AND PERIOPERATIVE MANAGEMENT

With advancements in CVD management, a host of new anticoagulant agents are available. Familiarity with these various medications, including an understanding of their mechanism of action, reversal agent, bioavailability, and half-life, is important to minimize perioperative morbidity. The most common agents will be discussed in this section, acknowledging that we are unable to provide a comprehensive review of all anticoagulation options in this chapter.

Aspirin irreversibly inhibits cyclooxygenase-1 (COX-1) and subsequently impairs platelet function. The effects of aspirin last the duration of the platelet life span, from 8 to 10 days. Continuation of low-dose aspirin (81 mg) through the perioperative period is safe in patients undergoing major abdominal surgery, without an increased risk of major postoperative bleeding complications (83). Dedicated studies investigating bleeding complications in the setting of high-dose aspirin (325 mg), however, are limited. If chosen to discontinue prior to surgery, high-dose aspirin should be held for 7 days.

Clopidogrel is a platelet receptor inhibitor and most commonly used in patients with prior cardiac or vascular stents, or history of stroke. Due to its irreversible effects on platelet aggregation, when possible it should be discontinued 5–7 days prior to elective surgery. In specific settings where a major abdominal procedure with high risk of bleeding is required in a patient with a recent cardiac stent, bridging agents such as tirofiban may be used, as previously mentioned in the section "Cardiac Evaluation."

Warfarin inhibits vitamin K-dependent clotting factor synthesis, with a half-life of 36–42 hours. Most indications for anticoagulation have a therapeutic range between 2 and 3 or 2.5 and 3.5, and warfarin should be held 5 days before surgery, with the level rechecked the day prior to or morning of surgery. Ideally, the INR level should be 1.4 or less before major abdominal surgery to minimize bleeding complications. In the event of an emergent surgery, FFP can be administered as a reversal agent, acknowledging that FFP has an INR of 1.6. Postoperative resumption of anticoagulation should be at the discretion of the surgeon. For patients at high risk of clotting, bridging options with Lovenox injections or a continuous heparin infusion are effective options.

Heparin inactivates antithrombin III and can be administered as an IV infusion for therapeutic indications or subcutaneous injection for thromboembolic prophylaxis. With a half-life of 45 minutes, heparin infusions provide the advantage of implementing therapeutic anticoagulation with easier and faster reversibility if bleeding complications arise. Low molecular weight heparin (enoxaparin) has a half-life of 3–5 hours and is attractive for bridging of anticoagulation in the outpatient setting. Compared to enoxaparin, unfractionated heparin is cheaper, has a shorter half-life, and is safer to use in renal failure patients. However, enoxaparin has a lower risk of heparin-induced thrombocytopenia (HIT) and provides the flexibility of use in the ambulatory setting. For patients receiving enoxaparin twice daily, the evening dose the night prior to surgery should be held. Heparin infusions should be stopped 6 hours prior to surgery. If necessary, protamine sulfate can be used to reverse the effects of heparin products.

Rivaroxaban, Apixaban, and Dabigatran etexilate are oral agents that have been recently introduced as alternatives to traditional options for therapeutic anticoagulation. Rivaroxaban and apixaban inhibit Factor Xa, while Dabigatran etexilate is a direct thrombin inhibitor. Ease of administration and the lack of routine drug-level surveillance are attractive features of these new medications. These medications should be stopped at least 2 days prior to elective surgery, and resumed as soon as able. In situations that require a more specific description of the drug's impact on clotting, anti-Factor 10a levels can be measured. No reversal agent is currently available for Factor Xa inhibitors.

Although hemostasis is a key concern for any surgeon, timing of resuming anticoagulation should be coordinated with the patient's cardiologist or primary care physician to minimize the risk of thromboembolic events as well.

## HYPERCOAGULABLE CONDITIONS

Patients with thrombophilia conditions deserve specific attention regarding perioperative medical management. Hypercoagulable conditions, such as Factor V Leiden deficiency, antithrombin deficiency, and protein C and S deficiency, can lead to spontaneous thrombosis in the form of venous thromboembolism or arterial thrombosis. For patients on chronic anticoagulation, such as warfarin, therapeutic low molecular weight heparin or a heparin infusion can be used to bridge therapy in the perioperative setting, as noted in the section "Chronic Anticoagulation and Perioperative Management." It is important to remember that timing to resume anticoagulation in this population with inherent hypercoagulability (84) is often more critical compared to those on chronic anticoagulation for prevention of thrombotic complications related to atrial fibrillation. When therapeutic anticoagulation is suspended for an extended period of time, patients can experience significant complications, ranging from mesenteric thrombosis to limb-threatening ischemia.

## CONSIDERATIONS FOR EXTENDED THROMBOPROPHYLAXIS

Indications for extended thromboprophylaxis after surgery are well established in colorectal cancer patients but poorly defined otherwise. Extended thromboprophylaxis after abdominal surgery for colorectal cancer is recommended for 3–4 weeks, using enoxaparin (85). In a randomized study of 1-week versus 4-week prophylaxis for VTE events after laparoscopic colorectal cancer surgery, Vedovati and colleagues demonstrated a significant reduction of VTE events (9.7% versus 0%, $p = 0.001$) without increased bleeding risk in those receiving extended therapy (86).

Similar guidelines in other high-risk populations, including IBD and bariatric patients, are lacking but emerging as areas of interest. Aminian and colleagues recently introduced a risk assessment tool to guide indications for extended postoperative thromboprophylaxis after bariatric surgery. Based on ACS NSQIP data, the authors found that more than 80% of VTE events occurred after discharge, with the most significant predictors including congestive heart failure, paraplegia, dyspnea at rest, and reoperation (87). In addition, prior history of DVT and procedure-specific factors, including open approach, operating time more than 3 hours, and revision surgeries have been associated with more VTE events after bariatric surgery (84,88,89). A promising study by Raftopoulos compared administration of twice-daily enoxaparin 30 mg until hospital discharge versus 176 patients who also received enoxaparin 40 mg daily for 10 days following discharge after bariatric surgery (90). In the latter group, no VTE events occurred within 30 days of surgery compared to 4.5% in those not receiving postdischarge anticoagulation ($p = 0.006$). No significant difference in bleeding events or mortality was noted. These results are encouraging and may be relevant in the prevention of VTE events in morbidly obese colorectal surgery patients as well.

A recent review of NSQIP data similarly reported higher rates of VTE in IBD compared to colorectal cancer patients (2.7% versus 2.1%) (91). Additional studies have identified a 1.5- to 1.8-fold higher risk of VTE in IBD patients, with highest rates among ulcerative colitis versus Crohn patients, with an OR of 2.1 versus 0.96 (92,93).

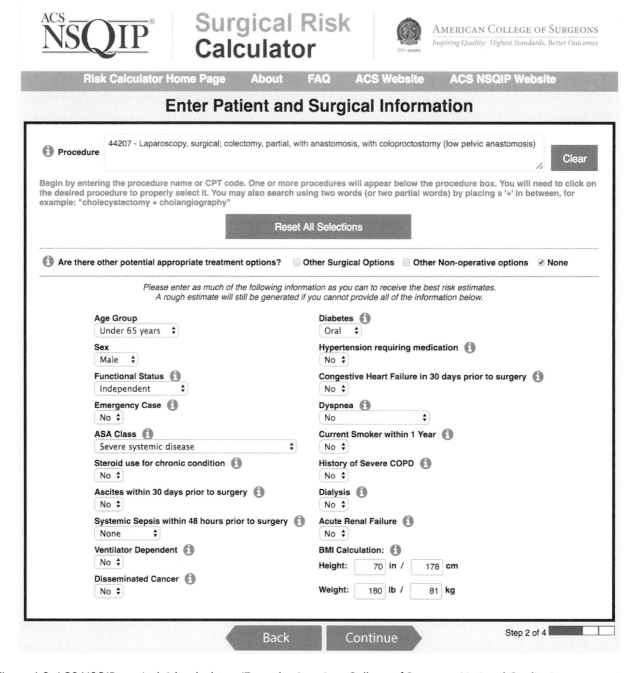

Figure 1.2 ACS NSQIP surgical risk calculator. (From the American College of Surgeons National Quality Improvement Program, http://riskcalculator.facs.org/RiskCalculator.) *(Continued)*

A recent study by Scarpa et al. evaluated VTE rates in patients undergoing major colorectal surgery and identified a significantly increased risk of VTE in ulcerative colitis patients (OR 7.4; 95% CI, 1.4–44.4; $p = 0.017$). Again, in this study DVT rates were higher in ulcerative colitis compared to colorectal cancer patients ($p = 0.009$) (94). Given the multitude of variables that contribute to VTE risk, development of a VTE risk calculator for colorectal surgery may help stratify and better select patients who will benefit from extended therapy.

## RISK ASSESSMENT TOOLS

During the initial encounter, a limited amount of time is available to evaluate and address each patient's pathology, review comorbidities, and have an informed discussion regarding surgical indications, alternatives, risks, and benefits of a proposed procedure. In the last decade, surgical risk calculators have been adopted as helpful adjuncts in this discussion and the informed consent process.

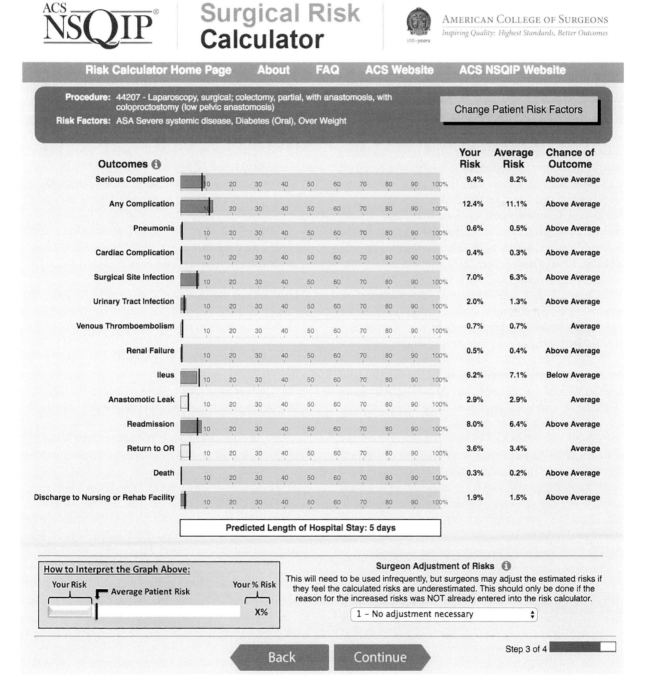

Figure 1.2 (Continued) ACS NSQIP surgical risk calculator. (From the American College of Surgeons National Quality Improvement Program, http://riskcalculator.facs.org/RiskCalculator.)

Traditionally, risk evaluation was based on physician experience and his/her interpretation of a patient's preexisting conditions. For example, the ASA Classification was developed by anesthesiologists to define a patient's operative risk by assessing comorbidities, and ranges from ASA I to VI. ASA class has been shown to be an accurate predictor of surgical outcomes (95), but predictive capacity of this classification depends heavily on clinical judgment and physician experience rather than objective measures.

Given these limitations, risk calculators such as POSSUM (Physiological and Operative Severity Score for enumeration of Mortality and Morbidity) were introduced to include objective measures into this estimation (96). POSSUM, first introduced in 1991, calculates complication and mortality rates using 12 physiologic and 6 operative variables. However, POSSUM and modifications of the tool including the Colorectal-POSSUM (CR-POSSUM) score have repeatedly overestimated mortality after colorectal cancer surgery (97).

In 2013, the ACS NSQIP Surgical Risk Calculator was introduced as a Web-based decision aid tool to facilitate the informed consent process (98). This tool calculates patient-specific, empirically derived risk estimates based on 21 patient-specific risk factors and the type of procedure. This tool was created from an updated, high-quality database recording demographics, comorbidities, and 30-day outcomes after surgery from more than 500 institutions in the United States and Canada. Measured outcomes include readmission, ileus, anastomotic leak, and the most common complications associated with colorectal surgery, as seen in Figure 1.2. Estimates of potential for discharge to skilled nursing or rehabilitation facilities are also calculated and can be an important component of the preoperative discussion. Furthermore, the Surgical Adjustment Score (SAS) allows the surgeon to subjectively adjust estimated risk based on clinical assessment of variables not yet measured with this tool. For example, the ACS NSQIP Surgical Risk Calculator currently does not assess hypoalbuminemia, a known predictor of postoperative complications, into calculated risk estimates. However, a recent study by Hu and colleagues demonstrated that addition of hypoalbuminemia as the 22nd factor in the calculator increased accuracy of morbidity and mortality estimates (99). Initial evaluation of the risk calculator's utility has been promising and highlights the opportunity for continued development with additional modifiers.

## CONCLUSION

Close attention to patient comorbidities in the preoperative setting is an essential component of surgical planning. A thorough history and physical exam are the foundation of this evaluation and will help guide additional testing, interventions, and consultations, when indicated. Ultimately, accurate assessment of these preexisting conditions helps optimize clinical outcomes, and along with risk calculators, allows the surgeon to have an educated, informed discussion with patients who present for surgery.

## REFERENCES

1. Kaplan EB et al. *JAMA*. 1985;253(24):3576–81.
2. Benarroch-Gampel J et al. *Ann Surg*. 2012;256(3): 518–28.
3. Davenport DL et al. *J Am Coll Surg*. 2007;204(6): 1199–210.
4. Maddox TM. *Mt Sinai J Med*. 2005;72(3):185–92.
5. Fleisher LA et al. *Circulation*. 2014;130(24):2215–45.
6. Lee TH et al. *Circulation*. 1999;100(10):1043–9.
7. Goldman L. *N Engl J Med*. 1994;330(10):707–9.
8. Gupta PK et al. *Circulation*. 2011;124(4):381–7.
9. Kirklin JW et al. *J Am Coll Cardiol*. 1991;17(3):543–89.
10. Breen P et al. *Anaesthesia*. 2004;59(5):422–7.
11. Hillis LD et al. *Circulation*. 2011;124(23):2610–42.
12. Levine GN et al. *Circulation*. 2011;124(23):e574–e651.
13. Kaluza GL et al. *J Am Coll Cardiol*. 2000;35(5): 1288–94.
14. Hawn MT et al. *JAMA*. 2013;310(14):1462–72.
15. Kristensen SD et al. *Eur Heart J*. 2014;35(35): 2383–431.
16. Fleisher LA et al. *Circulation*. 2014;130(24):e278–333.
17. Group PS et al. *Lancet*. 2008;371(9627):1839–47.
18. Fernandez-Bustamante A et al. *JAMA Surg*. 2017; 152(2):157–66.
19. Garibaldi RA et al. *Am J Med*. 1981;70(3):677–80.
20. Fujita T, Sakurai K. *Am J Surg*. 1995;169(3):304–7.
21. Smetana GW et al. *Ann Intern Med*. 2006;144(8): 581–95.
22. Canet J et al. *J Am Soc Anesthesiol*. 2010;113(6): 1338–50.
23. Gupta H et al. *Chest*. 2013;143(6):1599–606.
24. Wetterslev J et al. *Acta Anaesthesiol Scand*. 2000; 44(1):9–16.
25. Morton H. *The Lancet*. 1944;243(6290):368–70.
26. Schwilk B et al. *Acta Anaesthesiol Scand*. 1997;41(3): 348–55.
27. Frick W et al. *Tex Dent J*. 1994;111(6):21–3.
28. Theadom A, Cropley M. *Tob Control*. 2006;15(5): 352–8.
29. Mills E et al. *Am J Med*. 2011;124(2):144–54. e8.
30. Warner MA et al. (eds). *Mayo Clinic Proceedings* 1989 Jun 1;64(6):609–616. Elsevier.
31. Myers K et al. *Arch Intern Med*. 2011;171(11):983–9.
32. Wong J et al. *Can J Anesth/J Canadien d'anesthésie*. 2012;59(3):268–79.
33. Kaw R et al. *Chest J*. 2012;141(2):436–41.
34. Chung F et al. *Br J Anaesth*. 2012;108(5):768–75.
35. Feely MA et al. *Am Fam Physician*. 2013;87(6):414–8.
36. https://www.niddk.nih.gov/health-information/kidney-disease/chronic-kidney-disease-ckd. Accessed July 23, 2018.

37. Currie A et al. *Colorectal Dis.* 2014;16(11):879–85.
38. Metcalf AM et al. *Dis Colon Rectum.* 1987;30(7): 529–31.
39. Peng Y et al. *Medicine (Baltim).* 2016;95(8):e2877.
40. Neeff H et al. *J Gastrointest Surg.* 2011;15(1):1–11.
41. Ghaferi AA et al. *Ann Surg.* 2010;252(2):345–50.
42. Mansour A et al. *Surgery.* 1997;122(4):730–5; discussion 5–6.
43. Meunier K et al. *Dis Colon Rectum.* 2008;51(8): 1225–31.
44. Azoulay D et al. *J Am Coll Surg.* 2001;193(1):46–51.
45. Gervaz P et al. *J Am Coll Surg.* 2003;196(6):874–9.
46. Centers for Disease Control and Prevention. *National Diabetes Statistics Report, 2014: Estimates of Diabetes and its Burden in the United States.* Atlanta, GA: US Department of Health and Human Services. 2014.
47. Fransgaard T et al. *Colorectal Dis.* 2016;18(1):O22–9.
48. Yeh CC et al. *Diabetes Care.* 2013;36(10):3216–21.
49. Delamaire M et al. *Diabet Med.* 1997;14(1):29–34.
50. McConnell YJ et al. *J Gastrointest Surg.* 2009;13(3): 508–15.
51. Ata A et al. *Am Surg.* 2010;76(7):697–702.
52. Kwon S et al. *Ann Surg.* 2013;257(1):8–14.
53. Investigators N-SS et al. *N Engl J Med.* 2012;367(12): 1108–18.
54. Goodenough CJ et al. *J Am Coll Surg.* 2015;221(4): 854–61 e1.
55. Gustafsson UO et al. *Br J Surg.* 2009;96(11):1358–64.
56. National Center for Health Statistics (US. Health, United States, 2016: with Chartbook on Long-term Trends in Health.
57. Jung UJ, Choi MS. *Int J Mol Sci.* 2014;15(4):6184–223.
58. Must A et al. *Jama.* 1999;282(16):1523–9.
59. Martin ST, Stocchi L. *Clin Colon Rectal Surg.* 2011; 24(4):263–73.
60. Mullen JT et al. *Ann Surg.* 2009;250(1):166–72.
61. Wick EC et al. *Arch Surg.* 2011;146(9):1068–72.
62. Stein PD et al. *Am J Med.* 2005;118(9):978–80.
63. Huhmann MB, Cunningham RS. *Lancet Oncol.* 2005; 6(5):334–43.
64. Hu WH et al. *Nutr J.* 2015;14:91.
65. Bharadwaj S et al. *Gastroenterol Rep (Oxf).* 2016;4(2): 87–95.
66. Braga M et al. *Surgery.* 2002;132(5):805–14.
67. Thornblade LW et al. *Dis Colon Rectum.* 2017;60(1): 68–75.
68. Higgins PD et al. *Clin Gastroenterol Hepatol.* 2015; 13(2):316–21.
69. Ismael H et al. *Am J Surg.* 2011;201(3):305–8; discussion 8–9.
70. Slieker JC et al. *Arch Surg.* 2012;147(5):447–52.
71. Eriksen TF et al. *Colorectal Dis.* 2014;16(5):O154–60.
72. Bouguen G, Peyrin-Biroulet L. *Gut.* 2011;60(9): 1178–81.
73. Lazarev M et al. *Inflamm Bowel Dis.* 2010;16(5): 830–5.
74. Syed A et al. *Am J Gastroenterol.* 2013;108(4): 583–93.
75. Norgard BM et al. *Aliment Pharmacol Ther.* 2013; 37(2):214–24.
76. Waterman M et al. *Gut.* 2013;62(3):387–94.
77. Willems MC et al. *PLOS ONE.* 2013;8(9):e76348.
78. Dean PG et al. *Transplantation.* 2004;77(10):1555–61.
79. Yoshioka Y et al. *Surg Today.* 2014;44(7):1300–6.
80. Eveno C et al. *Clin Res Hepatol Gastroenterol.* 2011; 35(2):135–9.
81. Deshaies I et al. *J Surg Oncol.* 2010;101(2):180–3.
82. Gordon CR et al. *Ann Plast Surg.* 2009;62(6):707–9.
83. Mantz J et al. *Br J Anaesth.* 2011;107(6):899–910.
84. Jamal MH et al. *Surg Endosc.* 2015;29(2):376–80.
85. Bergqvist D et al. *N Engl J Med.* 2002;346(13): 975–80.
86. Vedovati MC et al. *Ann Surg.* 2014;259(4):665–9.
87. Aminian A et al. *Ann Surg.* 2017;265(1):143–50.
88. Finks JF et al. *Ann Surg.* 2012;255(6):1100–4.
89. Chan MM et al. *Surg Obes Relat Dis.* 2013;9(1): 88–93.
90. Raftopoulos I et al. *Surg Endosc.* 2008;22(11): 2384–91.
91. Gross ME et al. *Dis Colon Rectum.* 2014;57(4):482–9.
92. Wilson MZ et al. *Ann Surg.* 2015;261(6):1160–6.
93. Nguyen GC, Sam J. *Am J Gastroenterol.* 2008;103(9): 2272–80.
94. Scarpa M et al. *Int J Colorectal Dis.* 2009;24(9): 1049–57.
95. Menke H et al. *Int Surg.* 1993;78(3):266–70.
96. Copeland GP et al. *Br J Surg.* 1991;78(3):355–60.
97. Senagore AJ et al. *Dis Colon Rectum.* 2004;47(9): 1435–41.
98. Bilimoria KY et al. *J Am Coll Surg.* 2013;217(5): 833–42.
99. Hu WH et al. *Medicine (Baltim).* 2016;95(10):e2999.

# 2

# Preoperative bowel preparation

AARON L. KLINGER AND DAVID A. MARGOLIN

A 57-year-old man with a sigmoid colon cancer found via colonoscopy for a history of anemia and weight loss is awaiting surgery. The patient had a mechanical and oral antibiotic bowel preparation ordered. While you are seeing the patient in the preop holding area, he tells you that he took the oral antibiotics, but "I tried drinking that prep last night and after only half a glass I got sick and threw up. I just couldn't take it." Do you perform elective surgery?

## CASE MANAGEMENT

Yes. Multiple studies have demonstrated the safety of elective bowel surgery in the absence of a mechanical bowel preparation.

## INTRODUCTION

In 1887, Halsted published his landmark study, "Circular Suture of the Intestine" (1). Here he further supported the novel realization that microorganisms, not air exposure, lead to peritonitis and noted the high rate of death at the time following bowel surgery. He concluded that "the chief danger of infection of the peritoneal cavity is manifestly from the contents of the intestine, in case they find their way through the wound in the intestine or along the lines of suture." Since then the idea of cleaning the bowel to reduce bacterial burden and prevent infectious complications has been adapted into surgical dogma, but practice continues to be challenged.

Rates of surgical site infection (SSI) following elective colon and rectal resection remain among the highest of the general surgical procedures with estimates at 20% or higher

(2–4). This is due largely to the high concentration of aerobic and anaerobic bacteria that reside within the gut. Surgical wound infection has been shown to increase length of stay by 1 week and hospital costs by over $17,000 (4). Currently, to help mitigate these infectious complications, IV antibiotics with the addition of a preoperative bowel preparation consisting of mechanical bowel preparation (MBP), oral antibiotics (OAP), or a combination of the two have become common practice. The purpose of bowel preparation is to decrease the bacterial load in the gut in order to reduce rates of infectious complications including wound infection, abscess, and anastomotic leaks. Suggested secondary benefits of bowel preparation include ease of bowel handling (especially in minimally invasive surgery) and facilitation of intraoperative endoscopy. Those who question the benefits of preoperative bowel preparation note suboptimal patient compliance, associated patient discomfort, potential electrolyte imbalances, as well as the aspiration risk associated with consuming large volumes of liquid.

## SYSTEMIC ANTIBIOTIC PROPHYLAXIS

There is no debate regarding the importance of systemic antibiotic prophylaxis in colorectal surgery. In the 1860s Joseph Lister, having been made aware of the work of Louis Pasteur, began work on antiseptic techniques for wounds (5). He famously sprayed incisions, dressings, and instruments with carbolic acid in hopes of preventing infection. Experimentation with preoperative systemic antibiotic prophylaxis began in the 1940s following the release of penicillin, a time when SSI following colon surgery was as high as 90% (6). Use of perioperative penicillin was common practice by the mid-1950s, and its use became expected by the general public. This prompted Altemeier to state in 1955 that "antibiotics are most effective prophylactically when used as adjuvants to careful and adequate surgery but not as substitutes for it." He noted that the evidence at the time supported the use of antibacterial agents in select conditions, including surgical procedures through contaminated areas such as the gastrointestinal tract, and warned of rising antibiotic resistance (7).

Song and Glenny, in their landmark review, evaluated 147 trials of antibiotic prophylaxis in colorectal surgery performed between 1984 and 1995. They showed that the infection rate of those receiving prophylaxis had improved significantly from 22% (mean rate 1965–1980) to 11% (1984–1995). Pooled data from four trials showed a much higher infection rate in patients receiving no prophylaxis than in those receiving any systemic antibiotics (40% versus 13%). They also concluded from their review of 17 trials that there is no benefit to multiple antibiotic doses compared with a single preoperative dose. Oral antibiotics alone were shown to be significantly worse at preventing SSI than oral antibiotics with additional systemic antibiotics (odds ratio [OR] 3.34). They concluded that oral antibiotics alone were inadequate prophylaxis, that the regimen chosen must provide adequate coverage of aerobic and anaerobic bacteria, and that parenteral antibiotic administration must be timed to assure that tissue concentration of antibiotics is sufficient at the time of bacterial contamination (8).

In addition to recommending combined OAP and MBP prior to colorectal surgery, the 2013 guidelines from the Surgical Infection Society strongly recommend the use of preoperative IV antibiotics (3). They note infectious complication rates as high as 30%–60% without antibiotics compared to <10% with prophylaxis. Pooled data analysis by this group also shows a significantly decreased mortality rate with the use of preoperative IV antibiotics (11.2% versus 4.5%). The authors echo that systemic antibiotics should offer coverage for both aerobic and anaerobic bacteria. Recommended regimens include a single dose of a second-generation cephalosporin with appropriate coverage (cefoxitin or cefotetan) or cefazolin plus metronidazole. Alterative regimens are provided for those in resistant communities or with allergies to recommended agents. It is noted that ertapenem has been shown to be superior to cefotetan at preventing SSI (18.1% versus 31.1%), but its use remains controversial due to concern of creating resistant organisms and potential for *Clostridium difficile* infection (increased, but not statistically significant rates have been reported). Systemic prophylaxis should be provided within 1 hour to the start of surgery, drugs with shorter half-lives may require re-dosing for longer operations. This can be avoided by using an antibiotic with a longer half-life.

To better determine the ideal prophylactic IV antibiotic regimen, Poeran et al. analyzed 90,725 patients receiving open colectomies at 445 hospitals between 2006 and 2013 (9). The overall SSI prevalence for the study was 5.2%. Although cefoxitin was the most commonly used preoperative antibiotic (42% of cases), they found ampicillin-sulbactam (OR 0.71), ertapenem (OR 0.65), and metronidazole with cefazolin (OR 0.56) all to be superior in preventing SSI. The authors confirmed lack of benefit to providing antibiotics beyond the day of surgery.

## MECHANICAL BOWEL PREPARATION

Physical clearance of the colonic lumen before surgery has been common practice for over a century. Historic preparations included extended period dietary restriction, cathartics, whole bowel irrigation, and enemas (6). Today several oral preparations are available for bowel cleansing. While these have U.S. Food and Drug Administration (FDA) indications for cleansing for colonoscopy and radiologic studies, none are approved for preoperative cleansing for surgery. Available preparations vary from large volume isomotic preparations to smaller hyperosmotic solutions. Osmotic agents include polyethylene glycol (PEG), sodium phosphate (NaP), sodium sulfate, sodium ascorbate, and sodium picosulfate.

PEG is an inert osmotically active polymer that is mixed with an electrolyte solution, typically to a volume of 4 L, which a patient is instructed to ingest over 2–3 hours. The added electrolyte content in concert with the osmotic activity of PEG prevents net absorption or excretion of water and electrolytes acting to clear bowel contents without causing significant fluid shifts or electrolyte abnormalities in most patients. Due to the potential for these imbalances, however, special care needs to be taken in elderly patients, patients with congestive heart failure, and patients with renal insufficiency. A modified, reduced volume prep consists of 2 L PEG solution taken with four bisacodyl tablets. While not FDA approved, some surgeons have begun using a "MiraLAX prep," which consists of over-the-counter electrolyte-free PEG solution dissolved in a sports drink (i.e., Gatorade). This prep with the addition of bisacodyl utilizes less volume than traditional PEG and is more palatable for patients, allowing for better compliance (10).

NaP is a sodium-based hyperosmolar oral laxative. Its use requires smaller volumes than PEG, which like the "MiraLAX prep" may result in better patient compliance. This regimen consists of 45 mL NaP in 240 mL clear liquids taken twice, 10 hours apart. Patients should be instructed to take their prep early so that they are not kept awake the night prior to their procedure. Alternatively, patients can take NaP in tablet form—4 tablets and 240 mL clear liquids are taken every 15 minutes until 28 tablets have been consumed. The FDA issued a black box warning in May 2006 regarding the use of oral NaP for bowel preparation in elderly patients, those with underlying kidney disease, those with dehydration, or those taking medications that alter renal perfusion (such as angiotensin-converting enzyme inhibitors, angiotensin receptor blockers, diuretics, and nonsteroidal anti-inflammatory drugs). This population is at an increased risk for development of acute renal failure, or nephrocalcinosis, secondary to fluid shifts, phosphate load, and decreased intravascular volume when taking NaP prep. This complication can be avoided by consuming a larger (2–3 L) volume of clear liquids while taking this prep. However, oral NaP solutions are not currently commercially available.

The efficacy of MBP in reducing infectious complications has recently been questioned. Multiple randomized controlled trials and meta-analyses have failed to show a benefit to MBP alone. In a 2011 Cochrane Review, Güenaga et al. compared 5,805 patients from 18 trials who underwent elective colorectal surgery (11). Of these, 2,906 received MBP, and 2,899 received no preparation. All patients received IV antibiotics. They found no significant difference between these groups in rates of anastomotic leakage or wound infection in low anterior resection or colonic resection.

Despite these findings, MBP remains common practice in colorectal surgery. A survey of members of the American Society of Colon and Rectal Surgeons (ASCRS) performed by Beck and Fazio in 1990 showed 100% of respondents using some form of mechanical (most commonly enemas and cathartics) and antibiotic preparation, most using combined oral and parenteral agents (12). A repeat survey in 1997 by Nichols again found 100% compliance with some form of MBP prior to elective colorectal surgery with the majority using PEG solutions. Eighty-seven percent of respondents used both oral and parenteral antibiotics (13). A 2005 survey by Lassen et al. of colorectal surgeons in five Northern European countries found over 90% using some form of mechanical prep prior to elective left colectomy (14). Finally, a survey of ASCRS surgeons in 2016 found that 94.3% of respondents used a mechanical bowel preparation always or selectively (15).

It is difficult to establish the true value of MBP in isolation of other factors. A common endpoint in most studies is SSI, which as discussed previously and in the following section is influenced by the use of oral and/or systemic antibiotics.

## ORAL ANTIBIOTIC BOWEL PREPARATION

Attempts to reduce the colon's bacterial load with poorly absorbed oral antibiotics have been made since the 1930s–1940s. At this time the mortality of colon surgery was 10%–12% with, as mentioned previously, 80%–90% of survivors experiencing a wound infection (6). It was noted that MBP reduced overall bacterial counts but did not alter the concentration of remaining colonies. Oral antibiotic preparation is aimed at clearing the colonic lumen of aerobic (*Escherichia coli*) and anaerobic (*Bacteroides fragilis*) species. In 1943 Firor and Poth showed preoperative oral sulfanilamide reduced mortality from peritonitis from 10% to 4%. Their protocol, like most of that era, consisted of a mechanical bowel preparation followed by a clear liquid or low residue diet and a week of oral antibiotics prior to surgery. It was agreed that oral antibiotics were not adequate alone without mechanically cleared bowel (16).

In 1972, Nichols and Condon developed a protocol consisting of a mechanical bowel preparation followed by 1 g doses of neomycin and erythromycin taken three times starting 19 hours prior to the time of surgery (administered at 19, 18, and 9 hours prior to surgery). With this preparation, they showed a SSI reduction from 43% to 9%. This is still the most common protocol used today (17). A modified version with equally efficacious outcomes substitutes erythromycin, which can have significant gastrointestinal side effects, with 500 mg of metronidazole (18).

These outcomes have been challenged, and several small trials have failed to show a benefit to OAP when broad-spectrum IV antibiotic prophylaxis is also administered. Furthermore, in a study in which all patients received IV antibiotics and MBP, Wren et al. found a higher rate of *C. difficile* infection in patients taking oral antibiotics (19).

As skepticism of the utility of MBP grew, surgeons questioned the utility of OAP alone. Like Poth and his contemporaries 70 years prior, Atkinson et al. hypothesized that oral antibiotics without MBP would not alter incidence of SSI (20). They reviewed 6,399 patients from the American College of Surgeons National Surgical Quality Improvement Program (ACS-NSQIP) who underwent elective segmental colon resection. They found a significantly lower rate of SSI (9.7%) in those taking oral antibiotics than in those who did not (13.7%); however, this study did not compare this to patients receiving combined oral/mechanical prep.

In 2010, Englesbe reviewed 1,553 elective colectomies performed over 16 months in 23 hospitals in Michigan (2). He compared infectious outcomes and ileus in patients receiving a combined (MBP + OAP) prep to MBP alone. Patients who received a combined prep were significantly less likely to develop surgical site infection (4.5% versus 11.8%), organ space infection (1.8% versus 4.2%), or prolonged ileus (3.9% versus 8.6%). There was no significant difference in *C. difficile* rate. Importantly, these groups were matched for various other factors, including use of parenteral prophylactic antibiotics. Scarborough and colleagues collected data from the 2012 Colectomy-Targeted ACS-NSQIP database (21). They compared 4,999 patients divided into four groups: no preparation, MBP only, OAP only, and combined prep. Unlike Atkinson, they found no significant benefit to either modality alone but noted significantly decreased rates of SSI (3.2% versus 9%), anastomotic leak (2.8% versus 5.7%), and length of stay (4 days versus 5 days) in combined mechanical/OAP prep patients compared to those receiving no bowel prep. A Cochrane Review of studies published between 1980 and 2007 including 43,451 patients was performed to determine the ideal antimicrobial prophylaxis for CRS. Their meta-analysis, in which all patients received MBP, showed a statistically significant decrease in SSI with receipt of combined oral and parenteral antibiotics compared to parenteral alone (relative risk [RR] 0.56) or oral alone (RR 0.56). However, the authors did state that while their review shows that antibiotics delivered within this framework can reduce the risk of postoperative surgical wound infection by as much as 75%, it is not known whether oral antibiotics would still have these effects when the colon is not empty (22).

The authors of this chapter performed a retrospective case-control study of the prospectively collected

Colectomy-Targeted ACS-NSQIP database from 2012 to 2015. We evaluated over 27,000 patients using doubly robust propensity score–adjusted multivariable regression and found that patients receiving IV antibiotics combined with MBP/OAP have reduced odds of SSI, organ space infection, wound dehiscence, and anastomotic leak than no preparation and lower odds of SSI than OAP alone. Importantly, unlike Wren, the authors found a reduction in *C. difficile* infections with the use of combined bowel preparation (23).

## SPECIAL CIRCUMSTANCES

Patients with partial large bowel obstruction create a unique and challenging population. These patients are at an increased risk for infectious complication, and the use of bowel prep would be ideal. Since large volumes will not be tolerated by mouth, PEG cannot be used. Endoscopically placed stents may allow for a bowel prep to be completed prior to operative intervention; however, the use of stenting is beyond the scope of this chapter. A "slow prep" with NaP or small volumes of PEG may be attempted in select patients; they must be well hydrated without uncorrected electrolyte abnormalities. A low threshold must be held to abort the bowel preparation or to operate. An initial dose of 15 mL of NaP or 17 g of PEG in 120 mL of water is given to a monitored and serially examined patient. Two additional doses are given at 4-hour intervals, at which point the doses of NaP can be increased to 30 mL if tolerated or PEG continued. Abdominal pain or emesis should be considered indications to cancel the prep and consider early operative intervention.

### SUMMARY

While the risk of infectious complications in colorectal surgery can never be completely eliminated, there are a variety of things that should be done to mitigate the risk:

1. Intravenous antibiotics are mandatory and should be given within 1 hour of skin incision. It is incumbent that surgeons be familiar with their hospital's antibiotograms so that they can choose the most efficacious drugs.

2. In addition, combined mechanical bowel preparation and oral antibiotic bowel preparation significantly reduce infectious complications, including *C. difficile* colitis, in elective colon and rectum resections.

## REFERENCES

1. Halsted WSMD. *Am J Med Sci.* 1887;188:436–460.
2. Englesbe MJ et al. *Ann Surg.* 2010;252(3):514–9, discussion 519–20.
3. Bratzler DW et al. *Surg Infect (Larchmt).* 2013;14(1): 73–156.
4. Hedrick TL et al. *Dis Colon Rectum.* 2013;56(5): 627–37.
5. Lister J. *Br Med J.* 1867;2(351):246–8.
6. Poth EJ. *World J Surg.* 1982;6(2):153–9.
7. Altemeier WA et al. *AMA Arch Surg.* 1955;71(1): 2–6.
8. Song F, Glenny AM. *Br J Surg.* 1998;85(9):1232–41.
9. Poeran J et al. *Dis Colon Rectum.* 2016;59(8): 733–42.
10. Siddique S et al. *Am J Gastroenterol.* 2014;109(10): 1566–74.
11. Guenaga KF et al. *Cochrane Database Syst Rev.* 2011; (9):CD001544.
12. Beck DE, Fazio VW. *Dis Colon Rectum.* 1990;33(1): 12–5.
13. Nichols RL et al. *Clin Infect Dis.* 1997;24(4):609–19.
14. Lassen K et al. *BMJ.* 2005;330(7505):1420–1.
15. Beck DE, McCoy AB. Perioperative management of the colorectal; surgery patient: Current status and an ASCRS survey. Submitted.
16. Firor WM, Poth EJ. *Ann Surg.* 1941;114(4):663–71.
17. Nichols RL et al. *Ann Surg.* 1972;176(2):227–32.
18. Pollock AV, Evans M. *N Engl J Med.* 1980;303(18): 1066.
19. Wren SM et al. *Arch Surg.* 2005;140(8):752–6.
20. Atkinson SJ et al. *Surg Infect (Larchmt).* 2015;16(6): 728–32.
21. Scarborough JE et al. *Ann Surg.* 2015;262(2):331–7.
22. Nelson RL et al. *Cochrane Database Syst Rev.* 2014;(5): CD001181.
23. Klinger AL et al. *Ann Surg.* 2017.

# 3

# Anesthesia and intraoperative positioning

W. DAVID SUMRALL, III AND DAVID E. BECK

## CHALLENGING CASE

A 47-year-old male is undergoing a transanal excision of a rectal villous adenoma under IV sedation and local infiltration of xylocaine. During the procedure, the patient complains of lightheadedness and numbness of the tongue. The anesthesiologist notices bradycardia and hypotension.

## CASE MANAGEMENT

Local anesthetic systemic toxicity is suspected. The patient should be moved to the supine position and supported with supplemental oxygen via mask. The patient's blood pressure is supported with IV fluid and epinephrine. Further treatment may require continued resuscitation and intralipid.

## INTRODUCTION

The American Society of Anesthesiologists (ASA) defines anesthesiology as a discipline within the practice of medicine that specializes in the (1) medical management of patients who are rendered unconscious and/or insensible to pain and emotional stress during surgical, obstetric, and certain other medical procedures; (2) protection of life functions and vital organs under the stress of anesthetic, surgical, and other medical procedures; and (3) management of problems in pain relief (1). This chapter discusses the various kinds of anesthesia used in colorectal surgery, including their relative benefits and risks. Anesthetic risks and enhanced recovery as managed by anesthesiologists (such as intraoperative opioid sparing, goal-directed fluid management, and new treatments for postoperative pain relief) will be reviewed. Finally, anesthetic considerations as they apply to the Surgical Care Improvement Project

(SCIP), including prophylactic antibiotic administration, temperature control, and the proper positioning of patients for colorectal surgery, will be reviewed.

## ANESTHETIC TECHNIQUE

Most anorectal operations involve only a relatively small external anatomic area. This allows for a number of anesthetic options to be the selection of which should be carefully undertaken. Techniques of regional and local anesthesia can provide excellent relaxation and comfort to the patient in most instances. Unfortunately, not all patients may agree to a technique other than general anesthesia anorectal operations. For these patients, general anesthesia is therefore the anesthetic of choice. Medically, however, the benefits of regional and local anesthesia may outweigh their disadvantages and may be safer than a general anesthetic. The selection of anesthetic technique must also take into consideration the comfort level of the perioperative team with the type of anesthetic selected. To make the choice that is in the best interest of the patient, one must be familiar with the options as well as their advantages, disadvantages, and complications.

### GENERAL ANESTHESIA

A patient's preference for general anesthesia may be based on a fear of the operation itself or a fear of the operating room. Some people's modesty makes them uncomfortable to be awake while they are exposed for an operation. Others worry that a local or regional anesthetic will wear off in the middle of the procedure, leaving them vulnerable to severe pain. They may also worry about repeated needle punctures. Still others simply do not want to know what occurs in an operating room and believe that anything less than a general anesthetic will make them too aware of the course of events. If these fears can be identified, they can frequently be addressed and overcome by careful consultation and agreement among all parties involved.

Potential disadvantages to a general anesthetic include the need for endotracheal intubation if the procedure is to be performed in the prone-jackknife position. Furthermore, there is a significant incidence of nausea and vomiting following general anesthesia, and patients with significant cardiac or pulmonary insufficiency may be at increased risk.

A distinct advantage of general anesthesia is total relaxation of the pelvic floor, which can be important when operating on complicated and high fistulas or when approaching the rectum for transanal excisions. Preoperative consultation with the surgeon is advisable to ascertain the nature and complexity of the surgical procedure. Local anesthesia is frequently inadequate in these instances. If regional anesthesia is contraindicated by a neurologic condition, a back injury, anticoagulation, infection at the site of needle entry, or for other reasons, general anesthesia may be the anesthetic of choice.

## LOCAL ANESTHESIA

The earliest local anesthetic used was cocaine (prepared in weak solutions and injected in high volumes) for field block at the turn of the nineteenth century (2). However, the toxicity of cocaine, its irritant properties, and its strong potential for physical and psychological dependence led to the development of alternative local anesthetics. Many of these—such as lidocaine—are still used today, as much as half a century after their introduction (3).

While there are relatively few instances in colorectal surgery where it is used as the sole anesthetic, local anesthesia still has a place. It requires, however, a cooperative patient who can remain immobile for both the infiltration of the local anesthetic, as well as for the actual procedure.

It is important to be cognizant of the patient's underlying health status and the position that the patient will be in for the procedure. A healthy patient in his or her mid-twenties can tolerate the prone-jackknife position much better than an obese geriatric patient with a pulmonary history who uses supplemental oxygen. Restlessness and inability to tolerate local anesthesia may be due to patient factors but also could be a result of sedation, including from self-administered medications when the procedure is performed in an office setting. Any degree of sedation blunts the body's response to hypoxia and hypercarbia, and while a restless patient may simply be a restless patient, there is always the possibility that the patient is agitated due to relative hypoxia or hypercarbia.

One must always keep in mind the possibility of local anesthetic systemic toxicity (LAST) when using these drugs. The typical doses used for local infiltration in colorectal procedures are far below the threshold needed for systemic toxicity (Table 3.1). However, unintended IV or intraarterial injection could result in systemic toxicity. As such, it is important to recognize the signs and symptoms of systemic toxicity when they first appear, as toxicity progresses in a dose-dependent fashion.

At lower plasma concentrations, the patient begins to experience central nervous system (CNS) toxicity characterized by lightheadedness, tinnitus, and numbness of the tongue. As plasma concentrations increase, the patient begins to experience CNS excitation, resulting in seizures, followed by unconsciousness, coma, and respiratory arrest. At higher plasma concentrations, cardiovascular (CV) toxicity occurs, as the local anesthetic blocks sodium channels of the myocardium.

Relative potency of the local anesthetic plays a role here. Lidocaine toxicity will result in bradycardia and hypotension prior to cardiac arrest, while the longer-acting, more potent bupivacaine often results in sudden cardiovascular collapse due to ventricular dysrhythmias. Maintenance of perfusion and ventilation through prolonged cardiopulmonary resuscitation (CPR) is the key, as the patient will not convert into a life-sustaining cardiac rhythm until the local anesthetic has had a chance to completely dissociate from the sodium channels of the conducting system of the heart. Cardiopulmonary bypass may even be considered. Dissociation of local anesthetic from sodium channels has been shown to take a considerable length of time, and prolonged, intensive, and continuous support is warranted.

Treatment of CNS toxicity, including the cessation of seizure activity, is with the use of benzodiazepines, propofol, or thiopental. Treatment of CV toxicity is supportive in nature and may require electric cardioversion, epinephrine, and magnesium (4). Systemic toxicity following local anesthetic administration is thankfully rare. More common, however, is inadequate analgesia following local anesthetic infiltration. This can be multifactorial in nature.

Table 3.1 Local anesthetic drugs

| Agent | Onset | Duration | Maximum dose | Maximum dose with epinephrine |
|-------|-------|----------|--------------|-------------------------------|
| Tetracaine | | | | |
| Lidocaine | 2–5 minutes | 30–45 minutes | 5 mg/kg | 7 mg/kg |
| Mepivacaine | | | | |
| Prilocaine | | | | |
| Bupivacaine | 30 minutes | 2 hours | 2 mg/kg | 4 mg/kg |
| Procaine | 5–10 minutes | 15–30 minutes | 10 mg/kg | |
| Liposomal bupivacaine | 30 minutes | 48–72 hours | 266 mg (with 133 mg bupivacaine) | 266 mg |

Inadequate analgesia resulting from insufficient quantities placed in the correct location is easily resolved with the addition of further local anesthetic at the site. Inadequate analgesia can also result from tachyphylaxis to local anesthetics, which is defined as repeated injection of the same dose of local anesthetic leading to diminishing efficacy. Additionally, inadequate analgesia can be a consequence of the tissue pH into which the local anesthetic is injected. Local anesthetics exist in both ionized and nonionized states; it is only in the nonionized state that local anesthetics can penetrate the nerve sheath, thus producing analgesia. In an acidic environment (i.e., an infected pilonidal cyst), more of the anesthetic is converted into the ionized state, leading to far less of the nonionized form available to produce analgesia. It is not uncommon for infected tissues to prove nearly impossible to be rendered totally insensitive despite more than adequate amounts of local anesthetic infiltration.

A perianal block (Figure 3.1) can be performed with the patient in either the prone or lithotomy position and provides relaxation of the sphincter as well as anesthesia. The anesthetic solution of choice is infiltrated in a fan fashion from the lateral positions to superficially encompass the anal margin. Emphasis should be placed in the posterolateral positions where the greatest concentration of nerves is found. A finger or retractor is placed within the canal. At the anterior, posterior, and lateral positions, anesthetic is injected submucosally or intramuscularly through the previously infiltrated tissue. The needle is held parallel to the finger, with care to avoid entering the canal.

A new formulation of liposomal bupivacaine (Exparel, Pacira Pharmaceuticals, Parsippany, New Jersey) has received approval from the U.S. Food and Drug Administration and can provide analgesia for up to 72 hours. It was approved for injection into the surgical site to produce postsurgical analgesia. The two pivotal studies leading to approval were in hemorrhoidectomy and bunionectomy patients (5,6). The drug is provided in a 20 cc vial that contains 266 mg of liposomal bupivacaine. It can be diluted up to 14 times if desired. Since its release, this drug has seen increasing adoption, but the reported experience has been limited to date (7). A series of four consecutive patients undergoing loop ileostomy closure were successfully managed with multimodality postoperative pain management (including liposomal bupivacaine, IV paracetamol, and ibuprofen) as 23-hour procedures. Utilization of local infiltration as part of a multimodality approach appears to have great potential.

## MONITORED ANESTHETIC CARE

Monitored anesthetic care (MAC) is defined by the ASA as "a procedure in which an anesthesiologist is requested or required to provide anesthetic services," and includes (1) the diagnosis and treatment of clinical problems during and immediately following the procedure; (2) the support of vital functions; (3) the administration of sedatives, analgesics, hypnotics, anesthetic drugs, or other medications necessary for patient safety; (4) physical and psychological comfort; and (5) the provision of other services as needed to complete the procedure safely (8). When it comes to the care of a patient undergoing MAC, all of the precautions and equipment needed to perform a safe general anesthetic must be present, as it is always possible that an escalation of care will be needed. While uncommon, it is possible that a patient cannot safely undergo a MAC for a specific procedure. Most commonly, this is due to the inability to safely prevent a patient from moving in response to painful stimuli without producing oversedation and/or apnea. Some patients, when sedated as part of MAC, appear either to move excessively in response to stimuli or to develop airway

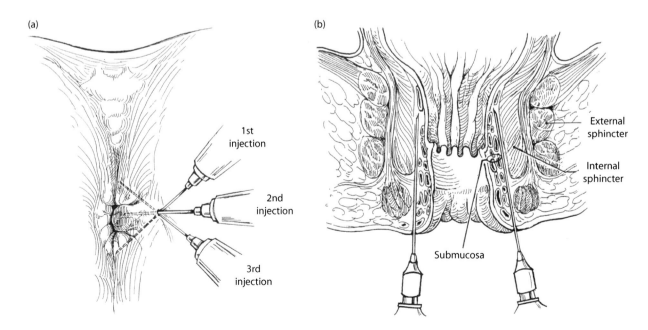

(a)

1st injection

2nd injection

3rd injection

(b)

External sphincter

Internal sphincter

Submucosa

Figure 3.1 Technique for anal block. **(a)** Perianal view of submucosal injection. **(b)** Sagittal view of injection of anal canal.

compromise, requiring further intervention and escalation of care by the anesthesiologist.

The same limits of positioning and patient tolerance that were discussed with local anesthetics apply to procedures under MAC as well. While most patients will be able to tolerate a lithotomy or prone position with mild sedation, others are unable to tolerate these positions without endotracheal intubation, positive pressure ventilation, and high inspired oxygen concentration. Additionally, there are those patients who are unable to understand or comply with the requirement to remain immobile. Young children, mentally challenged patients, or extremely ill patients are examples of poor candidates for MAC.

There is an erroneous perception on the part of patients—and even physicians—that a patient undergoing MAC is at decreased risk for serious anesthesia-related complications when compared to general anesthesia, that MAC is safer. This can best be appreciated by examining the ASA Closed Claims Project database. The ASA Closed Claims Project is a structured evaluation of all adverse anesthetic outcomes obtained from the closed claim files of 35 professional liability insurance companies in the United States. A 2006 review showed more than 40% of claims associated with MAC involved death or permanent brain damage, which was *similar* to the percentage seen in claims associated with general anesthesia (9). Respiratory depression was the most common (21%) damaging mechanism; nearly half of such occurrences were judged to be preventable through better monitoring.

Cardiovascular events comprised another 14% of the claims made in patients undergoing MAC, which was similar in frequency to that seen following general anesthesia. The average payment made to a plaintiff in these cases was $159,000. These data demonstrated that the significant risks of injury and death are similar among MAC and general anesthesia.

## REGIONAL ANESTHESIA

### Central neuraxial blockade

Regional anesthesia encompasses a wide variety of peripheral and central neuraxial blocks, many of which do not pertain to colorectal surgery. The most common regional anesthesia technique applied in colorectal surgery is the *spinal*, or *intrathecal*, blockade. The spinal block is relatively easy to place, has a fast onset of sensory and motor blockade, and has a predictable length of efficacy. This is a very old technique, dating back to the late 1800s, when it was performed using cocaine as the anesthetic agent, to the great amazement of surgeons of the day (2).

With the advent of newer local anesthetics, we can now tailor the duration of the spinal blockade to the projected length of the surgery by varying the type and amount of local anesthetic used. The goal is to provide adequate analgesia for the duration of the procedure, yet allow safe ambulation and encourage urination within a short time frame after cessation of surgery. There are three different densities

of the medications used: hyperbaric, isobaric, and hypobaric. Hypobaric local anesthetics are less dense than normal cerebrospinal fluid (CSF), which allows these medications to rise in the CSF following injection. This is commonly used for perineal procedures that will be performed in the prone jackknife position. The local anesthetic is injected into the intrathecal space, and the patient is immediately placed in the jackknife position to allow the hypobaric solution to drift upward, or caudad. After approximately 5 minutes, the spinal anesthetic will have "set up," meaning the uptake and distribution of the local anesthetic across nerve membranes have occurred. No further migration of the drug should occur at this point.

By adding a small amount of glucose to the local anesthetic used, the solution will become hyperbaric. The density of the solution will cause it to sink in relation to the CSF (10). An alternative approach to perineal analgesia performed in the prone jackknife position is performing the intrathecal block using a hyperbaric solution, then keeping patients in the sitting position for 5 minutes to allow the spinal anesthetic to sink caudad, thus blocking the lumbosacral nerves. Once the block has "set up," the patient is placed in the prone jackknife position. These two techniques have allowed the use of significantly less local anesthetic for the spinal anesthesia, compared to isobaric solutions, which have the same density as CSF. Isobaric solutions require a higher dose of local anesthetic to evenly distribute throughout the CSF, resulting in a larger volume needed to achieve the same blockade of the lumbosacral nerves. The benefits related to reducing the total amount of local anesthetic injected are a decreased risk of toxicity, along with providing adequate analgesia and allowing faster recovery of motor function.

A *caudal* anesthetic is the placement of a local anesthetic and/or narcotic into the epidural space from an approach through the sacral hiatus. This is typically performed in either the prone or lateral position. While uncommon in adults, this procedure is used frequently in children, where the caudal space is more easily accessible and a relatively safe and easy approach to infuse local anesthetic and/or narcotic for postoperative analgesia while still under general anesthesia.

The third and final type of central neuraxial block is the *epidural* anesthetic. While epidural anesthesia can be used as a single injection for colorectal procedures, it is more common to place a catheter within the epidural space to provide analgesia during and after the procedure. The location of the block is determined by the anesthesiologist based on several anatomic factors; however, a thoracic approach has been shown to be more effective in reducing postoperative ileus and early return of bowel and bladder function than a lumbar approach (11).

Most commonly, patients will receive a postoperative continuous infusion of a local anesthetic and narcotic mixture through the epidural catheter. In addition, they may be given the opportunity to provide themselves small amounts of analgesia through their epidural catheter on demand. This is termed *patient-controlled epidural analgesia* (PCEA), and it provides excellent pain control while minimizing the undesirable side effects typically seen with IV narcotics. Provided the patient does not manifest signs of systemic infection, the epidural catheter can remain in place for several days following surgery if needed to control pain. This benefit must be weighed against the risk of withholding anticoagulant prophylaxis and a possible resultant thromboembolic event.

While initial studies examining PCEA were performed using lumbar epidural, more recent studies have examined the impact of thoracic epidural analgesia on patients undergoing elective colorectal surgery. In 2001 Carli et al. reported 42 patients undergoing open large bowel resection, randomized to receive either an IV patient-controlled analgesia (IVPCA) morphine or a thoracic (T7-8) epidural with bupivacaine and fentanyl (11). Patients who received thoracic epidural had distinctly superior analgesia as compared to the IVPCA morphine group; time to first flatus and first bowel movement occurred, on average, 36 hours sooner in the epidural group, and time to readiness to discharge was the same in both groups. In 2007, Taqi et al. examined thoracic epidural analgesia compared to postoperative IV morphine for laparoscopic colectomy (12). Recovery from postoperative ileus occurred sooner in the epidural group by 1 or 2 days, and a full diet was resumed earlier. The epidural group experienced significantly less pain at rest, with coughing, and with ambulation. These studies demonstrate the effectiveness of thoracic epidural analgesia and its superiority in allowing early return of bowel function, ability to resume a full diet, and early ambulation, as compared to IV narcotics.

All three of these techniques—spinal, caudal, and epidural—have one thing in common: contraindications. Specifically, absolute contraindications to neuraxial techniques include patient refusal, infection at the planned site of needle puncture, elevated intracranial pressure, and bleeding diathesis. There are also several relative contraindications. Bacteremia raises the concern that the needle puncture site of the neuraxial block might allow an epidural abscess or meningitis to develop; however, a clinical scenario may exist where the need to avoid a general anesthetic might outweigh the small risk of such bacterial tracking into the neuraxial space.

While chronic back pain is not a contraindication to neuraxial techniques, patients with underlying neurological disease should be considered carefully, as neuraxial blockade might exacerbate their condition, such as in multiple sclerosis. The presence of cardiac disease also indicates that caution should be applied, as patients who receive a neuraxial block typically experience a sudden decrease in lower extremity vascular tone, leading to rapid vasodilation and a significant decrease in systemic vascular resistance. The resultant precipitous drop in systolic and diastolic blood pressure can be extremely dangerous in patients with severe coronary artery disease, aortic stenosis, and idiopathic hypertrophic subaortic stenosis (IHSS). It is still arguable whether the presence of IHSS or aortic stenosis is an absolute contraindication to neuraxial blockade, and many centers avoid them in the presence of these coexisting morbidities.

The final relative contraindication is abnormal coagulation status. Patients with abnormal coagulation—either due to endogenous factors such as liver disease or thrombocytopenia, or due to the administration of anticoagulants—must be considered carefully. Additionally, patients who are receiving or will be receiving anticoagulants postoperatively have different needs than patients who receive a general anesthetic alone. For spinal and caudal anesthesia, the greatest risk of spinal hematoma (a neurosurgical emergency) occurs at the time the block is placed. For epidural anesthesia, the risk of hematoma formation is just as great at the time of epidural catheter removal as during placement. As a result, certain guidelines should be instituted in order to reduce the risk of spinal hematoma formation upon removal of the epidural catheter.

Heparin is often administered perioperatively as prophylaxis against deep vein thrombosis (DVT) formation. While the effect of IV heparin administration is immediate, subcutaneous administration requires 1–2 hours to effect a change on coagulation. Small doses of heparin administered subcutaneously prior to surgery for DVT prophylaxis are not a concern in terms of risk of spinal hematoma formation (13). Postoperatively, subcutaneous DVT prophylaxis dosing twice daily of heparin while an epidural catheter is in place is acceptable. The catheter is removed 2 hours prior to the next heparin dosing to maximize safety.

Therapeutic heparin, however, is a different matter. Ruff et al. demonstrated that neuraxial procedures performed less than 1 hour after heparin therapy is discontinued resulted in a 25-fold increase in spinal hematoma (14). The effect is even more pronounced if the patient also received aspirin.

Low molecular weight heparin (LMWH) was introduced in 1993 as an alternative to heparin prophylaxis for prevention of DVT. There have been numerous reports of spinal hematoma in patients receiving LMWH with a neuraxial blockade. For patients receiving low-dose LMWH for thromboprophylaxis preoperatively, it is recommended that neuraxial anesthesia occur at least 12 hours after the last dose. In patients who are receiving high-dose LMWH, neuraxial anesthesia should be delayed for 24 hours after the last dose. Postoperatively, the typical prophylactic twice-daily dosing of LMWH should only begin 24 hours after the neuraxial block, and any epidural catheter should be removed prior to initiation of twice-daily dosing. Once-daily thromboprophylactic dosing, however, can safely occur with an epidural catheter in place, provided that the first dose occurs at least 8 hours following the initial blockade and that any epidural catheter is removed 12 hours after the last dose prior to its removal (12).

Warfarin therapy is another concern. Warfarin anticoagulation must be stopped 4–5 days prior to surgery, and the prothrombin time/international normalized ratio (PT/INR) assessed prior to surgery. Anticoagulation with warfarin can be used for thromboprophylaxis in patients with an indwelling epidural catheter, though the catheter should be removed while the INR is still less than 1.5. Typically, this is approximately 36 hours following the initial administration of warfarin. Neurologic and motor testing should be routinely performed on these patients (15).

All three of the neuraxial techniques have possible side effects. Patients can become hypotensive, as their systemic vascular resistance decreases. This is due to the sympathectomy caused by blockade of sympathetic fibers along the thoracic sympathetic chain. Rarely, patients can develop an unintentionally high spinal anesthetic, leading to bradycardia, apnea, and even loss of consciousness. This "high spinal" must be treated as a general anesthetic, with immediate securing of the airway with endotracheal intubation and supportive therapy until the local anesthetic is metabolized.

Some patients can experience mild back pain at the site of needle placement, especially when multiple attempts are needed to place the block. Postdural puncture headache (PDPH) can occur, typically following unintended dural puncture with an epidural needle—a "wet tap." These headaches are characterized by a slow leak of CSF from the puncture, leading to a headache that is strongest when standing and lessened when lying. They are often treated conservatively with oral fluid therapy, oral caffeine, and the recumbent position. If relief is not obtained after conservative treatment, an epidural blood patch can be performed. For this procedure, 20 mL of sterile, autologous blood is injected into the epidural space, resulting in thrombus formation, sealing of the dura, and cessation of CSF leak. If the diagnosis of PDPH is correct, there is typically immediate relief of symptoms. Epidural abscess and meningitis are possible if proper sterile technique is not used, or if systemic infection is present (10).

## Transversus abdominis plane block

The transversus abdominis plane (TAP) block is a relatively new procedure for blocking the abdominal wall afferent nerves by way of the lumber triangle of Petit. It can be performed using a landmark technique or under ultrasound guidance; 20 mL of 0.375% of bupivacaine or levobupivacaine is then injected into the transversus abdominis neurofascial plane (16–18). In a prospective, randomized controlled trial, McDonnell et al. reported patients undergoing large bowel resection who received the TAP block required 75% less morphine in the first 24 hours, and had significantly lower pain scores at all time points over the first 24 hours. Additionally, these patients experienced significantly less postoperative nausea and vomiting (16). This is an excellent block for patients having smaller abdominal procedures (e.g., ileostomy takedown/revision), on an outpatient basis.

## Ilioinguinal and iliohypogastric nerve block

These are field blocks of the terminal branches of the lumbar plexus, primarily from the L1 root. These blocks are relatively simple to perform and provide anesthesia in the inguinal and genital region. A 22-gauge needle is inserted

3 cm medial and 3 cm inferior to the anterior superior iliac spine, in a cephalolateral direction through the abdominal muscles until contact is made with the iliac bone. As the needle is removed, local anesthetic solution is injected. This is repeated one to two more times to cover a fan-shaped area, for a total of approximately 10–20 mL of local anesthetic (19).

## AWARENESS UNDER ANESTHESIA

Awareness under anesthesia is a rare complication of anesthesia, but one which has risen to prominence in the public eye recently. Studies of large numbers of patients in Sweden demonstrated an overall incidence of 0.16% (20). One can imagine that this would be a distressing event; the frequency of posttraumatic stress disorder in the 2 years following an incident of awareness under anesthesia approached 50%, even if the patient was not initially distressed by the incident. A similarly large study in the United States found an overall incidence rate for confirmed intraoperative awareness of 0.13%, and a rate of 0.24% of possible awareness (21). It has long been known that awareness occurs with greater frequency in emergent trauma surgery cases, cases involving cardiopulmonary bypass, and emergency cesarean sections. These are situations where patients may experience significant hypotension, requiring a reduction in volatile anesthetic agents below the level that ensures amnesia. If there is a question whether a patient has had an episode of awareness under anesthesia, it is imperative the anesthesiologist be contacted, and the patient reassured. Psychiatric evaluation is usually necessary to help the patient deal with the potentially distressing nature of this complication.

A device available that attempts to determine the depth of consciousness is the bispectral index (BIS), a monitor of anesthetic depth approved by the U.S. Food and Drug Administration. The frontal electroencephalograph is measured, processed using proven algorithms, and reported on an arbitrary scale of 0–100. On this scale, 100 equates to completely awake and responsive, and zero represents complete electrical silence of the brain. A BIS of less than 60 is generally considered a safe level to ensure adequate depth of anesthesia and lack of awareness under anesthesia. In the B-Aware trial, patients at high risk for awareness under anesthesia were randomized to two groups, either routine care or a BIS-guided anesthetic. While the incidence of awareness among even high-risk patients was very low, the risk of awareness was 82% lower in patients with BIS-guided anesthetics (22).

However, there is controversy surrounding the reliability of the BIS monitor. Use of the BIS monitor and maintenance within the proper depth of anesthesia (as indicated by the BIS algorithm) is still no assurance that the patient will not have an episode of awareness, as there are numerous reports to the contrary (23). Additionally, there are numerous conditions that can influence the BIS, causing BIS levels that are paradoxically high, such as ketamine administration or the use of halothane, or paradoxically low, such as following nitrous oxide termination (24). An analysis of the ASA Close Claims Project database demonstrates that between the years of 1961 and 1995 there were 79 claims for awareness made in the United States; 18 claims for awake paralysis, i.e., the inadvertent administration of a muscle relaxant to an awake patient, and 61 claims for recall under general anesthesia, i.e., recall of events while receiving general anesthesia. Most of the claims for awake paralysis represented substandard care; less than half of the claims for recall were the result of substandard care. The majority of patients experienced temporary emotional distress; 10% of patients were later diagnosed with posttraumatic stress disorder. The awareness of sound without pain was the most common intraoperative event; 21% of patients experienced pain while aware under anesthesia (25).

## INTRAOPERATIVE GOAL-DIRECTED THERAPY

With the introduction of enhanced surgical recovery programs, there has been renewed interest in optimizing surgical fluid regimens. The historical debate between liberal versus restrictive fluid regimens has been reevaluated, and the idea of individualized goal-directed therapy has been introduced and subjected to a number of randomized controlled trials. While untreated hypovolemia can be detrimental to patients, fluid overload can be just as (if not more) hazardous. By tailoring fluid administration to an individual patient's needs using a treatment algorithm based on closely monitored flow variables, postoperative recovery can be improved with reduced morbidity, less gastrointestinal dysfunction, and reduced hospital stay (26).

## INTRAOPERATIVE OPIOID SPARING

A recent development in general anesthesia techniques is opioid-sparing anesthetics. Opioids are known to be associated with some adverse side effects, including postoperative delirium, ileus, allergic reactions, and nausea. Opioid-sparing protocols attempt to use multimodal strategies to limit these side effects while still providing safe and comfortable care for the patient. Most guidelines use a combination of acetaminophen, ibuprofen, ketamine, lidocaine infusion, Decadron, dexmedetomidine, and local anesthetics. There are several studies that have shown great success adopting this technique (27).

## POSTOPERATIVE PAIN MANAGEMENT

A number of the pain management options have been grouped into multimodality pain management programs. Many of these include opioid-sparing techniques. Nonsteroidal anti-inflammatory drugs (NSAIDs) reduce the amount of opiates requested and administered to the patient and therefore opioid side effects (28). They are useful in treating mild to moderate pain. NSAIDs act by inhibiting the enzyme cyclooxygenase (COX), thereby blocking the production of prostaglandins resulting in an anti-inflammatory response. NSAIDs are classified by their selectivity of the COX isoenzymes. There is a risk of bleeding with these agents; use of NSAIDs is dependent on the individual patient's risk factors. Nonselective agents such as ibuprofen have an increased side effect profile (bleeding and antiplatelet effect); however, COX-1 inhibitors are preferred over selective COX-2 inhibitors such as celecoxib given the recent evidence of cardiovascular risks associated with COX-2 agents (28–30).

IV ibuprofen (Caldolor, Cumberland Pharmaceuticals, Nashville, Tennessee) is administered as 800 mg every 6 hours (31). In a prospective randomized study, Cataldo et al. compared the effect of intramuscular ketorolac in combination with PCA (morphine) to that of PCA alone. Narcotic requirements were decreased by 45% (32). They suggested that this combination may be particularly beneficial in patients especially prone to narcotic-related complications.

Acetaminophen is a centrally acting analgesic but lacks peripheral anti-inflammatory effects. Oral acetaminophen is widely used for acute pain relief. Acetaminophen is a common ingredient in many combination oral pain medications; it is vital to counsel the patient not to exceed the 4,000 mg daily maximum dose due to the risk of hepatotoxicity. Systematic reviews of randomized controlled trials (RCTs) confirm the efficacy of oral acetaminophen for acute pain (33). However, acetaminophen has a slow onset of analgesia and until recently the nonavailability of the oral route immediately after surgery limited its value in treating immediate postoperative pain. An IV form of acetaminophen is now commercially available (Ofirmev, Mallinkrodt Pharmaceuticals, St. Louis, Missouri). Acetaminophen's major advantage over NSAIDs is its lack of interference with platelet function and safe administration in patients with a history of peptic ulcers or asthma. Opioid-sparing effects have been associated with acetaminophen administered intravenously (34). A mixed trial comparison found a decrease in 24-hour morphine consumption when acetaminophen, NSAIDs, or COX-2 inhibitors are given in addition to PCA morphine after surgery with a reduction in morphine-related adverse effects. However, the study did not find any clear differences between the three nonopioid agents (35). A systematic review identified 21 studies comparing acetaminophen alone or in combination with other NSAIDs and reported increased efficacy with the combination of two agents than with either alone (35). Current dosing is 1000 g IV every 6 hours.

In patients undergoing major colorectal operations, Beck and colleagues compared 66 patients who received multimodality pain management to 167 patients managed with opioid PCA and found that the multimodality patients had lower pain scores, used less opioids, had less opioid-related adverse events, and had decreased lengths of postoperative hospital stay (average 1.8 days) (36). A sample multimodality pain management regimen is presented in Table 3.2.

Table 3.2 Sample multimodality pain management

**Preoperative**

Acetaminophen (paracetamol) 1000 mg IV in preop

Ibuprofen 800 mg IV in preop

**Intraoperative**

Liposomal bupivacaine 266 mg wound infiltration

**Postoperative**

Acetaminophen (paracetamol) 1000 mg IV every 6 hours until patient taking oral meds

Ibuprofen 800 mg IV every 8 hours until patient taking oral meds

PCA (morphine or Dilaudid) for severe pain (scale 6–10) until patient taking oral meds

Oxycodone 10 mg PO every 4 hours for moderate pain when taking oral medication

*Abbreviations:*  IV, intravenously; PCA, patient-controlled anesthesia; PO, by mouth.

# POSITIONING

## SUPINE

This is the most common surgical position; it results in the least hemodynamic and ventilatory changes and is frequently the best position for surgical exposure. The supine position is not perfect, of course, as it creates certain pressure points that, given time, result in ischemia over certain bony prominences, such as the heels, sacrum, and back of the head. The head should rest on a soft support to spread the pressure, decreasing the incidence of pressure points, thus preventing alopecia. Particular care must be given to the arms, including careful padding of the elbows and wrists. Abduction of the arms must not exceed 90° from the body to prevent compromising blood flow to the distal arm (37). Trendelenburg positioning while supine has several anesthetic implications, as it causes the diaphragm to move cephalad, causing increased airway pressures and possibly advancing the endotracheal tube into an endobronchial position.

Shoulder braces are sometimes used to prevent the patient from sliding off the table during extreme Trendelenburg positioning, though this can cause injury by compressing the brachial plexus (38). The most common upper extremity injury is to the ulnar nerve, which is three times more likely in men who undergo general anesthesia. This seems to occur despite padding of the extremity (39). Other nerves at risk due to positioning are illustrated in Figure 3.2.

## PRONE

Even when a procedure is planned in the prone position, induction of general anesthesia and intubation of the trachea should occur in the supine position. The patient is then turned prone, taking care to keep the cervical spine

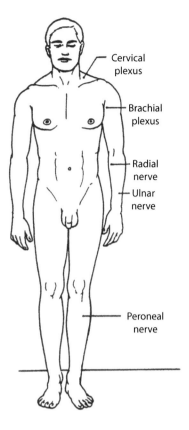

Figure 3.2 Nerves at risk for injury during positioning for a surgical procedure.

and head in line with the rest of the body. There are several different pillow types that allow for proper positioning of the head in a neutral position with the remainder of the body, while keeping the eyes, nose, and chin free from pressure. There is a low, but significant, risk that pressure on the eye or surrounding orbit will lead to increased intraocular pressure, decreased retinal artery blood flow, and resultant blindness, if the intraocular pressure exceeds systemic pressure. Although this is a rare complication associated with the prone position, it is, nevertheless, devastating. Extreme care must be taken to avoid this life-changing occurrence.

A soft but firm roll is placed under the hips of the prone patient. Placement is critical since positioning of the roll too far caudally will lead to poor exposure by not elevating the buttocks high enough to separate them. A low roll will also cause discomfort in the thighs during a local anesthetic and postoperatively from a general or regional anesthetic. A roll placed too far cephalad may restrict venous return through the inferior vena cava resulting in transient hypotension and the possibility of increased intraoperative bleeding. Excessive compression of the abdomen can also impair ventilation. Bean bags or chest rolls can improve ventilation. An additional roll is placed beneath each ankle to keep the toes off the surface of the operating table. All pressure points including knees, elbows, breasts, and male genitalia need to be carefully monitored and adequately padded.

The thorax should be supported with chest rolls that extend from the clavicle to the iliac crest. The arms can be placed at the side of the body in a neutral position, with careful padding of the elbows to prevent injury. Alternatively, the arms can be positioned alongside the head, taking care that the arms are not abducted greater than 90° to prevent injury to the brachial plexus (37,38). Great care must be taken to not inadvertently dislodge the endotracheal tube while prone, as it is exceedingly difficult to reintubate or mask ventilate a patient in the prone position.

The prone position has much to offer for most anorectal surgery. The entire operating teams including surgeon, assistant surgeon, and scrub nurse have a full and unobstructed view of the operative field. Thus, both the assistant and the nurse can always see the maneuvers of the surgeon, offering the best chance for improved efficiency; lighting of any type is enhanced. Anorectal anatomy is clearly delineated, and any bleeding automatically drains away from the operative field instead of onto the floor (39). Disadvantages include concern about the airway as mentioned.

## LATERAL DECUBITUS

The modified *left lateral or Sims position* has been championed by the Ferguson Clinic in their descriptions of hemorrhoidectomy technique (Figure 3.3) (40,41). This position allows an assistant easy access, but unless the patient is correctly positioned, the upper buttock, in a natural response to gravity, may coapt with the lower buttock, compromising visibility. Furthermore, the assistant usually has no opportunity to see any of the operation as the upper buttock retraction is most effectively accomplished from the contralateral side.

The patient is placed in a left lateral position with the buttocks extended beyond the side of the table. As shown in Figure 3.3, the patient's back is slightly flexed and angled across the table, which positions the head at the opposite side of the table to prevent the patient from falling off the side of the table. The legs can be positioned in a variety of ways: the left thigh and leg are extended straight to the bottom of the table and the right thigh and leg flexed on a pillow into a near knee-chest position or both legs can be flexed (with a small pillow between the legs for padding). The patient's arms can be crossed either in front of the head or under the forehead.

The left lateral position can be particularly useful for office examinations. Although the prone-jackknife position is probably the most popular position for rigid proctosigmoidoscopy

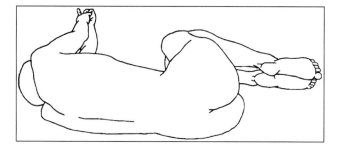

Figure 3.3 Modified left lateral or Sims position.

in the United States, this examination can also be performed with the patient in the left lateral position. The position is particularly suited to the pregnant patient, patients with severe chronic obstructive pulmonary disease, some amputees, and patients with spinal cord or other neurologic injuries. For local anesthetics, this position appears to eliminate complaints of pubic pain and low backache. It may limit visualization of the right posterior quadrant (42) but is a good alternative for sphincterotomies, fistulotomies, and pilonidal cysts being treated under local anesthetic.

Just as with prone positioning, it is imperative that the head be kept in a neutral position while turning the patient. Additionally, extra cushioning is needed under the head to keep the cervical and thoracic spines in line. An axillary roll needs to be placed just caudad to the dependent axilla in order to prevent compression injuries to the brachial plexus. It should not be placed in the axilla, as the purpose is for the weight of the thorax to be borne by the chest wall. The dependent arm is extended perpendicular to the body on a padded armboard, while the nondependent arm is similarly extended on an armrest suspended in such a way that the arm is not abducted greater than 90° from the body. Additionally, the arm should not be raised superior to the level of the deltoid. A pillow or cushion should be placed between the knees (37,38).

## LITHOTOMY

The lithotomy position is very common in colorectal surgery. The hips are flexed 80°–100° from the trunk, and the legs are abducted 30°–45° from midline. It is important that the legs always be moved simultaneously to prevent lumbar spine torsion, and that the legs be carefully padded to reduce the risk of injury. In a retrospective review of patients undergoing surgery in the lithotomy position, Warner et al. found that the most common lower extremity nerve injury was to the common peroneal nerve, accounting for 78% of nerve injuries. It was postulated that the cause was compression of the nerve between the leg support and the lateral head of the fibula (43).

While rare (1 in 8,720), the incidence of compartment syndrome of the lower extremities is markedly higher in the lithotomy position than in all other surgical positions. Compartment syndrome occurs when high tissue pressure builds within the closed space of the anterior compartment. Ischemia of the tissue in the compartment results in edema of the interstitium, thereby raising compartment pressure. Since perfusion is dependent on compartment pressure being lower than mean arterial pressure to allow tissue perfusion, any situation where increased compartment pressure and/or decreased arterial flow into the tissue can result in ischemia. The result is capillary endothelial damage and even greater interstitial edema. Unfortunately, it is not completely understood why some patients develop a compartment syndrome, while others do not. As a result, no safe maximum time limit can be defined (44). Early diagnosis and treatment with fasciotomy is imperative. Analysis of closed claims in cases of compartment syndrome due to the lithotomy position during colorectal surgery demonstrated an average indemnity payment of $426,000. Great care must be taken in the positioning and padding, as patients themselves cannot express any pain or discomfort they may be experiencing while under general or regional anesthesia.

## SURGICAL CARE IMPROVEMENT PROJECT

## PROCESS AND OUTCOME MEASURES

The SCIP of the United States is a national quality initiative involving the American Society of Colorectal Surgeons, the American College of Surgeons, the ASA, the American Hospital Association, the Association of Perioperative Registered Nurses, and a host of governmental agencies dedicated to improvement in health care (45). The goals of the SCIP partnership were to reduce the incidence of surgical complications by 25% by the year 2010 and to promote the use of evidence-based care processes known to reduce surgical complications.

Out of approximately 40 million major operations each year, postoperative complications account for up to 22% of preventable deaths among patients, depending on the complication. These complications accounted for 2.4 million additional hospital days and $9.3 billion in additional charges each year (46).

SCIP focuses on areas where the incidence and cost of the most common and preventable complications are high:

1. Surgical site infections
2. Adverse cardiac events
3. Venous thromboembolism
4. Postoperative pneumonia

Although not limited to anesthesia care, the anesthesiologist and colorectal surgeon must partner in attempts to meet the expectations set by the national SCIP initiative.

One such initiative is the administration of prophylactic antibiotics within 1 hour of surgical incision. Although not typically considered "anesthetic agents," antibiotics may best be given within 1 hour before incision if administered by the anesthesia provider. Frequent operating room and turnover delays may result in an antibiotic administration well before the 1 hour limit if given in the preoperative holding area. Late patient arrivals for same-day admit surgery or administrative paperwork delays may result in inadequate or insufficient time to infuse the antibiotic prior to going to the operating room, with the result of no antibiotic being given or being given only if the "missed dose" is noticed by someone in the operating room.

Although no longer reportable as public information, prophylactic antibiotic selection for surgical patients is monitored, as is discontinuation of the antibiotic within 24 hours after the surgery end time (48 hours for cardiac surgery patients). If an antibiotic is felt to be needed beyond the allowed 24 hours, the colorectal surgeon must document, in the medical record, the reason for continuation of the antibiotic.

Venous thromboembolism was discussed earlier in this chapter, and involvement of the anesthesiologist and associated regional anesthesia play a significant role here. As previously mentioned, an epidural catheter must be removed at an appropriate time surrounding the initiation and discontinuation of heparin, LMWH, or warfarin. The risks of inadequate venous thromboembolism prophylaxis must be weighed against the benefits of regional anesthesia for colorectal surgical patients.

Postoperative pneumonia is a complication where the cause is multifactorial. Ventilator management and weaning protocols for patients requiring postoperative mechanical ventilation may fall under the purview of the anesthesiologist.

## CONCLUSION

Although the sum total of anesthesia practice can hardly be related in a chapter, we have attempted in the preceding pages to highlight areas in anesthesia practice of which the colorectal surgeon should be aware. Improved patient satisfaction through reduction of postoperative pain, earlier ambulation, and quicker return of bowel function and diet will have a marked impact on surgical outcomes. Thoracic epidural anesthesia/analgesia is becoming a standard for many colorectal surgical procedures, whether as the sole anesthetic, or in conjunction with general anesthesia.

Awareness under anesthesia is a rare, but serious concern, highlighted more recently in the media and receiving much greater appreciation among surgical patients. Timely supportive care, including psychological counseling, may improve outcome and reduce the incidence of posttraumatic stress disorder. Oversedation resulting in hypoventilation, hypoxemia, and hypercarbia can produce devastating results. Extreme caution must be given to the patient who is restless, but sedated. Loss of airway is the ultimate disaster under general anesthesia and is a surgical, as well as anesthetic, emergency.

Proper positioning requires the vigilance of the anesthesia provider, the colorectal surgeon, and the operating room nurses. Severe nerve injuries can generally be avoided with the use of padding. Even with appropriate padding, there is an increased incidence of neurologic injury with the use of stirrups in the lithotomy position. Extra care must be taken with the patient in the prone position, as neck injuries from improper turning, endotracheal tube dislodgement, or perioperative blindness from periorbital pressure can all result in devastating outcomes.

Partnership of the surgeon and the anesthesiologist may help improve outcomes, reduce surgical site infections, improve perioperative cardiac morbidity and mortality, and reduce the incidence of venous thromboembolism. Whether in the office setting, outpatient center, or surgical hospital, safe anesthesia practice is paramount.

# REFERENCES

1. Stoelting RK, Miller RD. Scope of anesthesia practice. In *Basics of Anesthesia*, 5th Edition. Philadelphia, PA: Churchill Livingstone Elsevier, 2007, p. 11.
2. Hutson LR, Vachon CA. *Anesthesiology* 2005;103(4): 885–9.
3. Stoelting RK, Miller RD. Local anesthetics. In *Basics of Anesthesia*, 5th Edition. Philadelphia, PA: Churchill Livingstone Elsevier, 2007, pp. 123–34.
4. Barash PG et al. *Local Anesthetics in Clinical Anesthesia*, 5th Edition. Philadelphia, PA: Lippincott Williams and Wilkins, 2006, pp. 449–67.
5. Haas E et al. *Am Surg* 2012;78(5):574–81.
6. Golf M et al. *Adv Ther* 2011;28(9):776–88.
7. Cohen SM. *J Pain Res* 2012;5:567–72.
8. Stoelting RK, Miller RD. Choice of anesthetic technique. In *Basics of Anesthesia*, 5th Edition. Philadelphia, PA: Churchill Livingstone Elsevier, 2007, pp. 178–84.
9. Bhananker SM et al. *Anesthesiology* 2006;104: 228–34.
10. Stoelting RK, Miller RD. Spinal and epidural anesthesia. In *Basics of Anesthesia*, 5th Edition. Philadelphia, PA: Churchill Livingstone Elsevier, 2007, pp. 241–71.
11. Carli F et al. *Dis Colon Rectum* 2001;44(8):1083–9.
12. Taqi A et al. *Surg Endoscopy* 2007;21:247–52.
13. Liu SS, Mulroy MF. *Reg Anesth Pain Med* 1998;23:157–63.
14. Ruff RL, Dougherty JH. *Stroke* 1981;12:879–81.
15. Horlocker TT et al. *The Second ASRA Consensus Conference on Neuraxial Anesthesia and Anticoagulation*. http://www.asra.com/consensus-statements/RAPM-Anticoagulation.pdf
16. McDonnell JG et al. *Anesth Analg* 2007;104(1):193–7.
17. Rafi AN. *Anaesthesia* 2001;56(10):1021–6.
18. El-dawlatly AA et al. *Internet J Anesthesiol* 2006;16(2):1–3.
19. Stoelting RK, Miller RD. Peripheral nerve blocks. In *Basics of Anesthesia*, 5th Edition. Philadelphia, PA: Churchill Livingstone Elsevier, 2007, pp. 273–90.
20. Sandin RH et al. *Lancet* 2000;355:707–11.
21. Sebel PS et al. *Anesth Analg* 2004;99:833–9.
22. Myles PS et al. *Lancet* 2004;363:1757–63.
23. Rampersad SE, Mulroy MF. *Anesth Analg* 2005;100: 1363–4.
24. Dahaba AA. *Anesth Analg* 2005;101:765–73.
25. Domino K et al. *Anesthesiology* 1999;90(4):1053–61.
26. Noblett SE, Horgan AF. *Sen Colon Rectal Surgery* 2010;21:160–4.
27. Mulier JP. *Practical Implications 4th ESPCOP Meeting*, Bruges, December 2013.
28. Lowder JL et al. *Am J Obstet Gynecol* 2003;189: 1559–62; discussion 62.
29. Dajani EZ, Islam K. *J Physiol Pharmacol* 2008; 59(Suppl 2):117–33.
30. De Oliveira GS, Jr. et al. *Anesth Analg* 2012;114: 424–33.
31. Southworth S et al. *Clin Ther* 2009; 31(9): 1922–35.
32. Cataldo P et al. *Surg Gynecol Obstet* 1993;176: 435–8.
33. Toms L et al. *Cochrane Database Syst Rev* 2008: CD004602.
34. Maund E et al. *Br J Anaesth* 2011;106:292–7.
35. Ong CK et al. *Anesth Analg* 2010;110:1170–9.
36. Beck DE et al. *Ochsner J* 2015;15(4): 408–12.
37. Barash PG et al. Patient positioning. In *Clinical Anesthesia*, 5th Edition. Philadelphia, PA: Lippincott Williams and Wilkins, 2006, pp. 643–65.
38. Stoelting RK, Miller RD. Positioning and associated risks. In *Basics of Anesthesia*, 5th Edition. Philadelphia, PA: Churchill Livingstone Elsevier, 2007, pp. 291–303.
39. Goldberg SM et al. *Essentials of Anorectal Surgery*. Philadelphia, PA: JB Lippincott; 1980:80.
40. Ferguson JA et al. *Surgery* 1971;70:480–4.
41. Nivatvongs S. *Dis Colon Rectum* 1980;23:308–9.
42. Cheney FW et al. *Anesthesiology* 1999;90(4): 1062–9.
43. Warner MA et al. *Anesthesiology* 1994;81:6–12.
44. Beraldo S, Dodds SR. *Dis Colon Rectum* 2006;49: 1772–80.
45. "Medicare Quality Improvement Community" website. http://www.medqic.org accessed March 31, 2008.
46. Zhan C, Miller MR. *JAMA* 2003;290:1868–74.

# 4

# Sepsis

JENNIFER S. BEATY AND MORIAH E. WRIGHT

---

## CHALLENGING CASE

Five days after a subtotal colectomy with end ileostomy for medically refractory ulcerative colitis, your patient is febrile with tachycardia. Your patient also has leukocytosis with left shift and decreased urine output. Your patient rules in for sepsis criteria.

## CASE MANAGEMENT

Your patient is transferred to the intensive care unit (ICU), and the Surviving Sepsis Campaign Bundles are initiated. The patient receives a bolus of IV fluids, serum lactate is drawn, blood cultures are obtained, empiric antibiotics are initiated, and computed tomography (CT) scan of the abdomen and pelvis is performed. The study reveals intraabdominal abscess surrounding the rectal stump staple line, which appears amenable to drainage.

## INTRODUCTION

There are times in the postoperative period when patients do not follow a normal postoperative course. The patient may become septic, require transfer to the ICU, or require an unplanned operation. Since 1991, there have been increasing efforts to define the disease process of sepsis and improve upon its high mortality rate.

## SYSTEMIC INFLAMMATORY RESPONSE SYNDROME, SEPSIS, AND MULTIPLE ORGAN DYSFUNCTION SYNDROME

In 1991, the American College of Chest Physicians (ACCP) and the Society of Critical Care Medicine (SCCM) came together "to provide a conceptual and a practical framework to define the systemic inflammatory response to infection" (1). This is the origin of the concept of systemic inflammatory response syndrome (SIRS). This term came about because of recognition that a large number of clinical conditions not involving infection could still initiate an inflammatory response (1). Sepsis was defined as SIRS with a known source of infection (Table 4.1) (1). This was also the advent of multiple organ dysfunction syndrome (MODS), which describes a continuum of organ dysfunction (1). Changes in organ function over time can be viewed as an important prognostic indicator (1). These definitions were revisited in 2001 at the International Sepsis Definitions Conference (2). This included ACCP, SCCM, European Society of Intensive Care Medicine (ESICM), American Thoracic Society, and Surgical Infection Society (SIS) representatives. At this conference, the description of variables that may contribute to the diagnosis of sepsis was expanded without changing the definition of SIRS or MODS. In short, the committee felt that the signs and symptoms of sepsis were more varied than the initial criteria, but the existing concepts of sepsis, severe sepsis, and septic shock were robust and should remain as previously described (2).

## SEPSIS-3

In 2015, the SCCM and the ESICM met and determined new definitions for sepsis and associated conditions (3). This group sought to differentiate between uncomplicated infection and sepsis as well as to update the definitions of sepsis and septic shock to better reflect current understanding of pathobiology. The key concepts of sepsis include the following: it is the primary cause of death from infection; it is a syndrome shaped by pathogen factors and host factors with characteristics that evolve over time; organ dysfunction may be occult, and therefore, its presence should be considered in any patient presenting with infection and vice versa; the clinical and biological phenotype of sepsis can be modified by preexisting acute illness, long-standing comorbidities, medications, and interventions; and specific

Table 4.1 Sepsis definitions

| | 1991—ACCP/SCCM[a] | 2001—SCCM/ESICM/ACCP/ATS/SIS[b] | 2015—Sepsis-3[c] |
|---|---|---|---|
| SIRS | Two or more of the following:<br>• Temperature >38°C or <36°C<br>• Heart rate >90 bpm<br>• Respiratory rate >20 breaths/min or PaCO$_2$ <33 mm Hg<br>• White blood cell count >12,000/mm$^3$, <4,000/mm$^3$, or >10% bands | Unchanged | |
| Sepsis | SIRS with known source of infection | Infection with some of the following:<br>General variables<br>• Fever<br>• Hypothermia<br>• Heart rate >90/min<br>• Tachypnea<br>• Altered mental status<br>• Significant edema or positive fluid balance<br>• Hyperglycemia<br>Inflammatory variables<br>• Leukocytosis<br>• Leukopenia<br>• Normal WBC count with >10% bands<br>• Plasma C-reactive protein >2 SD above normal<br>• Plasma procalcitonin >2 SD above normal<br>Hemodynamic variables<br>• Arterial hypotension<br>• SVO$_2$ >70%<br>• Cardiac index >3.5 L/min/M$^{23}$<br>Organ dysfunction variables<br>• Arterial hypoxemia<br>• Acute oliguria<br>• Creatinine increase >0.5<br>• Coagulation abnormalities<br>• Ileus<br>• Thrombocytopenia<br>• Hyperbilirubinemia<br>Tissue perfusion variables<br>• Hyperlactatemia<br>• Decreased capillary refill or mottling | Life-threatening organ dysfunction caused by a dysregulated host response to infection.<br>Organ dysfunction can be described by an increase in SOFA score of two points or more. |
| Severe sepsis | Sepsis associated with organ dysfunction, hypoperfusion, or hypotension | Unchanged | Removed, felt to be redundant |

(Continued)

Table 4.1 (Continued) Sepsis definitions

| | 1991—ACCP/SCCM[a] | 2001—SCCM/ESICM/ACCP/ATS/SIS[b] | 2015—Sepsis-3[c] |
|---|---|---|---|
| Septic shock | Sepsis with hypotension despite adequate fluid resuscitation with perfusion abnormalities (lactic acidosis, oliguria, or acute alteration in mental status) | Unchanged | A subset of sepsis with profound circulatory, cellular, and metabolic abnormalities; associated with greater mortality than sepsis alone. Persisting hypotension requiring vasopressors to maintain MAP $\geq$65 mm Hg, serum lactate >2 mmol/L despite adequate volume resuscitation |
| MODS | Presence of altered organ function in acutely ill patient such that homeostasis cannot be maintained without intervention | Unchanged | Unchanged |

*Abbreviations:* ACCP, American College of Chest Physicians; ATS, American Thoracic Society; ESICM, European Society of Intensive Care Medicine; MAP, mean arterial pressure; MODS, multiple organ dysfunction syndrome; SCCM, Society of Critical Care Medicine; SD, standard deviation; SIRS, systemic inflammatory response syndrome; SIS, Surgical Infection Society; SOFA, Sequential Organ Failure Assessment; WBC, white blood cell.

[a] Bone RC et al. *Chest* 1992;101(6):1644–55.
[b] Levy MM et al. *Crit Care Med* 2003;31(4):1250–6.
[c] Singer M et al. *JAMA* 2016;315(8):801–10.

infections may result in local organ dysfunction without generating a dysregulated systemic host response (3). Sepsis is now recognized to involve early activation of pro- and anti-inflammatory responses, as well as major modifications in nonimmunologic pathways (cardiovascular, neuronal, autonomic, hormonal, bioenergetic, metabolic, and coagulation), all of which have prognostic significance (3).

Organ dysfunction severity can be described using a variety of scoring systems, but the most common one in current use, and the one recommended by Sepsis-3 is the Sequential Organ Failure Assessment (SOFA) (Table 4.2) (3). The baseline SOFA score is assumed to be zero in patients without preexisting organ dysfunction. A SOFA score greater than or equal to two reflects an overall mortality risk of approximately 10% in a general hospital population with suspected infection. It is important to note that SOFA is not intended to be a standalone definition of sepsis, and failure to meet two or more criteria should not lead to a deferral of investigation or treatment of an infection (3). It is also important to note that these updated definitions were not endorsed by the ACCP (4).

## EVALUATION AND DIAGNOSIS

## SEPSIS BUNDLES

The Surviving Sepsis Campaign (SSC) was developed to reduce mortality in severe sepsis. Specific measures should be completed in the workup and treatment of patients with

sepsis (5). Four measures should be performed within the first 3 hours (Table 4.3), including measuring serum lactate level, drawing blood cultures, initiating empiric antibiotics, and administering crystalloid bolus for hypotension of lactic acidosis (5). Three additional measures should be implemented within the first 6 hours (Table 4.3).

The International Multicentre Prevalence Study on Sepsis (IMPreSS) evaluated compliance with the SSC bundles and correlated compliance with mortality in 1794 patients (6). This is the first report of compliance with the 2012 SSC bundles. IMPreSS found the overall hospital mortality rate in sepsis to be 28.4% (6). Compliance with all of the evidence-based bundle metrics for the treatment of sepsis was low: only 19% compliance for 3-hour bundle and 35.5% for the 6-hour bundle. Patients whose care included compliance with all of the metrics in the 3-hour bundle had a 40% reduction in the odds of dying in the hospital (20% versus 31%, $p < 0.001$). Patients whose care included compliance with all metrics in the 6-hour bundle had a 36% reduction in odds of dying in the hospital (22% versus 32%, $p < 0.001$) (6).

In another recent study in 2014, Levy et al. evaluated 29,470 patients with sepsis and measured compliance with the SSC bundles and outcomes (7). If compliance with resuscitation bundle was high, mortality was 29%, as opposed to low compliance with resuscitation bundle, the mortality was 38.6% ($p < 0.001$) (7). Hospital and ICU length of stay decreased 4% for every 10% increase in compliance with resuscitation bundle. Increased compliance with SSC bundles corresponded to a 25% relative risk reduction in mortality rate. This study demonstrates performance metrics

Table 4.2 Sequential Organ Failure Assessment (SOFA) score

| System | Score | | | | |
|---|---|---|---|---|---|
| | 0 | 1 | 2 | 3 | 4 |
| **Respiration** | | | | | |
| $PaO_2/FiO_2$, mm Hg | $\geq$400 | <400 | <300 | <200 with respiratory support | <100 with respiratory support |
| **Coagulation** | | | | | |
| Platelets, $\times 10^3/\mu L$ | $\geq$150 | <150 | <100 | <50 | <20 |
| **Liver** | | | | | |
| Bilirubin, mg/dL | <1.2 | 1.2–1.9 | 2–5.9 | 6–11.9 | >12 |
| **Cardiovascular** | MAP $\geq$70 mm Hg | MAP <70 mm Hg | Dopamine <5 or dobutamine (any dose) | Dopamine 5.1–15 or epinephrine $\leq$0.1 or norepinephrine $\leq$0.1 | Dopamine >15 or epinephrine >0.1 or norepinephrine >0.1 |
| **Central nervous system** | | | | | |
| Glascow Coma Score | 15 | 13–14 | 10–12 | 6–9 | <6 |
| **Renal** | | | | | |
| Creatinine, mg/dL | <1.2 | 1.2–1.9 | 2.0–3.4 | 3.5–4.9 | >5 |
| Urine output, mL/day | | | | <500 | <200 |

*Source:* Adapted from Singer M et al. *JAMA* 2016;315(8):801–10.

can drive change in clinical behavior, improve quality of care, and may decrease mortality in patients with severe sepsis and septic shock (7).

In contrast to the IMPreSS trial and Levy's study, three recently completed, large multicentered randomized trials comparing early goal-directed therapy (EGDT) to usual therapy in academic and community hospitals did not demonstrate a survival benefit for EGDT. These trials include the 2014 ProCESS, the 2014 ARISE, and the 2015 ProMISe trials (8–10). In the ProCESS study, 1,341 patients diagnosed with sepsis in the emergency room were assigned to EGDT versus usual care (8). There were no differences in 90-day mortality, 1-year mortality, or need for organ support (8). The ARISE study randomized 1,600 patients

Table 4.3 Surviving sepsis campaign bundles

**To be completed within 3 hours:**
 1. Measure lactate level
 2. Obtain blood cultures prior to administration of antibiotics
 3. Administer broad-spectrum antibiotics
 4. Administer 30 mL/kg crystalloid for hypotension or lactate $\geq$4 mmol/L

**To be completed within 6 hours:**
 5. Administer vasopressors for hypotension not responding to initial fluid resuscitation
 • Maintain MAP $\geq$65 mm Hg
 6. If persistent hypotension after initial volume resuscitation (MAP $\leq$65 mm Hg) or if lactate >4 mmol/L,
 • Either
   • Repeat focused exam (after initial fluid resuscitation) by licensed independent practitioner including vital signs, cardiopulmonary, capillary refill, pulse, and skin findings
 • Or two of the following:
   • Measure central venous pressure (CVP), goal CVP $\geq$ 8 mm Hg
   • Measure central venous oxygen saturation ($S_{cvo2}$), goal $S_{cvo2} \geq$ 70%
   • Perform bedside cardiac ultrasound
   • Conduct dynamic assessment of fluid responsiveness with either fluid challenge or passive leg raise
 7. Remeasure lactate if initial lactate was elevated

*Source:* Adapted from Dellinger RP et al. *Crit Care Med* 2013;41:580–637.

diagnosed with sepsis in the emergency room to EGDT versus usual care. There were no significant differences in survival time, in-hospital mortality, duration of organ support, or length of hospital stay (9). The ProMISE study enrolled 1,260 with sepsis and randomized to EGDT or usual care. There was no difference in mortality between the groups, EGDT (29.5%) versus control (29.2%) (10). Interestingly, the EGDT group had higher costs, and the probability it was cost effective was only 20% (10). The true benefit of modern therapies for sepsis may lie in the early identification of those with the condition, which would ultimately lead to an early treatment, rather than a specific algorithm.

## INFECTION

## PREVENTION

Surgical prophylaxis has been a topic of discussion for many years. Guidelines from the Infectious Diseases Society of America (IDSA) were originally published in 1999, but they received an update in 2013 (11). This update included timing of preoperative antibiotic dosing. IDSA guidelines recommend dosing within 60 minutes prior to incision, and antibiotic agents with a prolonged administration time should be administered such that the dose is completed within 60 minutes of incision (11). For antibiotic selection and dosing, the ISDA provided guidance on agents for specific procedures as well as dosing for obese patients, the specifics of which are outside the scope of this chapter. Duration of prophylactic antibiotics should be no more than 24 hours after surgery, and this includes a lack of need for prophylaxis for the presence of indwelling drains or catheters (11).

## SURGICAL SITE INFECTION

Surgical site infection (SSI) is a common complication after any surgical procedure, the risk of which is delineated by patient factors as well as the type of procedure. One way the risk of SSI has been stratified is with the National Healthcare Safety Network wound classification system. This system divides wounds into four classes: clean, clean-contaminated, contaminated, and dirty or infected. Clean wounds include wounds without infection and without transection of the respiratory, biliary, gastrointestinal, genital, or uninfected urinary tracts. Clean-contaminated wounds involve transection of one of the above tracts. Contaminated wounds involve fresh open accidental wounds or operations with major break in sterile technique or gross spillage from the gastrointestinal tract. Dirty wounds include old traumatic wounds with devitalized tissue, existing clinical infection, or wounds associated with perforated viscera. With increasing contamination of the wound comes increased risk for SSI. Patient factors that contribute to an increased risk for SSI include extremes of age, nutritional status, obesity, diabetes mellitus, concurrent remote body-site infection,

tobacco use, altered immune response, corticosteroid use, recent hospitalization, length of preoperative hospitalization, and colonization with microorganisms (11).

*Superficial incisional SSI* occurs within 30 days postoperatively and involves skin or subcutaneous tissue of the incision and at least one of the following: purulent drainage from the superficial incision; organisms isolated from an aseptically obtained culture of fluid or tissue from the superficial incision; at least one of the following signs or symptoms of infection—pain or tenderness, localized swelling, redness, or heat; superficial incision is deliberately opened by a surgeon and is culture-positive or not cultured (a culture-negative finding does not meet this criterion); and diagnosis of superficial incisional SSI by the surgeon or attending physician (11). When stratifying by wound classification, the clean, clean-contaminated, contaminated, and dirty wound classifications had superficial SSI rates of 1.76%, 3.94%, 4.75%, and 5.16%, respectively (12).

*Deep incisional SSI* occurs within 30 days after the operative procedure if no implant is left in place or within 1 year if implant is in place and the infection appears to be related to the operative procedure, involves deep soft tissues (e.g., fascial and muscle layers) of the incision, and the patient has at least one of the following: purulent drainage from the deep incision but not from the organ/space component of the surgical site, a deep incision spontaneously dehisces or is deliberately opened by a surgeon and is culture-positive or not cultured and the patient has at least one of the following signs or symptoms—fever (>38°C) or localized pain or tenderness (a culture-negative finding does not meet this criterion); an abscess or other evidence of infection involving the deep incision is found on direct examination, during reoperation, or by histopathologic or radiologic examination; and diagnosis of a deep incisional SSI by a surgeon or attending physician (11). When stratifying by wound classification, the clean, clean-contaminated, contaminated, and dirty wound classifications had deep incisional infection rates of 0.54%, 0.86%, 1.31%, and 2.1%, respectively (12).

*Organ/space SSI* involves any part of the body, excluding the skin incision, fascia, or muscle layers, that is opened or manipulated during the operative procedure. Specific sites are assigned to organ/space SSI to further identify the location of the infection (e.g., endocarditis, endometritis, mediastinitis, and osteomyelitis). Organ/space SSI must meet the following criteria: infection occurs within 30 days after the operative procedure if no implant is in place or within 1 year if implant is in place and the infection appears to be related to the operative procedure, infection involves any part of the body, excluding the skin incision, fascia, or muscle layers, that is opened or manipulated during the operative procedure, and the patient has at least one of the following: purulent drainage from a drain that is placed through a stab wound into the organ/space, organisms isolated from an aseptically obtained culture of fluid or tissue in the organ/space; an abscess or other evidence of infection involving the organ/space that is found on direct examination, during reoperation, or by histopathologic or radiologic examination; and diagnosis of an organ/space SSI by a surgeon or attending physician (10). When stratifying by wound classification, the clean, clean-contaminated, contaminated, and dirty wound classifications had organ/space SSI rates of 0.28%, 1.87%, 2.55%, and 4.54%, respectively (12).

Management of SSI depends largely on the level of infection and the severity of illness. Superficial SSI is generally managed by opening the wound. Organ/space SSI is generally managed with drainage; further detail on management of this is provided in Chapter 9.

## TREATMENT

Despite the diversity of specific processes in these infections, the basic tenets of management of sepsis are similar: resuscitate patients who have SIRS, control the source of contamination, remove most of the infected or necrotic material, and administer antimicrobial agents to eradicate residual pathogens (13–15).

## SURVIVING SEPSIS CAMPAIGN 2012 INITIAL RESUSCITATION

### Fluid therapy in severe sepsis

Crystalloids are the initial fluid of choice in the resuscitation of severe sepsis and septic shock. SSC of 2012 recommends an initial fluid challenge in patients with sepsis-induced tissue hypoperfusion with suspicion of hypovolemia to achieve a minimum of 30 mL/kg of crystalloids (a portion of this may be albumin equivalent) (5). More rapid administration and greater amounts of fluid may be needed in some patients. The SSC recommends a fluid challenge technique be applied, wherein fluid administration is continued as long as there is hemodynamic improvement based on either dynamic (e.g., change in pulse pressure or stroke volume variation) or static (e.g., arterial pressure and heart rate) variables (5).

### Albumin use

The Saline versus Albumin Fluid Evaluation (SAFE) randomly evaluated 6,997 patients, comparing albumin and crystalloids. Albumin demonstrated a nonsignificant trend toward lower all-cause mortality at 28 days ($p = 0.09$) (16). The 2014 Albumin Italian Outcomes Sepsis (ALBIOS) trial randomized 1,818 patients and further investigated the use of albumin administration to maintain patients with severe sepsis or septic shock to a serum albumin level $\geq 3$ g/dL (17). There was no difference in survival at 28 and 90 days, although those treated with albumin had more favorable SOFA subscores and received fewer vasopressors or inotropes (17). The SSC of 2012 recommends albumin in the fluid resuscitation of severe sepsis and septic shock only when patients require substantial amounts of crystalloids. The

SSC specifically recommends against the use of hydroxyethyl starches for fluid resuscitation of severe sepsis and septic shock (5).

## Vasopressors

The goal when initiating vasopressor therapy is to maintain mean arterial pressure (MAP) of 65 mm Hg. All patients requiring vasopressors should have an arterial catheter placed as soon as practical if resources are available (5).

Norepinephrine is the first choice vasopressor, and epinephrine can be added to and potentially substituted for norepinephrine when an additional agent is needed to maintain adequate blood pressure (5,18–20).

Vasopressin 0.03 units/min can be added to norepinephrine with intent of either raising MAP or decreasing norepinephrine dosage. Low-dose vasopressin is not recommended as the single initial vasopressor for treatment of sepsis-induced hypotension, and vasopressin doses higher than 0.03–0.04 units/min should be reserved for salvage therapy (i.e., failure to achieve adequate MAP with other vasopressor agents) (5,20).

Phenylephrine is not recommended in the treatment of septic shock except in circumstances where norepinephrine is associated with serious arrhythmias, cardiac output is known to be high and blood pressure persistently low, or as salvage therapy when combined inotrope/vasopressor drugs and low-dose vasopressin have failed to achieve the MAP target (5).

Dopamine should be reserved as an alternative vasopressor agent to norepinephrine only in selected patients (e.g., patients with low risk of tachyarrhythmias and absolute or relative bradycardia). Low-dose dopamine should not be used for renal protection (5).

## Inotropic therapy

A trial of dobutamine infusion up to 20 micrograms/kg/min can be administered or added to vasopressor (if in use) in the presence of myocardial dysfunction as suggested by elevated cardiac filling pressures and low cardiac output, or ongoing signs of hypoperfusion, despite achieving adequate intravascular volume and adequate MAP (5).

## STEROID USE

The Annane Trial published in 2002 randomized 300 septic shock patients within 8 hours of diagnosis to receive 7 days of corticosteroids or placebo (21). The dose of hydrocortisone was 50 mg IV every 6 hours and fludrocortisone 50 microgram enterally per day. All patients had a short adrenocorticotropic hormone stimulation test at time of enrollment and were classified as responders (change in cortisol >9 microgram/dL) or nonresponders (change <9 micrograms/dL) (21). Among nonresponders, corticosteroid use was associated with a 10% absolute reduction in 28-day mortality (53% versus 63%), with no difference at 1 year (69% versus 77%). Corticosteroids were associated with more rapid reversal of shock.

However, the CORTICUS Trial (Corticosteroid Therapy of Septic Shock) by Sprung in 2008 evaluated 499 patients with septic shock in the past 72 hours. This was a multi-center, randomized, prospective, placebo-controlled trial (21). The hydrocortisone regimen was 50 mg IV every 6 hours for 5 days, then 50 mg IV every 12 hours (days 6–8), then 50 mg IV every 24 hours (days 9–11), then stop. No difference in mortality (39.2% versus 36.1%) was found (22). This study was not powered to assess for mortality, so type II error exists. However, time to reversal of shock (SBP >90 mm Hg without vasopressors for at least 24 hours) was quicker with hydrocortisone (3.3 versus 5.8 days) for both responders and nonresponders. Patients had high incidence of new infections occurring 48 or more hours after study drug (odds ratio [OR] 1.37, 95% confidence interval [CI] 1.05–1.79), hyperglycemia and hypernatremia (22).

The 2012 Surviving Sepsis Campaign guidelines for severe sepsis and septic shock only recommend using hydrocortisone 200 mg IV divided daily in septic shock if fluid resuscitation and pressors are not able to reverse hemodynamic instability (5).

# RECOMMENDATIONS FOR OTHER SUPPORTIVE THERAPY OF SEVERE SEPSIS

## Blood product administration

Once tissue hypoperfusion has resolved and in the absence of extenuating circumstances (myocardial ischemia, severe hypoxemia, acute hemorrhage, or ischemic heart disease), the SSC recommends the red blood cell transfusion occur only when hemoglobin decreases to <7 g/dL (5). In the setting of thrombocytopenia, prophylactic platelet administration is recommended when counts are <10,000 mm$^3$ in the absence of bleeding. If the patient has significant risk factors for bleeding, transfuse platelets prophylactically if <20,000 mm$^3$. If active bleeding is present or if surgery or an invasive procedure is planned, transfuse platelets to achieve counts >50,000 mm$^3$ (5). There is no current role for erythropoietin or antithrombin in the treatment of severe sepsis (5,23).

## Glucose control

A protocol should be used to manage blood glucose in ICU patients with severe sepsis, commencing insulin dosing when two consecutive blood glucose levels are >180 mg/dL (5). The Normoglycemia in Intensive Care Evaluation—Survival Using Glucose Algorithm Regulation (NICE-SUGAR) trial randomized 6,104 medical and surgical ICU patients to intensive glycemic control (target glucose 81–108 mg/dL) versus conventional glycemic control (target glucose ≤180 mg/dL) (24). Unexpectedly, the intensive glycemic control arm had a higher 90-day mortality and more hypoglycemic events. There was no difference between

medical or surgical ICU patients, and there were no differences in length of stay, duration of ventilator therapy, or need for renal replacement therapy (24). A 2012 follow-up publication by the authors demonstrated that excess mortality was due to moderate to severe hypoglycemia, especially in patients with distributive shock (25). This SSC approach should target an upper blood glucose ≤180 mg/dL rather than an upper target blood glucose ≤110 mg/dL. Blood glucose should be monitored every 1–2 hours until glucose values and insulin infusion rates are stable and then every 4 hours thereafter (5).

## Deep vein thrombosis prophylaxis

Patients with severe sepsis should receive daily pharmacoprophylaxis against venous thromboembolism with daily subcutaneous low molecular weight heparin. If creatinine clearance is <30 mL/min, use dalteparin or another form of low molecular weight heparin that has a low degree of renal metabolism (5). Intermittent pneumatic compression devices should also be used whenever possible. Septic patients who have a contraindication for heparin (e.g., thrombocytopenia, coagulopathy, or active bleeding) should not receive pharmacoprophylaxis but should receive mechanical prophylaxis (5).

## Nutrition

Administer oral or enteral (if necessary) feedings, as tolerated, rather than either complete fasting or provision of only IV glucose within the first 48 hours after a diagnosis of severe sepsis/septic shock (5). Avoid mandatory full caloric feeding in the first week, start low dose feeding (e.g., up to 500 calories per day), and advance as tolerated. Use IV glucose and enteral nutrition rather than total parenteral nutrition (TPN) alone or parenteral nutrition in conjunction with enteral feeding in the first 7 days after diagnosis of severe sepsis/septic shock. Use nutrition with no specific immunomodulating supplementation rather than nutrition providing specific immunomodulating supplementation in patients with severe sepsis (5).

## Setting goals of care

It is critical to discuss goals of care and prognosis with patients and their families. Incorporate goals of care into treatment and end-of-life care planning, utilizing palliative care principles where appropriate. Address goals of care as early as feasible, but no later than 72 hours into an ICU admission for sepsis (5,26,27).

## Other recommendations

There is no role for IV immunoglobulins or IV selenium for the treatment of severe sepsis (28,29). Bicarbonate therapy should not be used for the purpose of improving hemodynamics or reducing vasopressor requirements in patients with hypoperfusion-induced lactic acidemia with pH >7.15 (5). Stress ulcer prophylaxis with proton pump inhibitors should be used in patients with bleeding risk factors in severe sepsis. There are specific guidelines for mechanical ventilation of sepsis-induced acute respiratory distress syndrome (ARDS). These are outside the scope of this chapter.

## ANTIBIOTIC THERAPY

Current guidelines from the SIS and the IDSA recommend an antibiotic treatment course of 4–7 days, depending on clinical response (13–15). Observational studies show antimicrobial therapy is typically administered for 10–14 days (30–32). A newly published randomized Study to Optimize Peritoneal Infection Therapy (STOP-IT) trial compared two strategies guiding the duration of antimicrobial therapy for management of complicated intraabdominal infection (15). In this study, 518 patients with complicated intraabdominal infection were randomly assigned adequate source control to receive antibiotics until 2 days after the resolution of fever, leukocytosis, and ileus, with a maximum of 10 days of therapy (control group), or to receive a fixed course of antibiotics (experimental group) for 4 +/− calendar days (15). The primary outcome was a composite of surgical-site infection, recurrent intraabdominal infection, or death within 30 days after the index source-control procedure, according to treatment group. There was no significant difference between groups after fixed duration antibiotic therapy (approximately 4 days) compared to after a longer course of antibiotics (approximately 8 days) that extended until after the resolution of physiological abnormalities (15).

## Source control

A specific anatomical diagnosis of infection requiring consideration for emergent source control should be sought and diagnosed or excluded as rapidly as possible. An intervention should be undertaken for source control within the first 12 hours after the diagnosis is made. When source control in a severely septic patient is required, the effective intervention associated with the least physiologic insult should be employed (e.g., percutaneous rather than surgical drainage of an abscess, if possible). If intravascular access devices are a possible source of severe sepsis or septic shock, they should be removed promptly after other vascular access has been established.

## SURGERY IN THE SEPTIC PATIENT

With the success of damage-control surgery for the treatment of hemorrhagic trauma, it has been adapted to shock secondary to peritonitis. The structured approach of damage control is now a five-part process: ground zero is the initial evaluation or prehospital, part 1 is initial abbreviated laparotomy, part 2 is ICU resuscitation, part 3 is later definitive repair, and part 4 is definitive abdominal closure (33).

In the initial, abbreviated laparotomy to control intraabdominal sepsis, surgeons need to assess the degree of physiologic derangement early in the operation. If severe derangements exist, then the operative interventions need to be truncated. The primary aim in the operating room is to control the source of infection, resect nonviable bowel, close or divert bowel perforations, and wash out the abdomen. Initial surgical treatment focuses on source control using a combination of resection and/or wide drainage. Failure to achieve source control will lead to death. No definitive procedures should occur during this operation, including anastomosis and abdominal closure. An anastomosis is likely to fail in the setting of extreme physiologic derangement. The abdomen is quickly and temporarily closed, with the goal to contain the viscera, avoid potential injury and contamination, and control peritoneal effluent (34).

---

### KEY POINTS

- Early recognition of sepsis is critical.
- Compliance with SSC bundles may improve survival and should be implemented as routine order sets if not already in place.
- Infection source should be removed in the safest, least invasive method possible.
- If surgery is required to control sepsis, principles of "damage control surgery" should be followed.

---

## REFERENCES

1. Bone RC et al. *Chest* 1992;101(6):1644–55.
2. Levy MM et al. *Crit Care Med* 2003;31(4):1250–6.
3. Singer M et al. *JAMA.* 2016;315(8):801–10.
4. Simpson SQ. *Chest* 2016;149(5):1117–8.
5. Dellinger RP et al. *Crit Care Med* 2013;41:580–637.
6. Rhodes A et al. *Intensive Care Med* 2015;41:1620–8.
7. Levy MM et al. *Intensive Care Med* 2014;40:1623–33.
8. Yealy DM et al. *N Engl J Med* 2014;370(18):1683–93.
9. Peake SL et al. *N Engl J Med* 2014;371:1496–1506.
10. Mouncey PR et al. *N Engl J Med* 2015: doi: 10.1056/NEJMoa1500896
11. Bratzler DW et al. *Am J Health-Syst Pharm* 2013;70:195–283.
12. Ortega G et al. *J Surg Res* 2012;174(1):33–8.
13. Solomkin JS et al. *Surg Infec (Larchmt)* 2010;11:79–109.
14. Solomkin JS et al. *Clin Infec Dis* 2010;50:133–64.
15. Sawyer RG et al. *N Engl J Med* 2015;372:1996–2005.
16. Finfer S et al. *N Engl J Med* 2004;350(22):2247–56.
17. Caironi P et al. *N Engl J Med* 2014;370(15):1412–21.
18. De Backer D et al. *N Engl J Med* 2010;362:779–89.
19. De Backer D et al. *Crit Care Med* 2012;40:725–30.
20. Russell JA et al. *N Engl J Med* 2008;358:877–88.
21. Annane D et al. *J Am Med Assoc* 2002;288(7):862–71.

22. Sprung CL et al. *N Engl J Med* 2008;358(2):111–24.
23. Liumbruno G et al. *Blood Transfus* 2009;7:132–50.
24. The NICE-SUGAR Study Investigators. *N Engl J Med* 2009;360:1283–97.
25. Finfer S et al. *N Engl J Med* 2012;367(12):1108.
26. Nelson JE et al. *Crit Care Med* 2010;38:1765–72.
27. Lee Char SJ et al. *Am J Respir Crit Care Med* 2010; 182:905–9.
28. Werdan K et al. *Crit Care Med* 2007;35:2693–2701.
29. Angstwurm MW et al. *Crit Care Med* 2007;35:118–26.
30. Riccio LM et al. *Surg Infec (Larchmt)* 2014;15:417–24.
31. Guirao X et al. *J Antimicrob Chemother* 2013; 68(Suppl 2):ii37–44.
32. Samuelsson A et al. *Scand J Infect Dis* 2012;44:820–7.
33. Waibel BH, Rotondo MF. *Surg Clin North Am* 2012; 92:243–57.
34. Waibel BH, Rotondo MF. *Rev Col Bras Cir* 2012;39(4): 314–21.

# 5

# Intraoperative anastomotic challenges

DAVID E. BECK

## CHALLENGING CASE

A 28-year-old man is undergoing a restorative procto-colectomy using a double-stapled technique for the ileoanal anastomosis. During insertion of the stapler into the anus, the anal canal distal linear staple line is disrupted. What are your options?

## CASE MANAGEMENT

The initial action is to visualize the distal staple line using retractors. If the ends of the partially closed distal bowel can be visualized and grasped with clamps or traction sutures, the amount of residual bowel can be assessed. If adequate length is present, one option is to reclose the bowel with a linear stapler placed below the disrupted staple line. After the stapler is fired, the residual bowel end can be resected with scissors or a scalpel. A second option is to reclose the disrupted staple line with sutures placed from the abdominal side or placed intraluminally via a retractor (lighted Chelsea-Eaton, Hill-Ferguson, etc.) placed into the anal canal. If the defect and bowel are successfully closed, the anastomosis can proceed.

If the distal segment of bowel is impossible to visualize or close, a mucosectomy can be performed via the anus and a hand-sewn ileo-anal anastomosis can be performed, as described in Chapter 35. Most surgeons will create a diverting loop ileostomy when the anastomosis has been this challenging.

## INTRODUCTION

Colon and rectal surgery is a technique-oriented specialty with many procedures requiring an anastomosis to reestablish bowel continuity. Achievement of a successful anastomosis is related to a number of surgical principles, which can be divided into patient factors and surgeon factors (1–3). Patient-related factors, such as the patient's nutritional status and associated medical conditions or medications, are not under the operating surgeon's control and are discussed in other chapters. This chapter focuses on anastomotic principles and problems (e.g., leakage, ischemia, stenosis, and hemorrhage) that can be identified and managed during the procedure.

## PREANASTOMOTIC CONSIDERATIONS

### PREOPERATIVE DISCUSSION AND PLANNING

Prior to surgery, the surgeon should have a plan that includes the expected operative findings or pathology and restoration of intestinal continuity, if possible. If the preoperative findings are confirmed, the operation should proceed along an organized pathway. Unexpected findings will obviously require modifications. Prior to the procedure, the surgeon should also have a discussion with the patient, which includes these considerations with special emphasis on aspects of the anastomosis and the possible need for a temporary or permanent stoma should restoration of intestinal continuity be impossible or ill advised (4). Proximal diversion will reduce the clinical sequelae from an anastomotic dehiscence. This is more likely in patients receiving preoperative chemotherapy and/or radiation, with poor nutrition, associated infection, or comorbid conditions (steroid use, hypotension, etc.). The appropriate site for a potential stoma should be chosen preoperatively, with the assistance of an enterostomal therapist. The selection and marking of a stoma site provide another opportunity for dialogue between the surgeon and patient.

### OPERATIVE PRINCIPLES

The key to uncomplicated healing of an intestinal anastomosis depends on adherence to well-established principles as well as the specifics of the technique. The principles of intestinal anastomosis include the following: (1) appropriate access and exposure to the two ends of the bowel, (2) healthy bowel to be joined, (3) good blood supply, (4) gentle handling of the bowel, and (5) good apposition of ends with no tension on the anastomosis (5). Any compromise of these principles places the anastomosis at risk for complications.

Exposure and access to bowel ends is maximized by taking the time to set up and position retractors and intraabdominal packs. Headlights and lighted retractors minimize the frustration of inadequate overhead lights. Deep pelvic retractors such as the St. Mark's retractor or Fazio pelvic retractors assist the visualization of the distal rectum prior to anastomosis. Extending the midline incision to the symphysis pubis likewise allows maximum exposure of the distal rectum. Operating with poor lighting and inadequate exposure not only jeopardizes the anastomosis but also increases operating room time.

Techniques of intestinal anastomosis should also be performed following the principle of gentle bowel handling. Clamps should be used only when absolutely necessary with the least amount of closure required to occlude the lumen. Care should be taken to exclude mesenteric blood vessels within the intestinal clamp. Gingerly inserting appropriately sized intraluminal staplers prevents inadvertent splitting and tearing of bowel ends to be anastomosed. Excessive use of electrocautery at the anastomosis can cause unappreciated tissue necrosis with potential for disruption. Mobilization of intestinal ends is required for exposure, access, and freedom of tension on the anastomosis. However, during mobilization, it is important to preserve those blood vessels required for adequate anastomotic healing. For example, excessive skeletonization of the cut intestinal ends may compromise their blood supply.

Having two healthy ends of bowel to anastomose is ideal. In some cases (bowel obstruction, diverticular disease, radiation enteritis, and Crohn disease), this situation may not be possible and the plan to anastomose may be questioned. Optimizing patient nutrition, treating infection, and minimizing inflammation in the preoperative period may improve the bowel status. At operation, all diseased bowel is resected whenever possible to provide soft, pliable bowel ends for anastomosis.

## BOWEL PREPARATION

As described in Chapter 2, bowel preparation has undergone major changes over the last 70 years. Until the last decade, mechanical bowel preparation was a standard feature of elective bowel surgery, and the lack of a bowel preparation or poor results with a mechanical preparation was in many surgeons' views a contraindication to a primary anastomosis. Recent studies have failed to support the accepted view that bowel cleansing, in the presence of appropriate antibiotics, reduced the risk of anastomotic leak or wound infection (6). Case series and reports from the trauma literature suggested that good or better outcomes could be achieved in unprepared bowel with an anastomosis

(7,8). A Cochrane Review of five randomized trials showed equal or better morbidity or mortality in 576 patients with a mechanical bowel preparation and 583 patients without a mechanical preparation (9). An additional meta-analysis of seven randomized trials containing 1,454 patients showed no significant differences for wound infection and septic and nonseptic conditions (10). Certain situations, such as laparoscopic procedures, potential need for intraoperative colonoscopy, or avoidance of spillage from proximal stool loading after a low colorectal anastomosis, still require adequate mechanical bowel preparation. For other situations, many surgeons are minimizing or eliminating a mechanical bowel preparation in elective situations. The current evidence suggests that intraluminal contents should not be the primary factor in deciding if an anastomosis should be performed. Other options to consider with unprepared bowel are to perform a subtotal colectomy with ileocolonic or ileorectal anastomosis. This option has been shown to be a safe option for avoiding a stoma in left colon obstruction (11). Alternatively, intraoperative colonic lavage in some hands offers the ability to construct an anastomosis in patients with this condition (11–13).

Whatever the bowel preparation used, it is critical that spillage of intraluminal contents be avoided to minimize complications and neoplastic dissemination. Most surgeons agree that a clean, empty colon has less potential for spillage, but that cannot compensate for poor technique. Additional protection against spillage of residual intestinal contents is provided by controlling the ends of bowel used in the anastomosis. This can be accomplished by elevating the ends (with traction sutures) or by occluding the bowel proximal and distal to the anastomosis with tapes or noncrushing clamps (14).

## BOWEL STATUS

When intestinal surgery is being performed for urgent situations or even during certain elective operations, the first decision is whether or not an anastomosis is appropriate. Healing of an anastomosis is at risk in certain clinical situations. Traditionally, intestine that is unprepared, obstructed, irradiated, inflamed, or ischemic may not be suitable for anastomosis (15–17). However, other than ischemia, current evidence suggests that constructing an anastomosis is safe in selected cases of obstruction, irradiation, inflammation, and without bowel preparation (5,11,18,19). In addition to these local factors, patient factors such as malnutrition, diabetes, renal failure, chronic hepatic disease, anemia, shock, steroid use, and other immunocompromised states may place an anastomosis at risk for failure (4–6).

The safety of intestinal anastomosis in any particular clinical scenario thus depends on patient and intestinal factors that must be carefully weighed by the operating surgeon (5). Optimally, the bowel will have a good blood supply (documented by pink color, peristalsis, and pulsatile bleeding from the cut edge), lack edema, be free of tension (see the section "Obtaining Adequate Length"), and have adequate lumen for the type of anastomosis. The decision to perform an intestinal anastomosis ultimately depends on surgical judgment derived from an understanding of documented risks as well as knowledge of one's own ability and experience.

## EXPOSURE

The importance of adequate exposure cannot be overemphasized. Exposure is facilitated by patient position, adequate length of incision, appropriate choice of retractors, and lighting. If the possibility of a left-sided anastomosis exists, the patient should be placed in lithotomy position, using stirrups, after anesthesia is induced (Figure 5.1). Great care is taken to avoid pressure on the peroneal nerves and hips (20). The perineum should extend slightly over the end of the operating table to allow easy access for transanal stapled anastomosis, upward pressure on the perineum for exposure of the distal rectum, or a two-surgeon combined approach to hand-sewn coloanal anastomosis or abdominoperineal resection. Once the patient is correctly positioned, irrigation of the rectum should be performed to ensure the quality of the bowel preparation and to evacuate any remaining fecal residue. Leaving a large mushroom-shaped or Foley catheter in the rectum alerts the surgeon to the level of dissection in the low pelvis, prevents rectal distension and possible enterotomy during mobilization, and allows drainage of rectal contents, which minimizes luminal spillage.

The trend toward smaller incisions should be critically evaluated when planning a colorectal anastomosis (4). Pelvic exposure is greatly facilitated by incisions that extend to the pubic bone. The incision may require proximal extension if mobilization of the splenic flexure is required. The extent of this extension will depend on factors such as the patient's body habitus, disease process, and surgical technique. Adequate exposure with less generous incisions is often possible in thin patients or those with low splenic flexures, mobile colons, or left-sided Crohn disease (the splenic flexure that is contracted down into the abdominal cavity). Placement of the operating surgeon between the patient's

legs often improves visualization during splenic flexure mobilization. Adequate visualization is imperative for safe splenic flexure mobilization, and additional retraction or incision extension should be one of the first considerations if mobilization is difficult.

Different retractors are available to improve exposure. Those that are fixed to the bed, such as the Bookwalter, "Upper Hand," Omnitract, or Polytract (Teleflex. Inc, Morrisville, NC) make life easier for surgical assistants and provide a consistent view throughout the operation (4). When placing retractor attachments, the surgeon must be aware of the relation of the retractor to the femoral vessels, nerves, and iliac crests. Prolonged constant traction on the bowel may also be a problem, and consideration of relieving the pressure intermittently during long cases may be appropriate.

Finally, adequate lighting is extremely important during pelvic dissection as well as to provide a view of the anastomosis, deep in the pelvis. Equipment available to enhance vision includes headlights, lighted retractors, cautery instruments, and suction devices.

## OBTAINING ADEQUATE LENGTH

After the appropriate resection is completed, sufficient proximal and distal mobilization provides tension-free bowel ends for a secure anastomosis. Tension is rarely a problem for small bowel or ileocolic anastomosis. The small bowel mesentery has an avascular plane anterior to the aorta to the takeoff of the superior mesenteric artery. The right and left colon have a posteriolateral fusion plane anterior to Gerota fascia. This avascular plane can be opened using a lateral or medial approach.

Difficulty in obtaining tension-free bowel occurs more commonly with a left-sided (e.g., colorectal) anastomosis. Additional left colon length is obtained using the following maneuvers in this order: division of the lateral colonic attachments, division of the splenic flexure attachments, division of the inferior mesenteric artery at its aortic takeoff, and division of the inferior mesenteric vein at the inferior border of the pancreas (Figure 5.2) (4). If these maneuvers do not provide adequate bowel length, branches of the distal middle colic artery and veins may need division. Unfortunately, this last action may compromise the blood supply to the remaining colonic end. If this occurs, the ischemic bowel must be resected, and additional vessels will need to be divided to provide the required bowel length. In some cases the middle colic vessels will have to be divided proximally, and the blood supply of the residual colon will need to be based on the right and/or ileocolic artery. In most patients, these vessels will provide adequate blood supply to the proximal transverse colon or hepatic flexure, which can be made to reach the rectum with one of two techniques.

One method is to open a window in the ileal mesentery medial to the ileocolic artery and vein. The proximal transverse colon is brought through this window to reach the pelvis (Figure 5.3) (21). Another option is to completely mobilize the right colon and then rotate it counterclockwise. This

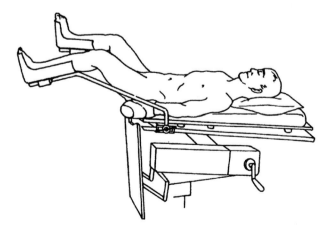

Figure 5.1 Stirrups for modified lithotomy position.

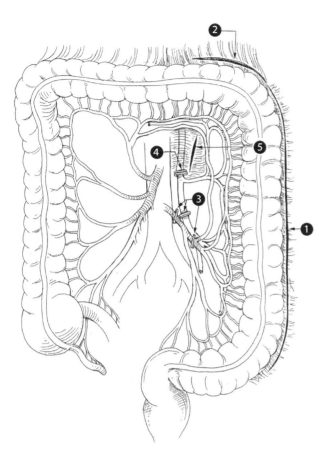

rotates the cecal tip to the right middle abdomen (pointed toward the liver), reverses the direction of the colon, and provides enough length for the hepatic flexure to reach the pelvis (Figure 5.4). As this maneuver moves the cecum to an abnormal position, it is important to remove the appendix, since development of appendicitis would produce confusing signs and symptoms.

In addition to a lack of tension, it is also critically important that the anastomotic site have a good blood supply. Before the anastomosis is constructed, the bowel should be routinely checked for viability (normal color and peristalsis and a pulsatile blood supply). Bleeding from divided appendices epiploicae (or marginal vessels) at the cut end of the proximal bowel intended for the anastomosis is frequently used to objectively confirm an adequate blood supply. In addition to the factors described previously, bowel used for an anastomosis must not be edematous, radiated, or ischemic. An appropriate resection should remove ischemic or radiated bowel, while edema of the residual bowel (e.g., associated with peritonitis) may mandate forgoing an anastomosis in favor of a diverting stoma.

## ANASTOMOTIC TECHNIQUE

In performing an anastomosis, surgeons have multiple options. Each technique has associated advantages and disadvantages, and the specific one favored by an individual surgeon depends more on training, personal experience, and perhaps blind faith than on the results of randomized, prospective studies. There has been no consistent scientific proof that one intestinal anastomotic technique is superior. Options range from the physical configuration of the anastomosis (end-to-end, side to side, end to side, side to

Figure 5.2 Operative techniques to obtain left colon length. (1) Division of lateral colonic attachments; (2) division of the splenic flexure; (3) division of the inferior mesenteric artery at its aortic takeoff and the inferior mesenteric vein; (4) second division of the inferior mesenteric vein at the inferior border of the pancreas; and (5) incision of splenic flexure mesentary. (From Rafferty JF. *Clin Colon Rectal Surg* 2001;14:25–31. With permission.)

(a)                                        (b)

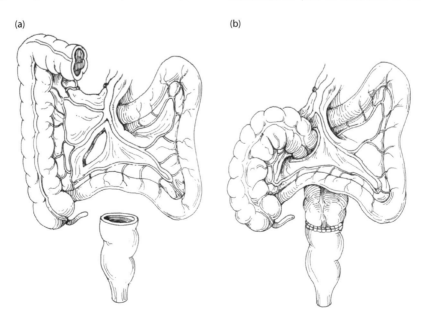

Figure 5.3 **(a)** Window in mesentary is created medial to the ileocolic artery and vein. **(b)** Transverse is brought through ileal mesenteric window to reach the pelvis.

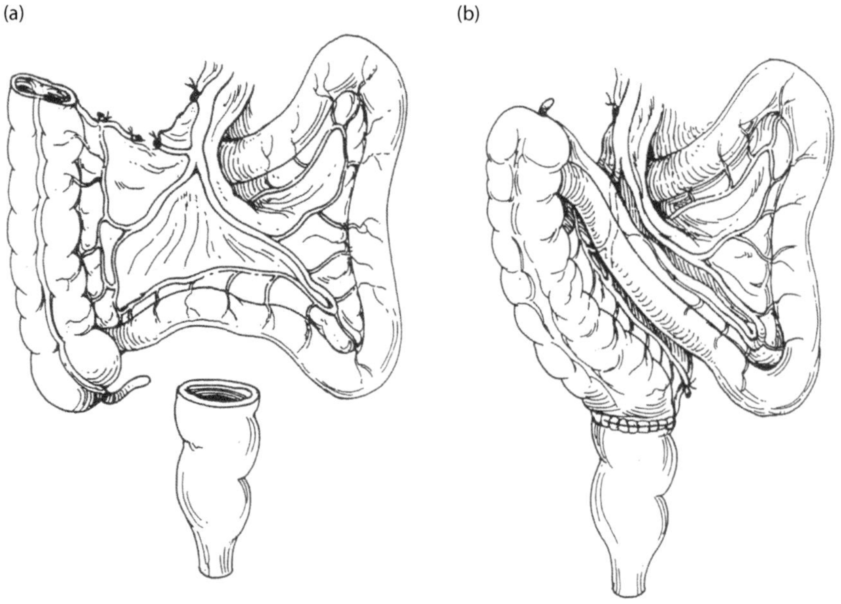

(a)                                                    (b)

Figure 5.4 **(a)** Right colon is mobilized, right colic vessels are divided, and appendix is removed. **(b)** The right colon is derotated to allow the hepatic flexure to reach the pelvis.

end, etc.) (Figure 5.5) and the method used to construct it: sutures, staples, a combination of these, and experimental methods such as compression devices or adhesives. Several of these merit discussion.

## STAPLES VERSUS SUTURES

Suturing has been used since the beginning of intestinal surgery. Different suture materials have shown some experimental differences, but the clinical difference is arguable. In general a stapled anastomosis usually takes less time but is more expensive (22,23). Blood flow may be higher with a stapled anastomosis, and in certain situations, such as a low colorectal anastomosis, the use of staples is technically easier (24). A final consideration is that any device can malfunction and lead to the need for use of additional staplers or conversion to a sutured anastomosis (5).

A meta-analysis of 13 trials comparing hand-sewn with stapled anastomoses showed similar mortality, leak rates, local cancer recurrences, and wound infections (25). This review revealed a higher rate of postoperative strictures with the stapled anastomosis, most of which were asymptomatic and easily managed with dilation.

Suture techniques, such as the number of layers or use of interrupted versus running sutures, have shown some clinical differences. An inverting anastomosis is superior to an everting technique. A number of investigators advocate a single-layer anastomosis because they believe it causes less narrowing of the lumen since a smaller amount of tissue is strangulated (26,27). A single-layer anastomosis is also felt to cause less devascularization, infection, and necrosis, while the continuous suture distributes tension more evenly around the lumen (27,28). In clinical practice, however, technical factors such as the correct placement of sutures,

correct tension of the suture, and secure knots appear to be more important than the experimental findings discussed previously. Experience, training, clinical judgment, and ability are major factors in a surgeon's choice of anastomotic technique; however, some of the reported experience with suturing merits additional comment.

An extensive experience using a running monofilament technique has been described by Max and colleagues (28). In a retrospective report of 1,000 single-layer continuous polypropylene intestinal anastomoses, the authors believed that this technique was quick, simple, economical, and safe. Although an intraoperative leak rate was not reported, their postoperative leak rate of 1% with the technique compares very favorably with others in reports using alternate techniques (28).

Six trials with 955 ileocolic participants were reviewed in a Cochrane Database Systemic review (29). The three largest prospective randomized trials comparing stapled versus hand-sewn methods for ileocolic anastomoses conducted between 1970 and 2005 showed fewer leaks with stapled anastomosis. All other outcomes—stricture, anastomotic hemorrhage, anastomotic time, reoperation, mortality, intraabdominal abscess, wound infection, and length of stay—showed no significant difference.

## END-TO-END

The use of surgical staplers has advantages in certain situations (e.g., the very low colorectal anastomosis), and they have enjoyed widespread clinical usage. These mechanical devices, however, do not compensate for improper or poor technique.

In an early survey of stapler complications by the American Society of Colon and Rectal Surgeons (ASCRS) published in 1981, 243 surgeons responded that they had

(a)

(b)

(c)

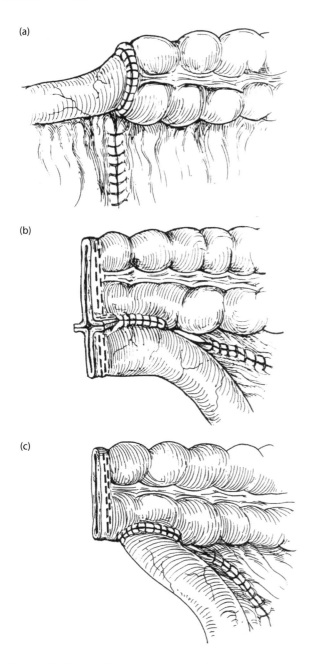

Figure 5.5 Types of anastomoses. **(a)** End-to-end anastomosis. **(b)** Side-to-side functional end-to-end anastomosis. **(c)** End-to-side anastomosis. (From Beck DE. In Beck DE, ed. *Handbook of Colorectal Surgery.* St. Louis, MO: Quality Medical, 1997, pp. 400–30. With permission.)

performed 3,594 end-to-end anastomoses (EEA) (30). Intraoperative complications were reported in 15.1% of patients. These complications included anastomotic leak (9.8%), tear during extraction (1.9%), anvil not extractable (1.2%), complete anastomotic failure that required conversion to another technique (0.9%), instrument failure (0.8%), and bleeding (0.5%). This report represents surgeons' early experience with the use of staplers, and therefore, the results must be evaluated in the proper context. Improvements in the instruments, anastomotic technique, and surgeon experience have resulted in fewer complications.

Early experience with 73 consecutive stapled end-to-end colorectal anastomoses by Gordon and Vasilevsky identified intraoperative complications in 19 patients (26%) (31). These included instrument failure (4), incomplete or inadequate "donuts" (5), bleeding (3), bowel injury associated with use of sizers (1), anvil extraction (1), anvil insertion (3), difficulty with stapler extraction (1), and anvil not extractable (1). The relative high incidence of these problems reflects the early learning curve with stapling instruments and the early developmental nature of the instruments used. Increased experience and advances in instruments have minimized the occurrence of these problems.

A prospective randomized multicenter study by Dochetry and colleagues described 652 patients who were randomized to a sutured ($n = 321$) or stapled large bowel anastomosis ($n = 331$) between 1985 and 1989 (32). During the study, 5 of the 331 patients (1.5%) randomized to a stapled anastomosis had an instrument or technical failure. Intraoperative anastomotic testing was not routinely performed, but postoperative radiologic leaks were identified in 14.4% of the sutured and 5.2% of the stapled colorectal anastomoses. Clinical anastomotic leakage was evident in 4.4% of the sutured patients and 4.5% of the stapled patients.

Proper technique is a critical component to obtaining a good anastomosis with a circular intraluminal stapler. To minimize problems, the largest diameter stapler that can be accommodated by both bowel ends should be used (33). As originally described, an intraluminal stapler entails usage of purse-string sutures to hold the bowel over the stapler cartridge and anvil during stapler closure. This purse-string suture can be placed by hand (with a baseball or in-and-out technique), with a fenestrated purse-string clamp (Purse String Device, Davis & Geck, Wayne, New Jersey), or with a stapling device (Purse String Instrument-65, U.S. Surgical Corp., Norwalk, Connecticut). To work properly, the sutures must be placed correctly (approximately 1–2 mm back from the bowel ends and 2–3 mm apart). If the sutures are placed too close, the bowel will not close tightly around the stapler shaft. This nonconstricting purse-string may be corrected by carefully cutting the bowel overlying the suture in two or more places to release additional suture to bunch up more of the bowel end. If the sutures are placed too far apart or some tear through, gaps in the bowel ends will appear when the suture is tightened. This can be repaired by use of a "Pulley Stitch" (Figure 5.6) (1,34). These interrupted 4-0 or 3-0 braided sutures (e.g., silk or braided polyester) hold the purse-string suture to the bowel ends and assist in pulling it tightly around the shaft. Finally, placement of sutures too near the bowel end results in their tearing through the bowel, while placing the sutures too far back from the bowel ends will produce an excessive bulk of tissue around the shaft.

If a purse-string clamp is used, it is important that the bowel be divided close to the clamp before the clamp is released. Leaving excess tissue adjacent to the clamp may result in too much tissue at the purse-string, which may prevent the stapler from closing and firing properly. Releasing

(a)

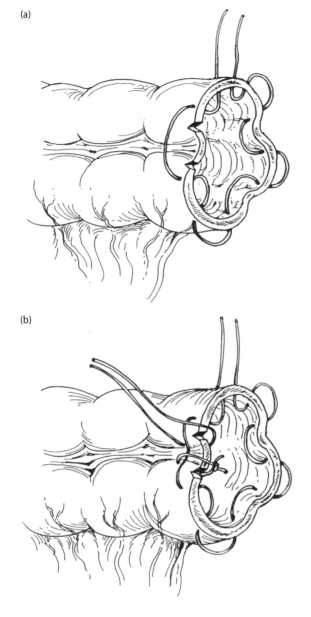

(b)

Figure 5.6 Repair of purse-string stitch. **(a)** Gap is identified in purse-string suture. **(b)** Gap is closed with "pulley" sutures.

the clamp before dividing the bowel may result in inadequate tissue to hold the purse-string. Difficulties in using the purse-string clamp low in the pelvis are minimized by the use of a double-armed suture (e.g., 2-0 monofilament polypropylene, double-armed TS-9, David and Geck, Wayne, New Jersey). Both needles are placed through the clamp, and the needles can be bent several times while the needle is withdrawn to allow the needles to be removed in the confined pelvis.

Many surgeons use clamps to hold the bowel ends while placing the purse-string or to hold the bowel open to assist placement of the anvil or stapler. Several problems can occur with use of these clamps. If the clamps are placed too far back from the bowel end and placed too tightly, an injury to the bowel wall can occur, which can produce a leak despite

a secure anastomosis. The use of open-ended clamps (e.g., Babcock clamps) allows for the possibility of placing the purse-string through the end of the clamp. If this occurs, the purse-string suture will need to be cut. Use of solid-ended clamps eliminates the chance of this happening. Large clamps increase the difficulty in inserting an anvil in bowel diameter close to the diameter of the anvil.

## Double staple

Another end-to-end stapling option involves a double-staple technique (35,36). With this method a linear staple line is placed across the distal bowel, and a circular stapler is inserted into this bowel (via the anus for a left-sided anastomosis). To avoid creating an ischemic area, the trocar of the circular stapler should exit adjacent or as close as possible to the linear staples. The anvil is placed in the proximal bowel and secured with a purse-string as described previously. When closed and fired, the circular stapler removes a portion of the crossed linear staple line to create the anastomosis. Concern was initially expressed about these crossing staple lines. However, subsequent experimental and clinical evidence has confirmed the relative safety of this method (37,38). The double-staple technique is helpful in anastomosing bowel ends of dissimilar size and in ultralow colorectal or coloanal anastomoses. Outside of these situations, the extra cost of using a stapler rather than a sutured purse-string argues more for the use of a purse-string.

With low distal staple lines, it can be challenging to insert the stapler into the anus and not disrupt the staple line. Distal staple line disruption can occur if the distal bowel is tenuous or under too much traction. If this occurs, several options are available. The initial action is to visualize the distal staple line. If the ends of the partially closed bowel can be grasped with clamps or traction sutures, the amount of residual bowel can be assessed. If adequate length is present, the bowel can be closed with a linear stapler placed below the disrupted staple line. After the stapler is fired, the residual bowel end can be resected with scissors or a scalpel. A second option is to reclose the disrupted staple line with sutures placed from the abdominal side or placed intraluminally via a retractor placed into the anal canal (39). If the bowel is successfully closed, the anastomosis can proceed. If the distal segment of bowel is impossible to close, a musectomy can be performed via the anus, and a hand-sewn coloanal or ileoanal anastomosis can be performed.

A serious problem associated with double stapling of the low rectum is the inadvertent creation of a rectovaginal fistula. This unfortunate complication results from incorporating the posterior wall of the vagina into the staple lines. Maneuvers to reduce this occurrence include an adequate dissection of the rectum off the posterior vagina, careful visualization of the bowel ends during closure of the stapler, and intravaginal palpation of the posterior vaginal wall prior to firing the stapler (1).

A variation of double stapling is triple stapling. In this anastomotic method, an extralinear stapler is used to close the bowel end after placement of the anvil into the proximal bowel. The anvil trocar is then advanced through the closed bowel. This technique has been suggested for intracorporeal laparoscopic techniques; however, it is costly and produces another linear suture line that must be incorporated into the final anastomotic staple line. The technique has not gained widespread acceptance due to the relative ease in placing the proximal purse-string.

Difficulty with anvil insertion in the proximal bowel lumen usually occurs when the stapler is too large for the diameter of the bowel. Experience or the use of scissors allows accurate selection of the correct size of circular stapler. Additional helpful techniques include the use of dilators or glucagon to overcome bowel spasm, lubrication of the anvil head (with betadine, saline, or blood), and distraction of the bowel ends with three small-ended forceps or clamps. Use of a recently developed low-profile anvil (CDH Ethicon-Endosurgery, Inc., Cincinnati, Ohio) has diminished this occurrence.

## Detachable staplers

For colorectal anastomosis, the circular stapler is usually placed through the anus. With currently available detachable head staplers, the flat stapler shaft may be difficult to pass atraumatically through the anal sphincter muscles. Khoury and Opelka, in 1995, described a technique to facilitate this maneuver (40). A Faensler or Chelsey-Eaton anoscope allows a gradual controlled dilation of the sphincters. After removal of the obturator, the stapler shaft can easily be passed through the anoscope (Figure 5.7). Once through the sphincter, the stapler must be inserted up to the resected end of the rectum. Knowledge of rectal anatomy, adequate mobilization of the posterior rectum, and selection of an appropriate size of stapler assist in accomplishing this advancement. Incorrect insertion can tear or split the rectum. Such an injury to the rectum mandates a very low or coloanal anastomosis to reestablish intestinal continuity.

A proctoscopic (or flexible endoscopic) examination of the rectum ensures an adequate lumen, confirms an adequate preparation and mobilization, and assists in identifying the apex of a Hartmann pouch.

Once the stapler is closed and fired, it must be removed. Stapler extraction from the anastomotic area may be aided with a traction stitch. Bowel spasm or a stapler misfire may cause extraction difficulty. Gentle traction and careful stapler manipulation usually allow it to be removed. If a misfire results in an inability to remove the stapler, it may be necessary to excise and reaccomplish the anastomosis.

## END TO SIDE AND SIDE TO SIDE (FUNCTIONAL END-TO-END)

An end-to-side or side-to-end (the proximal bowel is usually listed first) anastomosis is useful for joining bowel of different diameter. The size of the anastomosis is not limited by the bowel diameter. This configuration is often used for ileocolic or ileorectal anastomoses. A side-to-side anastomosis is frequently used to join bowel with a linear cutting stapler. Use of the bowel ends for a side-to-side anastomosis serves as a functional end-to-end anastomosis. A surgical atlas should be consulted for additional technical details.

A meta-analysis of studies published between 1992 and 2005 of end-to-end versus other anastomotic configurations in Crohn disease used eight studies including 661 patients (41). The authors conclude that a side-to-side anastomosis led to fewer anastomotic leaks and overall complications, a shorter hospital stay, and a perianastomotic recurrence rate comparable to end-to-end anastomoses.

## ANASTOMOTIC TESTING

All surgeons should test their anastomoses in some way. At a minimum, the anastomotic site is inspected and in some

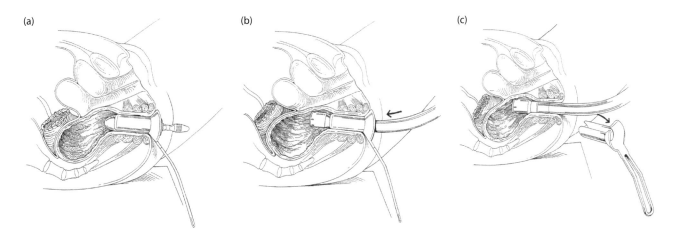

(a)  (b)  (c)

Figure 5.7 Anoscopic-assisted stapler insertion. **(a)** Faensler anoscope is inserted after gentle anal dilation. **(b)** The anoscope obturator is removed, and the circular stapler is inserted through the anoscope. **(c)** The anoscope is withdrawn and taken off the shaft of the stapler.

cases palpated. A visual inspection of a side-to-side anastomosis may be performed prior to closing the ends of the bowel. Gentle constriction of the bowel proximal or distal to the anastomosis will confirm a patent lumen and the absence of a gross leak. A more sensitive test can easily be performed in the colorectal anastomosis (which is at higher risk for a leak) (42–45).

The author prefers to test low colorectal anastomosis with intraluminal instillation of a dilute solution of providine-iodine (Betadine, Purdue Frederick Co, Norwalk, Connecticut). After the bowel is occluded above the anastomosis with finger pressure, the testing solution is instilled gently with a bulb syringe inserted into the anus. Any leak is readily apparent. Irrigation with this dilute providine-iodine solution also provides antimicrobial and tumoricidal activity. Others have suggested testing with a dilute solution of methylene blue (46). Larger volumes are infused via a rectal tube, and with care even ileocolic anastomosis can be tested for leaks with this technique. The optimal pressure recommended for detecting intraoperative leaks with air/water testing is 25–30 cm $H_2O$ (47,48). If an infusion system is used, the pressure can be controlled by the height of the infusion bag.

Some surgeons prefer to test their anastomosis with air (45). The pelvis is first filled with saline and the distal bowel (containing the anastomosis) is distended with air (instilled transanally). Any anastomotic defect will produce air bubbles. Unfortunately, with this method it is often difficult to accurately identify the location of the leak if any blood has mixed with the saline. The saline must also be removed before any identified leak can be repaired. Testing with air may be preferable for higher colorectal anastomosis as infused intraluminal fluid may not reach a higher anastomosis.

A proctoscope (or colonoscope) can also be used to inspect the colorectal anastomosis. Sufficient lumen size is usually confirmed by the lack of stenosis, hemostasis is confirmed, and the bowel can easily be distended with air.

Finally, some surgeons inspect the intraluminal stapler "donuts." The author has not found this to be helpful as complete donuts do not ensure the absence of a leak at the anastomotic site (e.g., due to a tear of the bowel or staple lines during stapler removal). Also, an incomplete donut may be produced with an intact anastomosis. Intraoperative testing as described above is more sensitive and specific.

Whatever method is used to inspect or test an anastomosis, it is important to act on any defect or leak identified. Options include suture reinforcement, reconstruction, or proximal diversion.

## CHALLENGES

### INADEQUATE ANASTOMOTIC LUMEN

Adequate luminal patency is important for several reasons. Bowel edema occurs in the perioperative period, and a marginal lumen may lead to a partial obstruction. The

anastomotic lumen can be sized by palpation or visually inspected. The ability to remove the anvil of a circular stapler confirms a lumen corresponding to the size of the stapler, while distal rectal anastomosis can be evaluated by a proctoscope. An alternative technique for colorectal anastomosis is an isoperistaltic side-to-side anastomosis (Figure 5.8).

## LEAKAGE

An accurate incidence of anastomotic leakage is difficult to determine. Few studies have reported the incidence of intraoperatively identified anastomotic problems. The incidence of leaks identified in the postoperative period is described in Chapter 6.

If a defective anastomosis is identified, it may be repaired in several ways. Additional sutures can approximate a small gap, or the anastomosis can be resected and completely redone using a stapler or hand-sewn technique. Another option is to replace purse-string sutures around the defective anastomosis and reinsert a new stapler through the lumen. The purse-string sutures are tightened, which should close the defect and hold the previously placed staples toward the stapler shaft. After closure and firing of the new stapler, the new donuts (which should also contain the old staples) are removed with the stapler (49). If the anastomosis is very low, the defect may also be repaired transanally.

## ANASTOMOTIC HEMORRHAGE

Hemorrhage can occur at both a staple and a suture line. Proper size staple height and correct tension of sutures

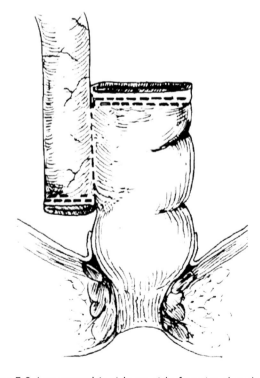

Figure 5.8 Isoparastaltic side-to-side functional end-to-end anastomotic technique.

minimize the occurrence of this problem. For side-to-side anastomoses performed with linear staples, care should be taken to avoid incorporating any portion of the mesentery in the staple line. Techniques to stop hemorrhage include cautery of the bleeding vessels or placement of a suture at the site of bleeding. Excessive cautery is to be avoided as the staple line has the potential to transfer the electrical energy to adjacent portions of the bowel. Reduction or stoppage of the bleeding may also be helped by digital compression or intraluminal instillation of an epinephrine solution (1-100,000 or 1-200,000 u/mL). Another option is submucosal injection of an epinephrine solution (50).

## PROXIMAL PROTECTION (STOMAS)

For high-risk anastomosis, a proximal diverting stoma is often used. A diverting stoma will not prevent an anastomotic leak but will reduce the septic morbidity and mortality associated with the leakage. A properly constructed loop stoma is almost totally diverting (51). However, if absolute total diversion is desired, a Prasad type of end-loop stoma may be constructed (52).

If diversion is needed, the author and editors prefer an ileostomy over a colostomy. A diverting colostomy following a colonic resection has several problems. A colostomy includes a larger stoma, and due to its proximal location, the ostomy output is loose or liquid and very odorous. If a significant colonic resection has been performed, the remaining colon length is often insufficient to easily reach the abdominal wall at a preferred stomal location. Closure of a loop colostomy puts the marginal blood supply to a more distal anastomosis at risk.

A loop ileostomy has several advantages (53). (1) It is easy to construct and close. As it is usually created in bowel removed from the anastomotic site, (2) tension and blood supply are rarely a problem. (3) Ileostomy output is liquid, has little odor, and (4) unless the mesentery is abnormally shortened, an ileostomy will reach almost any site on the abdominal wall.

## ADJUVANTS AND DRAINS

Due to the morbidity associated with leaks, several adjuvants have been used in cases where there is high risk of potential compromised anastomoses. Wrapping the anastomosis with omentum is a popular adjunct that is felt by many surgeons to prevent disruption. Unfortunately, there is no evidence to support this practice in humans (54,55). The use of foreign materials around the anastomosis has been shown to be harmful (56,57). Reinforcing sutures positioned around a stapled anastomosis, while not routinely necessary, may provide security, especially for low rectal anastomoses.

Controversy continues regarding the use of drains as an adjunct to intestinal anastomosis. The abdominal cavity cannot be adequately drained, but in cavities like the low pelvis it is possible. Proponents believe that the drain removes contaminated fluid and blood, and should a leak occur, it would be controlled. Opponents argue that the drain is dangerous as it allows bacteria a portal of entry and it may erode the anastomosis. Trials have clearly shown no benefit from drainage of intestinal anastomoses (58,59). Despite evidence to the contrary, the practice of closed suction drainage for low pelvic anastomoses the first few days postoperatively continues due to individual surgeon's beliefs (5). It should be emphasized that lack of enteric contents in a drain placed near an anastomosis does not preclude an anastomotic leak.

## SUMMARY

Adherence to established surgical principles and techniques should minimize anastomotic problems. Mechanical devices cannot overcome limitations in experience, skill, or judgment. Intraoperative identification of problems that occur permits correction with minimal morbidity.

## REFERENCES

1. Beck DE. Intraoperative anastomotic complications. In: Hicks TC, Beck DE, Opelka FG, Timmcke AE. (eds.) *Complications of Colon and Rectal Surgery*. Baltimore, MD: Williams and Wilkins, 1996, pp. 70–81.
2. Goligher JC. *Surgery of the Anus, Rectum, and Colon*, 5th Edition. London, UK: Balliere Tindall, 1984.
3. Steichen FM, Ravitch MM. *Surg Clin North Am* 1984; 64:425–40.
4. Rafferty JF. *Clin Colon Rectal Surg* 2001;14:25–31.
5. Sweeney WB. *Clin Colon Rectal Surg* 2001;14:15–23.
6. Delaney CP, Mackeiggan JM. Preoperative management—Risk assessment, medical evaluation, and bowel preparation. In Wolff BG, Fleshman JW, Beck DE, Pemberton JH, Wexner SD. (eds.) *ASCRS Textbook of Colorectal Surgery*. New York, NY: Springer-Verlag, 2007, pp. 116–29.
7. Demetriades D et al. *J Traum* 2001;50:765–75.
8. van Geldere D et al. *J Am Coll Surg* 2002;194:40–7.
9. Guenga KF et al. *Cochrane Database Syst Rev* 2003; 2:CD001544.
10. Slim K et al. *Br J Surg* 2004;91:1125–30.
11. Torralba JA et al. *Dis Colon Rectum* 1998;41:18–22.
12. Kressner U et al. *Eur J Surg* 1994;160:287–92.
13. Forloni B et al. *Dis Colon Rectum* 1998;41:23–7.
14. Wexner SD, Beck DE. Sepsis prevention in colorectal surgery. In Fielding LP, Goldnerg SM (eds.) *Operative Surgery*, 5th Edition. London, UK: Butterworth-Heineman, Ltd., 1993, pp. 41–6.
15. Irvin TT, Goliger JC. *Br J Surg* 1973;60:461–4.

16. Schrock TR et al. *Ann Surg* 1973;177:513–8.
17. Khoury GA, Waxman BP. *Br J Surg* 1983;70:61–3.
18. Hsu T-C. *Dis Colon Rectum* 1998;41:28–32.
19. Weiber S et al. *Eur J Surg* 1994;160:47–51.
20. Karulf R. Anesthesia and intraoperative positioning. In Hicks TC, Beck DE, Opelka FG, Timmcke AE. (eds.) *Complications of Colorectal Surgery.* Baltimore, MD: Williams and Wilkins, 1996, pp. 34–49.
21. Le TH et al. *Dis Colon Rectum* 1993;36:197–8.
22. Graffner H et al. *Dis Colon Rectum* 1984;27:767–71.
23. Fingerhut A et al. *Surgery* 1995;118:479–85.
24. Wheeless CR, Jr, Smith JJ. *Obstet Gynecol* 1983;62: 513–8.
25. MacRae HM, McLeod RS. *Dis Colon Rectum* 1998;41: 180–9.
26. Gambee LP et al. *Am J Surg* 1956;92:222–7.
27. Templeton JL, McKelvey ST. *Dis Colon Rectum* 1985; 28:38–41.
28. Max E et al. *Am J Surg* 1991;162:461–7.
29. Choy PY et al. *Cochrane Database Syst Rev* 2007, Issue 3. Art. No.: CD004320. DOI: 10.1002/14651858. CD004320.pub2.
30. Smith LE. *Dis Colon Rectum* 1981;24:236–42.
31. Gordon PH, Vasilevsky CA. *Surg Clin North Am* 1984; 64:555–66.
32. Dochetry JG et al. *Ann Surg* 1995;221:176–84.
33. Fazio VW. *Surg Clin North Am* 1988;68:1367–82.
34. Last MD, Fazio VW. *Dis Colon Rectum* 1985;28:979–80.
35. Cohen Z et al. *Dis Colon Rectum* 1983;26:231–5.
36. Griffen FD, Knight CD. *Surg Clin North Am* 1984;64: 579–90.
37. Julian TB, Ravitch MM. *Surg Clin North Am* 1984;64: 567–78.
38. Ravitch MM. *Surg Clin North Am* 1984;64:543–54.
39. Tan WS et al. *Tech Coloproctol* 2007;11:266–7.
40. Khoury DA, Opelka FG. *Dis Colon Rectum* 1995;38: 553–4.
41. Simillis C et al. *Dis Colon Rectum* 2007;50:1674–87.
42. Beard JD et al. *Br J Surg* 1990;77:1095–7.
43. Griffith JM, Trapnell JE. *J R Coll Surg Edinb* 1990; 35:35–6.
44. Yalin R et al. *Eur J Surg* 1993;159:49–51.
45. Davies AH et al. *Ann R Coll Surg Engl* 1988;70:345–7.
46. Smith S et al. *BMC Surg* 2007;7:15.
47. Gilbert JM, Trapnell JE. *Ann R Coll Surg Engl* 1988; 70:158–60.
48. Wheeler JM, Gilbert JM. *Ann R Coll Surg Engl* 1999; 81:105–8.
49. Makabeli G, Williams LG. *Dis Colon Rectum* 1984;27: 490–1.
50. Perez RO et al. *Tech Coloproctol* 2007;11:64–6.
51. Pearl RK, Abcarian H. Diverting stomas. In MacKeigan JM, Cataldo PA. (eds.) *Intestinal Stomas: Principles, Techniques, and Management.* St. Louis, MO: Quality Medical, 1993, pp. 107–26.
52. Prasad ML et al. *Arch Surg* 1984;119:975–6.
53. Williams NS et al. *Br J Surg* 1986;73:566–70.
54. Carter DC et al. *Br J Surg* 1972;129–33.
55. McLachlin AD, Denton DW. *Am J Surg* 1973;125: 134–40.
56. Trowbridge PR, Howes EL. *Am J Surg* 1967;113: 236–40.
57. Laufman H, Method H. *Surg Gynecol Obstet* 1948;86: 669–73.
58. Hoffmann J et al. *Dis Colon Rectum* 1987;30:449–52.
59. Sagar PM et al. *Br J Surg* 1993;80:769–71.

# 6

# Other intraoperative challenges

JESUS FLORES AND SHARON G. GREGORCYK

## CHALLENGING CASE

You are performing a laparoscopic sigmoid colectomy on a 45-year-old man with recurrent diverticulitis. The sigmoid colon is inflamed, the mesentery bleeds easily, and the dissection is difficult as the sigmoid colon is stuck down to the left pelvic sidewall. As you are dissecting the sigmoid colon free, you note sudden dark blood quickly pooling in the operative field. You suspect a major venous injury to the left external iliac vein. Despite aggressive suctioning, you struggle to find the venous injury.

## CASE MANAGEMENT

You alert the anesthesiologist of bleeding from the suspected venous injury. You push the bowel you were just mobilizing into the side wall to help hold pressure as you quickly convert your laparoscopic procedure to a hand-assisted or open procedure. The colorectal surgeon can face various intraoperative challenges in any given case. One must remain calm and recall sound clinical judgment and surgical principles in dealing with complications.

## PREOPERATIVE EVALUATION

The preoperative evaluation is the first step in planning any operation. It should start with a thorough history and physical exam, which may provide clues to intraoperative challenges. One may discover increased risks for bleeding, extensive adhesive disease, or unusual anatomical considerations.

Indicators for potential bleeding risk include easy bruising, heavy menses, bleeding gums with brushing teeth, or family history of coagulation disorders. The patient with hepatic disease, portal hypertension, or renal disease should arouse suspicion for bleeding tendencies. Medication lists are particularly important as many prescription and nonprescription medications increase the risk for intraoperative bleeding.

Medications with antiplatelet properties such as aspirin, nonsteroidal anti-inflammatory drugs, and clopidogrel should be stopped 5–7 days prior to surgery. Warfarin, a well-known, commonly used anticoagulant is best stopped 3–5 days before surgery (1). The surgeon should be familiar with the newer direct oral anticoagulants including rivaroxaban and apixaban (Factor Xa inhibitors) and dabigatran (direct thrombin inhibitor). Rivaroxaban should be held at least 24–48 hours prior to surgery, while the timing of when to stop apixaban and dabigatran ranges from 24 to 96 hours, depending on the patient's baseline renal function (2,3). For patients at a higher risk, such as those with a recent coronary stent, a recent (<3 month) history of venous thromboembolism, or mechanical cardiac valve in the mitral position, a discussion with the patient's treating physician is advised. The surgeon must remember that common supplements, such as garlic, gingko, ginseng, fish oil, and vitamin E, can also prolong bleeding time and should be stopped 1 week prior to surgery (4). One must be prepared to transfuse platelets or fresh frozen plasma in an antiplatelet therapy or anticoagulation patient requiring an emergency operation.

In obtaining the surgical history, the indication, type of operation, postoperative hospital course, and any complications are important. Reviewing relevant operative reports can provide information about a patient's anatomy and can help anticipate intraoperative challenges, such as adhesions or altered surgical planes. Abdominal abscesses, fistulae, and use of mesh are red flags for adhesions. On physical examination, a stiff, scarred abdominal wall is concerning for challenging adhesions.

## INTRAOPERATIVE HEMORRHAGE

Intraoperative hemorrhage can vary, from minimal intermittent oozing to major life-threatening exsanguination.

Even minimal intermittent oozing can be problematic, as it stains the tissues, absorbs light, and can quickly obscure the operative field laparoscopically. Use of electrocautery and energy devices, such as the Harmonic scalpel or Enseal (Johnson and Johnson), Ligasure (Covidien), or Thunderbeat (Olympus) can help reduce this problem. These instruments can be used for careful blunt or sharp dissection, and dividing the mesentery and major vessels, minimizing the need to repeatedly exchange instruments.

The surgeon must always be prepared for the possibility of bleeding during division of a major blood vessel, regardless of the method of transection and operative approach. During an open procedure, one can often grasp the vessel remnant and suture ligate it. During a laparoscopic or robotic procedure, the bleeding can stain the camera lens, fill the operative field quickly, and prevent viewing of the bleeding vessel. Preparing for this possibility before dividing a major vessel is essential. One strategy is to hold on to the proximal portion of the vessel, as it is being divided, so that it can be quickly occluded should bleeding start. This allows the deployment of hemoclips or an Endoloop (Johnson and Johnson) around the base of the bleeding vessel during minimally invasive procedures. It is important to have these supplies in the operating room in case they are immediately needed. Just as important is deciding what method to use to divide a major blood vessel. In older patients who may have calcified vessels, it may be safer to divide them with a linear cutting stapler with a vascular load than using an energy device. In Crohn patients with inflamed, thickened mesentery, it may be smarter to clamp, sharply divide, and tie the mesentery with sutures rather than use an energy device.

The spleen can be a major source of intraoperative bleeding. Its proximity to the colon and omentum, along with the frequent need to mobilize the splenic flexure during colorectal operations makes it vulnerable to injury. Techniques to minimize the risk of splenic injury include incising the correct plane, avoiding excessive traction, using an energy device, and strategically approaching the splenic flexure from different angles. If the splenic flexure cannot be fully mobilized using a straight laparoscopic approach, conversion to hand-assisted laparoscopic procedure can allow better traction, tactile feedback, and safe mobilization. These extra steps to avoid injury to this delicate organ can save the surgeon headaches from troublesome splenic bleeding.

The most common splenic injury is a capsular tear, which is usually controlled with electrocautery. This is true even with minimally invasive approaches. If brisk bleeding is encountered, the spleen should be packed off with gauze. Ray-Tec sponges offer the advantage of being x-ray detectable and helping estimate blood loss. The surgeon and operating room personnel need to keep count of the number of Ray-Tec sponges placed intraabdominally to ensure that no sponge is left inside the abdomen. Next, one must address the bleeding. The anesthesiologist should be notified of the splenic injury and potential for significant blood loss. This allows adequate resuscitation of the patient, placement of additional IV access, and early notification of the blood

bank, should transfusion be necessary. Communication with the rest of the operating room personnel is also essential. They should have topical hemostatic agents, additional suction devices, laparotomy sponges, a long laparoscopic instrument set, and an open laparotomy tray available in the room. Once the anesthesiologist is prepared, the gauze can be removed and the splenic injury assessed. Topical hemostatic agents, such as Avitene (Davol), Surgicel Nu-Knit (Ethicon), or Evicel fibrin sealant (Ethicon) can be used to stop bleeding from small splenic capsular tears. An argon beam coagulator can also be useful and is available for both laparoscopic and open procedures (5).

Despite best efforts, sometimes splenic injuries incurred laparoscopically cannot be controlled and require conversion to an open procedure to stop the bleeding. During an open procedure, the avascular splenic ligaments can be divided with electrocautery, allowing medialization of the spleen. Manual pressure can be held on the spleen or the splenic hilum to slow the bleeding. The surgeon must now decide whether to attempt repair or perform a splenectomy.

Different techniques for splenorrhaphy have been described. This includes partial splenectomy, mattress suture repair, use of argon beam coagulation, mesh wrap, or a combination. Mattress sutures can be placed directly over the splenic surface or over Teflon pledgets (6). The mesh wrap uses a polyglycolic mesh. A keyhole defect is made in the mesh, and the spleen is passed through the defect until the keyhole encircles the splenic hilum. The mesh is wrapped around the spleen and sutured to itself, creating a tamponade effect (7).

The surgeon should make an aggressive attempt to preserve the spleen. However, splenic preservation should not be undertaken in the face of ongoing uncontrollable hemorrhage or hemodynamic instability. In these two situations, a splenectomy is warranted to stop the bleeding and get the patient off the operating room table as soon as possible. The surgeon and the patient should be aware that splenectomy carries a 5% lifetime risk of overwhelming postsplenectomy infection (OPSI), primarily from encapsulated bacteria such as *Streptococcus pneumoniae*, *Haemophilus influenzae*, and *Neisseria meningitides* (8–10). Vaccinations against these bacteria are recommended in the 2-week postoperative period. Antibiotic prophylaxis and early aggressive treatment of infections should be considered in asplenic patients as OPSI carries a mortality rate as high as 50% (10). Early postoperative complications from splenectomy can include pneumonia, pancreatitis, and subphrenic abscess.

Another challenging situation the colorectal surgeon may face is hemorrhage in the pelvis. There are several potential sources of hemorrhage, including the internal iliac arteries and veins in the pelvic sidewalls, enlarged pelvic collateral vessels from portal hypertension, and the presacral venous plexus. Surgery in this area can be especially challenging due to the limited work space, presence of pelvic organs such as the uterus, a bulky rectal tumor, inflammation from abscesses, or absence of anatomical planes from previous pelvic surgery.

Should pelvic hemorrhage occur, immediate pressure should be placed over the area. The surgeon needs to identify the source of bleeding and make preparations to control it. This may require conversion to an open procedure. The pelvis can be packed with laparotomy sponges. The surgeon should ask for long instruments, lighted pelvic retractors, and possibly a second working suction device. As pelvic hemorrhage can be rapid and severe, the anesthesia team should be made aware of the situation early on. Cell saver use can allow for autotransfusion of blood. Once the anesthesia team has adequately resuscitated the patient, the packs can be removed and the pelvis assessed for a bleeding source.

The pelvic floor and sidewalls are lined by the endopelvic fascia. Dissection in the correct plane without violation of this fascia can prevent injury to and bleeding from the underlying vascular structures. Violation of the endopelvic fascia along the pelvic sidewall can lead to injury to one of the internal iliac veins, leading to profuse bleeding. Direct pressure over the area is applied. If a vascular surgeon is readily available, their expertise can prove very helpful (11). They can attempt suture repair of these thinned-walled vessels. If they are not immediately available, suture ligation may be the best option. Other useful instruments for this situation include clip appliers and laparoscopic instruments, which in an open case can allow extra length needed deep in the pelvis. Internal iliac artery injuries also warrant intraoperative vascular surgery consultation for repair. While an assistant holds pressure over the injured artery, the surgeon can help prepare the operative field and ask for a vascular instrument set while awaiting the vascular surgeon. In the rare case where an arterial injury is not immediately found in the operating room, postoperative angiography with embolization can be useful.

Violation of the endopelvic fascia covering the sacrum can lead to injury to the underlying presacral venous plexus. The anatomy and fragility of this plexus makes control of bleeding difficult (12). This plexus contains avalvular veins that can attain high pressures. The presacral veins communicate with the internal vertebral venous system through the basivertebral vein. They are thin walled and often retract into the sacral foramen after injury. Use of electrocoagulation or suture ligation to control this bleeding often results in increased bleeding (13). Direct pressure using laparotomy sponges to pack the pelvis should be used to gain control of the bleeding, allowing the anesthesia team to "catch up" with resuscitation. When possible, the specimen should be resected to optimize access to the pelvis. Sterile thumbtacks or hemorrhage occluder pins can be placed directly into the sacrum (midline) to occlude the bleeding site. If the bleeding does not stop but is sufficiently minimized, use of topical agents or repacking the pelvis may achieve complete hemostasis (14).

If the massive pelvic exsanguination still does not stop, one can attempt using rectus abdominis muscle fragment welding to stop it. This technique involves harvesting a 1.5–2 cm² fragment of rectus abdominis muscle, holding it in place with forceps to occlude the bleeding site, and applying electrocautery at 100 Hz to the forcep, which transmits to the muscle fragment to weld close the bleeding point (15). The muscle fragment may fall off, but the bleeding source is controlled as the underlying vessel has been coagulated (Figure 6.1).

Another described technique involves harvesting a $4 \times 2 \times 1$ cm piece of rectus abdominis muscle as a free flap and sewing it over the bleeding area to tamponade the presacral bleeding (16) (Figures 6.2 and 6.3).

In cases of severe pelvic hemorrhage that does not respond to any attempts, the pelvis should be tightly packed with laparotomy pads and the patient taken to the surgical intensive care unit (ICU) for resuscitation and correction of any coagulopathy, acidosis, hypothermia, and anemia. Successful balloon tamponade with a Sengstaken-Blakemore

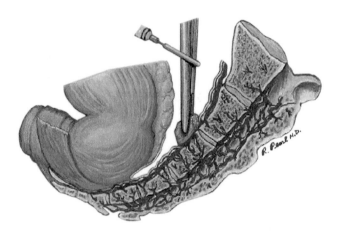

Figure 6.1 An overview of the operative technique of rectus abdominis muscle welding. A forceps is used to hold the muscle fragment over the bleeding point, occluding the vessel. Electrocautery is then applied to the forceps to weld closed the bleeding site. (From Harrison JL et al. *Dis Colon Rectum* 2003;46:1115–7.)

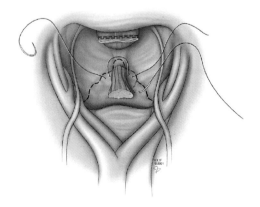

Figure 6.2 Two untied sutures were applied to adjacent tissue near the bleeding site. (From Harrison JL et al. *Dis Colon Rectum* 2003; 46:1115–7.)

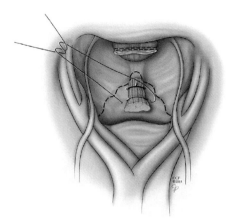

Figure 6.3 Sutures tied over the free muscle flap to provide tamponade. (From Harrison JL et al. *Dis Colon Rectum* 2003;46:1115–7.)

tube or a Bakri postpartum balloon has also been described. Packing requires a trip back to the operating room in 24–36 hours for removal of the pads. At this time, most bleeding will have stopped or become manageable. Another issue to be addressed, especially in the pelvis, is whether or not to proceed with an anastomosis. The patient's hemodynamic status influences this decision. Shock, pressor requirement, or multiple blood transfusions can lead to poor perfusion of the anastomosis resulting in a significantly increased risk of an anastomotic leak. Deterrents to an anastomosis in the pelvis include ongoing hypothermia, hypotension, coagulopathy, major blood loss, and increased time necessary to create the anastomosis.

With laparoscopic and robotic-assisted surgery, additional bleeding risk occurs at each trocar site. An abdominal wall vessel can be injured during trocar placement. Injury to the liver, spleen, aorta, inferior vena cava, and iliac vessels can occur with trocar placement, as well. Major vascular injury rates of 0.03%–0.1% and major abdominal organ injury rates of 0.08%–0.14% have been reported (17). The most commonly injured abdominal wall vessels during laparoscopic port placement are the inferior epigastrics, with an average incidence of approximately 0.1%. As the port can tamponade the bleeding, it is good practice to remove each port under direct laparoscopic visualization. Identifying and repairing an injury at this point prevents a subsequent return to the operating room. Typically, the abdominal wall vessel will be small and controlled with pressure or electrocautery alone. Should the bleeding persist, the incision may be enlarged and the vessel suture ligated. Alternatively, bleeding from a port site can be controlled laparoscopically by using a fascial closure device, such as an Endo Close (Covidien) or a Keith needle (18). The stitch is passed externally through the full thickness of the abdominal wall into the peritoneal cavity, grasped, and laparoscopically passed back out of the abdominal wall and tied. This can be repeated as needed to stop bleeding from port sites.

## DAMAGE CONTROL

Damage control laparotomy (DCL) was first described in the trauma literature and refers to an abbreviated resuscitative strategy where the primary goal is to rapidly control hemorrhage and contamination, restore normal physiology, and remove/debride frankly necrotic tissue (19,20). Laparotomy pads may be used to temporarily pack off and control massive hemorrhage. The abdominal wall is often closed temporarily with the use of a negative pressure wound therapy system, such as the wound V.A.C. (KCI) or ABThera system (KCI). Patients are subsequently transported to the ICU for continued resuscitation and correction of coagulopathy, hypothermia, and acidosis. Once the physiologic status has improved and stabilized, the patient is returned to the operating room for packing removal, reconstruction, definitive surgery, and abdominal wall closure. This strategy is now used by surgeons to treat patients in extremis needing resuscitation and stabilization before definitive treatment.

The surgeon must use sound judgment in deciding which patients would benefit from DCL over continued time spent in the operating room, as there is potential morbidity associated with leaving the abdominal wall open and multiple trips to the operating room. Previously proposed selection criteria include the inability to achieve hemostasis due to coagulopathy, long surgical procedures in unstable patients, inaccessible major venous injury, associated life-threatening injury in a second anatomical location, planned reassessment (24–72 hours) of abdominal contents, inability to close the linea alba fascia due to visceral edema, or concern for developing abdominal compartment syndrome (21–23).

The most common indications for DCL are related to hemorrhage, hemodynamic instability, and massive resuscitation. This is usually accompanied by the vicious cycle of hypothermia, coagulopathy, and acidosis, along with massive bowel wall edema. In the nontrauma venue, this may be the patient who has received large volume resuscitation for lower gastrointestinal or intraoperative hemorrhage or who has returned to the operating room for postoperative hemorrhage. During the operation, previously hemostatic sites may begin to bleed, signaling the onset of coagulopathy, which could be dilutional, consumptive, and/or hypothermia related. In this bleak scenario, it may be reasonable to pack the abdomen, apply an occlusive dressing, and take the patient to the ICU for aggressive rewarming, ongoing resuscitation, and optimization. Once the patient is stabilized and resuscitated, he or she is taken back to the operating room within 24–72 hours. Likewise, a patient may escape the coagulopathic and hypothermic effects of large volume resuscitation, but massive edema may manifest as increased pulmonary pressures or hemodynamic compromise from abdominal compartment syndrome when the fascia is closed (24).

Occasionally, massive bowel edema can prevent closure of the linea alba fascia. Attempting to close it in light of this edema can cause onset of abdominal compartment syndrome. This can be encountered when operating for bowel obstruction but can be worsened further when septic complications accompany the obstruction. Even after the obstruction is relieved, the bowel remains edematous from both the obstruction and the resuscitation. Serosal injuries can occur from massive dilation and edema. In this scenario, temporary closure of the abdominal wall with a negative pressure wound therapy system can allow for resolution of the systemic inflammatory response, edema, bowel dilation, and patient stabilization. The patient can then be brought back to the operating room at a later date, undergo assessment, any anastamoses, and definitive abdominal wall closure.

Abdominal compartment syndrome is defined as intraabdominal pressure (IAP) of 20 mm Hg or greater, indirectly measured by urinary bladder pressure, with or without abdominal perfusion pressure less than 50 mm Hg, and with single/multiple organ system failure that was not previously present (25). Abdominal compartment syndrome can be caused by increased intraabdominal volume, retroperitoneal volume, and/or restriction of abdominal wall expansion. As the IAP increases rapidly, physiologic derangement in multiple organ systems occurs. Pulmonary changes are usually the most prominent, with diaphragmatic elevation leading to decreased pulmonary compliance with decreased lung capacity, residual capacity, and volumes. Cardiovascular changes include decreased filling secondary to venous compression, decreased ventricular end-diastolic volumes, increased afterload, decreased contractility, and loss of cardiac output. Prerenal azotemia unresponsive to volume is characteristic, with oliguria leading to anuria due to decreased renal perfusion from low cardiac output, decreased glomerular filtration rate, and increased retention of sodium and water with renin production. Compression of the splanchnic vasculature leads to ischemia and translocation of bacteria. Hepatic insufficiency can also result. Intracranial pressure increases with decreased cerebral perfusion and decreased venous outflow (26).

Patients with high IAP and suspected abdominal compartment syndrome require a decompressive laparotomy. If when attempting to close the abdominal wall there is a sudden elevation in peak airway pressures, abdominal compartment syndrome should be suspected and definitive abdominal wall closure delayed. The objectives of temporary closure with a negative pressure wound therapy system are containment of the abdominopelvic viscera, control of peritoneal secretions, maintenance of tamponade, and facilitation of future abdominal wall closure (27).

Different negative pressure wound therapy systems can be employed. The surgeon can use a polyethylene sheet, which is perforated multiple times and placed over the abdominal viscera and underneath the abdominal wall peritoneum. Laparotomy pads are placed on top of the polyethylene sheet, and the sponge edges are tucked below the abdominal skin, fascia, and peritoneum. Jackson-Pratt or similar closed suction drains are placed on the towels and tunneled beneath the skin to exit away from the wound edge.

The abdominal skin is prepared with a tincture of benzoin and covered with an Ioban drape (3M) (28). The drains are kept to continuous wall suction. An alternative is to use a negative-pressure wound therapy system device such as the V.A.C. (KCI), which may be associated with a higher rate of primary delayed fascial closure (29) (Figures 6.4 and 6.5).

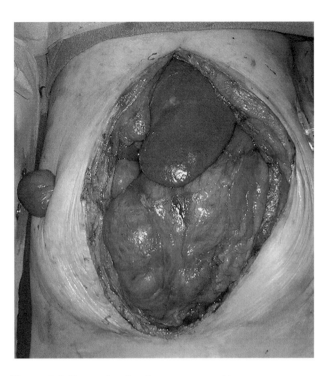

Figure 6.4 Example of a damage control laparotomy before placement of temporary closure device.

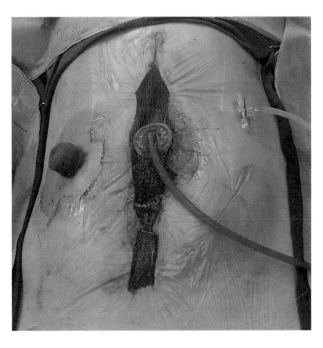

Figure 6.5 Example of a damage control laparotomy after placement of temporary closure device, with application of the V.A.C. (KCI) system. (Courtesy of Richard Fortunato, DO, Pittsburgh, PA.)

Patients should be brought back to the operating room for reassessment and possible abdominal closure within 72 hours (30). Careful planning, technique, and patient selection should minimize the colorectal surgeon's encounters with damage control situations. However, when confronted with suspect options and a dubious outcome, a DCL can turn an uncontrolled situation into a controlled second-look operation with more desirable options/outcomes.

## ADHESIVE DISEASE

Abdominal and pelvic adhesions resulting from prior abdominal surgeries or infections continue to be a source of frustration for patients and surgeons. Adhesions can make an operation challenging by preventing safe entry into the abdomen, requiring conversion to a formal laparotomy, and increasing the risk of hemorrhage and perforation (31). Particularly worrisome for adhesions are those patients with a history of multiple prior abdominal surgeries, bowel perforation, enterocutaneous fistulas, or intraperitoneal mesh.

An initial surgical objective is to safely enter the peritoneal cavity without causing bowel or vascular injury. This can be challenging in patients who have had previous abdominopelvic surgery. Sometimes, adhesions encountered during surgery are much less than initially anticipated, and other times, they are much worse. Multiple scoring systems for adhesions have been proposed. Adhesions can be categorized as shown in Table 6.1.

Patients who harbor significant adhesive disease are probably not candidates for laparoscopic or robotic surgery. In these patients, one strategy may be to look inside the peritoneal cavity with a laparoscope and assess the adhesions. The decision whether to proceed with a laparoscopic/robotic procedure or convert to an open procedure can then be made. A limited number of laparoscopic instruments can be initially opened to reduce costs until a final decision is made on the approach.

Placement of the initial camera port is considered critical in laparoscopic/robotic surgery, as it can be associated with gas embolism or injuries to bowel, bladder, or major vessels. Different options exist for abdominal entry during minimally invasive surgery. One approach is the open Hasson technique, where the rectus sheath and peritoneum are incised under direct visualization. The surgeon can then visualize and palpate for any bowel adhesions before placing the Hasson camera port. The abdomen is then insufflated with $CO_2$ gas. Another option is the closed Veress technique, where a Veress needle is inserted into the peritoneal cavity while lifting the abdominal wall for countertraction (32). The peritoneal cavity is then insufflated with $CO_2$ gas, and an optical viewing trochar, such as a Visiport (Covidien) or Endopath Optiview (Ethicon), is then placed under direct visualization. Alternatively, an optical viewing trochar can be placed initially without first insufflating the abdomen with a Veress needle. Ideally, the abdomen is entered in virgin territory away from any adhesions, which is particularly important in the two latter techniques described. One common location is in the left upper quadrant, also known as Palmer's point (33). Some advocate using a "peek-port" in patients who are high risk for conversion to an open procedure. A 7 cm incision is made and the abdomen is assessed. If the intraperitoneal conditions are favorable, the procedure is done using hand-assisted laparoscopic surgery (HALS). If not, the incision is converted to a formal laparotomy (34).

During an open procedure, one should attempt to enter the abdomen away from surgical scars. Upward retraction of the linea alba fascia can be done using Kocher clamps. The linea alba fascia is then incised slowly and sharply with a scalpel. Exposure and visualization are important to avoid injury and can be achieved by good positioning of the operating room surgical lights, frequent suctioning, dabbing with a laparotomy sponge, and use of appropriate handheld retractors. Different techniques for adhesiolysis exist. Most surgeons will lyse adhesions sharply with a scalpel or scissors. Thick adhesions close to bowel can be doubly clamped, divided sharply, and tied off with sutures. Judicious use of electrocautery and other energy devices is undertaken to minimize thermal spread and potential damage to adjacent bowel. Sharp scalpel dissection is especially useful when very dense adhesions of the bowel to the abdominal wall exist. Sometimes a distinct plane does not exist, and small pieces of peritoneum need to be excised sharply. More difficult or dense adhesions can be approached from different angles to help define the appropriate plane. Simpler adhesions can often be divided on either side or even behind the dense adhesion to help delineate the proper path of dissection. Placing one's fingers on either side of the adhesion and palpating can help stretch the adhesion to allow for easier division. The surgeon must use traction and countertraction to help expose adhesions and planes. One must be cautious about the amount of traction, as too much can lead to tears in the serosa and bleeding.

If an enterotomy occurs, it should be repaired immediately with absorbable sutures to minimize contamination. Serosal tears should also be repaired immediately to prevent enlargement. If the case is difficult and additional serosal tears or enterotomies are predicted, temporary closure and tagging the bowel with long cut sutures can be done. Once adhesiolysis is completed, the surgeon can run the bowel, easily identify the injured portion, and reexamine it.

Table 6.1 Grading system for bowel adhesions

| Grade | Description |
|---|---|
| 1 | Thin filmy adhesions |
| 2 | Adhesions that can be divided by blunt dissection |
| 3 | Dense adhesions that require sharp division |
| 4 | Dense adhesions, the division of which results in bowel injury |

*Source:* Adapted from Fazio VW. Personal communication, 1998.

A segment of bowel with extensive injuries may need to be resected and undergo primary anastomosis. When a loop of small bowel is firmly adherent to a vital structure such as a ureter or iliac vessel, an enterotomy can be intentionally created to separate the structures. The enterotomy can then be primarily closed, leaving a small piece of bowel wall adhered to the vital structure avoiding morbid injury. Mucosa left behind should be desiccated with electrocautery to prevent mucocele formation or malignant transformation.

The surgeon should always consider methods to minimize and prevent adhesion formation. This minimizes the risk of future bowel obstruction and makes future abdominal operations easier and safer. Adhesion formation is a local response of the peritoneum and abdominopelvic viscera to ischemia, desiccation, or trauma. They may form as a result of the primary disease process or due to contact with surgical instruments, staples, sutures, gloves, sponges, or other irritants. Several studies suggest that laparoscopic surgery leads to less adhesion formation than open surgery, by limiting bowel manipulation, lowering bleeding, and limiting exposure to irritants (35–38). Further support is found in laparoscopic-assisted ileocolic resection being associated with a reduced rate of bowel obstruction compared to open surgery (39,40). Adhesions to the anterior abdominal wall are minimal or absent (41) (Figures 6.6 and 6.7). We know that laparoscopic surgery does lead to adhesion formation, but to a lesser degree than open surgery.

Despite laparoscopic surgery advantages, bowel obstructions continue to occur frequently but in a different magnitude. In a report for the French Association for Surgical Research, Duron and colleagues noted that only 33% of postoperative bowel obstructions following various laparoscopic surgeries were due to multiple adhesions, while 17% were due to a single band (42). Intestinal incarceration in an abdominal wall defect or port site (Figures 6.8 and 6.9) was responsible for another 46%.

A report from the Western Pennsylvania Hospital describes unique mechanisms of bowel obstruction, such as an internal hernia, that are commonly associated with laparoscopic bariatric surgery (43). This is presumably due to decreased scar formation between the newly apposed peritoneal surfaces, which leaves defects open (44). A similar phenomenon may occur following laparoscopic colon resection. Obstructions from internal hernias are associated with a high incidence of bowel ischemia. High suspicion must be maintained and prompt surgical intervention undertaken. Fortunately, many of these can be identified and managed laparoscopically.

General principles to minimize adhesion formation include handling tissue gently, ensuring adequate hemostasis, minimizing bowel handling, avoiding desiccation, minimizing irritants, and avoiding infection and ischemia. Several studies have shown that routine closure of the peritoneum as a separate layer during open surgery, including via midline laparotomy and Pfannenstiel incisions, did not decrease the incidence of subsequent adhesions (45,46). Placing omentum over the bowel in the midline before

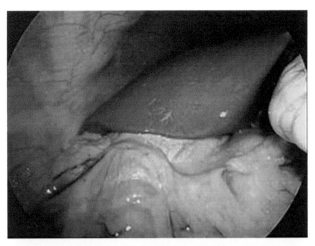

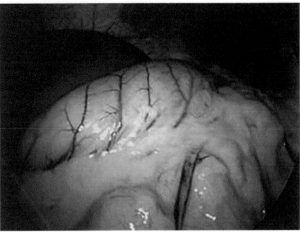

Figure 6.6 Laparoscopic images demonstrating lack of adhesions in a patient undergoing laparoscopic appendectomy for appendicitis 2 years after hand-assisted laparoscopic anterior resection sigmoid diverticulitis. (Courtesy of Thomas E. Read, MD, Pittsburgh, PA.)

closing the fascia is useful to avoid adhesions of bowel up to the abdominal wall. This maneuver may make subsequent reentry into the abdomen easier.

Adhesion barriers can be used to reduce the incidence of adhesions (47). The most well-known and studied is Seprafilm (Genzyme), a bioabsorbable membrane of sodium hyaluronate and carboxymethylcellulose (48–50). It significantly decreases the incidence and severity of adhesion formation after abdominal and pelvic surgery (52). These products should not be placed adjacent to the suture or staple line of newly created anastomoses as they may hinder the bowel's healing (51).

Special attention must be given to adhesions encountered in patients with an abdominal or pelvic malignancy. If the adhesions are between a malignant tumor and another structure, they should be treated as an extension of the malignancy and resected en bloc with the specimen. This may require partial resection of the abdominal wall or a loop of bowel. Not all adhesions encountered during cancer operations are malignant. Attention should be paid to the

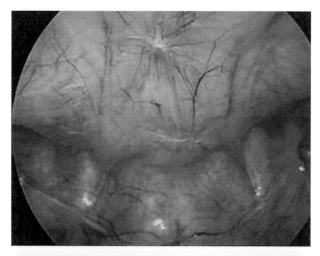

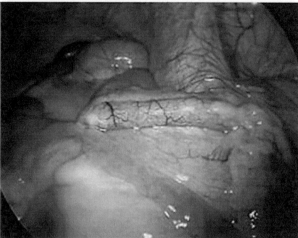

Figure 6.7 Laparoscopic images demonstrating lack of adhesions in a patient undergoing laparoscopic appendectomy for appendicitis 2 years after hand-assisted laparoscopic anterior resection for recurrent sigmoid diverticulitis. (Courtesy of Thomas E. Read, MD, Pittsburgh, PA.)

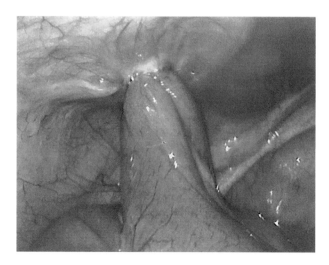

Figure 6.8 A port site hernia causing a bowel obstruction and injury to the bowel.

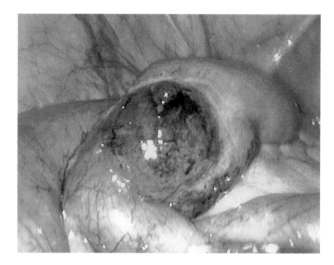

Figure 6.9 A port site hernia causing a bowel obstruction and injury to the bowel.

tumor extent, such as tumor growth through the full thickness of the bowel.

## INTRAOPERATIVE LESION IDENTIFICATION

Up to 22% of endoscopically unresectable colorectal tumors with benign histology on initial biopsy harbor invasive cancer. Adhering to oncological principles for these neoplasms is advised (52). Many of them will not be easily palpable during open surgery and may be even more difficult to find laparoscopically. For operative planning, accurate preoperative localization of the tumor is imperative to ensure removal of the tumor-containing bowel segment (53). Preoperative estimation of tumor location via colonoscopy alone is poor, unless the tumor is clearly noted to be in direct proximity to an unmistakable landmark such as the ileocecal valve or rectum (54,55).

Different methods to aid in the intraoperative localization of a colon or rectal polyp/mass have been proposed. The most commonly used technique, and now considered the gold standard, is preoperative endoscopic tattooing (56). The most commonly used dyes include India ink and SPOT (GI Supply), both of which are durable and long lasting. India ink needs to be diluted and sterilized before injecting. SPOT is available in a prepackaged sterile dilute suspension. Other dyes, such as methylene blue, indigo carmine, and indocyanine green, can be used, but these usually disappear within days. Endoscopic injection of India ink or SPOT in three or four quadrants of bowel adjacent to and distal to, but not through the tumor, is safe and reliable, and preferred in most centers (57,58) (Figure 6.10).

Another method used is preoperative colonoscopy with mucosal endoclip placement followed by an abdominal plain film (Figure 6.11). Preoperative endoclip placement can also be combined with intraoperative fluoroscopy or

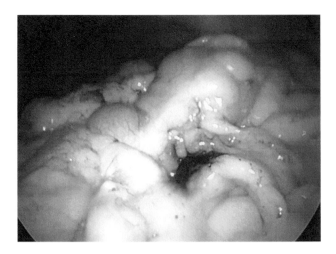

Figure 6.10 India ink injected endoscopically before laparoscopy provides excellent lesion localization.

intraoperative ultrasound (59). These techniques can be inaccurate due to clip migration or dislodgement. They also result in exposure to radiation and are user dependent and resource intensive. Additional methods include preoperative barium enema and computed tomography colonography.

With increasing use of robotics in colorectal surgery, many surgeons are using the da Vinci Firefly high-definition vision system to assess blood perfusion to the bowel when creating the anastomosis (60,61). This requires IV injection of indocyanine green (ICG) followed by switching to Firefly mode to assess perfusion. ICG can also potentially assist in real-time localization of colon and rectal lesions during robotic cases. ICG can be injected into the submucosal plane around the tumor at the beginning of the case, in a manner analogous to tattooing with India ink. Later, the da

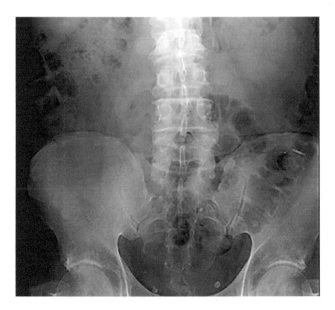

Figure 6.11 A plain film of the abdomen after endoscopic placement of clip (arrow) can provide valuable information about the location of the lesion and aid in preoperative planning.

Vinci Firefly mode can be activated and the area injected should fluoresce.

Due to the flexible nature of the colonoscope, the distance of the tumor from the anal verge cannot be accurately determined on colonoscopy. When the tumor is obviously within the colon or is palpable on digital rectal exam, this is not an issue. Unfortunately, and not uncommonly, a tumor reported by colonoscopy to be in the sigmoid colon is actually in the rectum. Surgeons should remember that a rigid proctoscope is useful to accurately measure the distance of the tumor from the anal verge. Accurate preoperative localization of rectal tumors is essential as it defines the operation to be performed and may influence the need for neoadjuvant therapy prior to surgery (62).

Careful preoperative evaluation and planning is the best way to ensure that the appropriate segment of intestine containing the pathology is resected. The most notable preventable cause is an assumption based on colonoscopic determination of a site that is not within the direct proximity to an unmistakable landmark such as the cecum or rectum. Occasionally, despite best efforts, localization attempts fail to identify lesions intraoperatively in up to 12% of cases (63). Failure to visualize a tattoo can result from its disappearance, especially when products other than SPOT or India ink are used. Additionally, failure to inject the product into the submucosal plane can result in dissemination of the ink, intraperitoneal injection, and imprecise localization. Techniques for proper injection have been described, including inserting the injection needle tangentially in the submucosa and injecting saline to develop the submucosal plane before ink injection (64,65).

The surgeon must be prepared to deal with the case where localization efforts have failed. Blind resection is not recommended unless the surgeon is absolutely confident of the lesion location from preoperative imaging. Mobilization of the flexures and dissection of the omentum off the transverse colon may reveal a hidden tattoo. During laparoscopy, placement of a hand port to allow palpation of the bowel wall can be used to try and palpate the mass. Even then, the lesion may be too small to palpate. Under such circumstances, intraoperative colonoscopy can allow for lesion localization (66). Intraoperative colonoscopy using $CO_2$ insufflation will minimize bowel distention, as $CO_2$ is absorbed at a much faster rate than room air. A serosal clip or suture can be placed laparoscopically at the localized site once it is found with intraoperative colonoscopy. Regardless of the localization technique, opening the resected specimen by the pathologist, or on a back table during the operation, is recommended to confirm that the lesion has been appropriately resected.

## TROUBLE WITH STOMA CREATION

Surgeons often consider intestinal stomas a minor part of a major operation, but they have a major impact on the patient postoperatively. The patient will have to learn to deal with its physiology, function, appearance, and maintenance. Hence, ideal stoma creation is essential. This involves choosing the correct location, identifying the appropriate segment of bowel to use, and correct construction. The surgical indication, patient's lifestyle, clothing preference, occupation, bowel function, body habitus, and surgical scars all influence the site chosen for stoma creation (67). Ideally, regardless of whether the stoma is temporary or permanent, a stoma should be created so that it will last a lifetime.

In elective cases, it is important to discuss the possibility of stoma creation with the patient and have the patient educated and marked by an enterostomal therapist (Wound, Ostomy, and Continence Nurse [WOCN]). In urgent situations or when an enterostomal therapist is not available, the surgeon must select and mark the stoma site, ideally before surgery. In emergent cases, such as for perforated diverticulitis with sepsis, preoperative marking may not be possible.

The surgeon must understand the "ostomy triangle," which is the area bounded by the anterior superior iliac spine, the pubic tubercle, and the umbilicus. The stoma ideally should be placed through the rectus muscle within the ostomy triangle, slightly below the umbilicus. It should be located 5 cm away from bony prominences, old scars, the belt line, midline incisions, and skin folds to allow proper stoma appliance fitting (67,68). The stoma marking should take place with the patient sitting, standing, and laying supine. In obese patients, preoperatively marking a location superior to the umbilicus will make creation of a stoma and its subsequent care much easier. The abdominal wall in the lower abdomen may be thicker due to a large pannus and obese patients may not be able to see their stoma to care for it. Patients with disabilities should be marked in the position they spend the most time in to facilitate appliance fitting/care.

The bowel brought up for the stoma has to have adequate length to allow it to traverse the abdominal wall and be matured without tension retracting it into the abdomen. It also has to be well perfused without compromise of the mesentery. Stoma creation can be challenging in many types of patients, particularly the obese, inflammatory bowel disease patients with thickened and shortened mesenteries, and those with edematous, dilated bowel.

Steps proposed to facilitate creation of an end colostomy or loop colostomy in a challenging situation include full splenic flexure mobilization, complete division of the lateral peritoneal attachments, ligation of the inferior mesenteric artery proximal to the origin of the left colic artery, high ligation of the inferior mesenteric vein, creating windows in the peritoneum in the medial and lateral aspects of the mesocolon, transection of medial peritoneal attachments at the base of the mesocolon, using an enlarged abdominal opening for the stoma, bringing the stoma through an Alexis wound retractor and then cutting out the retractor, and choosing a stoma location superior to the umbilicus (67–69). The surgeon should also consider if there is less

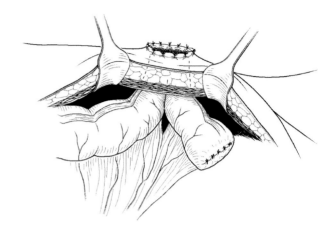

Figure 6.12 The "pseudo-loop" (end loop) colostomy can be employed in rare cases when no other stoma can reach the abdominal skin. (From Cataldo PA. *Clin Colon Rectal Surg* 2008;21:17–22.)

risk to creating a primary anastomosis with a diverting loop ileostomy than to constructing a difficult and poorly placed colostomy. In rare situations, it may be impossible to create a tension-free well-perfused colostomy despite the steps described above. In this case, an end-loop colostomy can be created, where an oversized abdominal wall opening is made and only a portion of the antimesenteric border of the colonic segment is incised and matured to the skin (Figure 6.12).

Similar steps for assisting in the creation of a well-perfused, tension-free loop ileostomy or end ileostomy in a difficult situation have been proposed: supraumbilical placement (especially in obese patients), mobilizing the small bowel mesentery to the base of the duodenum, ligation of ileocolic artery at its origin, creation of an oversized abdominal wall opening, creating windows in the small bowel mesentery overlying the superior mesenteric artery, bringing the stoma through an Alexis wound retractor and then cutting out the wound retractor, and creation of a noneverted ileostomy in an emergency case (69). Rarely, even with the above-mentioned steps, it may be impossible to create a viable ileostomy. An end-loop ileostomy can be used in this situation, created in a fashion similar to that described for an end-loop colostomy.

When creating a temporary stoma, the surgeon should plan strategically for the future and construct the temporary stoma so that it can be closed locally, if possible, without a laparotomy. For example, a patient undergoing a right colectomy for ischemia can have the terminal ileum and the antimesenteric corner of the stapled transverse colon brought out via a single opening on the right abdominal wall. The terminal ileum and the antimesenteric transverse colon corner staple lines are transected and matured. This allows future creation of an ileocolic anastomosis without the need for a formal laparotomy (Figure 6.13).

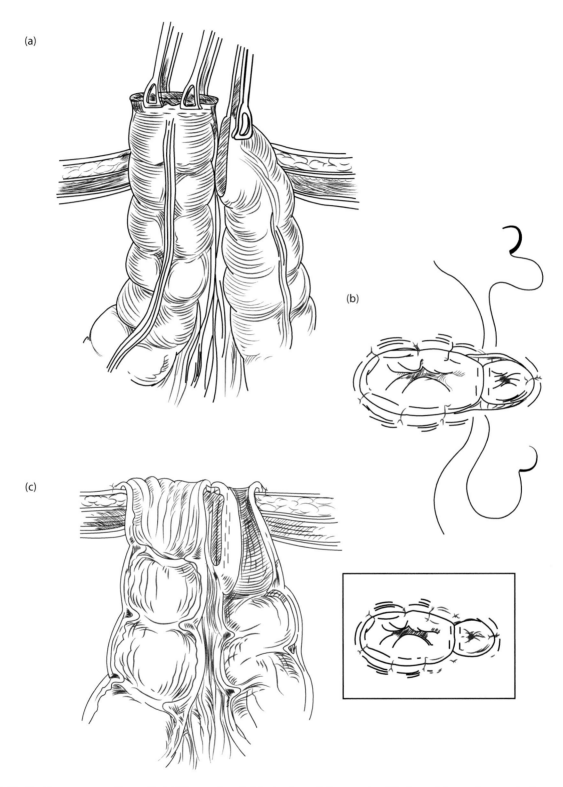

(a)

(b)

(c)

Figure 6.13 End-loop stoma (Prasad). **(a)** The entire divided edge of the proximal limb and the antimesenteric corner of the distal limb are gently drawn through the opening in the abdominal wall. After the abdomen has been closed, the staple line of the proximal limb is excised completely and only the antimesenteric corner of the distal staple line is removed. **(b)** The proximal limb is matured flush with the skin by suturing the deep dermal skin to full-thickness colon with absorbable sutures. Transition sutures may be placed to help mature the mucous fistula, which has the appearance of a "mini-stoma." **(c)** Sagittal view of the completed end-loop colostomy. Note the portion of the distal staple line in the subcutaneous tissue. (From Cataldo PA. *Clin Colon Rectal Surg* 2008;21:17–22.)

## CONCLUSIONS

The colorectal surgeon can be faced with any number of intraoperative challenges. Some of these can be anticipated, while others are only discovered during an operation. Proper preparation, calm reason, and sound surgical principles are the keys to optimizing the outcome.

## REFERENCES

1. Ansell J et al. *Chest* 2004;126(3 Suppl): 204S–33S.
2. Schulman S et al. *Circulation* 2015;132:167–73.
3. Sunkara T et al. *Health Serv Insights* 2016;9:25–36.
4. Ang-Lee MK et al. *JAMA* 2001;286(2):208–16.
5. Kwon AH et al. *Eur J Surg* 2001;167:316–8.
6. Holubar SD et al. *Arch Surg* 2009;144(11):1040–5.
7. Lange DA et al. *J Trauma* 1988;28(3):269–75.
8. Yorkgitis BK. *Am J Med* 2016;130(3):365e1–5.
9. Summary of Recommendations for Adult Immunization. The Advisory Committee on Immunization Practices. Department of Health and Human Services. Centers for Disease Control and Prevention. Available at www.immunize.org/catg.d/p2011.pdf. Accessed on January 7, 2017.
10. Hammerquist RJ et al. *Am J Health Syst Pharm* 2016; 73:e220–8.
11. Oderich GS et al. *J Vasc Surg* 2004;39:931–6.
12. Lou Z et al. *World J Gastroenterolog* 2013;19(25): 4039–44.
13. Filippakis GM et al. *Am Surg* 2007;73(4):410–3.
14. Celentano V et al. *Ann R Coll Surg Engl* 2014;96: 261–5.
15. Harrison JL et al. *Dis Colon Rectum* 2003;46:1115–7.
16. Remzi FH et al. *Dis Colon Rectum* 2002;45:1109–11.
17. Uranues S et al. *Langenbeck's Arch Surg* 2016;401: 909–12.
18. Chatzipapas IK, Magos AL. *Obstet Gynecol* 1997; 90(2):304–6.
19. Cotton BA et al. *Ann Surg* 2011;254(4):598–605.
20. Germanos S et al. *Int J Surg* 2008;6:246–52.
21. Moore EE et al. *World J Surg* 1998;22:1184–91.
22. Loveland JA, Boffard KD. *Br J Surg* 2004;91(9): 1095–101.
23. Voiglio EJ et al. *J Visc Surg* 2016;153:13–24.
24. Offner PJ et al. *Arch Surg* 2001;136:676–81.
25. Sugrue M. *Curr Opin Crit Care* 2005;11:333–8.
26. O'Mara MS et al. *Am Surg* 2003;69(11):975–7.
27. Schreiber MA. *Crit Care Clin* 2004;20:101–18.
28. Barker DE et al. *J Trauma* 2000;48:201–7.
29. Garner GB et al. *Am J Surg* 2001;182:630–8.
30. Abikhaled JA et al. *Am Surg* 1997;63:1109–12.
31. Maciver AH et al. *Int J Surg* 2001;9:589–94.
32. Taye MK et al. *J Clin Diagn Res* 2016;10(2):QC04–7.
33. Vilos GA et al. *J Obstet Gynaecol Can* 2007;29(5): 433–47.
34. Read TE et al. *Surg Endosc* 2009;23:477–81.
35. Gutt CN et al. *Surg Endosc* 2004;18:898–906.
36. Hiki N et al. *Br J Surg* 2006;93(2):195–204.
37. Kalff JC et al. *Ann Surg* 1998;228:652–63.
38. Schwarz NT et al. *Gastroenterology* 2004;126:159–69.
39. Alabaz O et al. *Eur J Surg* 2000;166(3):213–7.
40. Bergamaschi R et al. *Dis Colon Rectum* 2003;46: 1129–33.
41. Hasegawa H et al. *Br J Surg* 2003;90:970–3.
42. Durron JJ et al. *Arch Surg* 2000;135(2):208–12.
43. Papasavas PK et al. *Surg Endosc* 2003;17:610–4.
44. Higa K et al. *Obes Surg* 2003;13:350–4.
45. Kapustian V et al. *Am J Obstet Gynecol* 2012;206: 56.e1–4.
46. Gurusamy KS et al. *Cochrane Database Syst Rev* 2013;7:1–35.
47. Rajab TK et al. *J Surg Res* 2010;161:246–9.
48. Becker JM et al. *J Am Coll Surg* 1996;183:297–306.
49. Diamond MP. *Fertil Steril* 1996;66(6):904–10.
50. Nordic Adhesion Prevention Study Group. *Fertil Steril* 1995;63(4):709–14.
51. Beck DE et al. *Disc Colon Rectum* 2003;46(10): 1310–9.
52. Brozovich M et al. *Surg Endosc* 2008;22(2):506–9.
53. Larach SW et al. *Disc Colon Rectum* 1997;40:592–6.
54. Piscatelli N et al. *Arch Surg* 2005;140(10):932–5.
55. Yeung JM et al. *Colorectal Dis* 2009;11:527–30.
56. Ibrahim-Abdelaziz I et al. *J Clin Trials* 2015;6:227–30.
57. McArthur CS et al. *Surg Endosc* 1999;13(4):397–400.
58. Nizam R et al. *Am J Gastroenterol* 1996;91(9):1804–8.
59. Nagata K et al. *Surg Endosc* 2008;22(2):379–85.
60. Hellan M et al. *Surg Endosc* 2014;28:1695–702.
61. Whealon M et al. *Clin Colon Rectal Surg* 2016;29: 221–31.
62. McCormick JT, Gregorcyk SG. *Surg Oncol Clin N Am* 2006;15(1):39–49.
63. Feingold DL et al. *J Gastrointest Surg* 2004;8(5):543–6.
64. Cho YB et al. *World J Surg* 2007;31:1491–5.
65. Park JW et al. *Surg Endosc* 2008;22(2):501–5.
66. Zmora O et al. *Surg Endosc* 2002;16:808–11.
67. Cataldo PA. *Clin Colon Rectal Surg* 2008;21:17–22.
68. Beck SJ. *Clin Colon Rectal Surg* 2011;24:259–62.
69. Williams RS, Fazio VW. Challenging stomas. In: Fazio, Church, and Wu. (eds) *Atlas of Intestinal Stomas*, 2nd Edition. New York, NY: Springer Science+Business Media, LLC, 2012, pp. 273–84.

# 7

# Optimizing use of electronic health records

ALLISON B. McCOY AND GENEVIEVE B. MELTON-MEAUX

## CHALLENGING CASE

A 64-year-old woman presents to your office with a history of a symptomatic colon mass.

## CASE MANAGEMENT

Review of the patient's electronic health records documents a colonoscopy with a partially obstructing mass of the sigmoid colon and the pathology report with a moderately differentiated adenocarcinoma. She has no other significant medical problems. As you initiate an order set for a colonic surgery using an enhanced recovery after surgery pathway, the system identifies the patient's penicillin allergy and alerts you to modify your preoperative antibiotic selection.

## INTRODUCTION

In recent years, the United States has invested billions of dollars and other resources through the Health Information Technology for Economic and Clinical Health (HITECH) act to rapidly increase electronic health record (EHR) adoption nationwide (1). Implementation of EHRs has been reported to improve patient safety and reduce health-care costs by providing better access to information, clinical decision support (CDS), and more reliable communication. These systems require ongoing investment by health-care institutions and by clinician stakeholders, particularly around new protocols and pathways, as well as the addition at the individual or group practice level of personalized templates or other mechanisms to streamline documentation practices. In this chapter, we present an overview of EHRs and their functions. We also describe evidence for the role of EHRs in improved outcomes through implementation and use of these functions with emphasis on colon and rectal surgery examples.

## ELECTRONIC HEALTH RECORDS

The Centers for Medicare and Medicaid Services (CMS) define an EHR as "an electronic version of a patient's medical history, that is maintained by the provider over time, and may include all of the key administrative clinical data relevant to that persons care under a particular provider, including demographics, progress notes, problems, medications, vital signs, past medical history, immunizations, laboratory data and radiology reports" (2). Computer-based hospital information systems first began to appear in the late 1960s, largely as text-based systems intended to facilitate billing and reimbursement. In 1969, Lawrence Weed introduced the problem-oriented medical record, suggesting that medical records should be organized primarily by the medical problem, and that diagnostic and therapeutic plans should be linked to these problems (3). Over the next several decades, information systems implemented in clinical settings evolved to capture clinical information and improve patient outcomes through better information management and CDS. Since that time, EHRs have continued to evolve and become increasingly vital to modern patient care.

Contemporary EHRs can be classified as having basic or comprehensive electronic functions (Table 7.1). Basic EHRs include electronic clinical information; computerized provider order entry (CPOE) for medications; and viewing of lab reports, radiology reports, and diagnostic test results. In addition to these, electronic functions required for comprehensive EHRs include advance directives; CPOE for lab reports, radiology tests, consultation requests, and nursing orders; and viewing of radiology images, diagnostic test images, and consultant reports. As a result of the HITECH act, including incentive programs such as the meaningful use program, implementation of both basic and comprehensive EHRs has increased in recent years. In 2015, 96% of U.S. nonfederal acute care hospitals reported possession of EHR technology, 83.8% reported implementation of a basic EHR, and 40% reported implementation of a comprehensive EHR (4). Another common framework is the HIMSS Analytics Electronic Medical Record Adoption Model (EMRAM),

Table 7.1 Electronic functions required for hospital adoption of basic or comprehensive Electronic Health Records (EHRs)

| | Basic EHR | Comprehensive EHR |
|---|---|---|
| **Electronic clinical information** | | |
| Patient demographics | ✓ | ✓ |
| Physician notes | ✓ | ✓ |
| Nursing assessments | ✓ | ✓ |
| Problem lists | ✓ | ✓ |
| Medication lists | ✓ | ✓ |
| Discharge summaries | ✓ | ✓ |
| Advance directives | – | ✓ |
| **Computerized provider order entry** | | |
| Lab reports | – | ✓ |
| Radiology tests | – | ✓ |
| Medications | ✓ | ✓ |
| Consultation requests | – | ✓ |
| Nursing orders | – | ✓ |
| **Results management** | | |
| View lab reports | ✓ | ✓ |
| View radiology reports | ✓ | ✓ |
| View radiology images | – | ✓ |
| View diagnostic test results | ✓ | ✓ |
| View diagnostic test images | – | ✓ |
| View consultant report | – | ✓ |
| **Decision support** | | |
| Clinical guidelines | – | ✓ |
| Clinical reminders | – | ✓ |
| Drug allergy results | – | ✓ |
| Drug-drug interactions | – | ✓ |
| Drug-lab interactions | – | ✓ |
| Drug dosing support | – | ✓ |

Table 7.2 HIMSS analytics Electronic Medical Record Adoption Model (EMRAM)

| Stage | EMRAM cumulative capabilities |
|---|---|
| 7 | Complete electronic medical record, data analytics to improve care |
| 6 | Physician documentation (templates), full clinical decision support (CDSS), closed-loop medication administration |
| 5 | Full picture archiving and communication system (R-PACS) |
| 4 | Computerized provider order entry; clinical decision support (clinical protocols) |
| 3 | Clinical documentation, CDSS (error checking) |
| 2 | Clinical data repository (CDR), controlled medical vocabulary, clinical decision support (CDS), health information exchange (HIE) capable |
| 1 | All three ancillaries installed—Lab, rad, pharmacy |

Table 7.3 Top commercially available Electronic Health Record (EHR) vendors used for meaningful use attestations

| EHR vendor | Meaningful use attestations |
|---|---|
| Epic Systems Corporation | 166,215 |
| Cerner Corporation | 124,471 |
| Allscripts | 32,153 |
| athenahealth, Inc. | 21,068 |
| eClinicalWorks, LLC | 16,818 |
| GE Healthcare | 15,440 |
| NextGen Healthcare | 15,179 |
| Greenway Health, LLC | 8,469 |
| Medical Information Technology, Inc. (MEDITECH) | 5,344 |

which classifies EHRs using a similar paradigm around functionality and capabilities available within their EHR and other integrated health information systems and implemented by the particular organization (Table 7.2) (5).

Early adopters of EHRs were primarily large, academic, teaching facilities with locally developed, noncommercial systems. A systematic review of health information technology (HIT) and associated reported research in 2006 found that 24% of included studies came from four benchmark research institutions with locally developed EHRs (6): the Regenstrief Institute (Regenstrief Medical Record System) (7), Brigham and Women's Hospital/Partners Health Care (Brigham Integrated Computer System/Longitudinal Medical Record) (8), the Department of Veterans Affairs (Veterans Health Information Systems and Technology Architecture [VISTA]) (9), and LDS Hospital/Intermountain Health Care (Health Evolution through Logical Programming [HELP]) (10). More recently, the adoption and maturity of commercially available

EHRs have increased, in part due to the extensive efforts required by internal informatics personnel to meet criteria for the incentive programs introduced with the HITECH act. In fact, all of the four benchmark institutions previously identified are fully transitioned or in the process of transitioning to a commercially available EHR. While hundreds of commercially available EHR products have been developed, only nine vendors represent 40% of all attestations by providers who had met requirements for meaningful use incentives in 2016 (Table 7.3) (11).

## EVIDENCE FOR ELECTRONIC HEALTH RECORD USE

Since the advent of EHRs, extensive research has been conducted to evaluate their impact and potential value on improving outcomes such as health-care processes and quality, patient morbidity and mortality, patient and provider satisfaction, and costs. Much of the earliest research on EHRs included capabilities for identifying medication errors, which occurs in 4%–6% of orders using traditional manual checks, thus supporting the value of these systems for prevention of medication errors particularly through CPOE and CDS functionality. For example, one study demonstrated that this functionality was associated with a reduction of medication errors by 81% (12–18). Following these initial reports, most of the evidence for improved outcomes with EHRs has focused on health-care process and quality measures. CDS, in particular, through the alerts and reminders, has been effective at increasing preventive care and health maintenance compliance and publicly reported performance, clinical study ordering, and therapy prescribing (19,20).

Despite the great promise of improved safety through EHR use, evidence surrounding the effects on patient outcomes, including length of stay, morbidity, mortality, quality of life, and adverse events, remains mixed. Many institutions have reported positive effects, but many of these studies have been limited by weak study designs, small sample sizes, lack of significant findings, and limited generalizability due to study setting and subtle or significant differences in EHR configuration, making generalizability questionable (19,20). Recent reports have called for improved assessment and increased mechanisms to provide for scalability and external validity of EHR implementations to better understand and ultimately optimize EHR implementations to ensure improved outcomes (21).

Despite the large costs for implementation and maintenance of EHRs, some evidence also exists to support a positive return on investment for EHRs, in particular with implementation of CDS functionality to prevent costly adverse drug events. One study found high costs involved with implementing CPOE but greater projected financial benefit with a $28.5 million savings over 10 years, and CDS resulted in the greatest cumulative savings (22). A related study evaluated the return on investment of vendor CPOE systems implemented in four community hospitals and found modest returns, primarily due to lack of CDS (23). A study of EHRs in the ambulatory setting also found a positive return on investment beyond reduced adverse drug events, including savings in personnel and other indirect costs (24).

## CHALLENGES WITH ELECTRONIC HEALTH RECORD USE

Although many have found a return on investment with EHR implementations, high initial costs of implementing EHRs and ongoing high year over year maintenance are frequently reported as barriers to adoption by many health-care organizations (25–27). Costs of EHR implementation vary but generally include hardware, software, implementation assistance, training, and ongoing network fees and maintenance (28). With significant ongoing and increasing regulatory requirements and the need to provide

optimal, efficient, and safe care, health-care organizations are increasingly recognizing the key role of EHRs as a catalyst and lever to meet these goals. A 2011 study reported the cost of implementing EHRs to be $32,409 per provider through the first 60 days, in addition to $25,000 for one-time hardware costs, $7,000 per provider for individual hardware components, and $17,000 per provider annually for software and maintenance costs (29). Another report estimated the costs of implementation based on regional extension center experiences at $33,000 up front and $4,000 annually per provider for in-office EHRs and $26,000 up front and $8,000 annually per provider for software as a service (i.e., Web-based) EHRs (28).

Another frequently reported challenge with EHR use is poor fit with existing workflows (25–27). Specific workflow issues that have been identified include altered pace, sequencing, and dynamics of clinical activities; failure to support all required activities for all clinical personnel particularly for specialty care; reduced clinical situation awareness; and poor reflection of organizational policies and procedures (30). Further efforts by EHR vendors and researchers as well as information technology functions within health-care organizations are necessary to ensure that EHRs meet the needs of providers and other members of the care team, ultimately to facilitate and improve patient care without causing additional burdens.

Beyond this, another important challenge with EHRs is that in some cases they have facilitated errors and inefficiencies through unintended consequences, including more/new work, workflow issues, increasing or different system demands, altered communication, introduction of new kinds of errors, systems causing power shifts, and user dependence on the system (31). A large survey found widespread occurrence of these unintended consequences and highlighted the need for detection and management of these consequences to mitigate resulting errors. More recent efforts have continued to identify potential safety concerns or hazards with EHR implementations and called for new and improved approaches to identifying and reducing these safety issues (21,32,33).

In part due to the previously described challenges to implementation and use, provider satisfaction with EHRs, especially after initial implementation, is low (34,35). While it appears most providers would not want to return to the paper record, the burden of use of EHRs is cited as one of the greatest sources of provider burn-out and dissatisfaction (36). Because health-care providers and other clinicians such as nurses and other interdisciplinary staff are primary users of EHRs, their perceptions of EHRs are key for ensuring the successful and optimal integration of EHRs effectively into clinical practice (37). In one study, after implementing an EHR, clinicians' perceptions of productivity, patient care, clinical decision quality, easy access to patient information, time for patients, computer access, adequate resources, and ease of use decreased significantly (34). These findings support the hypothesis that improving implementations and optimizations of EHRs to meet the needs of providers and reduce errors may increase satisfaction and, ultimately, further increase health-care quality and safety overall. The medicolegal implications of EHRs are discussed in Chapter 15.

## ELECTRONIC HEALTH RECORD USE IN COLON AND RECTAL SURGERY

There are a number of examples of use of EHRs in surgical settings and colon and rectal surgery in particular, including CDS applications (38). A systematic review by Robertson and colleagues systematically describes the use of EHRs for surgical care broadly including a number of colon and rectal surgery examples (39). In the area of medication dosing support, EHRs have been demonstrated to be highly effective in both improving patient safety and reducing associated costs, including important examples like compliance with the Surgical Care Improvement Project for process metrics related to colon and rectal surgery care, including prophylactic antibiotic dosing and early Foley catheter removal (40–43). For busy surgeons, order facilitators including protocoled templates and preference lists can reduce the amount of time spent entering orders and leave more time for providing patient care. Order sets, collections of orders that are grouped by a specific clinical purpose, are frequently used in the inpatient to ensure adherence to guidelines or protocols (44). In surgical settings, order sets include those for admission to the colon and rectal surgery service or for postoperative care of patients (44,45).

Another prominent example where EHRs around order facilitators like order sets are mechanisms around colon and rectal surgery enhanced recovery after surgery (ERAS) programs. ERAS programs that include protocolized care like perioperative deep venous prophylaxis, early resumption of diet, and fluid restriction can be significantly aided and improved with standard EHR content and functionality and result in decreased length of stay, lower costs, and other improved outcomes (46). In addition, EHRs enable analysis, reporting, and registry implementation—often required by national flagship ERAS initiatives such as the American College of Surgeons and Agency for Healthcare Research and Quality Program for Improving Surgical Care and Recovery (ISCR), which is currently focused primarily on colon and rectal surgery procedures (47,48).

Point-of-care alerts and reminders prompt clinicians about drug-condition, drug-drug, and drug-allergy interactions; remind clinicians to assess specific care items; and notify clinicians about critical lab values or high-risk states. These reminders can be passive alerts that display additional text, change existing text colors, or show images, without interrupting the workflow, and can also be interruptive alerts, which require that providers acknowledge or respond to the alert before resuming order entry (49,50). Most examples of CDS usage in the literature for surgical patients are related to antibiotic dosing and timing (39). For colon and rectal diseases, alerts often prompt primary care providers to order or remind patients about cancer screening tests or to follow up with patients after abnormal screening test results (51–53).

EHR features around documentation, particularly operative notes, have also been described (39,54–58). This approach for increased structured information and templated documentation with key elements based off of evidence-based care are termed "synoptic reports." This documentation approach has been used extensively in pathology, as well as to some extent in radiology, and is considered best practice. Overall, studies around operative notes to date have been of marginal quality and have not been directly described with colon and rectal surgery procedures specifically. However, it does appear that EHR capabilities and focused initiatives around templated or synoptic operative reports can be effective for improving the inclusion of critical information including closure details, type of anesthesia, use of antibiotics, and type of dissection or approach.

Information display ensures that clinicians have up-to-date and necessary patient data to make decisions in providing care to the patients, such as showing recent laboratory test values during medication ordering. While specific examples for colon and rectal surgery have not been extensively described in the literature, knowledge about lab trends or cost of care is an important consideration for clinicians across all care settings.

Expert systems apply advanced logic or computational methods to assist clinicians in ordering, diagnosing, treating, and interpreting elements with the EHR. One example specific to colon and rectal surgery includes a study that applied statistical methods to predict outcomes for patients with diverticulitis (59). Another study evaluated a treatment planning system that suggests volume resuscitation and medication therapy, such as use of antibiotics and vasopressors, for surgical patients identified as having sepsis, and found that use of the CDS improved mortality in the observed patients (60).

Workflow support includes order routing, registry functions, medication reconciliation, automatic order termination, order approvals, free-text order parsing, and documentation aids. Registry functions are especially important for colon and rectal surgery, where appropriate patient follow-up is imperative for providing optimal care. For example, several studies have described reminders sent to patients, through mailed letters or telephone calls, to remind patients about completion of fecal occult blood tests (61–63).

## SUMMARY

Adoption of EHRs continues with significant impact on the practice of medicine including colon and rectal surgery. From most perspectives, it appears that this trend will continue, and as these technologies mature and organizations learn and implement best practices, their potential benefits and value will hopefully be increasingly realized, including improved outcomes. Utilization of these technologies has produced improvements in patient care but at a cost as described in this chapter. Several opportunities exist for EHRs to improve outcomes in colon and rectal surgery including best practices like ERAS.

## REFERENCES

1. Blumenthal D. *N Engl J Med.* 2010;362(5):382–5.
2. https://www.cms.gov/Medicare/E-Health/EHealth Records/index.html. Accessed July 23, 2018.
3. Weed LL. *N Engl J Med.* 1968;278(12):652–7.
4. Henry J et al. *Adoption of Electronic Health Record Systems among US Non-Federal Acute Care Hospitals: 2008–2015.* Washington, DC: Office of the National Coordinator for Health Information Technology, 2016. Report No.: 35.
5. *HIMSS Analytics.* 2017 [cited December 28, 2017]. Available from: http://www.himssanalytics.org/emram
6. Chaudhry B et al. *Ann Intern Med.* 2006;144(10):742.
7. McDonald CJ et al. *Int J Med Inf.* 1999;54(3):225–53.
8. Teich JM et al. *Int J Med Inf.* 1999;54(3):197–208.
9. Brown SH et al. *Int J Med Inf.* 2003;69(2):135–56.
10. Gardner RM et al. *Int J Med Inf.* 1999;54(3):169–82.
11. https://www.healthdata.gov/dataset/cms-medicare-and-medicaid-ehr-incentive-program-electronic-health-record-products-used. Accessed July 23, 2018.
12. Bates DW et al. *JAMA J Am Med Assoc.* 1995;274(1):29–34.
13. Lesar TS et al. *JAMA J Am Med Assoc.* 1997;277(4):312–7.
14. Bobb A et al. *Arch Intern Med.* 2004;164(7):785–92.
15. Reckmann MH et al. *J Am Med Inform Assoc JAMIA.* 2009;16(5):613–23.
16. Ammenwerth E et al. *J Am Med Inform Assoc.* 2008;15(5):585–600.
17. van Rosse F et al. *Pediatrics.* 2009;123(4):1184–90.
18. Bates DW et al. *J Am Med Inform Assoc JAMIA.* 1999;6(4):313–21.
19. Bright TJ et al. *Ann Intern Med.* 2012;157(1):29–43.
20. Jones SS et al. *Ann Intern Med.* 2014;160(1):48–54.
21. Committee on Patient Safety and Health Information Technology, Institute of Medicine. *Health IT and Patient Safety: Building Safer Systems for Better Care.* Washington, DC: The National Academies Press, 2012.
22. Kaushal R et al. *J Am Med Inform Assoc JAMIA.* 2006;13(3):261–6.
23. Zimlichman E et al. *Jt Comm J Qual Patient Saf.* 2013;39(7):312–8.
24. Grieger DL et al. *J Am Coll Surg.* 2007;205(1):89–96.
25. Poon EG et al. *Health Aff Proj Hope.* 2004;23(4):184–90.
26. DesRoches CM et al. *N Engl J Med.* 2008;359(1):50–60.
27. Linder JA et al. *AMIA Annu Symp Proc.* 2006;2006:499–503.
28. https://www.healthit.gov/providers-professionals/faqs/how-much-going-cost-me. Accessed July 23, 2018.
29. Fleming NS et al. *Health Aff (Millwood).* 2011;30(3):481–9.
30. Campbell EM et al. *J Gen Intern Med.* 2009;24(1):21–6.
31. Ash JS et al. *J Am Med Inform Assoc JAMIA.* 2007;14(4):415–23.
32. Singh H, Sittig DF. *BMJ Qual Saf.* 2016;25(4):226–32.
33. Sittig DF, Singh H. *Qual Saf Health Care* 2010;19(Suppl 3):i68–74.
34. Krousel-Wood M et al. *J Am Med Inform Assoc.* 2018 Jun 1;25(6):618–26.
35. Hanauer DA et al. *J Am Med Inform Assoc.* 2016;ocw077.
36. Friedberg MW et al. *Rand Health Q.* 2014;3(4):1.
37. Zhou L et al. *J Am Med Inform Assoc.* 2009;16(4):457–64.
38. McCoy AB et al. *Clin Colon Rectal Surg.* 2013;26(1):23–30.
39. Robinson JR et al. *J Surg Res.* 2016;203(1):121–39.
40. Jacques P S et al. *Surg Infect.* 2005;6(2):215–21.
41. O'Reilly M et al. *Anesth Analg.* 2006;103(4):908–12.
42. Schwann NM et al. *Anesth Analg.* 2011;113(4):869–76.
43. Thirukumaran CP et al. *Health Serv Res.* 2015;50(1):273–89.
44. Wright A et al. *Int J Med Inf.* 2012;81(11):733–45.
45. Hayman AV et al. *Am J Surg.* 2010;200(5):572–6.
46. Carmichael JC et al. *Dis Colon Rectum.* 2017;60(8):761.
47. Ban KA et al. *J Am Coll Surg.* 2017;225(4):548–557.e3.
48. https://www.ahrq.gov/professionals/quality-patient-safety/hais/tools/enhanced-recovery/index.html. Accessed July 23, 2018.
49. McCoy AB et al. *AMIA Annu Symp Proc,* Washington, DC. 2008, pp. 1051.
50. Lo HG et al. *J Am Med Inform Assoc JAMIA.* 2009;16(1):66–71.
51. McDonald CJ et al. *Ann Intern Med.* 1984;100(1):130–8.
52. McPhee SJ et al. *Arch Intern Med.* 1989;149(8):1866–72.
53. Singh H et al. *Am J Gastroenterol.* 2009;104(4):942–52.
54. Laflamme MR et al. *AMIA Annu Symp Proc,* Washington, DC. 2005, pp. 425–9.
55. Cowan DA et al. *Dermatol Surg Off Publ Am Soc Dermatol Surg Al.* 2007;33(5):588–95.
56. Park J et al. *J Am Coll Surg.* 2010;211(3):308–15.
57. Hoffer DN et al. *Int J Med Inf.* 2012;81(3):182–91.
58. Ghani Y et al. *Int J Surg Lond Engl.* 2014;12(5):30–2.
59. Chapman JR et al. *Ann Surg.* 2006;243(6):876–880. discussion 880–883.
60. Moore LJ et al. *Am J Surg.* 2010;200(6):839–44.
61. Ornstein SM et al. *J Fam Pract.* 1991;32(1):82–90.
62. Goldberg D et al. *Am J Prev Med.* 2004;26(5):431–5.
63. Mosen DM et al. *Med Care.* 2010;48(7):604–10.

# 8

# Postoperative anastomotic complications

TRACI L. HEDRICK

## CHALLENGING CASE

A 63-year-old morbidly obese woman undergoes a left nephrectomy with partial colectomy and primary anastomosis for a renal cell carcinoma involving the left colon through a left flank incision. On postoperative day 3 she develops tachypnea and tachycardia requiring transfer to the intensive care unit. At that time, an abdominal radiograph reveals dilated loops of bowel but no free air. Her white blood cell count is 11, and the rest of her labs are normal. She subsequently develops a fascial dehiscence after a deep cough on postoperative day 4 requiring exploration and closure with retention sutures. On postoperative day 6 she develops fever and worsening respiratory failure necessitating intubation. A computed tomography (CT) scan is performed demonstrating an anastomotic leak with contrast extravasation.

## CASE MANAGEMENT

She is taken to the operating room where a transverse loop colostomy is performed through a separate right upper quadrant incision. A percutaneous drain is placed under CT guidance into the fluid collection within the left paracolic gutter. She subsequently improves and is discharged on postoperative day 14.

## INTRODUCTION/BACKGROUND

Colorectal surgery is associated with significant morbidity owing to a multitude of different factors. The operations are complex, involve multiple quadrants, and are frequently associated with comorbid conditions including prior radiation or immunosuppression. Ultimately, much of the severe morbidity associated with colorectal surgery can be attributed to the construction of an anastomosis. Anastomotic leak (AL) is, in fact, the most common cause of death following colon and rectal surgery (1–3). Traditionally, it was thought that the biggest threat to the integrity of an anastomosis was tension and ischemia. However, modern research has called this into question as data continue to emerge citing the local microbiome as a critical factor in the development of an anastomotic leak (4,5).

Along with esophageal anastomoses, the colorectal anastomosis is among the highest-risk gastrointestinal anastomoses (6). The incidence of anastomotic leak following colorectal surgery ranges from 3% to 7% for colon anastomoses and up to 20% for distal rectal anastomoses (6,7). The incidence has remained stable over time despite the advent of minimally invasive surgery and improved perioperative care (6). The burden of anastomotic complications is far reaching, including effects on mortality, morbidity, costs, patient-reported outcomes, and oncologic outcomes. Development of an AL doubles the cost of index admission compared to those without a leak in patients undergoing gastrointestinal anastomoses ($16,085 versus $30,409, $p < 0.0001$) and prolongs length of stay by up to 7.3 days (6,8). Anastomotic leak (AL) can also have a significant impact on subsequent bowel function due to reduced distensibility and capacity secondary to fibrosis. Following an AL, patients report worse physical and mental scores, emotional stability, social function, and general health (9–12).

The development of an AL is also associated with higher rates of colorectal cancer recurrence and worse disease-free survival (13,14). Two large meta-analyses of 13,655 and 21,902 patients demonstrate significantly higher cancer-specific mortality and local recurrences in patients who suffered an AL (15,16). In addition to the alterations in the local inflammatory milieu, the delay or omission of adjuvant chemotherapy is thought to mediate the deleterious effects on oncologic outcomes (17,18).

# ANASTOMOTIC LEAK

## ETIOLOGIES

Traditionally, it was thought that the biggest threats to the integrity of an anastomosis were tension and ischemia. Vignali et al. demonstrated that local ischemia was associated with AL (19), which can occur through division of mesenteric arcades and stretching or twisting of mesenteric vessels (20–23). However, Shakhsheer et al. (4) randomized rats to undergo sham operation, segmental colon devascularization alone, colectomy alone, or segmental devascularization plus colectomy. The rats were sacrificed on postoperative day 6 and the anastomoses examined. There was no difference in tissue hypoxia noted in the rats with poor healing compared to those with well-healed anastomoses, suggesting that ischemia may not be the most critical factor in the developing anastomotic leak. Tension is intuitively associated with AL given that most distal rectal ALs are posterior, corresponding to the point of greatest mesenteric tension. However, there is very little research to actually demonstrate the deleterious effect of tension in the development of leak. Other important factors such as choosing correct staple height relative to tissue thickness (24), avoiding multiple intersecting staple lines (25), and minimizing the number of linear stapler firings on the distal rectum (26–29) appear to play a greater role in AL. Additionally, data continue to emerge citing the local microbiome as a critical factor in the development of an anastomotic leak (4,5). Matrix metalloproteinases (MMPs) and collagenases are part of the body's normal response to injury. However, these proteins have been implicated as important mediators of anastomotic leak. Animal studies have suggested that certain bacterial strains that produce these collagenolytic proteins (*Enterococcus*, *Pseudomonas*, or *Serratia* species) may contribute to the development of AL (30–32).

With regard to patient-related factors, location of the anastomosis is one of the most important risk factors for AL with distal rectal anastomoses having almost a five times increased risk compared to resection for colon cancer (15). In addition, male gender (33–36), chemoradiation (35,36), hypotension (37,38), diabetes, smoking, and atherosclerosis are known risk factors. Radiation seems to be timing related, with the most significant risk in the first 3 weeks following completion of radiotherapy (39). Malnutrition (defined as 10% or greater unintentional weight loss) is associated with increased postoperative morbidity. It is unclear whether preoperative nutrition support can negate these effects but it may help with surgical planning with regard to the construction of an anastomosis.

## PREVENTATIVE MEASURES

Dating back to trials from the 1970s, mechanical bowel preparation (MBP) combined with oral antibiotics has been shown to reduce surgical site infection (SSI) following elective colorectal surgery, including anastomotic leak (40,41). However, more recent trials and meta-analyses failed to demonstrate improvement in SSI or anastomotic leak with MBP (42,43). Based on these studies, MBP fell out of favor in the last decade (44).

Compared to the initial efficacy trials during the 1970s, the majority of recent trials included an MBP *without* the addition of oral antibiotics. In the absence of oral antibiotics, a mechanical cleansing results in liquid, bacteria-laden stool that is more likely to contaminate the operative field (45). In a 2009 Cochrane Review, Nelson et al. (46) concluded that oral antibiotics combined with a mechanical cleansing reduced the rate of SSI. In addition, data from large risk-adjusted national database studies including the National Surgical Quality Improvement Program and the Michigan Surgical Quality Collaborative-Colectomy Best Practices Project demonstrate significant reduction in infectious morbidity, including anastomotic leak, with the use of an MBP *when combined* with oral antibiotics (47–50).

Proximal diversion reduces the septic complications and the need for surgical intervention following anastomotic leak. However, it has also been shown to reduce the rate of AL. Meta-analyses show decreased rate of AL and need for reoperation with creation of a protective diverting stoma at the index operation (3,51,52).

Intraoperative inspection of the rectal anastomosis has evolved over time with the advent of modern technology. The basic air leak test with submersion of the anastomosis under fluid as air is insufflated transanally has been shown to reduce anastomotic leak rates (53). Whether the addition of endoscopy to visually inspect the anastomosis during the air leak test improves outcomes has not yet been formally studied. The use of fluorescence angiography has recently been postulated as a predictor of anastomotic vascularity that could theoretically reduce the risk of anastomotic leak. Several studies have suggested that it does affect surgical decision-making, but as of yet, none has demonstrated differences in AL rates (54,55). There is currently a multicenter prospective randomized controlled trial underway assessing the role of indocyanine green angiography in rectal resections for cancer (PILLAR III) (http://www.clinicaltrials.gov: NCT02205307).

## DIAGNOSIS/CLINICAL PRESENTATION

The classic presentation of an AL includes abdominal pain, fever, tachycardia, and a leukocytosis in the setting of peritonitis. However, AL can present along a continuum from low volume wound drainage to multisystem organ failure. Leaks present at varying time periods according to etiology and severity. Minor leaks generally take longer to recognize than major anastomotic dehiscences (56). Leaks attributed to technical issues are more likely to occur within the first 48 hours (57). The majority of ALs are diagnosed between the 7th and 12th postoperative days (58). Up to 12% are diagnosed 3 weeks after the index operation (58–60).

Early recognition of anastomotic leak can be difficult owing to poor specificity of the common signs and symptoms of AL, including abdominal pain and tachycardia. Certain biochemical markers have demonstrated promise in early detection. C-reactive protein (CRP) was shown to have a negative predictive value of 89%–97% for AL, with an area under the curve of 0.811 (61,62). Warschkow et al. (62) used CRP level (<135) as discharge criteria. In the PREDICS study, procalcitonin combined with CRP was highly predictive (area under the curve of 0.9) of AL on postoperative day 5 (63).

## IMAGING

CT is the most common test employed in the diagnosis of AL (Figure 8.1). While the specificity of CT is quite high (>84%), the sensitivity is only 68%–71% (64,65). Contrast extravasation is the most sensitive and specific sign, but it is unfortunately not always preset (64). The most common findings are extraluminal air and para-anastomotic collections with AL detection rates between 80% and 100% (66). The use of rectal contrast significantly increases the positive predictive value from 40% to 88%, $p = 0.0009$. This should be administered very carefully through a soft, small-bore catheter by an experienced member of the surgical team (67).

Postoperative pneumoperitoneum is a very common finding in the postoperative period in the absence of complications. It can be found in up to 44% of patients within the first 3–6 days after surgery, up to 30% in the second and third weeks following surgery, and up to 13% in the fourth postoperative week (68). In addition, fluid and inflammatory stranding are nearly always present in an early postoperative CT scan. For this reason, AL can be difficult to diagnose on CT in the first 3–4 days following surgery.

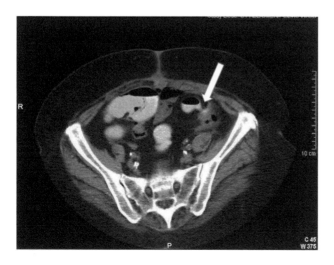

Figure 8.1 Demonstrates contrast extravasation from a left-sided anastomotic leak after administration of rectal contrast.

## DEFINITION

Colorectal surgery outcomes have become surrogate markers of institutional quality owing to the fact that colorectal surgery is a ubiquitous procedure that is performed at the majority of hospitals regardless of size, affiliation, and location. However, there has been a general lack of standardization surrounding the definition of AL (69). Frequently, the Centers for Disease Control and Prevention's definition for organ space infection is used to define AL. However, data suggest that organ space infection is an unreliable marker of AL based on a study by Rickels et al. (70) looking at the capture rates of anastomotic leak in both National Surgical Quality Improvement Program (which uses organ space infection to define AL) and a statewide registry, the Upstate New York Surgical Quality Initiative (UNYSQI). Only 25% of ALs following colorectal surgery were captured by National Surgical Quality Improvement Program using the organ space infection definition (70).

Several groups have produced standard definitions, classifying leaks into one of three grades based on severity and impact on clinical management (71,72):

- Grade A—asymptomatic or minor symptoms (for instance found on contrast enema prior to ileostomy reversal or a small fluid collection (<3 cm) adjacent to the anastomosis on CT. May respond to antibiotics. Does not require procedural intervention.
- Grade B—may have clinical signs of leak such as leukocytosis or fever but are nontoxic with normal vital signs. On CT scan there is a localized abscess that seems amendable to percutaneous drainage.
- Grade C—toxic in appearance with evidence of sepsis. Requires surgical intervention and often diversion.

## MANAGEMENT

Whatever the approach, the key to avoiding multisystem organ failure and death following anastomotic leak is the ability to rescue the patient early in the course so as to avoid the development of septic shock. This requires a high index of suspicion and an aggressive approach toward the management of anastomotic complications. Early recognition and intervention are key prior to development of significant contamination and subsequent fibrosis that will lead to sepsis and complicate the operative management. Management will depend on the clinical presentation and the severity of symptoms (Figure 8.2).

### Antibiotics

In general, abscesses less than 3 cm in size can be managed with antibiotics alone when the patient is clinically stable (73,74). Antibiotic regimens should cover gram-negative rods and anaerobic organisms. Possible choices include a β-lactam/β-lactamase inhibitor (piperacillin-tazobactam) or the combination of cefazolin and metronidazole.

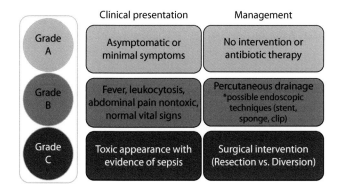

| Clinical presentation | Management |
|---|---|
| **Grade A** — Asymptomatic or minimal symptoms | No intervention or antibiotic therapy |
| **Grade B** — Fever, leukocytosis, abdominal pain nontoxic, normal vital signs | Percutaneous drainage *possible endoscopic techniques (stent, sponge, clip) |
| **Grade C** — Toxic appearance with evidence of sepsis | Surgical intervention (Resection vs. Diversion) |

Figure 8.2 Management of anastomotic leak according to severity and clinical presentation.

Traditionally, patients were treated with 7–10 days of antibiotics for intraabdominal infections. However, the Study to Optimize Peritoneal Infection Therapy (STOP-IT) trial demonstrated similar efficacy between patients with complicated intraabdominal infection *who had achieved adequate source control* randomized to a fixed course of antibiotics (4 days) versus antibiotics until 2 days after resolution of clinical signs of infection (up to a maximum of 10 days) (75). It is imperative to note that adequate source control is of the upmost importance, and there should be a very low threshold to repeat imaging following a course of antibiotic therapy for treatment of a small contained AL to assure that the inflammation has resolved. If it persists, therapeutic options should be considered, including percutaneous drainage or surgery.

## Drain

For abscesses greater than 3 cm in size, percutaneous drainage is a viable option with success rates up to 81%. For pelvic collections, this often requires a transgluteal approach. It is important that the entire collection be drained, as incomplete drainage is associated with high rates of failure (76). In addition to the size and resolution of the fluid collection, the quality of the drainage is also important. Pus is obviously more amendable to percutaneous drainage than stool, which results in a controlled colocutaneous fistula through the drain. Rarely, this can lead to a severe necrotizing infection along the course of the drain. My personal bias leans toward diversion rather than percutaneous drainage alone for fluid collections in the setting of contrast extravasation or when frank stool is encountered upon percutaneous aspiration.

Some advocate placing a transanal drain, such as a small Malecot catheter, through the anastomotic defect. The drain remains in place until the abscess cavity closes to the size of the drain upon instillation of contrast through the drain (77–79).

## Surgery

The operative management of anastomotic leak can be very challenging due to gross contamination, and severe inflammation. Traditional management of an anastomotic leak dictated either exteriorization of the leaking anastomosis or resection of the anastomosis with the creation of an end stoma and Hartmann pouch or mucus fistula (80). While certainly effective at controlling the leak, dissection around the anastomosis can prove difficult with the risk of injury to surrounding structures. In addition, restoration of intestinal continuity under these circumstances requires a subsequent major operation to reverse, and as a result, many end stomas are never reversed (81).

While resection of the anastomosis may seem desirable, it is not always feasible and, under certain circumstances, may be deleterious. Under these circumstances, a more desirable option may be drainage (either operatively or percutaneously) and proximal diversion. With diversion alone, less operative stress is placed on patients who are already critically ill. This "damage control" philosophy has proven successful in trauma situations and may be appropriate after the traumatic insult of an anastomotic dehiscence (82). This technique is safe, has a high rate of anastomotic salvage, and can often be reversed through a small peristomal incision (83,84). If the index operation was performed laparoscopically, diversion and drainage may be performed laparoscopically as well (85).

We published our own experience utilizing loop ileostomy with drainage as a treatment for patients with an anastomotic leak resulting in peritonitis or abscess (86). Our study included a variety of both intraperitoneal (85%) and extraperitoneal (15%) colon and rectal anastomoses. Proximal diversion and drainage were successfully utilized in 70% of patients requiring surgery for an anastomotic complication. Ultimately, 63% of patients treated with proximal diversion had restoration of their intestinal continuity, a percentage that is similar to that reported by Matthiessen et al. (59) and Eckmann et al. (87) following diversion for anastomotic leaks. Of the patients who underwent fluoroscopic evaluation for possible takedown, 92% had normal healing of their anastomosis. The algorithm in Figure 8.3 may assist with surgical decision-making.

Surgery is critical not only in the management of patients with overt sepsis and peritonitis, but also for patients with an intraabdominal abscess that does not promptly respond to catheter drainage.

## Endoscopic techniques

Based on the success in esophageal leaks, the use of covered stents as treatment for colorectal leaks has been described in several small case series (88–90). Counterdrainage of the accompanying abscess is required. There are different types of stents including self-expanding metal and plastic stents. They may be covered or uncovered. Stent migration is the major issue. The colorectal anastomosis must be an end-to-end anastomosis, and the distal end of the stent must be at least 5 cm above the anal verge. Therefore, stents are not effective for low anastomoses. Many of the stents are not large enough for colorectal anastomoses. Some have described the use of endoclips to secure the stent in

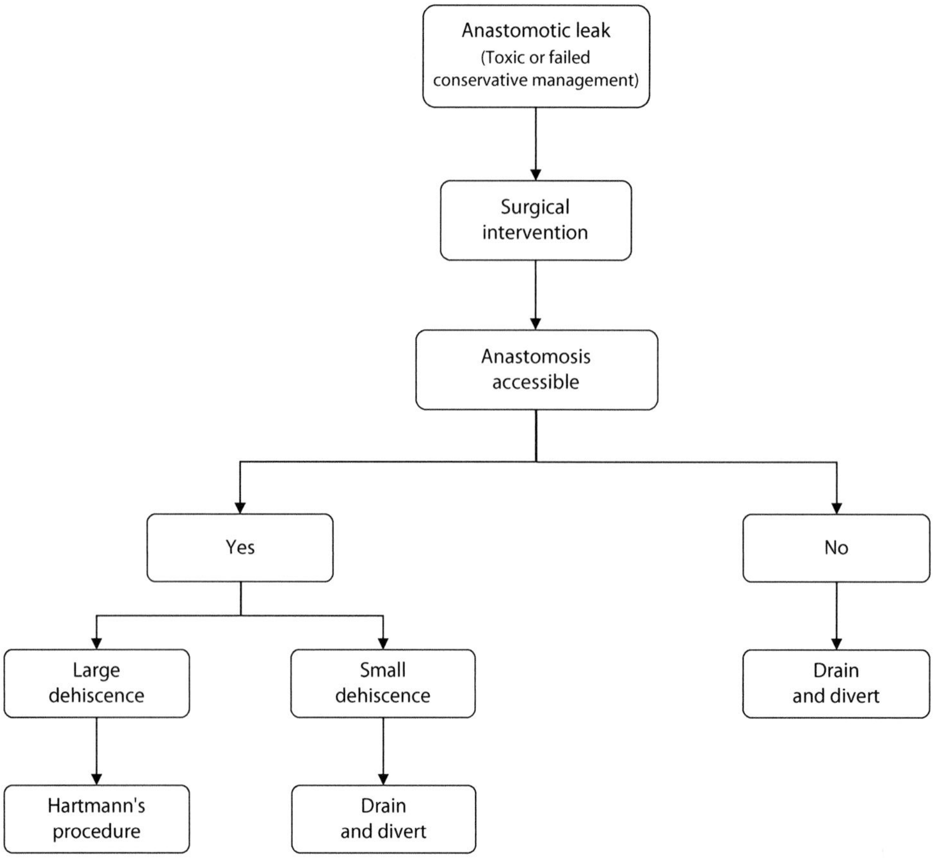

```
                    ┌──────────────────────────┐
                    │     Anastomotic leak      │
                    │    (Toxic or failed       │
                    │  conservative management) │
                    └────────────┬─────────────┘
                                 │
                    ┌────────────▼─────────────┐
                    │         Surgical          │
                    │       intervention        │
                    └────────────┬─────────────┘
                                 │
                    ┌────────────▼─────────────┐
                    │       Anastomosis         │
                    │        accessible         │
                    └────────────┬─────────────┘
              ┌──────────────────┴───────────────────┐
        ┌─────▼─────┐                           ┌─────▼─────┐
        │    Yes    │                           │    No     │
        └─────┬─────┘                           └─────┬─────┘
       ┌──────┴───────┐                               │
  ┌────▼────┐    ┌────▼────┐                    ┌─────▼──────┐
  │  Large  │    │  Small  │                    │   Drain    │
  │dehiscence│   │dehiscence│                   │ and divert │
  └────┬────┘    └────┬────┘                    └────────────┘
  ┌────▼─────┐   ┌────▼─────┐
  │Hartmann's│   │  Drain   │
  │procedure │   │and divert│
  └──────────┘   └──────────┘
```

Figure 8.3 Treatment algorithm for surgical management of anastomotic leak.

place, but that has not proven particularly effective. When deployed, the stents are generally left in place up to 60 days and then removed once the anastomosis heals. The partially covered stents seem to have less migration than fully covered stents. This technology has been described in patients with or without a diverting stoma (88–90).

Another innovative technique for the treatment of anastomotic leaks is endoscopic transanal vacuum-assisted rectal drainage (91–94). It was initially reported by Weidenhagen and Arezzo in separate reports with up to 79% success rate (91,95). The technique involves placement of a sponge via an introducer fitted over an endoscope through the anastomotic defect and into the presacral space. The placement of the sponge is verified endoscopically. It is exchanged every 48–72 hours and is downsized as the cavity decreases in size. Treatment is stopped when the cavity is less than 1 cm in size. It seems to be more effective if placed early when the rectum is more pliable prior to the development of associated fibrosis. It is important to note that a visible vessel in the presacral space is a contraindication to treatment. In addition, it has only been used in very distal anastomoses and in the setting of proximal diversion (83,91). It is important to note that although this technique has been described for several years, it has yet to become widely adopted.

Endoscopic clip application as a method to reapproximate the anastomotic dehiscence has also been described (96–100). Although the data are limited to small case series,

this technique seems better for small leaks less than 1.5 cm in size in the absence of a pelvic collection. It has also been used in conjunction with the transanal sponge technique once that cavity is small enough (101).

## ANASTOMOTIC LEAK WITH CUTANEOUS FISTULA

It is not uncommon for an AL to manifest as a colocutaneous fistula. The management of the colocutaneous fistula can globally be organized into three principle phases. The initial phase is the acute stabilization of the patient from a metabolic and sepsis standpoint in the first hours to days of presentation. This is followed by the development of an interim plan for wound care and nutrition. The final phase of treatment is the definitive management or closure of the fistula.

## CONTROL OF SEPSIS

Patients present along a continuum of severity depending on the volume of fistula output. Presentations range from a localized skin infection with a small underlying low-output fistula to septic shock with profound dehydration in patients with a proximal high-output fistula. Treatment of the fistula patient must be customized accordingly. In general, most fistulas resulting from colorectal surgery are low output fistulas that can be supported conservatively.

Source control is imperative to prevent intraabdominal sepsis. All patients who are suspected as having a fistula should undergo CT. These patients do not always manifest the usual signs of infection. Rather, they may present with weight loss, hypoalbuminemia, or jaundice (102). Any intraabdominal fluid collections must be adequately drained either percutaneously or surgically. Contrast injected into the cavity can give information regarding the size of the cavity and identify the location of the fistulous communication (102). At this point, the decision must be made whether to operate or manage the patient nonoperatively. This will depend on the timing of the leak. In general, this is best managed operatively within the first 7–10 days postoperatively. After this, the decision to operate will depend on the clinical presentation. Colocutaneous fistulas representing anastomotic leak may require proximal diversion if possible to facilitate closure.

## WOUND CARE

The fistula must be isolated from surrounding tissue to allow for nursing care, protection of the skin, or healing of the surrounding open wound. This also allows for quantification of the effluent, which is critical in the early stages of presentation for adequate replacement of the calculated volume loss. A stoma appliance can often be used to pouch most fistulas surrounded by intact skin. However, the enteroatmospheric fistula can be extremely challenging to isolate. A multidisciplinary team consisting of wound-care specialists, enterostomal therapists, and physicians is required to identify an effective wound-care system. Various strategies have been employed including wound-care managers, similar to very large stoma appliances that encompass the entire wound bed. The fistula effluent is isolated with closed suction drains, and the surrounding wound is managed with a wet to dry dressing.

The vacuum suction wound management system is utilized by many to isolate the fistula within the open wound, allowing for pouching of the fistula. However, caution must be used as the development of an enterocutaneous fistula has been described as a complication of wound vacuum management system in patients with open abdomens (103). If vacuum-assisted therapy is utilized within an open intraabdominal wound, caution is advised, and precautions should be taken to protect the underlying bowel.

Regardless of the interim wound management scheme, once the adjacent tissue within the surrounding open wound is granulated, skin grafting can be performed to allow for placement of a stoma appliance.

## ANTIMOTILITY AGENTS AND OCTREOTIDE

Volume reduction of effluent is not likely to facilitate spontaneous closure of the fistula. However, it does provide other significant advantages. Patients with low-volume (<200 cc/day) fistulas are unlikely to suffer electrolyte imbalance and volume depletion. Similarly, wound care is simplified by effluent volume reduction. The majority of patients with low-output fistulas can tolerate enteral nutrition (102). Therefore, significant effort should focus on antimotility therapy, including treatment with loperamide, diphenoxylate and atropine, tincture of opium, codeine, cholestyramine, and proton pump inhibitors.

## DEFINITIVE MANAGEMENT

Once the patient has been stabilized with source control, wound care, and nutritional support, a plan for definitive management of the fistula is imperative. Many low-volume colocutaneous fistula will close spontaneously over time in the absence of complicating factors such as radiation or a distal obstruction. Therefore, patience is of the upmost importance in this situation. Once it has been determined that surgery will be necessary, most surgeons wait at least 4–6 months from the inciting event. Definitive surgery is fraught with difficulty owing to prior inflammation and the common association with loss of abdominal wall domain (104). Tedious dissection upon entry to the abdomen is critical to prevent inadvertent enterotomies, which can be aided by using an alternative incision if possible or extending the incision superior to the prior incision into virgin territory. In cases of a large abdominal wall defect, component separation without or without biologic mesh is often necessary (104,105).

## ANASTOMOTIC STRICTURE

Anastomotic stricture is a common reason for failure of stoma reversal after low anterior resection with diverting loop ileostomy (106). The incidence of stricture has been reported in up to 15% of the patients following low anterior resection with diverting loop ileostomy (107). In most cases, anastomotic strictures develop as the result of an anastomotic leak, which may or may not be clinically appreciated at the original operation. Therefore, the same general principles for prevention and diagnosis apply. Anastomotic stricture related to Crohn disease represents an entirely different entity than sporadic postoperative strictures and is beyond the scope of this manuscript.

Many strictures are found at the time of contrast enema in anticipation of ostomy reversal. Other patients will have a delayed presentation, which may include changes in bowel habits, crampy abdominal pain, constipation or diarrhea, incontinence, and obstipation. The presentation can be insidious and surgeons must have a high index of suspicion to facilitate diagnosis and intervention prior to a complete obstruction. Diagnosis can be made endoscopically or radiographically on a contrast enema or CT scan with rectal contrast. Management depends on the severity of the stricture. Mild strictures, particularly on the right side, where the stool is liquid in character, may be successfully managed with a low-residue diet. Balloon dilation is an effective solution (108). Biraima et al. (108) report a single institution study of 76 patients over nearly 20 years with anastomotic stenosis. All patients were treated initially with balloon dilation. Balloon dilation was successful in 97% of the patients. The median number of dilations required was three. Recurrences were 11%, 11%, and 25% at 1, 3, and 5 years, respectively. Balloon dilation has also been combined with endoscopic incision of the fibrotic anastomotic tissue with successful results in small case series (109,110). Consideration can also be given to self-expanding metallic stents (90). Strictures that are refractory to balloon dilation require a surgical approach with revision of the anastomosis, if possible (111). If an anastomosis cannot be salvaged, the decision must be made whether to resect the anastomosis and bring up an end stoma or retain the anastomosis and simply divert above it. This decision obviously depends on each individual situation, and resection of the anastomosis will prove impossible for some patients. However, if possible, patients generally have fewer subsequent complications if the anastomosis can be resected and an end stoma can be created.

## CHRONIC ANASTOMOTIC SINUS

Chronic sinuses in low rectal anastomoses have been reported in up to 36% of anastomotic leaks (112). Of these, 8% are asymptomatic, found at contrast enema in evaluation for ileostomy takedown (113). These chronic sinuses represent a frustrating situation for both patients and surgeons alike. Some will close spontaneously with the elapse of additional time. However, they can adversely affect bowel function due to fibrosis with reduction in compliance (114). For patients with sinuses that do not heal spontaneously, many will result in the patient having a permanent stoma.

Some advocate for early intervention to prevent the development of a chronic cavity with resulting fibrosis (115). Marsupialization of the sinus has been reported using either an endoscopic stapler or cautery. Theoretically, this allows complete drainage of the cavity and incorporation of the sinus tract into the lumen of the bowel. Subsequently, with epithelialization of the cavity, the stoma can then theoretically be reversed (116,117). Transanal repair with flap closure via an endorectal advancement flap has also been described (118,119). If local measures fail, revising the anastomosis is an option. However, this can be a technically challenging operation with high rates of recurrent anastomotic problems (120).

## REFERENCES

1. Demetriades H et al. *Tech Coloproctol* 2004;8(Suppl 1):s72–5.
2. Isbister WH. *ANZ J Surg* 2001;71(9):516–20.
3. Matthiessen P et al. *Colorectal Dis* 2004;6(6):462–9.
4. Shakhsheer BA et al. *Int J Colorectal Dis* 2017;32(4): 539–47.
5. Krezalek MA, Alverdy JC. *Curr Opin Clin Nutr Metab Care* 2016. 23 [Epub ahead of print]
6. Turrentine FE et al. *J Am Coll Surg* 2015;220(2): 195–206.
7. Phitayakorn R et al. *World J Surg* 2008;32(6):1147–56.
8. Hammond J et al. *J Gastrointest Surg* 2014;18(6): 1176–85.
9. Ashburn JH et al. *Dis Colon Rectum* 2013;56(3): 275–80.
10. Hallbook O, Sjodahl R. *Br J Surg* 1996;83(1):60–2.
11. Marinatou A et al. *Dis Colon Rectum* 2014;57(2): 158–66.
12. Nesbakken A et al. *Br J Surg* 2001;88(3):400–4.
13. McArdle CS et al. *Br J Surg* 2005;92(9):1150–4.
14. Smith JD et al. *Ann Surg Oncol* 2013;20(8):2641–6.
15. Mirnezami A et al. *Ann Surg* 2011;253(5):890–9.
16. Lu, ZR et al. *Dis Colon Rectum* 2016;59(3):236–44.
17. Espin E et al. *Br J Surg* 2015;102(4):416–22.
18. Smith JD et al. *Ann Surg* 2012;256(6):1034–8.
19. Vignali A et al. *Dis Colon Rectum* 2000;43(1):76–82.
20. Boyle NH et al. *J Am Coll Surg* 2000;191(5):504–10.
21. Kashiwagi H. *Surg Today* 1993;23(5):430–8.
22. Konishi T et al. *J Am Coll Surg* 2006;202(3):439–44.
23. Sheridan WG, Lowndes RH et al. *Dis Colon Rectum* 1987;30(11):867–71.
24. Chekan E, Whelan RL. *Med Devices (Auckl)* 2014;7: 305–18.
25. Zilling T, Walther BS. *Dis Colon Rectum* 1992;35(9): 892–6.
26. Ito M et al. *Int J Colorectal Dis* 2008;23(7):703–7.
27. Kawada K et al. *Surg Endosc* 2014;28(10):2988–95.
28. Park JS et al. *Ann Surg* 2013;257(4):665–71.
29. Qu H, Liu Y et al. *Surg Endosc.* 2015;29(12):3608–17.
30. Shogan BD et al. *Surg Infect (Larchmt)* 2014;15(5): 479–89.
31. Shogan BD et al. *Sci Transl Med* 2015;7(286):286ra68.
32. Shogan BD et al. *J Gastrointest Surg* 2013;17(9): 1698–707.
33. Kirchhoff P et al. *Patient Saf Surg* 2010;4(1):5.
34. Lipska MA et al. *ANZ J Surg* 2006;76(7):579–85.
35. Midura EF et al. *Dis Colon Rectum* 2015;58(3):333–8.
36. Trencheva K et al. *Ann Surg* 2013;257(1):108–13.
37. Kologlu M et al. *Surgery* 2000;128(1):99–104.
38. Posma LA et al. *Dis Colon Rectum* 2007;50(7):1070–9.
39. Pettersson D et al. *Br J Surg* 2010;97(4):580–7.
40. Nichols RL et al. *Ann Surg* 1973;178(4):453–62.
41. Clarke JS et al. *Ann Surg* 1977;186(3):251–9.
42. Dahabreh IJ et al. *Dis Colon Rectum* 2015;58(7): 698–707.
43. Rollins KE et al. *World J Gastroenterol* 2018;24(4): 519–36.
44. Gustafsson UO et al. *Clin Nutr* 2012;31(6):783–800.
45. Mahajna A et al. *Dis Colon Rectum* 2005;48(8):1626–31.

46. Nelson RL et al. *Cochrane Database Syst Rev.* 2009;(1):CD001181. DOI: 10.1002/14651858. CD001181.pub3
47. Englesbe MJ et al. *Ann Surg* 2010;252(3):514–9, discussion 519–20.
48. Kim EK et al. *Ann Surg* 2014;259(2):310–4.
49. Moghadamyeghaneh Z et al. *J Am Coll Surg* 2015; 220(5):912–20.
50. Morris MS et al. *Ann Surg* 2015;261(6):1034–40.
51. Chude GG et al. *Hepatogastroenterology* 2008; 55(86–87):1562–7.
52. Huser N et al. *Ann Surg* 2008;248(1):52–60.
53. Nachiappan S et al. *Surg Endosc* 2014;28(9):2513–30.
54. Kin C et al. *Dis Colon Rectum* 2015;58(6):582–7.
55. Jafari MD et al. *J Am Coll Surg* 2015;220(1):82–92 e1.
56. Paliogiannis P et al. *Ann Ital Chir* 2012;83(1):25–8.
57. Baker RS et al. *Obes Surg* 2004;14(10):1290–8.
58. Hyman N et al. *Ann Surg* 2007;245(2):254–8.
59. Matthiessen P et al. *Ann Surg* 2007;246(2):207–14.
60. Morks AN et al. *Colorectal Dis* 2013;15(5):e271–5.
61. Singh PP et al. *Br J Surg* 2014;101(4):339–46.
62. Warschkow R et al. *Ann Surg* 2012;256(2):245–50.
63. Giaccaglia V et al. *Ann Surg* 2016;263(5):967–72.
64. Kauv P et al. *Eur Radiol* 2015;25(12):3543–51.
65. Kornmann VN et al. *Int J Colorectal Dis* 2013;28(4): 437–45.
66. Daams F et al. *World J Gastrointest Surg* 2014;6(2): 14–26.
67. Habib K et al. *Int J Colorectal Dis* 2015;30(8):1007–14.
68. Chapman BC et al. *J Surg Res* 2015;197(1):107–11.
69. Bruce J et al. *Br J Surg* 2001;88(9):1157–68.
70. Rickles AS et al. *Surgery* 2013;154(4):680–7; discussion 687–9.
71. Chadi SA et al. *J Gastrointest Surg* 2016;20(12): 2035–51.
72. Peel AL, Taylor EW. *Ann R Coll Surg Engl.* 1991;73(6): 385–8.
73. Elagili F et al. *Dis Colon Rectum* 2014;57(3):331–6.
74. Siewert B et al. *AJR Am J Roentgenol* 2006;186(3): 680–6.
75. Sawyer RG et al. *N Engl J Med* 2015;372(21): 1996–2005.
76. Khurrum Baig M et al. *Tech Coloproctol* 2002;6(3): 159–64.
77. Thomas MS, Margolin DA. *Clin Colon Rectal Surg.* 2016;29(2):138–44.
78. Sirois-Giguere E et al. *Dis Colon Rectum* 2013;56(5): 586–92.
79. Thorson AG, Thompson JS. *Dis Colon Rectum.* 1984; 27(7):492–4.
80. Alves A et al. *J Am Coll Surg* 1999;189(6):554–9.
81. Parc Y et al. *Dis Colon Rectum* 2000;43(5):579–87; discussion 587–9.
82. Parr MJ, Alabdi T. *Injury* 2004;35(7):713–22.
83. Blumetti J, Abcarian H. *World J Gastrointest Surg* 2015;7(12):378–83.
84. Longo J et al. *J Contin Educ Nurs* 2011;42(1):27–35.
85. Joh YG et al. *Dis Colon Rectum* 2009;52(1):91–6.
86. Hedrick TL et al. *Dis Colon Rectum* 2006;49(8): 1167–76.
87. Eckmann C et al. *Int J Colorectal Dis* 2004;19(2): 128–33.
88. Abbas MA. *JSLS* 2009;13(3):420–4.
89. Lamazza A et al. *Endoscopy* 2013;45(6):493–5.
90. Lamazza A et al. *Am J Surg* 2014;208(3):465–9.
91. Arezzo A et al. *Dig Liver Dis* 2015;47(4):342–5.
92. Glitsch A et al. *Endoscopy* 2008;40(3):192–9.
93. Kuehn F et al. *J Gastrointest Surg* 2016;20(2):237–43.
94. Smallwood NR et al. *Surg Endosc* 2016;30(6): 2473–80.
95. Weidenhagen R et al. *Surg Endosc* 2008;22(8): 1818–25.
96. Mennigen R et al. *World J Gastroenterol* 2014;20(24): 7767–76.
97. Mizrahi I et al. *J Gastrointest Surg* 2016;20(12): 1942–9.
98. Sulz MC et al. *World J Gastroenterol* 2014;20(43): 16287–92.
99. Weiland T et al. *Surg Endosc* 2013;27(7):2258–74.
100. Brunner W et al. *Surg Endosc* 2015;29(12):3803–5.
101. Chopra SS et al. *Surgery.* 2009;145(2):182–8.
102. Joyce MR, Dietz DW. *Curr Probl Surg* 2009;46(5): 384–430.
103. Bee TK et al. *J Trauma* 2008;65(2):337–42; discussion 342–4.
104. Hodgkinson JD et al. *Colorectal Dis* 2017;19(4): 319–30.
105. Atema JJ et al. *World J Surg.* 2017;41(8):1993–9.
106. Haksal M et al. *Ann Surg Treat Res* 2017;92(1):35–41.
107. Kim MJ et al. *Surgery* 2016;159(3):721–7.
108. Biraima M et al. *Surg Endosc* 2016;30(10):4432–7.
109. Truong S et al. *Endoscopy* 1997;29(9):845–9.
110. Tan Y et al. *Int J Colorectal Dis* 2016;31(5):1063–4.
111. Maggiori L et al. *Int J Colorectal Dis* 2015;30(4): 543–8.
112. van Koperen PJ et al. *Colorectal Dis* 2011;13(1):26–9.
113. Blumetti J et al. *World J Surg* 2014;38(4):985–91.
114. Blumetti J et al. *Colorectal Dis* 2012;14(10):1238–41.
115. Verlaan T et al. *Colorectal Dis* 2011;13(Suppl 7):18–22.
116. Stewart BT, Stitz RW. *Dis Colon Rectum* 1999;42(2): 264–5.
117. Whitlow CB et al. *Dis Colon Rectum* 1997;40(7): 760–3.
118. Fleshman JW et al. *Int J Colorectal Dis* 1988;3(3): 161–5.
119. Wexner SD et al. *Dis Colon Rectum* 1989;32(6): 460–5.
120. Genser L et al. *Dis Colon Rectum* 2013;5:747–55.

# 9

# General postoperative complications

J. MARCUS DOWNS AND KRISTINA K. BOOTH

## CHALLENGING CASE

A 56-year-old man underwent surgery 3 years ago for perforated diverticulitis, when a Hartmann procedure was performed. Six months later, he underwent colostomy closure. This operation was complicated by a ureteral injury at the pelvic brim, which was repaired primarily over a double-J stent. Over the past year, he has had three admissions for small bowel obstruction, which quickly resolved with nasogastric suction and IV fluids. He has multiple hernia defects at his midline wound, as well as a hernia at his colostomy site. He weighs 110 kg, and prior to this he had no medical problems. He also has left hydronephrosis, which is on the side of his ureteral injury.

## CASE MANAGEMENT

This patient required surgery for his recurring small bowel obstruction felt to be related to his multiple hernias. After induction of anesthesia, a cystoscopy was performed, and ureteral stent placement was attempted. This was unsuccessful, and retrograde ureterogram showed a completely obstructed ureter. The planned hernia surgery was not performed, and he was awoken. The next day, he underwent a percutaneous nephrostomy and ureterogram. The ureterogram showed only the proximal two-thirds of his ureter to be patent. With the nephrostomy tube in place, it was determined that the left kidney function was only 8% of normal. With this finding, ureteral reconstruction was felt not to be indicated. He returned to the operating room 3 weeks later for hernia repair. At that time, he was found to have a simple hernia at his stoma site, which was easily reduced, and multiple midline defects, two of which had incarcerated loops of small bowel. The hernias were repaired primarily

with biologic mesh underlay. He recovered uneventfully, going home on his fifth postoperative day. He returned 2 days later with severe pain, nausea, and vomiting with imaging suggesting small bowel obstruction. Initial treatment with nasogastric suction failed to improve his pain, and he was returned to the operating room the next day where he was found to have obstruction related to an internal hernia defect caused by his remaining momentum. This was corrected, and the abdominal wall once again reconstructed. His kidney has been left to involute.

This patient represents a spectrum of postoperative complications commonly related to colon surgery: hernia, bowel obstruction, and ureteral injury. He also represents the unfortunate truth that not all repairs are successful.

## INTRODUCTION

With surgery too often come complications. As surgeons, we decide upon whom to operate. We prepare our patients for surgery, operate, and care for our patients through recovery. Our approach to complications should be to minimize their occurrence, recognize their presence, and optimize their treatment. In this chapter, we discuss the postoperative problems of pain, bleeding, infection, deep vein thrombosis, nausea and vomiting, prolonged ileus, injury to normal organs, and retained foreign bodies. In Chapter 10, enhanced recovery after surgery (ERAS) protocols are presented. The elements of ERAS protocols typically include preoperative, intraoperative, and postoperative components. Often added is an additional bundle of elements specifically addressing surgical site infections (SSIs). As we discuss complications in this chapter, we break the discussion of each complication into the same time frames.

Surgical outcomes are measured incessantly. Each of us receives quarterly, if not monthly, reports on our length of stay, surgical volume, and SSIs. Patients having complications have prolonged lengths of stay (1,2). We have all seen our own numbers go from high to low, from one quarter to the next, with no change in our treatments. Rather than using the following information to improve our averages, search each section for ways to improve the care of our next patient.

## PAIN MANAGEMENT

Adequate pain control during the postoperative time frame can be both elusive to the patient and frustrating to the provider. Lack of pain control can lead to complications related to poor mobility, such as atelectasis and deep vein thrombosis (DVT); however, liberal use of opioids for pain control also leads to respiratory depression, ileus, and constipation (3). Each patient interprets pain differently and can enter the clinical encounter with varying expectations on pain management. Providers must balance easier opioid-based pain control options with their potential side effects including prolonged length of stay. In addition to shorter lengths of stay, reducing opioid prescriptions can prevent their diversion and reduce narcotic abuse (4). While an opioid-free recovery may not be possible in all patients, a narcotic-sparing regimen can provide good pain control and reduce length of stay as part of enhanced recovery pathways (5–7).

Treating pain begins before surgery. The first preoperative task is patient education. Patient's expectations should be addressed, and information provided. Patients should be coached that we want and expect them to be comfortable and to be mobile, but that pain control does not mean being pain free. Emphasis on preemptive pain control has mitigated the use of excess opioids in postoperative care by providing a prophylactic barrier for painful stimuli. A multimodal approach can be started in preoperative care and continued postoperative for a well-rounded strategy. Nonsteroidal anti-inflammatory drugs and cyclooxygenase-2 (COX-2) inhibitors can be used preoperatively and carried throughout the patient's recovery. Care should be taken to ensure adequate kidney function. There has been some hesitance in their use due to concerns of bleeding, but this seems not to be the case (8). There may be an association between Ketorolac use and anastomotic leak, particularly in nonelective cases (9,10). In addition, Etoricoxib, a COX-2 inhibitor, has been associated with risk of complications after colorectal surgery (9). Gabapentin, used preoperatively and scheduled postoperatively, can reduce opioid use and improve analgesia (11). Gabapentin may be associated with respiratory depression, and so intraoperative narcotics should be reduced. This problem is more prominent in elderly patients (11,12). In patients with normal liver function, preemptive and scheduled acetaminophen can be most helpful in decreasing pain levels during recovery (13). The use of these medications appears to be synergistic, as they each contribute a different mechanism of pain control.

A team-based approach to minimizing opioid use is paramount. This again serves to decrease opioid-induced complications and decrease the need for opioids postoperatively. Minimizing incision length is one aspect that can decrease trauma and thus decrease pain. This is an important benefit of minimally invasive surgery, which should be pursued if possible. Injection of local anesthetic at the site of port placement prior to incision is helpful. Intraoperative lidocaine infusion has been shown to reduce postoperative narcotic requirements. This has been demonstrated in both open and laparoscopic colectomy (14,15). It is unclear what the optimal duration of therapy should be (16).

Many conflicting reports have been presented surrounding various tools used to provide analgesia (13). Continuous preperitoneal analgesia was compared directly to epidural analgesia and found inferior in many aspects, including pain scores, length of hospital stay, and functional recovery for open surgeries (17). However, the benefits of epidural use in laparoscopic surgery appear to be minimal and may actually slow recovery. Patient-controlled analgesia (PCA) has been compared to epidurals with conflicting results (13,18). PCA has the benefits of self-titration, immediate action, and high patient satisfaction scores, but the downside includes the systemic effects of the opioid medication. Due to their localized site of action, epidurals do omit the effects of system opioids from the equation. However, epidurals have a failure rate of about 12%, can induce hypotension, can add potential procedural-related complications, and can even delay discharge in some instances (13,18). The use of epidurals in minimally invasive surgery does not seem to be justified given the risk profile and limited benefit. The use of epidurals in laparoscopic colorectal surgery within an enhanced recovery pathway appears to prolong length of stay compared to PCA use (18). The use of transverses abdominis plane (TAP) blocks has gained popularity as a reasonable alternative to epidurals and the cumbersome preperitoneal analgesia. TAP blocks have been shown to reduce pain and length of stay (19,20). The addition of a TAP block to an enhanced recovery pathway results in further reduction in length of stay and can be delivered under laparoscopic guidance (19).

Ketamine is a dissociative anesthetic agent. It has also been used in postoperative pain management (21). Ketamine has also been incorporated into ERAS pathways following cholecystectomy (22).

Adequate pain control is essential for optimizing patient outcome. Optimal pain control in colorectal surgery requires a multiple modality approach and should minimize narcotic use. The optimal pharmacologic cocktail has yet to be defined. The addition of local anesthetics epidurally, preperitoneally, locally, or via TAP will all reduce narcotic requirements, though epidural use may prolong length of stay. Additional information is presented in Chapter 10.

## BLEEDING

Minimizing bleeding complications begins well before surgery. A thorough history and physical exam must be completed on every patient. This includes specific inquiry into the patient's history of bleeding, easy bruising, known coagulopathy, medications expected to impair hemostasis, and family history of bleeding disorders. The patient evaluation is then looked at in the context of the proposed surgical procedure and the expected bleeding risk. Patients with no identified risk factors undergoing procedures with low bleeding risks, such as colonoscopy or anorectal surgery, require no laboratory evaluation. Low-dose aspirin may be continued.

Patients suspected of increased bleeding risk should have preoperative lab testing to include complete blood count, platelet count, prothrombin time, partial thromboplastin time, and international normalized ratio. Abnormalities that cannot be explained or corrected should trigger formal hematologic evaluation, as should known or suspected coagulopathies. Anticoagulants should be stopped prior to surgery. If this cannot be safely done, switching to heparin or enoxaparin prior to surgery and holding it the day of the procedure should be considered. Such decisions should be made in conjunction with the patient's primary care physician. In short, coagulopathies should be corrected prior to surgery.

Abdominal operations carry a higher risk of bleeding than anorectal or endoscopic procedures. Each patient should be typed and screened. Should problematic bleeding occur, the blood bank then already has a sample for crossmatching. A positive antibody screen suggests that crossmatching blood will be more difficult, and should be followed with a discussion with the blood bank to ensure blood is available, if needed. Of course, not every abdominal operation carries the same bleeding risk. Patients anemic to begin with, or when significant blood loss is expected, may require crossmatching prior to surgery. Massive blood loss may lead to coagulopathy and the need for blood component therapy. Many hospital blood banks have treatment protocols when massive transfusion is required (23). Work with your blood bank to establish one if none yet exists at your hospital.

While all benefit from the same preoperative evaluation, endoscopic, abdominal, and anorectal cases present differing challenges with regard to intraoperative bleeding. It is clear that increased transfusion leads to worse outcomes in patients with colorectal cancer (24). The unique challenge posed in endoscopy is the inability to apply direct pressure to bleeding points. The tools available to control bleeding endoscopically include injection of epinephrine, electrocautery, and application of hemostatic clips. Electrocautery may be either monopolar or bipolar. Monopolar electrocautery should be used judiciously due to concern for full-thickness injury. This risk is lessened with bipolar cautery (Bicap). Clips are particularly useful when larger polyps are removed.

Intraabdominal surgery presents several areas of bleeding risks of particular importance in colorectal surgery. These are pelvic bleeding, the spleen, and bleeding associated with the middle colic vessels. Life-threatening bleeding in the pelvis is usually due to injury to the presacral veins. When

such bleeding occurs, it is important to apply pressure, and pause. This is the time to give anesthesia time to "catch up" with fluids. This is not because the patient was behind in fluids, but that the occurrence of the bleeding often results in a massive, sudden blood loss. Now is the time to obtain blood, if already crossed, or to send blood for crossmatch, if this has not already been done. It is also a time to ensure needed materials are in the room. Techniques often used include electrocautery, topical hemostatic agents, sacral thumbtacks, and muscle fragment welding (Figure 9.1). Also reported is the use of tissue expanders, cyanoacrylate adhesives, and endoscopic tacking devices. When these fail, or coagulopathy occurs, the pelvis may be packed, the wound temporarily closed, and the patient taken to the intensive care unit for resuscitation, rewarming, and correction of coagulopathy. The patient is then returned to the operating room in 24–48 hours, by which time the bleeding has usually ceased.

The second area at risk of bleeding in colon surgery is the spleen. Meticulous dissection technique while mobilizing the splenic flexure is the best way to avoid this complication. A useful technique in mobilizing this flexure is to initiate the dissection medially at the ligament of Treitz, divide the inferior mesenteric vein, develop the plane posterior to the mesocolon out to the abdominal wall, and cephalad to the pancreas. This maneuver eases the identification of the proper plane as the peritoneal reflection and lienocolic ligament are divided.

The third area at risk of bleeding is at the base of the middle colic vessels, where anatomic variants can present increased bleeding risk, especially as the hepatic flexure is

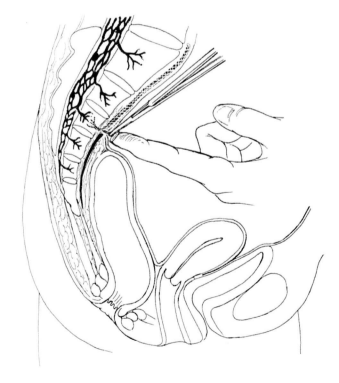

Figure 9.1 Thumbtack occlusion of a bleeding basivertebral vein.

mobilized medially. Bleeding here usually requires suture ligation, taking care to protect the superior mesenteric vein.

Control of bleeding in anorectal surgery is rarely problematic intraoperatively unless the patient has portal hypertension and/or a coagulopathy. These should be known before surgery as their presence may modify the operation performed. Patients with advanced liver disease or coagulopathy and bleeding hemorrhoids should be treated with suture ligation rather than excisional hemorrhoidectomy to minimize bleeding complications.

Management of postoperative bleeding differs by type of surgery. Bleeding after endoscopic procedures should be managed initially as any lower gastrointestinal bleed. Ongoing bleeding demands repeating colonoscopy. Reprepping is usually not required. The bleeding source is usually apparent and controlled with application of hemostatic clips. If the site is found but covered with a blood clot, the clot should be irrigated away to reveal the underlying bleeding site, which should then be clipped. Rectal bleeding following colectomy should be treated similarly, with colonoscopy performed liberally. The two most common sources of bleeding are at the anastomosis and ischemic colitis.

Postoperative bleeding in the abdomen often requires reexploration and evacuation of clotted blood. Often no discrete bleeding site is found. Bleeding in the pelvis after a difficult dissection may be addressed by angiographic embolization.

Some bleeding after anorectal surgery is expected. Excessive bleeding demands evaluation. This can be done with either a proctoscope or anoscope, and irrigation of blood from the rectum. If a bleeding site is identified, it can be addressed with injection of epinephrine or oversewing. This may require returning to the operating room.

Patient outcomes are improved by reducing bleeding complications. This is accomplished by the combination of a thorough preoperative evaluation, careful surgical technique, and recognition and treatment when these complications occur.

## INFECTION

Infection is an embedded element of colorectal surgery. While clean surgery regularly reports infection rates around 1%, colorectal surgery regularly experiences numbers closer to 10%. One cannot operate in this field without an extensive knowledge of surgical infections. If we are to improve our patient's outcome, we must improve this dimension of care.

Infections account for approximately one million hospital days per year, and add $1.6 billion in direct costs (25). Improving patient outcomes in colon and rectal surgery demands every effort to keep postoperative infections to a minimum. In this section, we discuss SSIs associated with abdominal surgery. Pneumonia and urinary tract infections are dealt with separately. As before, this discussion is broken down into preoperative, intraoperative, and postoperative elements.

One immediate problem is that of defining when SSI occurs. When surgeons use Centers for Disease Control and Prevention criteria to find infection, there is significant interobserver variability (26). In another study, wound photographs were examined to determine infection rates. Experienced surgeons found rates ranging from 6.2% to 14% looking at the same wounds (27). They recommend using the ASEPSIS system for wound evaluation (28). The ASEPSIS score awards points for the presence of exudate, erythema, purulent exudate, tissue separation, treatment with antibiotics, incision and drainage, debridement, and isolation of bacteria to define wound infection (Table 9.1). Using this tool, there was 96% agreement in defining infection (27,29).

SSIs in colorectal surgery also vary by diagnosis. In a National Surgical Quality Improvement Program study of almost 25,000 colorectal operations, Pendlimari et al. found infection rates for colorectal surgery ranging from 8.9% for surgery for benign colon neoplasms to 17% for rectal cancer surgery (30). In this study the rate of organ space infections varied from 2.5%, also for benign colon neoplasms, to 7.7% for ulcerative colitis. Operations involving additional organ resections increase the incidence of SSIs (31).

Patients bring to us not only their colorectal problems, but their other health problems as well. Often these cannot be modified. In the case of urgent surgery, little can be changed. With the luxury of time, patients can be prepared for surgery. Three areas deserve particular attention: glucose control, remote infections, and smoking cessation.

Diabetic patients have a higher rate of SSIs than nondiabetics undergoing colorectal surgery. Ata et al. using National Surgical Quality Improvement Program data from 2005–6, showed rates of 15.4% in diabetics compared to 11% in nondiabetics (32). Improved glucose control results in fewer infectious complications. This can be assessed preoperatively by measuring hemoglobin A1C. If over 8% on preoperative lab testing, it can be improved with several weeks of focused therapy, possibly improving postoperative complications. Postoperative glucose levels should be kept under 140 mg/dL. One mechanism of increased wound infections may be seen at the molecular level, where tissue fluid sampled from surgical wounds showed reduced levels of urokinase-type plasminogen activator as well as its receptor in diabetic patients. Plasminogen helps wound healing by proteolytic degradation of extracellular matrices (33).

Perioperative glycemic control requires modification of regular medications. Glucose should be checked three times a day the day prior to surgery. Clear liquids containing sugar should be avoided. Basal insulin dosage should be reduced by two-thirds on the day prior to surgery. Stop mealtime insulin the day before and the day of the procedure. Patients taking Metformin should continue this the day before and the day of surgery. Those taking sulfonylurea should stop this the day before and the day of the procedure. Patients taking Humulin 70/30 should take one-half their

Table 9.1 ASEPSIS score

| ASEPSIS wound score | | Proportion of wound affected | | | | |
| --- | --- | --- | --- | --- | --- | --- |
| Wound characteristic | 0 | <20 | 20–39 | 40–59 | 60–79 | >80 |
| Serous exudate | 0 | 1 | 2 | 3 | 4 | 5 |
| Erythema | 0 | 1 | 2 | 3 | 4 | 5 |
| Purulent exudate | 0 | 2 | 4 | 6 | 8 | 10 |
| Separation of deep tissues | 0 | 2 | 4 | 6 | 8 | 10 |

Points are scored for daily wound inspection.

| Criterion | Points |
| --- | --- |
| Additional treatment: Antibiotics | 10 |
| Drainage of pus under local anaesthesia | 5 |
| Debridement of wound (general anaesthesia) | 10 |
| Serous discharge* | daily 0–5 |
| Erythema* | daily 0–5 |
| Purulent exudate* | daily 0–10 |
| Separation of deep tissues* | daily 0–10 |
| Isolation of bacteria | 10 |
| Stay as inpatient prolonged over 14 days | 5 |

*Note:* Category of infection: total score 0–10 = satisfactory healing; 11–20 = disturbance ot healing; 20–30 = minor wound infection; 31–40 = moderate wound infection; >40 = severe wound infection.

* Given score only on five of seven days. Highest weekly score used

normal dose the day prior to surgery. Carbohydrate loading as done in many enhanced recovery pathways should not be done in diabetics (34).

Remote infections increase the risk of SSIs and should be resolved prior to surgery, if possible. Particular attention should be paid to skin infection at the site of proposed incisions.

Smoking cessation should be discussed with the patient prior to surgery. This can lower the odds of both pulmonary and wound complications. This should occur at least 4 weeks before surgery (35).

Other factors increasing the incidence of SSIs include obesity, pulmonary comorbidities, obstruction, wound class, abdominoperineal resection, and prolonged operating time (31).

Proper skin preparation lowers the incidence of wound complications. Hair should be clipped rather than shaved, and this should be done the day of surgery. Cleansing with chlorhexidine or soap the evening before surgery and the morning of is helpful. There does not seem to be any difference between chlorhexidine and iodine povacrylex in SSIs following colorectal surgery, or any difference in preps with or without isopropyl alcohol (36).

The topics of mechanical bowel preparation and nonabsorbable oral antibiotics have come almost full circle in the past 40 years. The combination of mechanical bowel prep along with oral neomycin and erythromycin was popularized by Nichols and Condon (37). This combination was shown to reduce wound complications and overall infections from 43% down to 9% (38,39). The concentration of bacteria in the gut was shown to undergo a 4–5 log decrease with oral antibiotics and mechanical bowel preparation

(40). Nevertheless, oral antibiotic use declined. Two factors contributing to this decline were the nausea experienced by some patients with the antibiotics, leading to the substitution of metronidazole for erythromycin, and to the favorable reports of primary repair of traumatic colon wounds using only intravenous antibiotics. This was followed by articles questioning the need for mechanical bowel preparation (41,42). Later studies showed significant improvement in SSIs with the combination of oral and IV antibiotics (43,44). Adding mechanical bowel preparation to IV antibiotics reduces ileus compared to IV antibiotics alone. The addition of oral antibiotics reduces the odds ratio of SSI to 0.39, as well as lowers leak rate and decreases mortality (45). This is the only regimen recommended in the ASCRS Textbook of Colon and Rectal Surgery (46). An additional discussion of bowel preparation was presented in Chapter 2.

Appropriate IV antibiotics should be administered within 1 hour of the skin incision. Repeat dosing may be needed intraoperatively depending on antibiotic chosen and length of surgery. Antibiotic choices include cefazolin plus metronidazole, cefoxitin, levofloxacin plus metronidazole, and ertapenam. The antibiotic should be given within 1 hour of the start of surgery, at which time adequate tissue levels should be present (47,48). There is no benefit to extending IV antibiotics beyond the first 24 hours after surgery.

Intraoperative care is critical to minimizing postoperative infections. Meticulous surgical technique will decrease the chances of leaving behind devitalized tissue. In colorectal surgery, particular care is needed to avoid spillage of bowel contents and converting a clean contaminated wound to a dirty wound. Interestingly, wound contamination does not always correlate with the development of SSI (49). Instruments contaminated should not be reused or replaced on the clean back table. Wound protectors may be helpful (50–52). Results with topical antibiotics applied to the wound are mixed.

Closed suction drains are often used in abdominal surgery in attempts to prevent or control infection. They are appropriately used when draining an abscess. They are inappropriately used in attempts to drain the peritoneal cavity, or to protect an anastomosis. They should be used when ureteral or bladder surgery is performed in conjunction with colon resection. Leaving a drain in the pelvis following pelvic dissection in order to evacuate accumulated blood is reasonable, in which case the drain should be removed when drainage is clear.

Diversion of the fecal stream from a distal anastomosis is commonly used in colorectal surgery in an attempt either to prevent infection or to mitigate damage should infection or anastomotic leak occur. A loop ileostomy is most commonly used. There are wide-ranging opinions regarding the use of diverting ileostomies. They are most favorably viewed when performed at the time of creation of ileal pouch anal anastomosis and coloanal anastomosis. They are commonly used following proctectomy with low pelvic reconstruction. When used in this setting, the height of the anastomosis from the anal verge, previous pelvic irradiation, and technical difficulty of the anastomosis are all factors to be considered in deciding to divert. Operations involving both construction and closure of stomas carry with them an increased risk of wound infection, which must be weighed against the potential benefit of diversion. Of course, stoma closure requires another operation, with additional cost and risk to the patient.

There is some evidence to support glove, gown, and instrument change for wound closure, and this is a common element in treatment bundles intending to reduce SSI. A wound vacuum-assisted closure applied over the closed skin may also reduce superficial wound infections.

Enhanced recovery pathways (ERPs) are covered in Chapter 10 and are mentioned here because they result in reduced risk of SSI, among other benefits (53). The bundling of care elements within a single pathway reduces unwanted variability in patient care. In concert with ERPs, and specifically directed toward reducing infectious complications, many institutions are adding specific SSI bundles of care. While these are not standardized, they share with ERPs a division into preoperative, intraoperative, and postoperative components. Common preoperative components include mechanical bowel prep with oral antibiotics, chlorhexidine skin wipes, patient education, appropriate selection and timing of antibiotics, and standardized catheter placement. Intraoperative elements may include limiting operating room traffic, a separate closing tray, wound protectors, maintenance of body temperature, glove or gown change at closing, and euglycemia. Postoperatively attention remains on euglycemia and normothermia, patient and staff handwashing, wound cleansing with Hibiclens, and dressing removal

within 48 hours (5,54,55). While it is clear that such bundles reduce SSIs, it is not clear which are essential elements (56). Within a given bundle, increasing compliance results in increased effectiveness (57).

Not all care bundles have been effective in reducing SSIs (58). Redraping, rescrubbing, and changing instruments make no difference in infection in the absence of additional elements (59).

Optimal postoperative care can also lessen infectious complications. Maintaining normothermia both before and after surgery is helpful (60).

Oxidative burst function of neutrophils is one of the primary defenses against SSI. As this is so, improving tissue oxygenation should reduce SSIs. Measurement of oxygen saturation at the thenar eminence using near-infrared spectroscopy has been shown to correlate with SSI (61). Results of supplemental oxygen to reduce infections have been mixed. Belda et al. reported a 50% reduction in wound infection rate with increased $FiO_2$ (62). When Kurz et al. randomly assigned patients to either 30% or 80% $FiO_2$ during surgery and for 1 hour following, no change in SSI rate was found (63).

After surgery, the focus evolves from preventing to identifying and treating infectious complications. Organ space infections, anastomotic leaks, superficial wound infections, and enteric infections are of particular importance in colorectal surgery. One tool emerging as possibly useful in predicting postoperative infections is C-reactive protein (CRP). This is an interleukin-6-dependent acute phase protein produced by the liver. It is increased in infections and in inflammatory diseases. Its level is dependent on its synthesis rate and duration of the inflammatory stimulus (64). It has been evaluated as a tool for predicting infections following surgery for colorectal cancer (65). An elevated level on postoperative day 3 (POD3) (greater than 170 mg/L) predicted both increased length of stay and 30-day mortality (65). A separate study showed that CRP elevation on POD4, in this case, 125 mg/L, had a 82% sensitivity for predicting septic complications. Its negative predictive value was 95.8% (66). It may be a useful tool for evaluating patients for early discharge. CRP is a better tool than procalcitonin, another inflammatory marker, in predicting infection after colorectal surgery (67).

Organ space infections are usually evident from 4 to 7 days after surgery and are found when the patient evidences some combination of fever, white blood cell elevation, ileus, and malaise. A computed tomography (CT) scan with oral and IV contrast is the most useful test for identifying these complications, though their usefulness in the first week after surgery is limited due to the inability to distinguish postoperative fluid collections from purulence. Treatment is usually drainage of the abscess by interventional radiology, and antibiotics. Antibiotic choice is initially broad spectrum, with narrowed coverage as culture results are available. Reoperation is necessary when radiologic drainage cannot be performed. This can sometimes be done laparoscopically (68).

Superficial wound infections are common and are usually treated by opening all or part of the wound and with wound care.

Anastomotic leaks are covered in Chapter 8.

*Clostridium difficile* infection (C-Diff) occurs with greater frequency in colorectal surgery than in most other surgical procedures. It occurs in about 2% of patients following colorectal surgery (69). It is more common following emergency procedures, in inflammatory bowel disease, and with increased injury scores. It results in increased complications, increased intensive care unit admissions, increased length of stay, and increased 30-day readmissions. It can progress to fatal colitis, and so it is a risk to the index patient. It is a leading cause of hospital-acquired infections and therefore presents a public health risk as well. C-Diff should be considered in our patients when they have unexplained diarrhea, particularly when accompanied by white blood cell elevation. When suspected, the patient should be placed in contact isolation, and stool studies submitted. Prevention is dependent on proper hygiene to avoid spreading it from patient to patient. Handwashing between patient contacts and wearing gloves during patient exams are critical to containment of this pathogen. Treatment varies with disease severity with metronidazole being the usual first-line treatment, with fidaxomicin or vancomycin for recurrent or persistent disease. Fecal transplant is highly effective and increasingly available.

## POSTOPERATIVE PULMONARY COMPLICATIONS

Postoperative pulmonary complications occur in about one in five patients undergoing abdominal surgery (70). Risk factors include American Society of Anesthesiologists (ASA) II or higher, chronic obstructive pulmonary disease (COPD), congestive heart failure, smoking, dependent functional status, alcohol use, impaired sensorium, weight loss, and sleep apnea.

Pulmonary complications related to COPD may be improved by preoperative antibiotic therapy to treat infection, such as bronchitis, bronchodilator therapy, and glucocorticoids in selected patients (70).

Preoperative assessment should include screening for obstructive sleep apnea. This should be considered in patients who are obese, have metabolic syndrome, or snore (71). Neck circumference greater than 17 inches in men and 15 inches in women is also a risk factor. Patients with sleep apnea have an increased risk of intensive care unit stay after surgery. Continuous positive airway pressure should be used postoperatively in abdominal cases. Consideration should be given for overnight observation in anorectal cases (72).

Smoking clearly increases the risk of postoperative complication, and these can be reduced by smoking cessation prior to surgery. In order to be beneficial, smoking should be stopped at least 4 weeks prior to surgery (35).

Intraoperative measures to reduce postoperative pulmonary complications include short-acting rather than long-acting neuromuscular blockade and local or regional anesthesia. Laparoscopic surgery is accompanied by a decreased incidence of pulmonary complications compared to open surgery (70,72).

Postoperative maneuvers decreasing pulmonary complications include early ambulation and avoidance of nasogastric tubes.

A bundle of steps meant to reduce postoperative pulmonary complications has been developed and can be included in postoperative recovery pathways. This bundle includes early ambulation, deep breathing and incentive spirometry, elevating the head of the bed, protocol-based pain control, and twice daily oral hygiene with chlorhexidine. These steps are reported to reduce postoperative pulmonary complications by 81% (73).

## URINARY TRACT INFECTIONS AND URINARY RETENTION

Catheter-associated urinary tract infection (CAUTI) is considered a preventable infection. The presence of a CAUTI is now used as a negative quality measure, and hospital incidence rates are reportable and are public information. A CAUTI does have negative effects on the patient, as bacteremia, longer hospital stays, and higher mortality have all been associated with CAUTIs. Preoperatively, symptomatic urinary tract infections (UTI) should be addressed and treated. Intraoperative use of catheters is up to the discretion of the surgeon, but most anorectal cases do not require catheterization. The modifiable risk factor most closely related to CAUTI is length of catheterization. While it is unclear if prolonged catheterization is a cause of CAUTI, the presence of a catheter for more than 2 days is associated with increased rates of UTI. Emphasis on early removal of urinary catheters has decreased this occurrence. Implementation of ERAS and an SSI bundle, which includes removal of the catheter by POD2 has decreased UTI rates from 7.4% to 2.8% (5). Most patients can have the catheter removed in less than 24 hours, but as pelvic surgeries have a higher rate of postoperative urinary dysfunction, it is acceptable to leave the catheter in until POD2 or POD3.

The downside of early catheter removal is the risk of postoperative urinary retention. The rate of urinary retention for colon surgery is 2%–5%; however, this increases to 24%, and in some reports as high as 41%, when referring to rectal or pelvic surgery (74,75). Anorectal surgery also carries a risk of urinary retention of 17% (76). Other risk factors include older age, male sex, lung disease, low rectal cancers, additional pelvic procedures, increased operative time, and poor pain control (74–76). One goal of surgeons should be to decrease the risk of urinary retention, which will prevent repeated catheterization and prolonged catheterization, thus decreasing the risk for CAUTI (74,75). This starts preoperatively and is carried through the operative and postoperative recovery by minimizing the volume of perioperative fluid administration; this has been shown to lower the risk of urinary retention (74). This holds true for both anorectal and abdominal surgeries. Larger amounts of fluid resuscitation may correspond to increased bladder distention that results in poor contractility of the detrusor and is followed by retention (77).

## RETAINED SURGICAL ITEMS

Many resources and brainstorming have been used to help keep surgical items from being retained in our patients. This event is uncommon, occurring 1:8,801 but is still a source of anxiety for all surgeons (78). The risk is not equal in every case. Acknowledging and being aware of the cases that are higher risk for retained foreign bodies can be the first step in prevention. These risk factors are obesity, emergency surgery, changes in the planned surgery, multiple surgical teams being involved in the case, and both increased surgical time and increased blood loss (78,79). Sponges are the most commonly retained surgical item and thus garnish the majority of the attention. The abdominal cavity is the operative site where most incidences of retained foreign bodies occur (78,80).

Intraoperative prevention takes active participation of the surgical teams and system policies focused on this potential complication. Surgeon-specific practices to prevent leaving a sponge in a wound are to avoid using smaller Ray-Tecs; in large open cases, placing hemostats on the sponge; not using radiolucent objects; audibly saying "lap in" and "lap out" to keep the team accountable; and doing one more exploration of the abdominal cavity before the final closure. An instrument and sponge count should be completed before the fascia is closed. The surgical count, which should be done before the case starts, at close of fascia, at close of skin, and anytime there is personnel change, should be documented and communicated to the whole team. Ideally, those performing the counting should be afforded the utmost concentration to avoid distraction.

It is important to remember that a correct surgical count does not guarantee that no instruments were left behind, and the surgeon must always be vigilant to the possibility of leaving an object behind. In fact, up to 87% of cases with retained surgical objects occur with correct counts (79,81). If the count is wrong, several steps can help to look for the missing object. Be sure to check the trash, the floor, and of course the surgical field. Magnetic rollers can be used to pick small needles off the floor. Intraoperative x-rays can be used to visualize the abdominal cavity for any radiopaque objects left behind (Figures 9.2 through 9.4). Many hospitals have policies in place that these closing x-rays must be done for high-risk cases, such as incorrect count, two surgical teams operating, morbidly obese patients, and patients returning to the operating room with an open abdomen. Some hospitals have obtained other devices to help mitigate

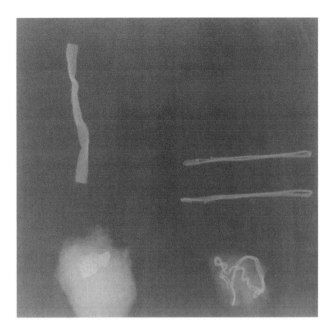

Figure 9.2 Radiograph demonstrating radiopaque markers. Left to right. Laparotomy sponge, Ray-Tec sponge. The upper image is flattened, whereas the lower image demonstrates the radiologic view when the item is crumpled.

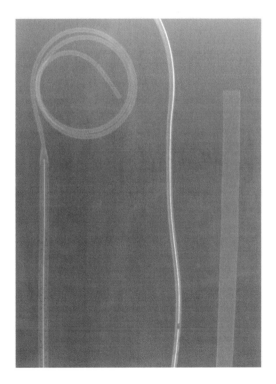

Figure 9.3 Radiograph of (left to right) Jackson-Pratt drain, Penrose drain, nasogastric tube.

this problem, such as radiofrequency scanners and barcoded sponges.

Retained surgical instruments can be devastating for the patient. These foreign bodies can be found incidentally on subsequent imaging or during investigation for infectious

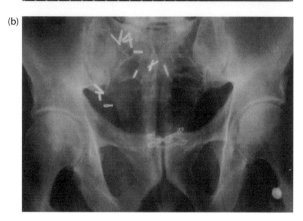

Figure 9.4 **(a)** CT scan of patient with a retained Ray-Tec sponge. Image is the inferior cut of the study. The upper edge of the Ray-Tec marker is demonstrated as white dotted lines between the bladder (filled with contrast) and the sacrum. **(b)** Pelvic radiograph of the same patient demonstrating Ray-Tec marker in pelvis.

or inflammatory symptoms. Finding this on imaging generally mandates surgical exploration to remove the objects, though it is thought that some small needles may be left. This does carry significant morbidity to the patient. These events are costly to the health-care system as well, with estimates that each incident costs over $200,000 in medical and liability costs (81). With ample attention, retained surgical instruments should truly be a never event.

## INJURY TO NORMAL ORGANS

Potential injury to normal organs is a common section in obtaining informed consent. Particular areas of importance in colorectal surgery are the ureters, spleen, and pelvic nerves (82).

Ureteral injury, as sustained in our challenging patient previously described, is reported to occur in 0.2% of colorectal resections (83). Our goal is to reduce the incidence of this complication as much as possible. Preoperative imaging is almost always done prior to surgery for both malignant and benign indications. Reviewing these studies prior

to surgery may also provide helpful information about ureteral anatomy. The ureters may be displaced due to previous surgery, tumor, or inflammation. The collecting system may be duplicated, or hydroureter may be present. Each of these should be known prior to surgery. Consideration should be given to placement of ureteral catheters in selected cases. While not shown to reduce the incidence of injury, they may be useful guides to dissection and may facilitate identification of ureteral injury.

When ureteral injury is suspected, methylene blue can be administered to allow easier visualization of a urine leak. The most important thing one can do to improve surgical outcomes when ureteral injury occurs is to recognize that injury has occurred. When detected postoperatively, repair requires additional surgery. Repair primarily over double-J stent, if possible. For distal injuries, ureteroneocystostomy may be required. Urology consultation should be obtained.

Ureteral injury identified postoperatively is usually evidenced by some combination of oliguria, abdominal distension, excessive drain output, or serum creatinine elevation. When injury is suspected, a CT scan with IV contrast can either demonstrate ureteral integrity or reveal the site of injury. Management depends on site of injury. Stent placement, either retrograde or prograde, can occasionally be used for injuries other than transection. Reoperation with either primary repair or reimplantation is the most common treatment. Less common treatments are intestinal interposition and crossed ureteroureterostomy. Urinary diversion with percutaneous nephrostomy is appropriate if, for some reason, immediate repair cannot be undertaken. Additional information on urologic injuries and their management is presented in Chapter 41.

Splenic injury has been mentioned earlier under bleeding complications. It is less likely to occur in laparoscopic cases compared to open (84) but deserves particular mention due to its occasional occurrence during colonoscopy. Injury is almost never detected during the procedure. Symptoms can range from left upper quadrant pain from capsular tears to hypotension and shock for severe injuries. Patients should be advised after colonoscopy to call if abdominal pain occurs. Evaluation should include exam, vital signs, and hemoglobin. CT should be performed if injury is suspected. Management is as usual for splenic injury.

Injury to pelvic splanchnic nerves often occurs with pelvic surgery and should be discussed with the patient if rectal dissection is contemplated. Meticulous sharp dissection will decrease injury to the nerves. Symptoms of injury include urinary retention and alteration of sexual function, particularly in males.

## DEEP VEIN THROMBOSIS

Sudden postoperative death from pulmonary embolism is a dramatic and memorable event. This can be seen after an uneventful course in a patient ready to go home. Years later we see patients wearing compressive stockings to control the swelling from postphlebitic syndrome. Each of these are sequelae from DVT, a complication our patients are at particular risk of sustaining. Virchow triad defines thrombotic events as associated with stasis, hypercoagulability, and endothelial damage.

The incidence of DVT in colorectal surgery patients is 1.2%. Pulmonary embolus occurs in 0.7% of patients undergoing colorectal surgery. Of these, 40% are diagnosed within the first week after surgery. About one-third are diagnosed after discharge. DVT prolongs length of stay from 6 days to 17 days. It is more common in open than in laparoscopic surgery, and with longer operations (85). In patients undergoing surgery for cancer, the venous thromboembolism (VTE) risk is between 2.4% and 3.4% (86).

DVT is increased in prolonged surgery, pelvic surgery, surgery for inflammatory conditions, and malignancy. Most of our patients have one or more of these characteristics. In addition, our patients may have the added risk factors of immobility, COPD, sepsis, anemia, and hypoalbuminemia. The Caprini VTE risk scoring system is a tool for assessing VTE risk (87). It assigns points for the above risk factors, and others. A score greater than or equal to five defines a high-risk patient. This number is reached with a 45-year-old patient with no other risk factors who undergoes a laparoscopic partial colectomy of more than 45-minutes duration. Low-risk patients have a very low risk of VTE (88). In short, colorectal patients undergoing major surgery are at significant risk of DVT. Improving outcomes requires minimizing the incidence of DVT as well as its recognition and management.

We should recognize that we deal with patients at high risk of DVT. Many risk factors our patients share cannot be changed. We can reduce the incidence of DVT by appropriate prophylaxis and early ambulation. Prophylaxis in high-risk patients may be either unfractionated heparin, low molecular weight heparin, or fondaparinux (87,89). All patients undergoing abdominal surgery should have compression stockings and/or prophylaxis. There has been debate regarding the timing of the first dose of heparin, with concern raised about increased risk of intraoperative bleeding if given prior to surgery. The bleeding risk associated with preoperative dosing is low and should not prevent its use in high-risk patients. Compression stockings should be continued until the patient is fully ambulatory. Recent data support the continued usage of heparin (or enoxaparin) for 1 month after discharge in patients with either cancer or inflammatory bowel disease. Antiplatelet therapy reduces the risk of recurrent thromboembolism (90).

One difficulty with DVT is detection, as symptoms may be minimal. Leg swelling and calf tenderness are signs of DVT. Duplex study of the lower extremity should be done when DVT is suspected. Pulmonary embolism (PE) should be suspected in patients with shortness of breath, hypoxia, hypotension, or tachycardia. When suspected, CT angiography is indicated.

Treatment for DVT and pulmonary embolism is anticoagulation. Timing depends on degree of suspicion and imaging availability. If there is a high degree of suspicion, begin parenteral anticoagulation while awaiting confirmation of DVT. For intermediate suspicion, withhold anticoagulation until imaging, if that can be accomplished within 4 hours. If the degree of suspicion is low, withhold anticoagulation if imaging will be done in 24 hours or less (91). This is usually initiated with heparin. Vena cava filter placement should be considered in patients having massive emboli (in whom additional emboli could be fatal) or in patients in whom anticoagulation is contraindicated. Duration of treatment is dependent on the patient's other medical problems but is generally for 6 months.

A related topic is that of dealing with the patient already anticoagulated and needing either surgery or colonoscopy. In general, reversal of anticoagulation before either surgery or colonoscopy is indicated. In high-risk patients, enoxaparin is substituted prior to surgery and then held the day of surgery. Patients on low-dose aspirin do not need to hold this prior to colonoscopy.

Portomesenteric venous thrombosis occasionally follows colorectal surgery. It is usually detected on CT and is treated with anticoagulation. It is more common in younger patients, the obese, and following restorative proctocolectomy. It is also more prevalent in patients with ulcerative colitis, or with postoperative thrombocytosis (92).

## NAUSEA AND VOMITING

Immediately following anesthesia up to 30% of patients will experience troublesome nausea and vomiting that can greatly influence their initial recovery (93). The biggest predictor of this problem is the presence of a history of postanesthesia nausea and vomiting. Many factors, including surgical trauma, influence this occurrence. Routine placement of a nasogastric tube does not mitigate this nausea and is not recommended. Total IV anesthesia and avoidance of inhaled anesthetic agents reduces postoperative nausea and vomiting (94). The most headway in this subject has been with prophylactically administering antiemetics to decrease this unpleasant side effect. Ondansetron can decrease postoperative nausea when given before induction of anesthesia (95). Dexamethasone, as a preemptive agent, has reduced postoperative nausea and vomiting in multiple randomized clinical trials (95,96). Dexamethasone and ondansetron can be used together with potentially synergistic effects (93). Gabapentin is a common element of enhanced recovery pathways due to its role in lessening narcotic usage, but it also has an antiemetic effect (97).

## ILEUS

Traditionally, bowel function was expected to return around POD3 for laparoscopic surgery and POD5 for open surgery.

More recent experience has demonstrated that bowel function may be retained in some patients, especially when components of ERAS are adopted. Ileus occurs when there is failure of bowel peristalsis by an expected amount of time. Patients will have distention, inability to tolerate intake by mouth, abdominal discomfort, and nausea and vomiting. Return of bowel function is often the limiting factor in hospital discharge. Many ERAS elements are directed toward the goal of restoring and preserving gastrointestinal motility. Nevertheless, postoperative ileus occurs 3%–32% of the time following colorectal surgery (98).

Risk factors are inconsistently identified across studies but likely include older age, male patients, malnutrition, increased body mass index, larger wound size, increased opioid consumption, and increased blood loss or need for blood transfusion (3,98,99). Prevention should focus on optimizing the modifiable risk factors when the luxury of elective surgery presents itself.

Ileus can be influenced by the extent of surgical trauma; thus, intraoperative prevention involves use of minimally invasive surgery when possible, and gentle handling of tissues to minimize surgical stress. Intraoperative normothermia may also help. Limiting IV fluids preoperatively can prevent ileus, as higher amounts of fluid have been linked to postoperative ileus (99), likely by causing increased bowel edema.

Mitigating the effects of opioids by use of preemptive and multimodal pain control will again be vital to preventing yet another complication (3). Early mobilization is traditionally felt to be important in stimulating bowel function. Early postoperative feeding decreases time to return of bowel function and decreases postoperative ileus. Sham feeding with gum will help to stimulate the autonomic reflexes to produce bowel motility (100). However, in a randomized controlled trial, this utility lost its effect in patients who were fed early (101). Alvimopan, a peripheral mu-opioid antagonist, can be given immediately preoperative and scheduled postoperative to decrease the incidence of ileus. Other prokinetic agents have also been used with less success in colorectal surgery than in upper gastrointestinal surgery, such as metoclopramide and methylnaltrexone.

When symptoms persist for more than 5–7 days, a possible etiology should be thoroughly sought. Postoperative complications, particularly infection, can cause paralysis of the intestine. Dehydration, UTIs, pneumonia, and intraabdominal abscess are often identifiable causes of ileus. Other considerations are adhesions and strictures causing mechanical obstruction (102). Treating the underlying causes, intravenous fluid (IVF), nasogastric tube decompression, and patience are the mainstays of treatment.

## TIME OUT AND WRONG SITE SURGERY

We are obliged to pause before beginning any invasive procedure and confirm the patient, proposed procedure, administration of antibiotics, and any particular needs unique to the case. This is the ideal time to ensure all needed materials are available. Confirm availability about needed staplers, suture, stoma appliances, etc. A preoperative protocol including time out reduces the incidence of wrong site surgery (103). The addition of a preoperative check list is associated with decreased mortality as well (104). Asking early will prevent waiting later. Preoperative history, consent, and imaging should be concordant, or discrepancies reconciled.

One area unique to colorectal surgery is localization of neoplasia. When the lesion is in the right colon, this is rarely a problem. Rectal lesions are sometimes found at surgery not to be where anticipated. This is more likely to occur when the endoscopy was not performed by the operating surgeon. A lesion in the rectum thought to be in the sigmoid raises obvious problems. This situation can be avoided by always performing a proctoscope exam on patients prior to going to the operating room. Lesions between the rectum and hepatic flexure can also present problems with localization. This is particularly so with large benign polyps, which may not be palpable, and in minimal access surgery, where palpation is not easily done. Tattooing can be used to help localize the lesion intraoperatively, though this is less helpful with rectal lesions (105). Another tool that is useful in rectal lesions is preoperative endoscopic injection of indocyanine green just distal to the lesion. SPY Fluorescence Imaging System or Firefly illumination can then help localize the lesion and define the site of division (106). Lesions can also be marked with a clip at the time of colonoscopy. A abdominal x-ray can then clearly demonstrate the location of the lesion. This is particularly helpful in villous lesion and in minimal access surgery.

## FUTURE DIRECTIONS

Enhanced recovery pathways provide a framework within which we describe our plan for patient care. The pathways contain many specific elements, and the framework enhances the probability of each patient receiving the intended optimal care. Our task is to refine the pathway and then to comply with pathway elements. As many are fairly well established, they need only be applied. Our patient's outcome will improve to the extent we provide to each patient the care we intend for all. By lessening unintended and nonbeneficial variation in care, we can expect our patients to do better. Internal audits within our hospitals are necessary to ensure we are actually doing that which we intend for our patients.

## CONCLUSION

Improving outcomes remains our perpetual goal. Choosing measurements to define improvement is more difficult. We frequently use length of stay as a measure, assuming that reduced length of stay while holding the line on emergency room return and readmission is an improvement in outcome. We also use return to normal activities as a definition of recovery with earlier return being synonymous with improved outcome. One measure of recovery in oncology patients is the time recovery has progressed to allow chemotherapy to be administered. By this standard, recovery after laparoscopic surgery is significantly improved over open surgery. Return to intended oncologic treatment has been promoted as a measurement of recovery most important to the patient (107). However defined, to obtain the best outcome for our patients, we need to be thoughtful in our approach, uniform in our intent, and meticulous in our technique. We must look to ourselves for technique, to our hospitals for adherence to our planned care, and to our surgical community for continual refinement of the care plan we intend to follow.

## REFERENCES

1. Keller DS et al. *Surg Endosc* 2014;28(1):74–9.
2. Chand M et al. *Int J Surg* 2016;25:59–63.
3. Barletta JF et al. *Ann Pharmacother* 2011;45(7–8): 916–23.
4. Wick EC et al. *JAMA Surg* 2017;152(7):691–7.
5. Keenan JE et al. *J Am Coll Surg* 2015;221(2): 404–14.e1.
6. Miller TE et al. Enhanced Recovery Study Group. *Anesth Analg* 2014;118(5):1052–61.
7. Roulin D et al. *Br J Surg* 2013;100(8):1108–14.
8. Gobble RM et al. *Plast Reconstr Surg* 2014;133(3): 741–55.
9. Zittel TT et al. *Dis Colon Rectum* 2013;56(6):761–7.
10. Hakkarainen TW et al. *JAMA Surg* 2015;150(3):223–8.
11. Mishriky BM et al. *Br J Anaesth* 2015;114(1):10–31.
12. Cavalcante AN et al. *Anesth Analg* 2017;125(1):141–6.
13. Chestovich PJ et al. *Surg Clin North Am* 2013;93(1): 21–32.
14. Herroeder S et al. *Ann Surg* 2007;246(2):192–200. Erratum in: *Ann Surg* 2009;249(4):701. Dijkgraaf, Omarcel G W [corrected to Dijkgraaf, Marcel G W].
15. Ahn E et al. *Int Surg* 2015;100(3):394–401.
16. Khan JS et al. *J Clin Anesth* 2016;28:95–104.
17. Jouve P et al. *Anesthesiology* 2013;118(3):622–30.
18. Hübner M et al. *Ann Surg* 2015;261(4):648–53.
19. Keller DS et al. *J Am Coll Surg* 2014;219(6):1143–8.
20. Favuzza J et al. *Surg Endosc* 2013;27(7):2481–6.
21. Bell RF et al. *Cochrane Database Syst Rev* 2006;(1): CD004603. Review. Update in: *Cochrane Database Syst Rev* 2015;7:CD004603.
22. Zhu J et al. *Int J Surg* 2018;49:1–9.
23. Johansson PI et al. *Blood* 2014;124(20):3052–8.
24. Halabi WJ et al. *Am J Surg* 2013;206(6):1024–32; discussion 1032–3.
25. de Lissovoy G et al. *Am J Infect Control* 2009;37(5): 387–97.
26. Hedrick TL et al. *Surg Infect (Larchmt)* 2014;15(4): 372–6.
27. Hedrick TL et al. *Dis Colon Rectum* 2015;58(11): 1070–7.
28. Underwood P et al. *Diabetes Care* 2014;37(3):611–6.
29. Wilson AP et al. *J Hosp Infect* 1990;16(4):297–309.
30. Pendlimari R et al. *J Am Coll Surg* 2012;214(4):574–80; discussion 580–1.
31. Kwaan MR et al. *Surg Infect (Larchmt)* 2015;16(6): 675–83.
32. Ata A et al. *Am Surg* 2010;76(7):697–702.
33. Akinci B et al. *J Diabetes Complications* 2014;28(6): 844–9.
34. Thompson RE et al. *Curr Diab Rep* 2016;16(3):32.
35. Mills E et al. *Am J Med* 2011;124(2):144–154.e8.
36. Kaoutzanis C et al. *Dis Colon Rectum* 2015;58(6): 588–96.
37. Nichols RL, Condon RE. *Surg Gynecol Obstet* 1971; 132(2):323–37.
38. Goldring J et al. *Lancet* 1975;2(7943):997–1000.
39. Clarke JS et al. *Ann Surg* 1977;186(3):251–9.
40. Bartlett JG et al. *Ann Surg* 1978;188(2):249–54.
41. Pineda CE et al. *J Gastrointest Surg* 2008;12(11): 2037–44.
42. Gravante G et al. *Int J Colorectal Dis* 2008;23(12): 1145–50.
43. Fry DE. *Surg Infect (Larchmt)* 2008;9(6):547–52.
44. Bellows CF et al. *Tech Coloproctol* 2011;15(4):385–95.
45. Kiran RP et al. *Ann Surg* 2015;262(3):416–25. discussion 423–5.
46. Steele SR et al. *The ASCRS Textbook of Colon and Rectal Surgery.* 3rd edition, New York: Springer International Publishing, 2016.
47. Wilson SE et al. *Surg Infect (Larchmt)* 2008;9(3): 349–56.
48. Ho VP et al. *Surg Infect (Larchmt)* 2011;12(4):255–60.
49. Lauscher JC et al. *Langenbecks Arch Surg* 2012; 397(7):1079–85.
50. Cheng KP et al. *Colorectal Dis* 2012;14(6):e346–51.
51. Edwards JP et al. *Ann Surg* 2012;256(1):53–9.
52. Baier P et al. *Int J Colorectal Dis* 2012;27(9):1223–8.
53. Thiele RH et al. *J Am Coll Surg* 2015;220(4):430–43.
54. Cima R et al. *J Am Coll Surg* 2013;216(1):23–33.
55. Wick E et al. *J Am Coll Surg* 2012;215(2):193–200.
56. Keenan JE et al. *JAMA Surg* 2014;149(10):1045–52.
57. Waits SA et al. *Surgery* 2014;155(4):602–6.
58. Anthony T et al. *Arch Surg* 2011;146(3):263–9.
59. Ortiz H et al. *Arch Surg* 2012;147(7):614–20.
60. Wong PF et al. *Br J Surg* 2007;94(4):421–6.
61. Govinda R et al. *Anesth Analg* 2010;111(4):946–52.
62. Belda FJ et al. Spanish Reduccion de la Tasa de Infeccion Quirurgica Group. *JAMA* 2005;294(16):2035–42. Erratum in: JAMA 2005 December 21;294(23):2973.
63. Kurz A et al. *Br J Anaesth* 2015;115(3):434–43.
64. Guirao X et al. *Surg Infect (Larchmt)* 2013;14(2): 209–15.

65. Platt JJ et al. *Ann Surg Oncol* 2012;19(13):4168–77.
66. Ortega-Deballon P et al. *World J Surg* 2010;34(4): 808–14.
67. Facy O et al. *Ann Surg* 2016;263(5):961–6.
68. Vennix S et al. *J Laparoendosc Adv Surg Tech A* 2013; 23(9):739–44.
69. Aquina CT et al. *Dis Colon Rectum* 2016;59(4):323–31.
70. Sachdev G, Napolitano LM. *Surg Clin North Am* 2012;92(2):321–44, ix.
71. Kaw R et al. *Br J Anaesth* 2012;109(6):897–906.
72. American Society of Anesthesiologists Task Force on Perioperative Management of patients with obstructive sleep apnea. *Anesthesiology* 2014;120(2): 268–86.
73. Wren SM et al. *J Am Coll Surg* 2010;210(4):491–5.
74. Kin C et al. *Dis Colon Rectum* 2013;56(6):738–46.
75. Changchien CR et al. *Dis Colon Rectum* 2007;50(10): 1688–96.
76. Toyonaga T et al. *Int J Colorectal Dis* 2006;21(7): 676–82.
77. Joelsson-Alm E et al. *Scand J Urol Nephrol* 2009; 43(1):58–62.
78. Gawande AA et al. *N Engl J Med* 2003;348(3):229–35.
79. Lincourt AE et al. *J Surg Res* 2007;138(2):170–4.
80. Cima RR et al. *J Am Coll Surg* 2008;207(1):80–7.
81. Regenbogen SE et al. *Surgery* 2009;145(5):527–35.
82. Kaafarani HM et al. *J Am Coll Surg* 2011;212(6): 924–34.
83. Halabi WJ et al. *Dis Colon Rectum* 2014;57(2):179–86.
84. Isik O et al. *Surg Endosc* 2015;29(5):1039–44.
85. Moghadamyeghaneh Z et al. *J Gastrointest Surg* 2014;18(12):2169–77.
86. De Martino RR et al. *J Vasc Surg* 2012;55(4):1035–1040.e4.
87. Gould MK et al. *Chest* 2012;141(2 Suppl):e227S–e277S. Erratum in: *Chest* 2012 May;141(5):1369.
88. Qadan M et al. *Ann Surg* 2011;253(2):215–20.
89. Khorana AA. *Oncologist* 2007;12(11):1361–70.
90. Coleman DM et al. *Curr Probl Surg* 2015;52(6): 233–59.
91. Kearon C et al. *Chest* 2016;149(2):315–52.
92. Robinson KA et al. *Surg Endosc* 2015;29(5):1071–9.
93. López-Olaondo L et al. *Br J Anaest* 1996;76(6): 835–40.
94. Habib AS et al. *Anesth Analg* 2004;99(1):77–81.
95. Gan TJ et al. Department of Anesthesiology, Duke University Medical Center. *Anesth Analg* 2003;97(1):62–71, table of contents.
96. Henzi I et al. *Anesth Analg* 2000;90(1):186–94.
97. Achuthan S et al. *Br J Anaesth* 2015;114(4):588–97.
98. Vather R, Bissett IP. *Int J Colorectal Dis* 2013;28(10): 1385–91.
99. Vather R et al. *Surgery* 2015;157(4):764–73.
100. Parnaby CN et al. *Int J Colorectal Dis* 2009;24(5): 585–92.
101. Lim P et al. *Ann Surg* 2013;257(6):1016–24.
102. Masoomi H et al. *J Am Coll Surg* 2012;214(5):831–7.
103. Algie CM et al. *Cochrane Database Syst Rev* 2015;(3): CD009404.
104. Haynes AB et al. *Ann Surg* 2017;266(6):923–9.
105. Conaghan PJ et al. *Colorectal Dis* 2011;13(10):1184–7.
106. Handgraaf HJ et al. *Minim Invasive Ther Allied Technol* 2016;25(1):48–53.
107. Aloia TA et al. *J Surg Oncol* 2014;110(2):107–14.

# 10

# Care paths and optimal postoperative management

## BENJAMIN D. SHOGAN AND HEIDI K. CHUA

### INTRODUCTION TO CARE PATHS

Care paths refer to evidence-based structured multidisciplinary protocols allowing patients to progress through a set pathway until discharge criteria are met. Care paths originated in the 1990s based on emerging evidence on the optimization of perioperative surgical care (1). Originally popular in Europe, they have rapidly spread and are increasingly becoming the standard of care across the globe.

Many synonyms exist for care paths: fast-track protocols, enhanced recovery after surgery (ERAS), integrated pathways, multidisciplinary pathways of care, and care maps all represent different flavors of care paths. Although there are no definitions that define a certain care path, specific specialties tend to use distinctive verbiage. For example, ERAS is generally used in reference to colorectal or gastrointestinal surgery, whereas care maps are often used in nursing or cardiac procedures. Regardless, for the purposes of this review, despite the name used in the literature we consider all care paths similar. In clinical practice, the actual name that defines the pathway is of little importance in comparison to the elements that make up the protocol.

All care paths have four common elements: timeline, categories of care and interventions, discharge criteria, and compliance recording. A timeline allows each patient to undergo the specific intervention on a consistent schedule. Categories of care include preoperative, intraoperative, and postoperative interventions. Different interventions have been described for each phase of care, and they may be hospital specific and dependent on hospital resources, patient demographics, and institutional footprint (Table 10.1). Discharge criteria are a set of milestones each patient must achieve prior to hospital dismissal. Developing predetermined criteria for discharge allows for consistency across multiple providers. Importantly, discharge criteria do not need to differ compared to those used for conventional postoperative care (1). Last, protocol compliance recording is an undervalued but necessary component of care. Although care paths are made up in part by clinical guidelines or algorithms, care paths significantly differ as they are used in a multidisciplinary fashion over the entire spectrum of all phases of care. Prospective data recording of each element of the care path allows for analysis of compliance, efficiency, and outcomes. This allows care paths to continually evolve and improve patient care over time, whereas algorithms remain static.

### BENEFITS OF CARE PATHS

The goals in development of care paths are decreased postoperative complications and sooner return of bowel function to promote a safe earlier hospital discharge without readmission. Multiple randomized control trials have supported these outcomes. Zhuang et al. published the results of a meta-analysis and systematic review on 13 randomized controlled trials comparing enhanced recovery protocols with traditional care in elective colorectal surgery. They reported that enhanced recovery was significantly associated with a decrease in primary hospital stay ($-2.44$ days; $p < 0.0001$), total hospital stay ($-2.39$ days; $p = 0.0003$), and total complications (relative risk [RR] $0.71$; $p = 0.00006$). There was no difference in readmissions, surgical complications, or mortality (2). A consequence of early discharge is hospital and patient cost. Pritts et al. reported that nearly \$7,000 was saved for every patient undergoing a small or large bowel resection after a care path was implemented compared with those who underwent a traditional postoperative protocol (3).

Care path protocols not only affect length of stay, but also have been shown to be associated with decreased postoperative complications. A recent meta-analysis and systematic review of randomized trials of ERAS or FTS protocols focusing on health care–associated infections was recently

Table 10.1 Components of a colorectal surgery care path

| Preoperative | Intraoperative | Postoperative |
|---|---|---|
| Patient education | Fluid management | Ambulation |
| Optimizing overall health | Minimally invasive | Oral intake/ nutrition |
| Nutritional assessment | Temperature control | Fluid management |
| Labs/x-rays/tests | Drain usage | Pain management |
| Bowel preparation | Pain management | Discharge criteria |
| Reduction of fasting state and/or nutritional supplementation | | |
| Pain management | | |

published (4). Compiling data from nearly 4,200 patients, these authors reported that compared to conventional controls, ERAS/fast-track surgery (FTS) was associated with a significant reduction in postoperative lung infections (RR 0.38), urinary tract infections (RR 0.42), and surgical site infections (RR 0.75).

Why care paths are associated with better outcomes remains to be defined but is certainly multifactorial. Teamwork is a critical component of any care path protocol, and establishing a successful program requires buy-in from a diverse multidisciplinary team. Development and implementation of care path thus creates a culture of teamwork and safety that is independently associated with better patient outcomes (5,6).

Emerging evidence has shown that care path protocols may play a role in decreasing systemic stress and inflammation (7). In a prospectively collected cohort of patients undergoing both open and laparoscopic colon resection, patient care paths inhibited release of postoperative inflammatory mediators, therefore playing a protective role on the immune system (8). Further investigation is needed to determine if decreased systemic inflammation is the underlying cause of improved outcomes in care path protocols. Studies attempting to delineate which parts of the protocol are responsible for the blunted immune response are needed.

## ELEMENTS OF CARE PATHS

Implementing an enhanced recovery protocol can be extremely daunting and often meet with resistance. Many of the aspects of enhanced recovery may be novel to some practitioners and in some instances directly counter current practice. We suggest an evidenced-based approach, explaining the rationale behind the concept of enhanced recovery

and the benefit of each individual component, allowing each discipline to contribute ideas specific to their specialty.

Health-care elements combine to form care paths. Separately, each element can have positive effects on patient outcomes, but when combined into a care path the impact can be dramatic (9). It is not critical for every intervention in the care path to have a beneficial impact. Polle et al. showed that despite patients only completing an average of 7.4 of 13 predefined fast-track modalities, the fast-track pathway still had a significant positive impact on length of stay and patient satisfaction (10). Even though the optimal arrangement of elements to be included is yet to be fully elucidated, we suggest that an optimal care path include elements that cross all phases of care. As stated earlier, the number and type of interventions used within a care path will be hospital specific and determined by local factors, such as hospital resources, specialties present within the health-care system, and the recommendations of the local multidisciplinary team (Table 10.1). In the following sections, we discuss the most common interventions within a care path (Table 10.2).

## PATIENT EDUCATION

We begin patient education during the preoperative clinic. The concept of care paths should be explained to the patient. Carli et al. investigated the effects of preoperative education and counseling on patients undergoing laparoscopic colorectal surgery (11). During a clinic visit, patients were informed of milestone setting, multimodality analgesia, early postoperative oral intake, early mobilization, and expected discharge on postoperative day three. Although

Table 10.2 Current enhanced recovery protocol at Mayo Clinic

**Preoperative**
- Education with surgeon and ostomy nurse
- Mechanical bowel prep with oral neomycin and metronidazole
- Gabapentin 600 mg

**Intraoperative**
- Intrathecal opioid injection at discretion of anesthesiologist
- Net even fluid balance

**Postoperative**
- Early ambulation
- Low-residue diet starting immediately after surgery
- Intravenous ketorolac scheduled for 24 hours transitioned to oral ibuprofen
- Oral oxycodone as needed
- Rate of 40 mL/h then saline lock at 8 a.m. on morning after surgery
- Foley catheter removed at 8 a.m. on morning after surgery
- 400 mg magnesium oxide twice per day for 3 days starting on postoperative day 1

we cannot conclude that it was directly related to education, the authors reported that 95% of patients could be discharged within the fourth postoperative day.

Preoperative ostomy teaching is mandatory. For all patients undergoing surgery where creation of an ostomy is a possibility, a preoperative visit by a certified wound, ostomy, and continence (WOC) nurse is necessary. The preoperative visit should not be limited to those undergoing permanent ostomy, as many ostomies thought to be temporary at the time of creation are never reversed. During the visit with the WOC nurse, expectations of life with an ostomy are delineated as well as care and troubleshooting. Further, the WOC nurse marks the patient for the optimal stoma placement based on body habitus and patient flexibility. Preoperative visits with a certified WOC compared to other health-care providers are associated with a significantly higher postoperative quality of life (12,13).

## FEEDING: PREOPERATIVE CARBOHYDRATE TREATMENT AND EARLY FEEDING

Preoperative fasting is the standard of care to prevent aspiration during general anesthesia and endotracheal intubation. Recently, it has been shown that postoperative insulin resistance induces postoperative hyperglycemia that is associated with overall complications, wound healing complications, and increased length of stay, calling the long-standing "NPO after midnight" into question (14,15). To combat postoperative insulin resistance, practitioners have begun to explore the use of preoperative administration of oral or IV high-dose carbohydrates instead of a conventional preoperative fast. In 15 randomized patients, insulin resistance was better maintained in patients given a preoperative carbohydrate-rich drink (16). Noblett et al. randomized 36 patients to three groups: group 1 underwent conventional fasting, group 2 was given preoperative water, and group 3 was given a high-carbohydrate drink (96 grams carbohydrate) the night before and then again 3 hours prior to elective colorectal surgery (17). Results showed that the carbohydrate group had a significantly lower length of stay (mean 7.5 days; $p < 0.01$) compared to the water group (mean 13 days) or the fasting group (10). Time to first flatus, bowel movement, and complication rate was similar between the three cohorts. Thus, it is unclear the reason for the delayed discharge in the no-carbohydrate cohorts. Interestingly, in the fasting group, grip strength was significantly decreased compared to preoperative values, whereas there was no significant difference in the carbohydrate or water group.

A Cochrane Review of 1,976 patients in 27 trials comparing preoperative carbohydrate treatment (at least 45 grams of carbohydrate) to placebo or fasting in elective surgery was recently performed (18). The authors noted that there was a very small but significant reduction in length of stay (0.30 days, 95% confidence interval [CI] 0.56–0.04) with no significant change in the incidence of aspiration or postoperative complications. The authors did comment that lack of blinding in the majority of included studies significantly limited their conclusion. Together, their remains only limited evidence to suggest that preoperative carbohydrate loading is a critical part of a care path.

The time to resume feeding postoperatively has been extensively studied. Historically, oral intake was held until the passage of flatus or bowel movement. These recommendations were largely based on surgical dogma and were not scientifically sound. Over the last decade, investigations have proved that early feeding prior to clinical evidence of bowel function is safe and not associated with an increased need for nasogastric decompression or increased minor or major complications (19). Quite the opposite was, in fact, noted, with early feeding shown to be beneficial. In Dag et al., patients were stratified into starting a liquid diet on postoperative day one compared with waiting until the passage of flatus. Those patients in whom oral intake was initiated early decreased time to tolerating solid food (2.48 versus 4.77 days) and decreased hospital length of stay (5.55 versus 9 days) (20). Nearly 90% of patients in the early feeding group tolerated the early feeding schedule. Although routinely done, initiating feeding with clear liquids and advancing as tolerated to solid food showed no benefit in a randomized trial on gastrointestinal and vascular patients comparing clear liquids versus solid food as the first postoperative diet (21). This finding is of particular importance as elective colorectal patients prefer simple solid foods rather than clear fluids as their first diet (22). Besides patient safety and comfort, early feeding has been shown to decrease complications and promote bowel function. In a meta-analysis of 15 studies comparing feeding during the first 24 hours postoperatively compared to a traditional feeding schedule, there was a 45% decrease in the relative odds of postoperative complications (odds ratio 0.55, CI 0.35–0.87; $p = 0.01$) in the early feeding group (23). Furthermore, very early feeding may also be associated with prevention of postoperative ileus. Patients who were fed immediately after surgery had a significantly decreased time to passage of flatus and passage of first defecation (24). In our practice, we routinely start every patient on low residue diet the evening of surgery.

## BOWEL PREPARATION

The utility of preoperative mechanical bowel preparation (MBP) has long been under question. Several recent studies have failed to provide evidence of the benefit of MBP. A 2011 Cochrane Systematic Review found no difference in anastomotic leak rate, complication rate, or mortality in patients undergoing colon or rectal excision (25). An update to this analysis was published 5 years later, again failing to show clear evidence of the benefit of MBP (26). As the authors noted, significant limitations exist in analysis of this pooled dataset, specifically the variability of the type of bowel preparation and lack of reported details on location of colon resection; therefore, they cannot rule out a modest 30%–50% benefit of MBP. Nevertheless, most care paths have chosen to omit MBP as an intervention.

There are emerging data that anastomotic leak may have an infectious cause rather than technical failure (27,28). Given this concept, there has been resurgence in the interest in adding oral antibiotics to the traditional MBP. Using the National Surgical Quality Improvement Program (NSQIP) database, Scarborough et al. reported that the addition of oral antibiotics resulted in a significantly decreased incidence of surgical site infection (3.2% versus 9%; $p < 0.001$), anastomotic leak (2.8% versus 5.7%, $p = 0.001$), and hospital readmission (5.5% versus 8; $p = 0.03$) compared to patients who received no preparation (29). In our institution, we have chosen to change practice to include MBP with oral antibiotics (neomycin and metronidazole) in all patients undergoing a bowel resection. This may be the one component of the care path that is most variable in application.

## FLUID MANAGEMENT

Fluid administration during the intraoperative and postoperative period has become a cornerstone of current care paths. IV fluids are necessary to maintain tissue perfusion during general anesthesia and postoperatively when oral intake is minimal. Traditional fluid administration focuses on replacing all fluid loss in the operating room, including blood loss, insensible losses, and third spacing. This fluid strategy is associated with an increase of 3–6 kg of increased postoperative weight, which, in turn, can lead to interstitial and pulmonary edema (17). Furthermore, supplemental fluid is associated with poor wound healing and anastomotic leak, potentially secondary to changes in tissue perfusion pressures (30,31).

Two main strategies have been developed to limit the amount of perioperative fluids given: restrictive fluid therapy and goal-directed fluid therapy. Restrictive fluid strategies attempt to replace only the fluid that is lost intraoperatively and maintain a zero-fluid balance. Kressner et al. conducted a double-blinded randomized trial of fluid restriction as part of a fast-track protocol in colorectal surgery (32). In the restricted cohort, patients received 5% buffered glucose solution at 2 mL/kg/h from induction of anesthesia until skin closure, then 1 mL/kg/h until the morning after surgery at which time IV fluids were stopped. The standard fluid group received 500–1,000 mL Ringer lactate solution prior to the induction, 5 mL/kg/h of Ringer lactate solution during surgery, followed by 10% glucose solution at 1 mL/kg/h until the morning after surgery. Results showed that the restrictive cohort received significantly less IV fluids (3,050 mL versus 5,775 mL; $p < 0.001$) and gained an average of two fewer kilograms over the first three postoperative days. Although the length of hospital stay was similar between the two groups, the proportion of patients with complications was significantly lower in the restrictive group (39% versus 57%; $p = 0.027$). A systematic meta-analysis confirmed these results (33). Compiling 3,861 patients, patients in the standard fluid therapy group had a significantly higher risk of pneumonia (RR 2.2%, 95% CI 1–4.5), pulmonary edema (RR 3.8%, 95% CI 1.1–13), and increased hospital stay (2 days, 95% CI 0.5–3.4).

Despite the positive impact on morbidity, patients on a restrictive fluid strategy are at an increased risk for reversible acute kidney injury. Because a strict restrictive fluid strategy does not fully take into account patient hemodynamics, it may not be suitable for every patient. Goal-directed strategies have therefore been developed where the amount of fluid is tailored to reach certain goals such as stroke volume or cardiac output (34). Hemodynamic monitoring may be achieved by arterial line, central line, Swab-Ganz catheter, or esophageal echocardiography. In one such protocol, 108 patients were randomized to conventional fluid administration left to the discretion of the anesthesiologist, while the other cohort's fluid administration was based solely on predetermined esophageal Doppler perimeters. Goal-directed therapy resulted in a reduced hospital stay, fewer postoperative complications, and early toleration of full diet (35). A recent multicenter randomized trial was performed comparing goal-directed via esophageal Doppler to near maximal strove volume to a restrictive zero-balance strategy in patients undergoing elective colon surgery (36). Interestingly, goal-directed therapy provided no additional benefit over a zero-balance strategy in terms of major, minor, or cardiopulmonary complications.

Although clear that both goal-directed fluid strategies and restrictive strategies are better than traditional fluid administration, the optimal fluid management remains to be defined. In an effort to develop a consensus on perioperative fluid management in colorectal surgery, the Perioperative Quality Initiative was formed, supported by the American Society of Enhanced Recovery and Evidence-Based Perioperative Medicine. In a consensus statement published in 2016, they recommend 13 evidence-based strategies for fluid management (37). Among these are the recommendations to have access to clear fluids up to 2 hours prior to surgery to prevent dehydration and the use of hemodynamic monitoring equipment when available to guide intraoperative fluid management or perform a restrictive strategy. Currently, our strategy is to maintain an intraoperative net zero balance with all IV fluids stopped on the morning after surgery.

## ANALGESIA

Postoperative pain control is critical to promote early ambulation, improve patient pain scores, and increase satisfaction. Much has been learned regarding the mechanisms and pathophysiology of acute pain, and a detailed review is outside the scope of this chapter. Prior to this understanding, many centers used single-modality opioid-based analgesia, usually with a patient-controlled device (PCA). It is well known that opioids cause slowing of the gastrointestinal track leading to ileus, respiratory depression, confusion, and sedation. Contemporary pain management used in care path is best undertaken in a multimodality approach with the goal being to minimize the use of narcotics.

Regional anesthesia can be given preoperatively as an epidural or spinal and can be delivered with either an opioid or local anesthetic. No preferred regimen currently exists, but all regimens have shown a benefit in elective colorectal surgery. Six trials comparing the effect of epidural analgesia on laparoscopic colorectal surgery were reported in a meta-analysis (38). Although there was no significant change in length of stay, time to return of bowel function and postoperative pain scores were significantly decreased with the epidural pathway. The authors noted no significant adverse events in all the trials related to the regional anesthetic. Similarly, when patients were given a spinal injection of bupivacaine and morphine versus IV morphine, those in the spinal anesthetic cohort had significantly decreased opioid use and better pain control (19). In our practice, we work collaboratively with a pain specialists service to determine if the patient is a candidate for a regional anesthetic, and if so we recommend its use.

Pharmacological adjuncts are the cornerstone of postoperative multimodality therapy. In a large meta-analysis of 52 controlled trials comparing nonsteroidal anti-inflammatory drugs (NSAIDs), acetaminophen, and cyclooxygenase-2 inhibitors to morphine, it was shown that the nonopioid medications were associated with a significant reduction on morphine intake, pain intensity, and postoperative nausea/emesis (39). Importantly, NSAIDs did increase the risk of postoperative bleeding from 0% to 1.7% (number needed to harm = 59). The addition of acetaminophen to an NSAID regimen further decreases opioid dependence for pain control by up to 30% compared to either used independently (40).

Other adjuncts may also play a role in reducing opioid use, although the data are less clear. Gabapentin and pregabalin, calcium channel blockers that can reduce opioid channel neurotransmitter release, have been studied in a variety of perioperative settings. As described by Dauri et al., in 6 of 10 randomized trials, gabapentin was shown to provide better postoperative analgesia when given preoperatively compared to placebo, but 14 trials did not show any benefit on postoperative nausea or emesis (41). Magnesium is a glutamate receptor found on nerve cells and has also been studied in lowering opioid requirements. There is no standard dosing for magnesium, and various studies have reported both oral and/or IV dosing schemes. Nevertheless, it has been shown that perioperative magnesium reduces postoperative pain and opioid consumption without increased toxicity (42). Looking at the entire body of evidence, it is our current practice to give all patients gabapentin (600 mg patients aged 18–59; 300 mg patients greater than 59) preoperatively, scheduled ketorolac for the first 24 hours after surgery that is then transitioned to ibuprofen, scheduled acetaminophen, and 400 mg magnesium oxide twice per day for 3 days starting on postoperative day 1.

At the editors' institution (Ochsner Clinic Foundation Hospital, New Orleans, Louisiana), a slightly different multimodality approach to postoperative pain management is used and includes the following elements (43). Preoperatively, acetaminophen 1,000 mg IV and ibuprofen 800 mg IV are given. Intraoperatively, liposomal bupivacaine 266 mg and Marcaine 75 mg (0.25%) are infiltrated at the level of the transversalis fascia just lateral to the rectus sheath with direct or laparoscopic visual control and in the subdermal space of all incisions. Postoperatively, patients receive acetaminophen 1,000 mg IV every 6 hours and ibuprofen 800 mg IV every 8 hours until they are able to take oral medications. Intermittent injections or PCA (morphine or dilaudid) are available for severe pain (scale 6–10) until the patients are taking oral medications. When oral medications are tolerated, the acetaminophen and ibuprofen are switched to oral forms, and oxycodone 10 mg orally every 4 hours is available for moderate pain. As epidurals are time consuming, expensive, and do not always work, their use in our institution for abdominal colorectal surgery has been abandoned. A retrospective review of our early experience (compared to historical controls) demonstrated a shorter hospital stay, lower opioid consumption, and better pain scores (44).

## EARLY AMBULATION AND USE OF URINARY CATHETERS

Other common elements of care paths include early ambulation and early catheter removal. Early mobilization is significantly associated with a decrease in pneumonia and venous thrombosis rates (45). Although routinely cited, it is not well supported that ambulation decreases the rate of postoperative ileus. In fact, recently it was shown that adherence to an intensive ambulatory program consisting of dedicated staff assistance compared to usual care of "targets" provided no benefit in terms of postoperative complication rate, return of bowel function, or length of stay (46). Nevertheless, there is little harm in early ambulation, and we strive for at least five walks per day.

Indwelling Foley catheters are significantly associated with urinary tract infections (UTIs), and patients who have their catheters in place longer than 48 hours postoperatively are twice as likely to develop a UTI (47). Furthermore, an indwelling catheter is often a reason cited for decreased ambulation. In our practice, unless needed for strict fluid management or the presence of a urogenital procedure, we remove all Foley catheters in the morning of postoperative day 1. If the patient is subsequently unable to void spontaneously, he or she will undergo intermittent catheterization until able to pass urine spontaneously.

## CARE PATHS DURING EMERGENCY SURGERY

While originally designed for elective procedures, care paths have started to become routinely used during emergency colorectal surgery. Wisely et al. (48) showed that there was a significant change in management toward ERAS principles in emergency abdominal surgical patients following introduction of an ERAS program in elective patients (46). Specifically, post-ERAS patients received less IV fluids, spent less time with an indwelling Foley catheter, and spent less time on a narcotic PCA. Emergency patients placed on a care path may also experience a similar benefit as compared to elective patients. Although limited by a small sample size ($n = 60$), it was shown that a comprehensive care path in the emergency setting is associated with shorter hospital stays (5.5 days versus 7.5; $p = 0.009$) and decreased time to first flatus (1.6 days versus 2.8; $p = <0.001$). Further studies are needed to define which subsets of emergency surgical patient care paths are safe and feasible.

## PUTTING IT TOGETHER

Care paths are multidisciplinary protocols used to optimize patient care. When compared to traditional perioperative care, care paths lead to decreased patient complications and decreased hospital stays with no increased readmissions. In this chapter, we reviewed the relevant literature for the most commonly cited elements of care paths. As it remains unclear which elements are most impactful, when designing a care path, it is imperative to choose elements that are feasible and reproducible at the specific institution. In this way, compliance and efficiency can be documented, allowing for continuous recalibration to optimize future patient outcomes.

## REFERENCES

1. Kehlet H, Wilmore DW. *Br J Surg* 2005;92(1):3–4.
2. Zhuang CL et al. *Dis Colon Rectum* 2013;56(5): 667–78.
3. Pritts TA et al. *Ann Surg* 1999;230(5):728–33.
4. Grant MC et al. *Ann Surg* 2017;265(1):68–79.
5. Pronovost PJ et al. *J Crit Care* 2008;23(2):207–21.
6. Bliss LA et al. *J Am Coll Surg* 2012;215(6):766–76.
7. Watt DG et al. *Medicine (Baltimore)* 2015;94(36): e1286.
8. Wang G et al. *J Gastrointest Surg* 2012;16(7): 1379–88.
9. Wilmore DW, Kehlet H. *BMJ* 2001;322(7284):473–6.
10. Polle SW et al. *Dig Surg* 2007;24(6):441–9.
11. Carli F et al. *Can J Anaesth* 2009;56(11):837–42.
12. McKenna LS et al. *J Wound Ostomy Continence Nurs* 2016;43(1):57–61.
13. Maydick D. *Ostomy Wound Manage* 2016;62(5): 14–24.
14. Ljungqvist O et al. *Proc Nutr Soc* 2002;61(3):329–36.
15. van den Berghe G et al. *N Engl J Med* 2001;345(19): 1359–67.
16. Svanfeldt M et al. *Br J Surg* 2007;94(11):1342–50.
17. Noblett SE et al. *Colorectal Dis* 2006;8(7):563–9.
18. Smith MD et al. *Cochrane Database Syst Rev* 2014; 14(8):CD009161.
19. Wongyingsinn M et al. *Br J Anaesth* 2012;108(5): 850–6.
20. Dag A et al. *Clinics (Sao Paulo)* 2011;66(12):2001–5.
21. Jeffery KM et al. *Am Surg* 1996;62(3):167–70.
22. Yeung SE, Fenton TR. *Dis Colon Rectum* 2009;52(9): 1616–23.
23. Osland E et al. *JPEN J Parenter Enteral Nutr* 2011; 35(4):473–87.
24. Fujii T et al. *Int Surg* 2014;99(3):211–5.
25. Güenaga KF et al. *Cochrane Database Syst Rev* 2011; 7(9):CD001544.
26. Dahabreh IJ et al. *Dis Colon Rectum* 2015;58(7): 698–707.
27. Shogan BD et al. *J Gastrointest Surg* 2013;17(9): 1698–707.
28. Shogan BD et al. *Sci Transl Med* 2015;7(286): 286ra68.
29. Scarborough JE et al. *Ann Surg* 2015;262(2):331–7.
30. Arkiliç CF et al. *Surgery* 2003;133(1):49–55.
31. Shandall A et al. *Br J Surg* 1985;72(8):606–9.
32. Abraham-Nordling M et al. *Br J Surg* 2012;99(2): 186–91.
33. Corcoran T et al. *Anesth Analg* 2012;114(3):640–51.
34. Noblett SE et al. *Br J Surg* 2006;93(9):1069–76.
35. Pearse RM et al. *JAMA* 2014;311(21):2181–90.
36. Brandstrup B et al. *Br J Anaesth* 2012;109(2):191–9.
37. Thiele RH et al. *Perioper Med (Lond)* 2016;5:24.
38. Khan SA et al. *Surg Endosc* 2013;27(7):2581–91.
39. Elia N et al. *Anesthesiology* 2005;103(6):1296–304.
40. Ong CK et al. *Anesth Analg* 2010;110(4):1170–9.
41. Dauri M et al. *Curr Drug Targets* 2009;10(8):716–33.
42. De Oliveira GS et al. *Anesthesiology* 2013;119(1): 178–90.
43. Beck DE. Perioperative care. In Beck DE, Wexner SD, Raferty J, Jayne D (eds). *Gordon and Nivatvong's. Principles and Practice of Surgery for the Colon, Rectum, and Anus.* 4th Edition. Thieme. In press.
44. Beck DE et al. *Ochsner J* 2015;15(4):408–12.
45. Wren SM et al. *J Am Coll Surg* 2010;210(4):491–5.
46. Fiore JF et al. *Ann Surg* 2017;266:223–31.
47. Wald HL et al. *Arch Surg* 2008;143(6):551–7.
48. Wisely JC, Barclay KL. *ANZ J Surg* 2016;86(11): 883–8.

# 11

# Limitations of anorectal physiology testing

THOMAS E. CATALDO AND SYED G. HUSAIN

## CHALLENGING CASE

A 65-year-old woman and her 30-year-old daughter both present to your office with complaints of fecal incontinence. Both are gravida 3 para 3, all vaginal deliveries, and have had at least one delivery of a child of 3.6 kg or more. Both have required an assistance device for delivery of one child. Both report fecal soiling for the last year. The older woman reports progressive uncontrolled passage of flatus and occasional identification of stool in her undergarments that she was unaware of having passed. The daughter reports incontinence to moderate amounts of stool despite attempts to delay defecation. There is additional incontinence associated with athletic activity.

## CASE MANAGEMENT

Both patients are examined. The younger patient has reduced tone and squeeze. An anterior defect is found but the sphincter muscles appear to contract with squeeze. The older patient also has poor sphincter tone and no squeeze. Both patients are offered a trial of increased fiber and Imodium, which fails to resolve their symptoms and are scheduled for physiologic testing. Anal manometry in the younger patient confirms the physical exam and intra-anal ultrasound confirms an anterior sphincter defect. The patient is offered an overlapping sphincteroplasty. Manometry on the older patient confirms low resting and squeeze pressures. Ultrasound does not identify any sphincter defects. The patient is offered a sacral nerve stimulator.

## INTRODUCTION

Normal function of the anus and rectum resulting in comfortable passage of stool under voluntary control is a complex balance of a number of competing factors and requires intricate correct performance of enteric and colonic physiology, rectal, anal, and pelvic sensory and motor nerves, as well as anatomically intact and functioning anal and pelvic musculature. Disruption of any of these factors may result in fecal incontinence. On the other end of the spectrum, the patient may suffer difficult, painful, or incomplete evacuation. Anorectal dysfunction is often devastating to the patient resulting in emotional distress and social isolation.

Fecal continence is defined as the ability to defer defecation until a socially appropriate time and place. Incontinence has a number of definitions, from simply involuntary passage of stool to inability to control passage of solid, liquid, or gas. In a 2001 consensus conference report, fecal incontinence is defined as, "recurrent uncontrolled passage of fecal material for at least one month in an individual with a developmental age of at least four years" (1). Reported prevalence varies from 1.4% to 18%, with rates as high as 45% in elderly, debilitated, or psychiatrically impaired institutionalized adults (1–3). The numbers are generally accepted as underreported due to patients' unwillingness to come forward due to associated social and cultural stigma.

Constipation is as difficult to define. It may be as subjective as any difficulty or infrequency in passing stool as perceived by the patient. The Rome II criteria define constipation as two or more of the following for at least 3 months: straining more than 25% of the time, hard stools more than 25% of the time, incomplete evacuation more than 25% of the time, or two or fewer bowel movements in a 7-day period (4).

A problem inherent to all anorectal physiology (ARP) testing is the scarcity of "normal" values for comparison. There is relative paucity of literature describing ARP testing on the normal population, and almost all of the available studies are composed of a small group of subjects.

## PHYSIOLOGY OF FECAL CONTINENCE

Normal fecal continence relies on a number of mechanisms. The first of which is normal enteral and colonic motility and fluid transport physiology resulting in manageable stool volume and consistency. Stool consistency may be the most important characteristic that influences fecal continence (5). Some patients may be continent to solid stool but not to liquid or gas. The rectum needs to maintain adequate reservoir capacity. In addition, the rectum, anus, and pelvic musculature must have adequate ability to sense and differentiate the presence of solid, liquid, and gas and to differentiate between these. Additionally, it is postulated that the vascular cushions or hemorrhoids create a controllable seal as a rectal "corpus cavernosum." This is supported by the identification of leakage in some patients after otherwise uncomplicated hemorrhoidectomy (5). On a mechanical level, defecation occurs when the pressure within the rectum exceeds the pressure or resistance provided by the anus. For normal defecation, this relies on the controlled increase in rectal pressure combined with simultaneous relaxation of the anus and straightening of the rectum through relaxation of the pelvic muscles.

For normal defecation to occur, the rectum must also possess correct mechanical properties of capacity and distensibility. It must be able to sense the need to empty and the qualities of the contents within it. Disease processes or injuries that limit the ability of the rectum to distend to accept stool and air from the sigmoid colon will alter the urge to defecate, and the ability to defer defecation. Conversely, a chronically distended capacious rectum may lose the ability to sense when it is full and thereby overflow. Both cases might present as incontinence. Alternatively, if the body cannot differentiate between solid, liquid, or gas, or if the mechanism by which this is sampled is altered, the result is often fecal soiling.

A battery of devices and tests has been developed to investigate many aspects of normal and altered defecation. Much work remains to fully elucidate the source and thereby the solutions to disordered defecation.

## THE ANORECTAL PHYSIOLOGY LAB

A battery of devices and tests have been developed to investigate many aspects of normal and altered defecation. Many centers have collected the equipment to accomplish these tests (Figure 11.1). Work remains to be done to fully elucidate the source and thereby the solutions to disordered defecation.

## INVESTIGATIONS FOR INCONTINENCE: MANOMETRY

Manometry is a technique to measure the pressures that exist within the anal canal and the pressures the anus is capable of achieving voluntarily. Over many years a variety of catheters, pressure detectors, and recording apparatuses have been developed. In addition, different operator techniques have been developed making standardization of results difficult. Throughout the 1960s a variety of catheters were developed with different numbers of open-tipped channels and microballoons. The number of channels varied, and they were

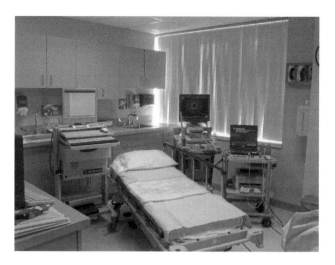

Figure 11.1 Typical anorectal physiology lab with manometry, transanal ultrasound, pudendal nerve terminal motor latency testing, biofeedback, storage, and equipment for sterilization.

arranged radially or in a spiral orientation. Water within the channels was either static or continuously perfused. Initial continuous recordings were made with pen and ink on polygraph devices. State-of-the-art manometers contain solid-state micropressure transducers mounted within the catheter itself (Figure 11.2a,b). In addition to more reliable and reproducible data, the catheters are more easily and reliably cleaned from patient to patient. Pressure data are recorded continuously to computer-based software that assists in creating the interpretation and the report. One critical observation of the water-perfused systems is that the patient may react to the sensation of water dripping from the anus with increased tone. Scrupulous technique may avoid this.

Because various technologies and methods exist for measuring anal canal pressures, no universally accepted set of normal values exists. Simpson et al. addressed this issue in a study comparing five different catheters and techniques of manometry in both normal and incontinent patients (6). Although their sample size was small, 10 normal and 11 patients with incontinence, the authors found no significant difference between five commonly employed devices. They were a water-perfused end-hole catheter, a catheter water perfused with four radially arranged side holes, a water-filled microballoon, a microtransducer, and an air-filled portable microprocessor-controlled device.

## SPHINCTER PRESSURE MEASUREMENT

Although written consent is not required as the patient is fully awake, at our institution we obtain full informed consent and confirmation of patient identity, condition being evaluated, and the patient's understanding of the tests he or she is about to undergo. The patient takes one or two small-volume cleansing enemas at home prior to the exam. Anal canal pressures are measured with the patient lying comfortably in the left lateral decubitus position with knees and hips

(a)

(b)

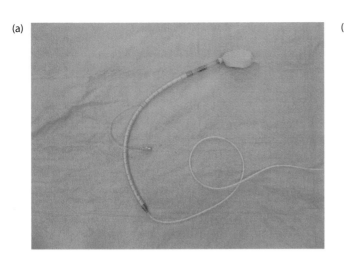
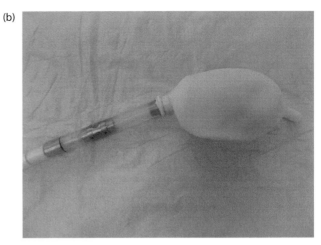

(c)  Squeeze #1

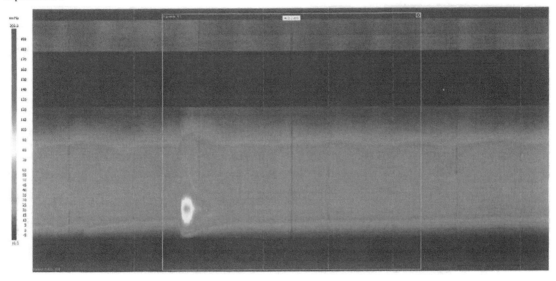

Squeeze #1

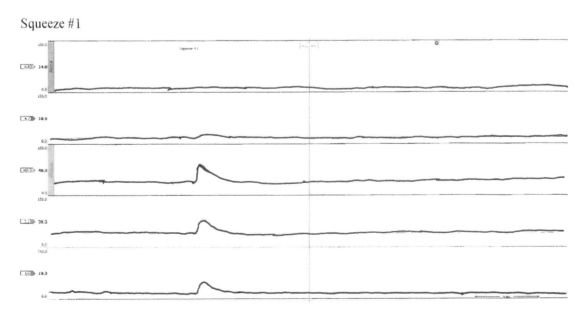

Figure 11.2  **(a)** Manometry catheter, with balloon. **(b)** Manometry catheter, detail microtransducers. **(c)** Manometry tracing, computer display.

flexed 90°. Some emphasis is placed on comfort and relaxation as anxiety, talking, and anything that increases the intraabdominal pressure may affect the results. We employ stationary pull-through technique. The catheter is placed transanally with the measuring points (balloons, holes, or microtransducers) to a distance of 6 cm above the anal verge. Measurements are taken in the anterior, posterior, and left and right lateral positions (Figure 11.2c). Pressures are recorded at relaxation and at maximum "squeeze" for 10 seconds. The patient must be instructed to try to isolate squeeze of the anus and not employ the gluteal and other accessory muscles. The catheter is repositioned 1 cm distally, and the process is repeated. The process is repeated in step-wise fashion until the entire canal has been tested. An alternative to this "station pull-out" technique is recording pressures during a continuous pull-out of the catheter at a controlled steady rate. Some modern catheters have transducers extending the length of the anal canal that allow for simultaneous pressure measurements and obviate the need for withdrawing the catheter. The following parameters are recorded: length of the anal high-pressure zone, mean resting tone, and maximum squeeze pressure.

In an effort to study the symmetry and detailed overall pressure profile of the anal sphincter, pressure vectography, a technique that provides graphical representation of the radial pressure profile of the anal canal, was developed.

## THE RECTOANAL INHIBITORY REFLEX

The presence or absence of the rectoanal inhibitory reflex (RAIR) is identified by rapid distention of the rectum by insufflation of the balloon at the tip of the catheter with 10 cc of air. Simultaneous recordings taken in the middle of the anal canal high-pressure zone are made for 10 seconds. If the RAIR is present, a slight contraction of the external sphincter followed by a reflex relaxation of internal sphincter and resultant decrease in anal canal pressure should be observed. Balloon insufflation may be repeated with more air at 10 cc increments up to 60 cc until a reflex is observed.

## RECTAL CAPACITY AND SENSATION

The balloon at the end of the catheter may also be filled with water in an incremental fashion to assess rectal sensation and compliance. Measurements are made at the minimum volume of first rectal sensation, the volume required to produce a sustained feeling of the need to defecate, and a maximum volume that creates significant discomfort or an irresistible need to defecate.

## VALUE AND LIMITATIONS OF MANOMETRY FOR INCONTINENCE

Anal manometry has become a staple in the evaluation of fecal incontinence. Though routinely performed in many centers, manometry lacks standardization of technique, data collection, and methods of interpretation. This makes it extremely difficult to compare data obtained at different centers. The range of accepted normal values is wide. Furthermore, normal values change for gender, parity, age, and numerous other factors. Despite the fact that the newer catheters are more comfortable and easier to maintain, the test remains mildly invasive and uncomfortable for the patient.

There are several technical caveats that may lead to considerable alteration in results. Patients with megarectum may require a higher volume to illicit RAIR and may be falsely labeled as RAIR negative if the usual volume of 30–40 cc is used to illicit RAIR (7). The balloon material can influence the results as latex balloons tend to deform along their axis, resulting in a falsely elevated rectal compliance (8). Rectal compliance testing depends entirely upon the patient's input; thus, the patient's psychological status plays a very important role in data acquisition during this test (7). Furthermore, the results of rectal compliance may differ if the test is performed on "prepared," that is, after enema evacuation, versus unprepared rectum (7). The rate at which water is injected into the balloon may also affect the rectal sensitivity testing (9). Thus, it is recommended that slow filling should be accomplished at a rate of 1 mL/s (7). Whatever the method used, the same technique should be applied to all patients in order to obtain reproducible and comparable results.

Caution should be exercised while making treatment decisions based on manometric findings, as normal or abnormal values in incontinent patients do not necessarily correlate with severity of symptoms. In a large prospective study, Lieberman et al. evaluated 90 incontinent patients, including 6 males with a specific goal at determining what impact physiology testing including manometry had on treatment and outcome. After appropriate history and physical exam, patients were selected for medical or surgical management. Following this determination, they underwent ARP testing including manometry, pudendal nerve terminal motor latency (PNTML), and transanal ultrasound (TAUS). Overall, only 9 (10%) had a change in their management plan. Based on the results of these tests, 5 of 45 patients initially assigned to medical management were offered surgery instead. Three of 45 patients assigned to undergo surgical treatment were switched to the medical group. Almost all of these alterations in management were based on TAUS. Manometry was found to be abnormal in one-third of both management groups, and there was no correlation between manometric results and change in management plan. There did not appear to be an association between manometry, TAUS, and PNTML results (10). In an elaborate study of 350 patients including 80 controls, Felt-Bersma et al. (11) found that the most significant difference between continent and incontinent patients was maximum squeeze pressure. However, the authors surmised that continent function could not be predicted based on anal manometry alone and suggested that these results should only be interpreted in conjunction with other tests.

Although it creates a rather striking and impressive graphical representation of anal canal pressure profile, pressure vector diagrams have been shown to be of questionable clinical value for sphincter evaluation (12). A study by Yang et al. (12) could not demonstrate any correlation when vectoral analysis was compared to needle electromyography (EMG) and ultrasonography.

Anorectal manometry remains of value for objective preoperative documentation of anal tone function or muscle weakness. It is also useful in excluding patients from surgery (2). Perhaps the biggest merit of manometry is its ability to diagnose short-segment Hirschsprung disease and pelvic floor dyssynergia.

## ELECTROMYOGRAPHY

EMG is the measurement of the electrical activity generated by muscle fibers during contraction or at rest. In 1930 Beck first described anal sphincter EMG (13). Specifically, the EMG measures activity in a motor group or those muscle cells innervated by a single axon. Muscles whose nerves have been damaged will demonstrate altered activity. Myography has been used to map the perianal area for muscular activity and thereby detect sphincter defects. EMG is also used to demonstrate nerve conduction and appropriate activation and relaxation used in biofeedback therapy.

### Concentric needle EMG

A concentric needle electrode is two insulated electrodes, one within the other. With the needle inserted into the muscle to be observed, in this case the external sphincter or the pelvic floor, the electrical potential from one electrode to the other is recorded. Information collected includes amplitude, duration, and frequency, as well as the number of phases. Amplitude is proportional to the number of muscle fibers activated. Normal values are an amplitude of less than 600 µV and duration less than 6 microseconds (14,15). Longer duration or spreading of the signal can indicate dispersion of the motor unit potential (MUP). This may represent denervation or demyelinization, or simply aging. The sum of the activity of many muscle cells creates a shape to the MUP. Normal MUPs are bi- or triphasic. In general, more phases within the action potential indicated denervation and reinnervation. However, four or more phases have been reported in normal muscle in up to a quarter of the time.

### Single-fiber EMG

Individual muscle fiber action potentials can be recorded with a single-fiber EMG. The recording area of the needle is much smaller, 25 µm. In normally innervated external anal sphincter muscle, only a few fibers will be activated by a single motor group axon. However, when damage occurs, denervated muscle fibers are recruited by surviving axons. The number of muscle fibers and thereby signal density within the recording area of the needle increases, resulting in a more

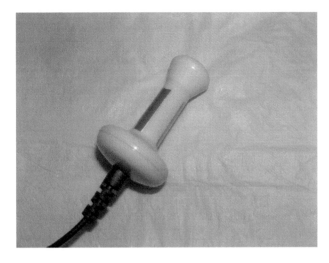

Figure 11.3 Anal plug, surface EMG electrode for biofeedback.

polyphasic signal. The test is performed by taking multiple readings requiring multiple skin punctures around the anus.

### Surface EMG/biofeedback

Measurement of muscular activity through the insulation of the skin is far more imprecise but less painful than needle EMG. Surface EMG is valuable for documentation of overall activity, especially during attempted voluntary rest, inhibition, or contraction of a muscle. Surface EMG is helpful to document paradoxical sphincter activity as part of the diagnosis of disordered defecation. Two self-adhering surface electrodes can be applied on opposite sides of the anus over the subcutaneous portion of the external sphincter, with a grounding electrode placed at a distance on the patient. Alternatively, a plug electrode is employed within the anal canal (Figure 11.3). Surface measurement of muscle activity is more valuable if the muscle is being artificially activated by stimulating the nerve. When the time of nerve stimulation is known and the time of muscle activity is measured, nerve conduction velocity can be assessed. A specific application of nerve stimulation and surface EMG is measurement of the PNTML.

## PUDENDAL NERVE TERMINAL MOTOR LATENCY

The pudendal nerve arises from the second, third, and fourth sacral nerve roots bilaterally and passes along the inferior pubic rami through Alcock's canal. Prolonged labor or the use of forceps for delivery may injure the pudendal nerve as it exits from the canal. The conduction time of the nerve can be measured by stimulating the nerve transrectally and observing the time to electrical activity of the external anal sphincter. A St. Mark's electrode attached to a gloved finger provides both stimulation and measurement (Figure 11.4a–c). An absent trace may indicate injury to the nerve, whereas a prolonged PNTML is interpreted to indicate nerve injury and repair.

(a)

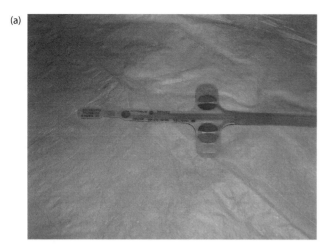

(b)

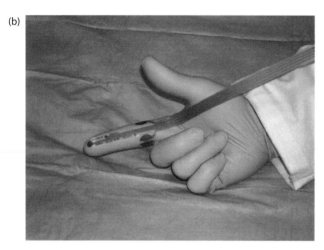

(c)

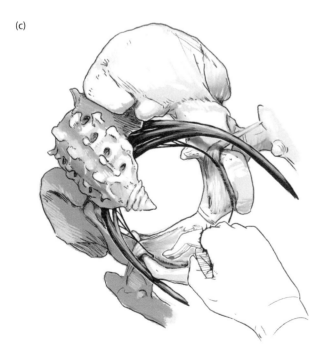

Figure 11.4 **(a)** St. Mark's electrode. **(b)** Electrode on gloved finger to be placed transanally. **(c)** St. Mark's electrode is inserted into anus with the finger tip directed toward Alcock's canal.

## LIMITATIONS OF ELECTROMYOGRAPHY IN INCONTINENCE

The EMG delineation of an anatomic sphincter defect has been largely supplanted by imaging studies such as ultrasound and pelvic magnetic resonance imaging (MRI). Concentric needle EMG and single-fiber EMG testing are uncomfortable, or in some cases, frankly painful for the patient. The equipment is expensive and difficult to master. Results are variable based on the cooperation of the patient, the experience of the examiner, and the patience of both (16). Surface EMG is mildly uncomfortable to the patient and technically challenging to perform. Identification of the nerve trace can be subjective. Pudendal nerve latency testing is operator dependent. Since PNTML measures the fastest remaining fibers, a normal latency time does not exclude injury. The latency values obtained are also affected by the distance between the electrode and the pudendal nerve; the shortest latencies are obtained by placing the electrode as close to the nerve as possible (9). This is usually accomplished with subtle movements of the electrode-bearing finger inside the anal canal while observing waveforms for the shortest latency thus generated in response to repeated electrical stimuli. This trial-and-hit method results in significant patient discomfort in many cases. There is some bilateral crossover innervation of the sphincter; therefore, a unilaterally abnormal test does not preclude normal function. Earlier studies indicated that significantly abnormal bilateral results were predictive of poor outcome with sphincter repair (17–19). However, other authors have not found PNTML to be helpful in this regard (10,20). Increased pudendal nerve terminal velocities have been previously associated with patients with idiopathic incontinence (21). Newer literature, however, suggests that this association might not be entirely true. Ricciardi et al. (22) showed that only a small percentage of patients with idiopathic fecal incontinence had associated pudendal neuropathy.

### Transanal ultrasonography

High-quality circumferential images of the anal sphincter complex can be obtained using TAUS. Although a number of probes are available, the most commonly used for evaluation of the anal sphincter is a rotating probe that creates a 360°, two-dimensional (2D) transverse image. The transducer generally used is a combined 7 or 10 MHz transducer, rotating within a water-filled rigid cap covered with a balloon or condom. Newer probes are fully self-contained. They still require protection with a condom and some type of interface media such as gel or water (Figure 11.5).

In many outpatient ARP labs, the procedure is performed in the left lateral decubitus position in conjunction with anal manometry. For a patient scheduled to undergo multiple ARP studies the same day, we follow a policy of performing manometry initially followed by other investigations as the sphincter stretch induced by 12 mm sonogram probe may produce erroneous manometric findings. As such, the patient may have had limited preparation with a small volume enema. This is not

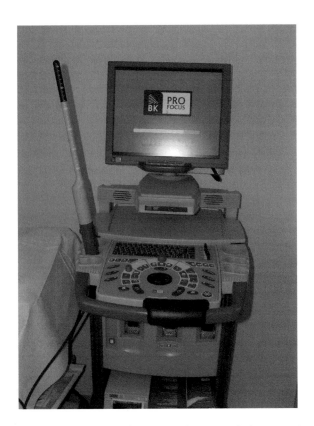

Figure 11.5 B&K 3D self-contained transanal ultrasound. Computer console and probe.

required for TAUS alone. Some authors prefer the prone or lithotomy positions, feeling that the lateral position deforms the anatomy (23). The clinical significance of this is unclear. TAUS can distinguish the internal and external sphincters individually, with an intact internal sphincter representing a continuous hypoechoic band. The external sphincter is more heterogenous but distinctly more hyperechoic. Although images can be taken throughout the anal canal, images are traditionally documented and preserved at proximal, mid, and distal anal canal. Defects in either the internal or external sphincters are identified as a disruption in the continuous ring. The external sphincter naturally splits proximally as it extends to the levator sling and the pelvic floor musculature. Disrupted tissue heals with a scar that appears amorphous, more echogenic than the internal sphincter, but less so than the external. It is seen bridging the gap in the defect between the disrupted ends of the sphincters. The presence of a sphincter defect on TAUS correlates well with a history of obstetrical trauma, as well as with physical exam and manometric findings (10,20,24). Interobserver agreement is excellent, and when an anatomic defect is present, TAUS sensitivity approaches 100% (25), specifically for internal anal sphincter defects in the mid anal canal. Different techniques have been employed to either improve or make easier definition of the anal anatomy. Some authors claim anal squeeze and relaxation improve the yield of the sonographic exam, while others have no benefit (23). A finger placed in the posterior wall of the vagina used to measure the thickness of the perineal body has been shown to aid in the evaluation of anterior sphincter defects (25).

Global deficiencies or thinning of the sphincters rather than defects are more difficult to define with TAUS. The internal sphincter is normally between 2 and 4 mm. Since it is more distinct on TAUS, excessive thickness or thinness can be identified. One elusive objective is to identify atrophy of the external sphincter, as this correlates with poor outcome from sphincter repair (26).

Three-dimensional (3D) axial endosonography is now available. The probe spirals and moves through the sphincter at a fixed rate collecting a 3D block of echo-data that can be represented on a computer screen and evaluated through any plane through the block.

In a study involving 33 women with suspected sphincter injury, two different observers compared 2D TAUS with 3D evaluation. There was an identifiable improvement in the confidence of the examiner in detecting sphincter defects with 3D evaluation over 2D images. Interobserver correlation was also improved by 3D evaluation but not to a significant degree (27). Nevertheless, 3D TAUS has not been indisputably demonstrated to be more sensitive or specific than transverse planar TAUS.

## LIMITATIONS OF ULTRASOUND IN INCONTINENCE

Ultrasound is the most important test in the evaluation of fecal incontinence with few limitations. Anorectal ultrasound entails a significant learning curve (28), and results are operator and experience dependent. The external sphincter is less distinct than internal sphincter and smaller, <90°, defects are harder to demonstrate (29). Patients with minimal symptoms and limited defects may not require surgery; therefore, the clinical significance of a defect is determined by the combination of physical exam, ARP testing, and TAUS. The presence of atrophy of the external sphincter is similarly hard to prove. This is due to the fact that atrophic external sphincter becomes replaced with fat, making sonographic delineation of the sphincter from the surrounding fat tissue more difficult (30). Many investigators believed that 3D ultrasound, by virtue of its superior resolution, may result in improved identification of external sphincter atrophy. However, a comparative study showed no correlation between 3D TAUS and MRI in 18 incontinent women with MRI evidence of sphincter atrophy (31).

### Biofeedback for fecal incontinence

Biofeedback is a process by which the patient is given an auditory or visual representation of anorectal information, pressure, or muscle activity, which he or she cannot otherwise perceive or correctly interpret. Techniques of biofeedback have successfully been used in the treatment of fecal incontinence for over 25 years. The practice parameters of the American Society of Colon and Rectal Surgeons give a grade "B" recommendation for its use as a first-line therapy and in patients who have incomplete success after sphincter repair (2).

## LIMITATIONS OF BIOFEEDBACK FOR INCONTINENCE

Despite some encouraging earlier reports describing success of biofeedback in the management of incontinence, the Cochrane system review of treatments for incontinence in 2006 did not support its use (32). The authors reported, "The 11 trials reviewed were of very limited value because they were generally small, of poor or uncertain quality, and compare different combinations of treatments." Overall success with biofeedback varies from 65% to 89% (2,33,34). Two large randomized controlled trials included more than 100 subjects. Both concluded that biofeedback provided no additional benefit over office counseling therapy, such as advice, education, dietary modification, digital guidance, and medication. Despite the lack of demonstrated benefit, both trials showed improvement in severity of symptoms, fecal incontinence scores, and quality of life (35–37). These benefits were seen in both the treatment and control groups, indicating the role of patient motivation and ongoing medical involvement in the treatment of fecal incontinence. The most important predictors of success were completion of the program and age over 60 years. Higher body mass index was associated with a worse outcome.

## Summary: Value and limitations of ARP testing for evaluation of fecal incontinence

The perceived value of ARP testing in the evaluation and management of fecal incontinence varies greatly depending on the perspective of the examiner and the expectations of the patient. The most frequently employed tests include anal manometry, TAUS, and PNTML. Techniques and normal values are not universally accepted. Abnormal results do not equate with specific disease, injury, or symptomatology. TAUS and MRI provide excellent anatomic definition to aid in the planning of surgical intervention. At best, manometry serves for documentation of preoperative function and may assist in patient selection for surgery. PNTML is still controversial as to its role in the treatment of fecal incontinence.

## Investigations for constipation and disordered defecation

Constipation is one of the common ailments presented to the colorectal surgeon. It usually entails unsatisfactory defecation resulting from decreased frequency of defecation or difficulty in passing stools or both. Prevalence in the general population in the United States has been reported to be as high as 2%–15% (38,39). Women are affected two to three times more commonly than men with incidence increasing with age. As with incontinence, the etiology is multifactorial and complex. Etiologic factors associated with constipation include lifestyle issues and medications, especially narcotics, antidepressants, and calcium channel blockers. Pelvic outlet obstruction (puborectalis dysfunction or rectocele) is also a common underlying abnormality. Other causes include neurologic or endocrine dysfunction, for example, Parkinson disease, diabetes mellitus, and hypothyroidism. Finally, dysfunction of the enteric nervous system seen in Hirschsprung and Chagas diseases and psychological factors may also play an important role in the pathogenesis.

Refractory constipation that fails to respond to dietary modification and conservative management warrants a formal workup. From a management perspective, constipation is usually referred to as either slow transit constipation or obstructed defecation. The initial history and physical examination, in most cases, are able to indicate if the patient is experiencing slow transit constipation versus obstructed defecation. Colonic transit studies are usually the first tests to be ordered in cases where slow transit is suspected to be the underlying etiology, whereas in patients with obstructed defecation, a defecogram should be offered as the initial diagnostic study. However, studies have shown that there is little, if any, correlation between these two diagnostic modalities, and the clinical picture does not necessarily reciprocate the radiological findings (40).

### DEFECOGRAPHY

Since the 1960s, continuously recorded fluoroscopy has been used to evaluate the dynamic function of the pelvic floor. Defecating proctography or cinedefecography is a method whereby semisolid radiopaque contrast material is placed retrograde into the rectum and lateral images are obtained in real time. Creating a realistic "pseudo stool" has been a challenge. A commercially available product was available but was transiently taken off the market. Many institutions create their own contrast as needed using a combination of barium and potato starch. At the authors institution, we use a unique recipe based on breadcrumbs. The material must be thick enough to simulate stool but able to be passed transanally.

Once the enema is administered, the subject is seated in a lateral orientation on a radiolucent commode. Prior to defecation, measurements are made of the angles of the proximal and distal rectum. In women the vagina may be delineated with a tampon soaked with water-soluble contrast, and in certain circumstances the small bowel is opacified with oral contrast. If further delineation is required, sterile water-soluble contrast can be place intraperitoneally to define the lower peritoneal reflection; furthermore, in patients with suspected cystocele, instillation of dye into the bladder may increase the diagnostic yield of the study.

The anorectal angle is created in part by the tone and function of the puborectalis muscle. Measurements are taken as the patient is sitting at rest, during forced contraction, straining without defecation (Valsalva maneuver), and during defecation. Perineal descent is defined as the change in distance of the line drawn perpendicularly from the anorectal junction to the pubococcygeal line. This line is drawn from the tip of the coccyx to the posterior-inferior margin of the pubic ramus. In addition, perianal skin can be marked with a metal marker and the motion or descent of the perineum measured.

Normal reported values vary widely. One author offers a broad range, 70°–140° at rest, 100°–180° defecating, and 75°–90° squeezing (41,42); where another is more specific, 92° ± 1.5° resting and 137° ± 1.5° straining (5). The change in the angle may be more important than the absolute numbers. In our practice, the test is of most value if the surgeon reviews the study with the radiologist while the test is being performed.

Abnormal findings include perineal descent of more than 3 cm while resting or more than 3 cm while straining. Paradoxical contraction of the puborectalis and disordered defecation is indicated by an observed ascent of the perineum or a static or more acute anorectal angle during attempted defecation. Additional findings may include internal intussusception to frank prolapse, rectocele, or enterocele. Small, <2 cm rectoceles are commonly seen in asymptomatic patients and are regarded as a normal finding.

## LIMITATIONS OF DEFECOGRAPHY IN CONSTIPATION

It must be remembered that defecography is not a "physiologic" study, as the study is not performed in response to a natural desire to defecate; instead patients are asked to evacuate in a rather alien, uncomfortable environment. Among other criticisms regarding defecography are poor interobserver agreement (43,44). To complicate issues further, abnormal defecographic findings are common in asymptomatic patients (45,46). The significant degree of overlap between defecographic findings in patients with constipation and asymptomatic controls raises questions regarding the cause-and-effect relationship between clinical symptoms and defecographic findings. One of the radiological signs frequently documented during these studies is contrast retention within the rectoceles. The clinical significance of this "barium trapping" seen has also been questioned (47).

In a study by Shorvon et al., one-half of asymptomatic subjects had some aspect of mucosal prolapse and intussusception, and 17 of 21 women demonstrated some degree of rectocele (48). In addition, prior to that work, no work had employed normal, healthy volunteers as controls, and "normal" was determined retrospectively by lack of anatomic abnormality. Other studies were performed in patients undergoing barium enemas for other, nonanorectal conditions (45,48,49). Anorectal angle assessment and its interpretation should be performed with utmost caution. As eluded to earlier, there is a wide variation in normal values for anorectal angle, and many investigators believe that it is the change in angle rather than the absolute values that serve as a useful guide to therapy (7).

Patients with urge incontinence may frequently show increased threshold for urge to defecate. It is unclear if this finding is the result rather than the cause of constipation (9), and the clinical implication of this finding remains uncertain. Abnormal puborectalis function noted at defecography has also been a topic of considerable debate. Many normal individuals have been shown to have puborectalis abnormalities on defecograms (50); thus, the clinical relevance of these findings is questionable, and therapeutic decisions should be based on clinical rather than mere abnormal findings on radiological studies.

## Colonic transit studies

Colonic transit studies play a pivotal role in the assessment of constipation. The majority of colorectal surgeons agree that transit studies supply the most pertinent information out of all the physiology testing modalities available for constipation (51). The most widely accepted technique involves ingestion of a commercially available capsule containing 24 radiopaque rings followed by x-ray at days 3 and 5. A normal study entails passage of more than 80% of the rings. The mean colonic time has been shown to be 31 hours in males and 39 hours in females (15). Based on the location of retained rings, abnormal studies may be labeled as "outlet obstruction" if 20% or more rings are retained at day 5 in the rectosigmoid region or "colonic inertia" if more than 20% rings are dispersed throughout entire colon. Clinical efficacy of colonic transit studies to detect segmental bowel motility remains controversial (9). No bowel prep is administered prior to the study, and patients are directed to avoid using laxatives and promotility agents, including dietary fiber.

## Small bowel transit studies

Since it is generally accepted that slow transit constipation is overwhelmingly attributed to colonic dysfunction, small bowel transit studies are infrequently requested. However, when clinical suspicion exists, such as patients with gastroparesis and dilated small bowel on plain x-rays, small bowel motility studies should be undertaken before undertaking a surgical intervention. Several techniques are available to assess small bowel transit. Nondigestible carbohydrates are broken down into hydrogen and fatty acids upon reaching the colon. Hydrogen and fatty acids are then absorbed into the bloodstream. Therefore, the interval between ingestion of substrate and increments in exhaled hydrogen levels estimate small bowel transit. Similarly, orally administered sulfasalazine is broken down by colonic bacteria into mesalazine and sulfapyridine and then absorbed. Colonic transit can be measured by serum detection of sulfapyridine. Radionucleotide scintigraphy has also been used to assess small bowel transit function. However, the clinical application of these tests is limited by their complexity and variation in bacterial flora in different subjects.

### MAGNETIC RESONANCE IMAGING

MRI of the pelvic floor is the newest addition to the diagnostic armamentarium available for pelvic floor evaluation. MRI obviates the exposure to radiation. One technique involves filling the rectum with ultrasound gel. Images can be obtained in a "static" manner or in the form of dynamic pelvic MRI, which involves having the patient perform maneuvers similar to those performed during conventional defecography. During these maneuvers, multiple images are obtained, which are then viewed as a cine loop. MRI provides excellent spatial orientation of the sphincter complex and provides superior delineation of the surrounding structures. MRI appears to be superior to ultrasonography in discerning external sphincter abnormalities (30). Additionally, dynamic MRI defecography appears to be superior to conventional defecography in the evaluation of descending perineum syndrome as it provides excellent spatial assessment of pelvic floor musculature (52).

## LIMITATIONS OF MRI IN CONSTIPATION

Dynamic pelvic floor MRI shares similar limitations as conventional MRI: cost, claustrophobia, and availability. There are, however, some specific limitations related to the diagnostic modality. Studies comparing dynamic MRI with conventional defecography have yielded conflicting results. Healy et al. (53) found significant correlation between dynamic MRI findings and defecography in 10 patients examined employing both techniques. On the contrary, Matsouka et al. (54), in their study of 22 patients, reported defecography to be more sensitive than dynamic MRI and recommended against the routine use of this expensive modality. Most centers perform pelvic floor imaging with patient in supine position. Patients are asked to strain in a position that is far from physiologic and raises concerns regarding the reliability of the test. The influence of patient positioning has been investigated. Bertschinger et al. (55) performed a prospective comparison of 38 patients who underwent closed MRI in supine position followed by open MRI in a sitting position. Four rectal descents, two enteroceles, four small cystoceles, and four small anterior rectoceles were missed at supine MRI. The clinical significance of these findings, however, remains questionable. As mentioned earlier, the lack of "normal controls" makes it difficult to assess the efficacy of this test.

## Balloon expulsion test

The balloon expulsion test is an infrequently used method to test motor defecatory function of the rectum. There is a complete lack of standardization of methods used in various anorectal manometry laboratories. Various size balloons have been used for this purpose. Commonly, 50–100 cc deformable balloons are used. Alternatively, smaller, more rigid balloons may also be employed. The impact of size and compliance of balloon on the final interpretation of the test is unclear. In general, it is easier to evacuate larger balloons (56). Many investigators believe that the volume of the balloon should be individualized to induce a constant desire to defecate. Consequently, the use of lower volumes may result in false-positive results (57). There is a wide variation in what is considered to be a normal test. The inability to expel the balloon in a sitting position within 30–60 seconds is considered abnormal in most centers. Balloon expulsion has been shown to be of importance in differentiating between constipation caused by slow transit from that caused by pelvic floor dyssynergia (57).

## Biofeedback for constipation

Biofeedback training is widely utilized to teach relaxation of the pelvic floor in patients with pelvic floor dyssynergia. A critical review of the available literature by Heymen et al. (58) including 38 studies showed that mean success rate with pressure biofeedback was 78% compared to mean success rate of 70% seen with EMG feedback. The authors surmised that despite the reported success rates, quality research is lacking.

The most controversial area involving biofeedback training for constipation is the questionable durability of the results. Ferrara et al. (59) reported a clear loss of benefits over time despite initial success.

### PATIENT PERSPECTIVE

Inherent to the evaluation of fecal incontinence is the patient's feelings of shame, embarrassment, and discomfort. These sensations are felt by the incontinent patient, resulting in depression and social isolation. A number of quality-of-life tools have been developed to quantify the results of evaluation and treatment of fecal incontinence. No one tool is universally accepted, and these tools have been difficult to validate (60,61).

In addition, the testing incontinent patients are subjected to may be embarrassing and uncomfortable. Deutekom et al. conducted a cohort study of 240 consecutive patients undergoing evaluation of fecal incontinence in 16 Dutch centers. Each patient underwent manometry, defecography, TAUS, PNTML, and MRI. Two hundred forty of the 270 self-administered questionnaires were returned. Patients were asked to evaluate anxiety, discomfort, embarrassment, and pain. Answers were scaled from 1 (not 0), none, to 5, severe. Results were also summarized as total test burden. Overall test results were surprisingly low, with average scores in each category not exceeding 2. Overall, MRI was the most preferred and least uncomfortable test. Defecography was the most inconvenient and uncomfortable. Anorectal combined testing, manometry, PNTML, and TAUS, also scored low for discomfort and overall test burden but more so than MRI (62).

## CONCLUSION

Physiological studies of anorectal function can provide valuable information in carefully selected cases. While performing these studies, one should be cognizant of the fact that these procedures can be embarrassing, and at best are far from the patient's usual habits. It is unnerving for many patients to perform the act of defecation in the presence of an audience, and it is conceivable that "performance anxiety" may lead to results that are not truly representative of actual patient status. Thus, these studies should be interpreted with a grain of salt. Despite the plethora of literature available, the clinical usefulness of these tests remains vague, and there is limited evidence that anorectal imaging guides management in pelvic floor disorders (63). There are multiple well-designed studies, which, unfortunately, report conflicting results. We therefore recommend that the most decisive factor governing treatment decisions is history and physical exam. Physiology testing should always be used as an adjunct rather than a primary determinant.

# REFERENCES

1. Whitehead WE et al. *Dis Colon Rectum.* 2001;44: 131–144.
2. Tjandra JJ et al. *Dis Colon Rectum.* 2007;50: 1497–1507.
3. Person B et al. *Surg Clin N Am.* 2006;86(4):969–86.
4. Thompson WG et al. *Gut.* 1999;45(Suppl 2):ii43–7.
5. Gordon PG. Anatomy and physiology of the anorectum. In Fazio VW, Church JM, Delaney CP (eds). *Current Therapy in Colon and Rectal Surgery*, 2nd Edition. Philadelphia: Elsevier-Mosby, 2005, pp. 1–9.
6. Simpson RR et al. *Dis Colon Rectum.* 2006;49:1033–8.
7. Wexner SD et al. Setting up a colorectal physiology laboratory. In Corman ML (ed.). *Colon and Rectal Surgery*, 5th Edition. Philadelphia, PA: Lippincott, Williams and Wilkins, 2005, pp. 129–67.
8. Madoff RD et al. *Int J Colorectal Dis.* 1990;5(1):37–40.
9. Barnett JL et al. *Gastroenterology.* 1999;116(3):732–60.
10. Liberman H et al. *Dis Colon Rectum.* 2001;44:1567–74.
11. Felt-Bersma RJ et al. *Dis Colon Rectum.* 1990;33(6): 479–85.
12. Yang YK, Wexner SD. *Int J Colorectal Dis.* 1994;9(2): 92–5.
13. Beck A. *Phlugers Arch.* 1930;224:278–92.
14. Ferrara A et al. *Tech Coloproctol.* 2001;5:13–8.
15. Smith LE, Blatchford GJ. Physiologic testing. In Wolff BG, Fleshman JW, Beck DE et al. (eds). *The ASCRS Textbook of Colon and Rectal Surgery.* New York, NY: Springer, 2007, pp. 40–56.
16. Timmcke AE. Limitations of anal physiologic testing. In Hicks TC, Beck DE, Opelka FG, Timmcke AE (eds). *Complications of Colon and Rectal Surgery.* Baltimore, MD: Williams and Wilkins, 1996, pp. 419–30.
17. Jacobs PPM et al. *Dis Colon Rectum.* 1990;33(6): 494–7.
18. Laurberg S et al. *Br J Surg.* 1998;75:786–8.
19. Wexner SD et al. *Dis Colon Rectum.* 1991;34:22–30.
20. Buie WD et al. *Dis Colon Rectum.* 2001;44:1255–60.
21. Kiff ES, Swash M. *Br J Surg.* 1984 August;71(8):614–6.
22. Ricciardi R et al. *Dis Colon Rectum.* 2006 June;49(6): 852–7.
23. Frudinger A et al. *Abdom Imaging.* 1998;23:301–3.
24. Nazir M et al. *Dis Colon Rectum.* 2002;45:1325–31.
25. Zetterstrom JP et al. *Dis Colon Rectum.* 1998;41: 705–13.
26. Briel JW et al. *Br J Surgery.* 1999;86:1322–7.
27. Christensen AF et al. *Brit J Radiol.* 2005;78:308–11.
28. Badger SA et al. *Int J Colorectal Dis.* 2007 October; 22(10):1261–8.
29. Dobben AC et al. *Int J Colorectal Dis.* 2007;22:783–90.
30. Terra MP, Stoker J. *Eur Radiol.* 2006;16:1727–36.
31. West RL et al. *Int J Colorect Dis.* 2005;20:328–33.
32. Norton C et al. *Cochrane Database Syst Rev.* 2006;(3).
33. Jensen L, Lowry A. *Dis Colon Rectum.* 1997;40: 197–200.
34. Heyman S et al. *Dis Colon Rectum.* 2001;44:728–36.
35. Solomon MJ et al. *Dis Colon Rectum.* 2003;46:703–10.
36. Pager CK et al. *Dis Colon Rectum.* 2002;45:997–1003.
37. Norton C et al. *Gastroenterology.* 2003;125:1320–9.
38. Stewart WF et al. *Am J Gastroenterol.* 1999 December; 94(12):3530–40.
39. Sonnenberg A, Koch TR. *Dis Colon Rectum.* 1989;32(1): 1–8.
40. Infantino A et al. *Dis Colon Rectum.* 1990 August; 33(8):707–12.
41. Moieira H, Wexner SD. Anorectal physiologic testing. In Beck DE, Wexner SD (eds). *Fundamentals of Anorectal Surgery*, 2nd Edition. Philadephia, PA: WB Saunders, 1998, pp. 37–53.
42. Finlay IG et al. *Int J Colorectal Dis.* 1998;3:67–98.
43. Penninckx F et al. *Int J Colorectal Dis.* 1990 May;5(2): 94–7.
44. Ferrante SL et al. *Dis Colon Rectum.* 1991 January; 34(1):51–5.
45. Bartram CI et al. *Gastrointest Radiol.* 1988;13(1):72–80.
46. Turnbull GK et al. *Dis Colon Rectum.* 1988;31(3):190–7.
47. Halligan S, Bartram CI. *Dis Colon Rectum.* 1995;38(7): 764–8.
48. Shorvon PJ et al. *Gut.* 1989;30:1737–49.
49. Roe AM et al. *J Roy Soc Med.* 1986;79:331–3.
50. Jones PN et al. *Dis Colon Rectum.* 1987;30(9):667–70.
51. Karulf RE et al. *Dis Colon Rectum.* 1991;34(6):464–8.
52. Healy JC et al. *Br J Surg.* 1997;84(11):1555–8.
53. Healy JC et al. *AJR Am J Roentgenol.* 1997;169(3): 775–9.
54. Matsuoka H et al. *Dis Colon Rectum.* 2001;44(4):571–6.
55. Bertschinger KM et al. *Radiology.* 2002;223(2):501–8.
56. Azpiroz F et al. *Am J Gastroenterol.* 2002;97(2):232–40.
57. Minguez M et al. *Gastroenterology.* 2004;126(1):57–62.
58. Heymen S et al. *Dis Colon Rectum.* 2003;46(9):1208–17. Review.
59. Ferrara A et al. *Tech Coloproctol.* 2001;5(3):131–5.
60. Wexner SD et al. *Dis Colon Rectum.* 1993;36:139–45.
61. Rockwood TH et al. *Dis Colon Rectum.* 2000;43:9–17.
62. Deutekom M et al. *Brit J Radiology.* 2006;79:94–100.
63. Bharucha AE, Fletcher JG. *Gastroenterology.* 2007; 133(4):1069–74.

# 12

# Limitations of colorectal imaging studies

ANDREW C. MATTHEWS AND CHARLES C. MATTHEWS

## CHALLENGING CASE

A 53-year-old women presents to the emergency room with fever and left lower quadrant abdominal pain and tenderness. Her temperature is 39°C, and her white blood cell count is 17,000 cells per cubic milliliter. What is the best radiologic test to confirm her diagnosis?

## CASE MANAGEMENT

A computed tomography (CT) scan of the abdomen and pelvis will evaluate her to confirm the diagnosis of acute diverticulitis. In the absence of acute diverticulitis, it may very well provide another explanation for her symptoms.

## INTRODUCTION

Diagnostic imaging examinations are an important component of the overall evaluation of diseases of the colon and rectum. Today, multiple modalities are available to examine the abdomen and colon including plain radiographs, contrast studies under fluoroscopy, nuclear medicine (NM) scintigraphy, computed tomography (CT), positron emission tomography (PET), magnetic resonance imaging (MRI), and ultrasound. This chapter focuses on two cross-sectional modalities—CT and MRI—with particular application to specific clinical problems. Diagnostic imaging examinations have variable accuracy—some findings are diagnostic while others are helpful in the differential diagnosis but are not specific. Understanding the strengths and limitations of each exam is important for the clinical physician to properly select what is best for the patient.

## CONVENTIONAL IMAGING OF THE ABDOMEN AND PELVIS

Classic radiographic examination of the colon includes plain radiographs of the abdomen and single and double barium contrast enemas under fluoroscopy. The fluoroscopic examinations are almost an art form, requiring real-time interaction including the patient, the fluoroscope, the instillation of barium contrast, and the radiologist. Both of these modalities are projection techniques, rendering a three-dimensional (3D) object into a two-dimensional (2D) image, and have limited soft tissue contrast resolution (1).

Plain radiographs of the abdomen have limited diagnostic value. In a study of 1,000 consecutive emergency department patients, Ahn et al. evaluated the diagnostic finding of plain radiographs and CT examinations in the setting of nontraumatic abdominal pain. This retrospective review of the radiology reports excluded 129 patients in whom a final diagnosis was not reliably established. The review included 871 patients with abdominal radiographs and 188 patients with abdominal CT scans. The overall findings on plain radiographs were nonspecific in 68%, normal in 23%, and abnormal (specific diagnosis) in 10%. The radiographs had the highest sensitivity for detection of foreign bodies (90%) and bowel obstruction (49%). The radiographs had 0% sensitivity for appendicitis, pyelonephritis, pancreatitis, and diverticulitis. The overall findings on CT scans were normal in 20% and abnormal (specific diagnosis) in 80%. CT had the highest sensitivities for bowel obstruction (75%), urolithiasis (68%), and pancreatitis (60%). These results demonstrate greater diagnostic yield with a CT exam (2) (Figures 12.1 and 12.2).

Multiple clinical trials have evaluated the performance of double-contrast barium enema (DCBE), CT colonography (CTC), and optical colonoscopy (OC) for the detection of polyps and masses in the colon. Rockey et al. reported a series of 614 patients who had all three examinations. Their data indicated sensitivity for the detection of colonic

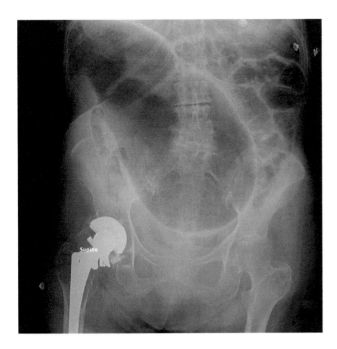

Figure 12.1 Radiograph. Cecal volvulus. Markedly distended cecum with pneumatosis in wall.

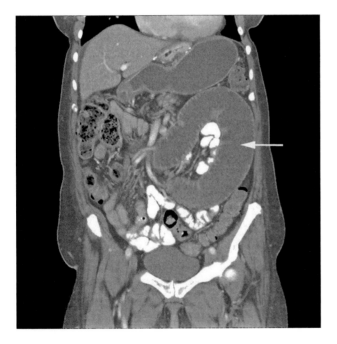

Figure 12.2 CT. Small bowel obstruction, S/P Roux-en-Y gastric bypass. Coronal image demonstrates fluid-filled and obstructed biliary limb in mid-abdomen.

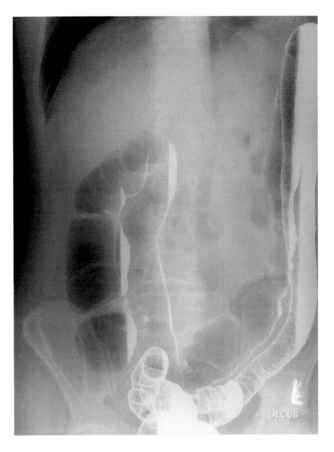

Figure 12.3 Radiograph. Double-contrast barium enema. Decubitus view demonstrates layering of barium liquid and air distending the colon.

both CTC and OC. Their data indicated a sensitivity of 90% for CTC for colonic lesions 10 mm or greater. Sensitivity decreased with decreasing size of lesion (4) (Figure 12.3).

## CROSS-SECTIONAL IMAGING

Cross-sectional imaging modalities include ultrasound, PET, CT, and MRI. All of these came into clinical practice in the 1970s and 1980s. CT and MRI were recognized as such great advances in medicine that the inventors of each were awarded the Nobel Prize in Medicine (Cormack and Hounsfield for CT in 1979 and Lauterbur and Mansfield for MRI in 2003) (5).

Cross-sectional imaging such as CT demonstrates additional anatomic information with improved soft tissue contrast providing the advantage of showing pathology in the colonic wall and adjacent structures. The routine transverse images can be supplemented with multiplanar reformations in the coronal and sagittal planes. Today, the images are routinely acquired at 5 mm or thinner sections. Nonionic iodinated contrast agents are routinely given intravenously to enhance solid organs and vascular structures; the images are typically acquired around 70 seconds postinjection for maximal enhancement of solid organs such as the liver.

lesions 10 mm or greater as follows: DCBE, 48%; CTC, 59%; and OC, 98% (3). Because of the low sensitivity of DCBE, its continued use to screen for polyps is controversial (1). Others have similarly reported very high sensitivity for OC but better sensitivity for CTC. For example, the National CT Colonography Trial of the American College of Radiology Imaging Network reported their results of the multicenter trial involving 2,531 asymptomatic patients undergoing

Gastrointestinal (GI) contrast is also routinely given by mouth to opacify the stomach and intestines. GI contrast agents are usually 2% preparations of barium sulfate or nonionic iodinated contrast; they are given 60–90 minutes before the exam to allow transit through the intestines. The basic CT scan is performed after the IV contrast injection, but additional series may be done before IV contrast and after several minutes of delay. CT evaluation of the GI tract has high sensitivity for detection of pneumoperitoneum and leaks of oral contrast from the GI tract. Significant CT limitations include low sensitivity for early and superficial mucosal abnormalities of inflammatory bowel disease and depth of tumor invasion in the colon wall (6).

## INFLAMMATORY AND INFECTIOUS BOWEL DISEASES

Inflammatory and infectious diseases of the colon have numerous possible etiologies. These are usually regarded as various types of "colitis." The principal pathologic processes are infection, inflammatory bowel disease, and ischemia. Other inflammatory processes that are not usually considered colitis are diverticulitis, epiploic appendagitis, stercoral colitis, and radiation enteritis. Infectious colitis may require a stool culture for accurate diagnosis. Inflammatory bowel disease has two major forms—Crohn disease and ulcerative colitis. The typical presentation is cramping abdominal pain, fever, leukocytosis, and change in bowel habit, usually diarrhea. The prevalence in the general population in the United States is low—approximately 10–12 per 100,000 for ulcerative colitis and 20–40 per 100,000 for Crohn disease. For both diseases, most patients are young adults (7).

Several general observations and patterns are helpful in the CT diagnosis of bowel diseases. The length of diseased colon is an important feature. Focal disease may represent neoplasm, diverticulitis, epiploic appendagitis, and infection. Segmental disease usually indicates some type of colitis—Crohn disease, ischemia, infection, or ulcerative colitis. Diffuse disease usually indicates infection or ulcerative colitis. Certain locations have a predilection for involvement by certain processes: examples include amebiasis and Crohn disease in the cecal region, ischemia in the splenic flexure region, and ulcerative colitis and stercoral colitis in the rectum. Enhancement patterns are also helpful—the target or double halo pattern is typically benign with possibilities including infection, inflammatory bowel disease, edema, and ischemia (7,8).

## CT AND MRI ENTEROGRAPHY

More advanced CT exam protocols have been developed to better evaluate inflammatory bowel disease. The technique commonly used today is termed *CT enterography*. The major features of the technique are (1) excellent vascular enhancement with IV contrast, (2) bowel distension with low or neutral density oral contrast, and (3) thin-section reconstructions in the transverse and coronal planes. The

details vary among published protocols (9–12). Excellent vascular enhancement is performed with 125–150 mL nonionic IV contrast at a flow rate of 4 mL/s. The timing of the scan varies from 30 (arterial phase) to 70 (portal venous phase) seconds following the start of the injection. Many protocols use a single phase between these times, the enteric phase at 45 seconds (10). High-level vascular enhancement is necessary to demonstrate mural hyperenhancement, wall stratification ("target sign"), and engorged vasa recta ("comb sign") (9). The neutral density oral contrast is given to distend the bowel lumen and aids visualization of mucosal enhancement; this would be obscured by the traditional high-density oral contrast. A large volume of oral contrast is administered, typically 450 mL at 60 and 40 minutes and 225 mL at 20 and 10 minutes prior to the exam for a total of 1350 mL. A commonly used agent is VoLumen by E-Z-EM (11). Images are typically reconstructed from a helical acquisition at 2.5 or 3 mm thickness; thin sections improve the demonstration of small structures (Figure 12.4).

Paulsen et al. from Mayo Clinic reported their experience with over 700 cases of CT enterography. The most common indication was suspected Crohn disease, and this was confirmed in about half of the patients. They report that mural hyperenhancement, mural stratification, bowel wall thickening (>3 mm), stranding in the mesenteric fat, and engorged vasa recta correlate with active inflammation. A minority of their patients also demonstrated associated pathology outside the bowel, such as fistula and abscess or both (12). Another study from Mayo Clinic evaluated small bowel enhancement characteristics and sensitivity and specificity by comparing to endoscopic and histologic results. The study involved 42 patients undergoing CT enterography. Exams were performed with 150 mL of IV contrast delivered at 4 mL/s with a 45-second delay. Their

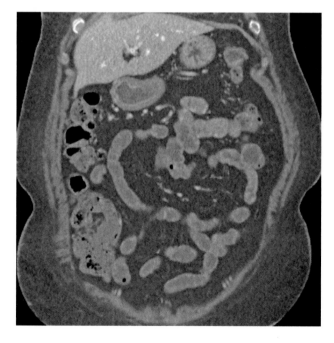

Figure 12.4 CT enterography. Normal small bowel.

study concluded that jejunal attenuation is greater than ileal attenuation, and collapsed bowel has a greater attenuation than distended bowel. The most sensitive appearance of Crohn disease was mural enhancement (73%–80%) followed by mural thickening. The most specific findings of active disease were the comb sign of engorged vasa recta and increased attenuation of perienteric fat (10). Similar findings were also reported by Baker et al. from the Cleveland Clinic study of 630 patients undergoing CT enterography (11) (Figures 12.5 and 12.6).

Concerns about radiation exposure have been raised in the evaluation of patients with suspected or confirmed Crohn disease, particularly considering the chronic nature of the disease and the typical young age of the patients (13). A review in the *New England Journal of Medicine* by Brenner and Hall reports a dramatic increase in the widespread utilization of CT scans in the U.S. population from 1980 to 2006, estimated at 62 million scans in 2006. They estimated the lifetime risk of death from a single abdominal CT exam for a 50-year-old person at around 0.01%. The risk for a 20-year-old is about six times higher (14).

DelGaizo et al. from Mayo Clinic reported multiple techniques to reduce effective dose in CT enterography. These include the following: (1) reduce scan length to shortest possible, (2) reduce tube voltage to 100 kV, (3) reduce tube current based on patient size, and (4) utilize automated

(a)

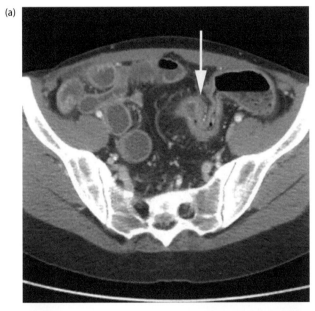

(b)

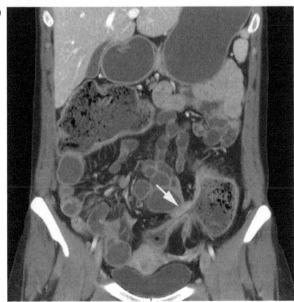

Figure 12.5 CT enterography. Crohn disease with obstruction. **(a)** Mural thickening and enhancement, engorged vasa recta, and stranding of adjacent fat. **(b)** Segmental stricture causing obstruction.

(a)

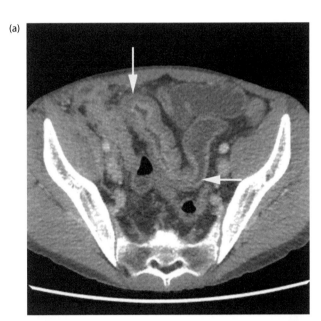

(b)

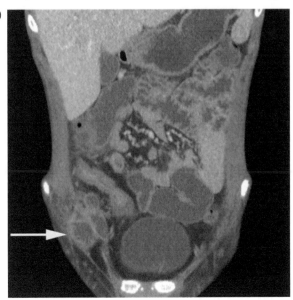

Figure 12.6 CT enterography. Crohn disease with fistula and abscess. **(a)** Mural enhancement and thickening of terminal ileum. **(b)** Adjacent abdominal wall abscess.

exposure control. These techniques will reduce the total exposure, noting that image noise will increase with reduced dose (13). A trade-off or balance has to be reached to lower the dose as low as possible while maintaining diagnostic image quality. In recent years, new methods of image reconstruction termed *adaptive statistical iterative reconstruction* (ASIR) have allowed a lower-dose CT exam with equivalent image quality. Kambadakone et al. from the Massachusetts General Hospital investigated the use of ASIR technology to achieve a low-dose CT enterography exam using an ASIR setting of 30%. The images obtained were evaluated as optimal diagnostic quality, and the radiation dose was reduced to 34% (15). In our practice, we use more aggressive dose reduction with ASIR 40%.

With a goal of reducing the risk of radiation exposure, MRI enterography has been developed and evaluated in comparison to CT. The major benefits of CT enterography are better spatial resolution, fewer motion artifacts, increased availability, lower cost, and shorter exam time. The principal detraction for CT enterography is radiation exposure. MRI enterography advantages include better tissue contrast resolution, better evaluation of perianal disease, better distinction between acute and chronic disease, and no radiation exposure. Similar to CT, the MRI enterography techniques utilize oral contrast for bowel distension and IV contrast (gadolinium based) for bowel wall enhancement. Most MRI protocols also use antiperistaltic agents. Multiplanar, multisequence images are obtained prior to IV contrast; exact sequences are variable and machine dependent. Most protocols use a liver acquisition volume acceleration (LAVA) type sequence around 15 and/or 60 seconds following injection of IV contrast (16).

Comparing CT and MRI enterography, Siddiki et al. from Mayo Clinic reported on a series of 30 patients with suspected Crohn disease. MRI and CT enterography showed excellent and similar sensitivities, 91% and 95%, respectively ($p = 0.32$). CT was evaluated with higher image quality. The authors concluded MRI enterography may be the preferred imaging exam for patients with small bowel Crohn disease who may be undergoing multiple exams (17).

A more recent study on MRI and CT enterography by Masselli et al. reported on 150 patients with suspected small bowel disease. Their findings indicated sensitivity of MRI enterography for all small bowel disease was significantly higher compared to CT at 93% and 76%, respectively ($p = 0.0159$). The sensitivities for detecting inflammatory bowel disease, however, were not significantly different (MRI, 100%; CT, 96%; $p > 0.99$). MRI performed significantly better for the detection of neoplastic disease (18) (Figures 12.7 through 12.9).

## DIVERTICULITIS

Diverticular disease is a common condition in the United States with increasing frequency by age, approximately <5%

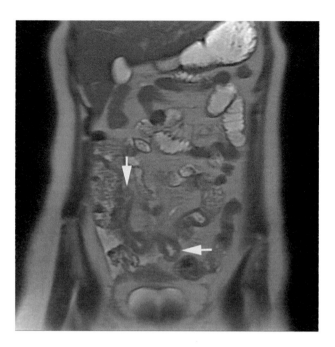

Figure 12.7 MRI enterography. Crohn disease. Precontrast T2-weighted coronal image demonstrates thickening of terminal ileum.

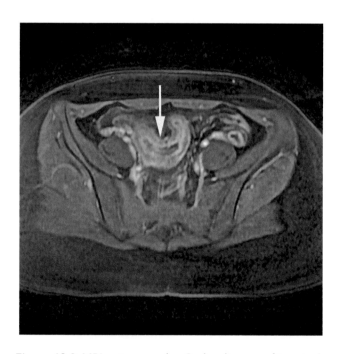

Figure 12.8 MRI enterography. Crohn disease of terminal ileum. Postcontrast T1-weighted image shows thickened wall with increased enhancement and mural stratification.

under age 40 increasing to >65% by age 85. Acute diverticulitis is the most common complication of the disease, beginning as a localized infection in a segment involved with diverticulosis. The inflammation extends to the adjacent pericolic area. Complications include perforation, abscess, and fistula formation (19). Zaidi and Daly found in their series of patients at an urban medical center in the United

(a)

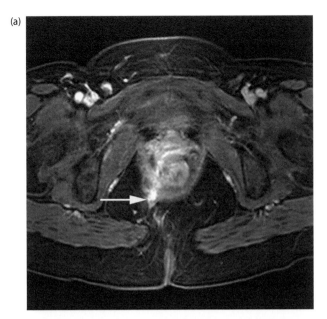

(b)

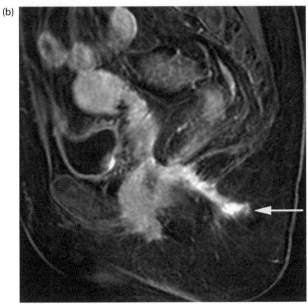

Figure 12.9 MRI. Crohn disease with perianal fistula. **(a)** Short T1 inversion recovery (STIR) sequence shows fistula from perianal area to ischiorectal fossa. **(b)** In sagittal plane, shows fistula extending to buttock cleft.

States that a high percentage of patients, 54%, with acute diverticulitis were 50 years of age or younger and that 21% were 40 or younger. Their conclusion suggests a rising frequency of diverticulitis in younger and obese patients in the United States (20).

Before the development of CT, barium enema was the imaging test used to confirm the clinical diagnosis. The ability of CT to diagnose diverticulitis was recognized early in the development of this diagnostic tool. Hulnick et al. in 1984 described the findings and advocated the routine use of CT in patients with signs and symptoms of diverticulitis (21). Kircher et al. reported on the individual signs of

diverticulitis on helical CT in their series of 312 patients at the Massachusetts General Hospital. They found the most sensitive findings for diverticulitis were bowel thickening (96%) and fat stranding (91%). Less frequent but highly specific signs were fascial thickening and inflamed diverticula. The diverticulitis was located in the sigmoid colon in 55%, in the junction of the descending and sigmoid colon in 17%, and in the descending colon in 16% (22). Abdominal CT is generally considered the preferred imaging test for evaluating patients with possible acute diverticulitis. Besides its high accuracy for diverticulitis, CT is also an accurate test for diagnosing alternative conditions including appendicitis (19) (Figure 12.10).

(a)

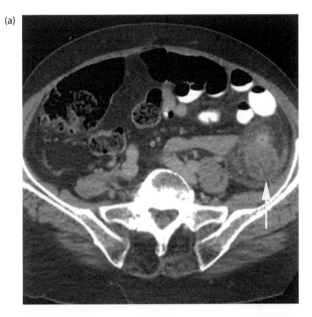

(b)

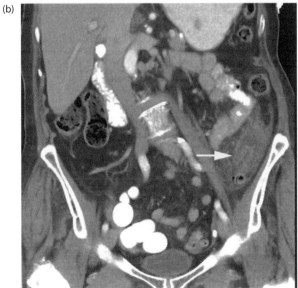

Figure 12.10 CT. Acute diverticulitis. **(a)** Axial image shows marked thickening of descending colon with inflammation of adjacent fat. **(b)** Coronal image shows segmental involvement of descending colon.

Abscess development is a recognized complication of diverticulitis that may be treated with antibiotics, interventional radiology percutaneous drainage, and/or surgery. Siewert et al. found abscesses in 30 (17%) of their 181 patients with CT diagnosis of diverticulitis. Twenty-two (73%) of those 30 patients had abscesses less than 3 cm in size and were successfully treated with antibiotics alone ($p < 0.001$). Patients with abscesses larger than 4 cm can be managed with CT-guided abscess drainage followed by referral for surgical treatment. The majority of patients with the larger abscesses underwent surgery after resolution of symptoms (23) (Figure 12.11).

In the CT assessment of diverticulitis, some features overlap with findings of colon cancer. Chintapalli et al. reported their retrospective and prospective results in a series of 58 patients with diverticulitis ($n = 27$) or colon cancer ($n = 31$). They found the most specific findings for diverticulitis were pericolonic inflammation ($p < 0.01$) and length of segment greater than 10 cm ($p < 0.012$). The most specific signs for colon cancer were presence of lymph nodes ($p < 0.001$) and luminal mass ($p < 0.003$) (24). As the CT features of acute diverticulitis can overlap those of colon cancer, professional societies such as the American College of Gastroenterology have previously recommended patients have follow-up colonoscopy to rule out cancer. Sai et al. performed a literature review for patients with a CT diagnosis of acute diverticulitis who had surgery, colonoscopy, or barium enema within 24 weeks. From the articles in the literature, the pooled data identified 771 patients that met the criteria. Colon cancer

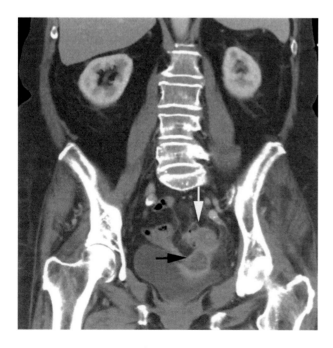

Figure 12.11 CT. Acute diverticulitis with abscess. Acute diverticulitis (white arrow) with adjacent 3 cm abscess (black arrow) and inflammation of bladder dome. Patient was successfully treated with IV antibiotics.

was found in 14 patients for a prevalence of 2.1%. The same authors calculated from Surveillance, Epidemiology, and End Results (SEER) Program data a prevalence of colon cancer in the general population of U.S. adults older than 55 years at 0.68%. They concluded the broad recommendation of follow-up colonoscopy to exclude colon cancer is not justified (25). deVries et al. reviewed pooled data from nine published series including 2,490 patients with diverticulitis. Follow-up colonoscopy was performed in 1,468 patients (59%); colorectal cancer was found in 17 patients for a prevalence of 1.16%. They concluded routine colonoscopy follow-up is not necessary unless there are clinical signs of colon cancer or a patient over 50 years of age has not had screening colonoscopy (26). In another review article on radiologic and endoscopic imaging in the diagnosis and follow-up of colonic diverticular disease, Flo et al. also concluded the role of colonoscopy after acute diverticulitis remains controversial. While many practice guidelines from professional societies advise follow-up colonoscopy, this is mainly supported by expert opinion and a lack of robust scientific evidence. Systematic reviews show that colonoscopy is generally not necessary (19).

## GASTROINTESTINAL BLEEDING

Acute and chronic GI bleeding has a variety of etiologies and involves multiple medical specialties in diagnosis, management, and treatment. In 2009, the hospitalization rate for GI bleeding in the United States was approximately 60.6/100,000 for upper GI bleeding and 35.7/100,000 for lower GI bleeding. The overall hospitalization rate decreased in the 2000s (27). The ligament of Treitz divides the classification into upper GI bleeding proximal to this level and lower GI bleeding distal to it. The most common causes of upper GI bleeding are erosions or ulcers and variceal bleeding. The most common causes of lower GI bleeding are diverticular disease, angiodysplasia, and neoplasm (28). Investigation of GI bleeding is routinely performed with esophagoduodenoscopy (EGD) and colonoscopy. When neither of these endoscopic examinations has provided a diagnostic cause for the bleeding, it is considered obscure GI bleeding (29). Patients typically become symptomatic with tachycardia and hypotension when the acute blood loss exceeds approximately 500 mL in a day. Most bleeds will stop spontaneously with supportive measures (28). In the era prior to the development of CT, catheter-directed angiography and nuclear medicine (NM) were used to diagnose causes of obscure GI bleeding. In a paper published in 1971, Rosch et al. reported on 21 patients with acute GI bleeding that were treated with selective arterial infusion of the vasoconstrictors epinephrine and pitressin. The GI bleeding was successfully controlled in the majority, though not all, of patients (30). In another sentinel paper from the 1970s, Bookstein et al. reported their results from transcatheter embolization in seven patients with lower GI bleeding. They used Gelfoam and Ivalon for the embolic agents to achieve control of bleeding in five of the patients;

the other two re-bled from angiodysplasia after several months (31). In a report from a larger and more contemporary series of 102 patients with acute nonvariceal GI bleeding, Koo et al. achieved a clinical success rate in 77% (78/102) using *N*-butyl-2-cyanoacrylate (NBCA) as the embolic agent. Bowel infarction was a complication experienced by two patients. Cancer-related bleeding was associated with increased clinical failure. NBCA is widely used as an embolic agent in many other clinical settings besides GI bleeding (32).

In recent years, CT has developed as a mainstream tool for the noninvasive diagnosis of acute GI bleeding, particularly for obscure bleeding. Two exam protocols have been used—CT enterography and CT angiography (29,33,34). Lee et al. reported a sensitivity of 55% and positive predictive value of 100% for identifying the source of GI bleeding with CT enterography. Diagnostic yield was higher in massive bleeding. CT enterography requires 8 hours of patient preparation time for fasting and the administration of a neutral type of oral contrast agent (29). However, CT angiography requires no special preparation and is suited for use in the emergent setting. CT angiography is performed as a three-phase examination with initial noncontrast series, then postcontrast arterial and portal venous phases. This exam needs to be performed on a modern scanner, typically a 64 detector helical unit with thin sections approximately 1 mm, depending on vendor specifications. Importantly, no oral contrast is given. IV contrast is administered as a dose of 100–125 mL at a high flow rate of 4–5 mL/s to achieve high levels of vascular enhancement. GI bleeding is diagnosed when extravasation of contrast is identified in the bowel lumen. Noncontrast images are very important to reveal opaque material that is often present in the GI tract and which may mimic extravasation of contrast. The venous phase helps confirm GI bleeding with increased volume and dispersion of the extravasated contrast in the bowel lumen compared to the arterial phase. CT angiography has a reported lower limit for the detection of bleeding at a rate of approximately 0.5 mL/min. Of course, false-negative exams can occur in the setting of intermittent bleeding (34) (Figures 12.12 and 12.13).

Nuclear medicine scintigraphy with Technetium-99m-labeled red blood cells (RBCs) is also a mainstream test for the detection of GI bleeding with reported sensitivity to detect bleeding at 0.1 mL/min. Strengths of the exam include noninvasive modality and prolonged observation time to detect intermittent bleeding. Weaknesses of the exam include less accessibility for the test in off-hours and inaccuracy in localizing the site of bleeding (35). In a retrospective study of 45 CT angiography and 90 RBC examinations for suspected lower GI bleeding, Feuerstein et al. found that CT angiography and RBC scintigraphy showed active bleeding in 38% of cases each. However, the site of bleeding was accurately localized in 30% of RBC scintigraphy cases compared to 53% of CT cases ($p = 0.008$). Time to complete the exam after placement of the order was significantly shorter for CT at 1 hour 41 minutes compared to

(a)

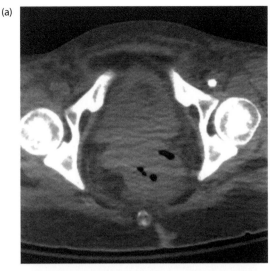

(b)

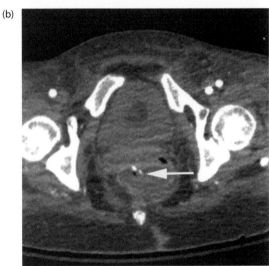

(c)

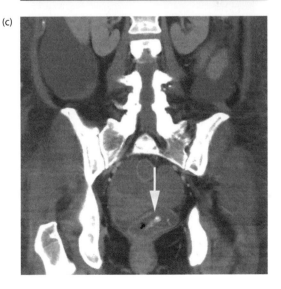

Figure 12.12 CT angiogram. Rectal bleeding. **(a)** Initial noncontrast image shows fluid in rectum. **(b)** Arterial phase shows extravasation of contrast at anterior wall of rectum. **(c)** Coronal image confirms active bleeding with pooling of contrast in rectal lumen. Colonoscopy diagnosed a bleeding ulcer at this site.

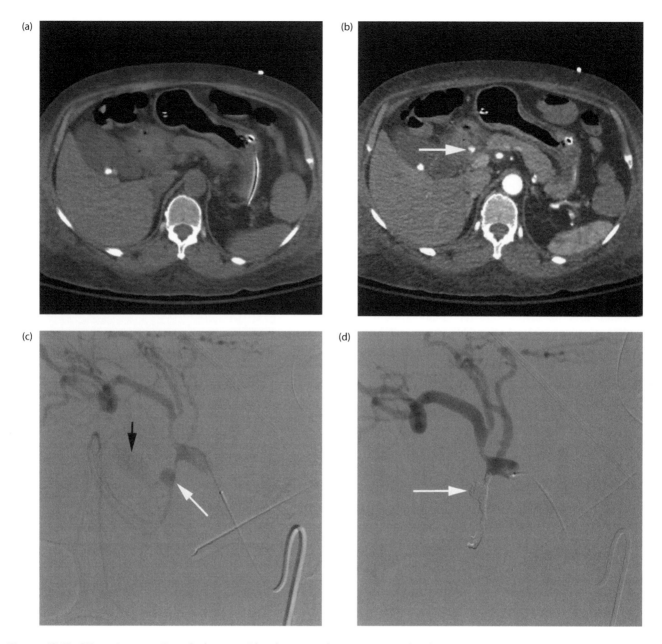

Figure 12.13 CT angiogram; IR embolization. Bleeding pseudoaneurysm in duodenum. **(a)** Precontrast image. **(b)** Arterial phase image shows pseudoaneurysm of gastroduodenal artery without active bleeding. **(c)** Catheter angiogram demonstrates the pseudoaneurysm (white arrow) with active bleeding (black arrow) into duodenal lumen. Massive blood loss required a 13-unit blood transfusion during procedure. **(d)** Angiogram shows successful embolization with microcoils.

3 hours 9 minutes for RBC scintigraphy ($p < 0.001$). These two advantages for CTA have important implications in the treatment of the bleeding source (36).

Today, a variety of embolic agents are now in clinical use for transcatheter treatment of GI bleeding. These include microcoils, polyvinyl alcohol particles, Gelfoam, NBCA, and embucrylate. A combination of agents is often employed. Reported technical (angiographic cessation of bleeding) and clinical (no bleeding for 30 days) success rates are variable. Some reported results for clinical success rates range from 68% to 82% for upper GI bleeding and 81% to 91% for lower GI bleeding (28) (Figure 12.14).

## RECTAL CANCER STAGING

Advances in surgical techniques for the treatment of primary rectal cancer have generated a need for equal advances in preoperative imaging. High-resolution MRI has become the essential imaging modality in the preoperative evaluation of all rectal tumors, with MRI found to be superior to transrectal ultrasound (TRUS) and CT in preoperative imaging (37). TRUS and MRI have comparable accuracy in terms of T and N staging, but the limited field of view and operator dependence of TRUS yields MRI as the better alternative (38,39). CT lacks the detailed evaluation of

(a)

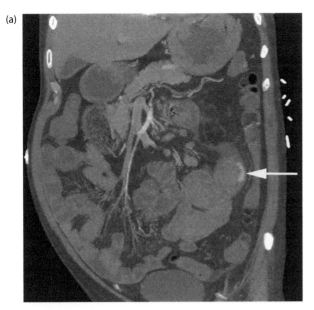

(b)

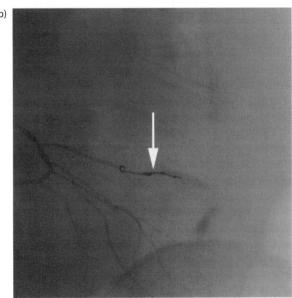

Figure 12.14 CT angiogram; IR embolization. **(a)** CT angiogram shows active bleeding from jejunal ulcer. **(b)** IR embolization image demonstrates embolization with microcoils.

the rectum and surrounding structures, as provided by the other modalities.

Although MRI can suggest the initial diagnosis of cancer, its utility is the evaluation of previously histologically diagnosed rectal tumor to preoperatively assess depth of tumor invasion in regard to the muscularis propria (T1–3), local involvement of adjacent structures (T4) including the mesorectal fascia (MRF), and the morphology of pelvic lymph nodes. MRI acts to guide surgical planning and/or indicates the use of neoadjuvant treatments as a means to achieve curative treatment with negative margins on surgical resection. Its full potential as an imaging tool requires a detailed clinical history, prior colonoscopy, and details of the rectal tumor (40).

## IMAGING TECHNIQUE

Adequate evaluation of rectal tumors relies on high-resolution T2-weighted images and a detailed clinical history including tumor location (low, mid, or high). Although 3.0 Tesla magnets yield improved spatial recognition and signal-to-noise ratio, studies have not yielded significant differences in diagnostic accuracy between 1.5 T and 3.0 T magnets (37). Typically there is no significant patient preparation prior to the examination, although antispasmodics can be used to reduce bowel motion. Similarly, rectal gel is another optional component to help define small or polypoid tumors. Body or endorectal coils can be used for image acquisition. Endorectal coils typically generate more detailed evaluation of the rectal wall, but cost and patient factors limit their use.

The essential portions of the examination are the high-resolution T2-weighted sequences. Typically, this involves a T2-weighted fast spin echo sequence with 3 mm slices. Initial sagittal T2-weighted images from pelvic sidewall to sidewall are acquired for planning the orthogonal slices (Figure 12.15a). It is important to know the tumor location to accurately identify and plan the tumoral axis in which the orthogonal slices will be based. The tumoral axis will be used to plan axial orthogonal images perpendicular to the tumor. Proper angulation is crucial to avoid volume averaging and correctly identify tumor borders (Figure 12.15c). Additional coronal T2-weighted images are obtained, which provide valuable information on the relationship of low rectal tumors to the anal sphincter (41).

Additional but nonessential sequences include T1, diffusion-weighted, and postgadolinium sequences. T1 sequences are useful for the evaluation of incidental osseous lesions in the pelvis such as metastases. Diffusion-weighted images have shown promise in detecting colorectal tumors (42) and in detecting lymph nodes, although they are not highly specific in differentiating malignant versus hyperplastic benign nodes (43). The use of IV gadolinium contrast has not typically been included in rectal tumor MR evaluation, and current studies suggest no added benefit of contrast material in assessing tumor penetration through the rectal wall and into the MRF (44). Other studies have suggested a benefit of gadolinium enhancement in detecting tumors and malignant lymph nodes (45,46). Currently, however, it appears gadolinium is not crucial or necessary in the evaluation of rectal cancers.

## IMAGING INTERPRETATION

The radiologist's duty is to convey numerous important findings to the colorectal surgeon to guide surgical planning or neoadjuvant treatment. The multitude of facts pertaining to the lesion is best conveyed through a structured report, as recent studies have shown the benefit of a structured report in improving the quality of MRI reports in rectal cancer staging (47). Information on the report should include tumor location, tumor type (mucinous or not),

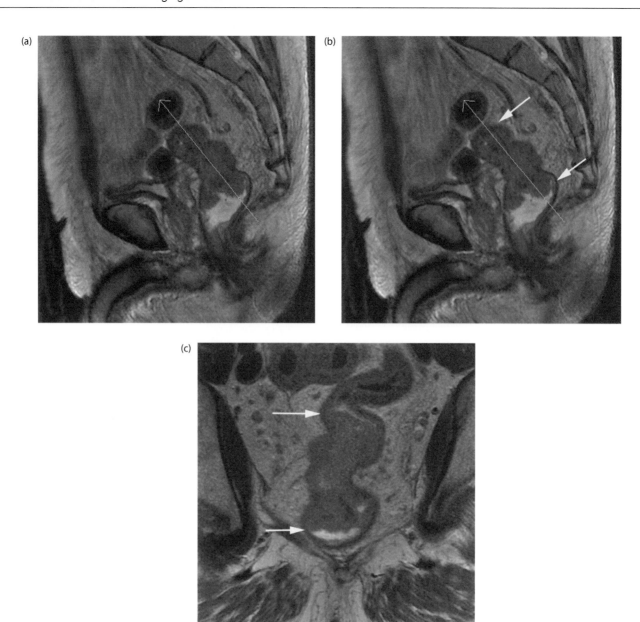

**Figure 12.15** MRI. **(a)** Sagittal T2-weighted image of the pelvis demonstrates planing of the tumoral axis with an arrow running down the length of the rectal tumor. Axial and coronal orthogonal images will be based off this new "tumoral axis." **(b)** Arrows depict the extent of the tumor, which straddles the peritoneal reflection as the tumor is identified above the level of the urinary bladder. **(c)** Coronal orthogonal T2-weighted image shows the rectal tumor in plane.

relationship to the muscularis propria and MRF, involvement of adjacent organs, and morphology and location of pelvic lymph nodes. The structured report at our institution was developed as a collaborative effort among the radiology and colorectal departments to ensure inclusion of pertinent information (Figure 12.16).

## T-STAGING

The utility of MRI over other modalities, namely, CT and TRUS, is the detailed evaluation of the rectum and surrounding structures, such as the MRF, in determining initial local extent of disease. Prior to imaging, the location of the tumor has usually been established by direct visualization

via colonoscopy/sigmoidoscopy as low (within 5 cm of the anorectal verge), mid (between 5 and 10 cm from the anorectal verge), or high (between 10 and 15 cm from the anorectal verge). Although likely diagnosed histologically, the lesion should first be characterized as mucinous or not, as mucinous tumors usually present at a more advanced stage (48). This is simply accomplished as mucinous tumors present with higher intrinsic T2 signal intensity than nonmucinous tumors (49). MRI is then utilized to determine the T-stage of the lesion (Figure 12.17).

A rectal tumor, if not mucinous, typically demonstrates an intermediate signal between the generally mildly hyperintense submucosa and hypointense muscularis propria on T2-weighted images (40). Diffusion-weighted imaging

**PELVIS MRI RECTAL MASS PROTOCOL**

*Technique:* Multiplanar FSE T2 sequences were performed.
Overall image quality:[Adequate Suboptimal Nondiagnostic]

*Results:*

*Tumor Location:* Tumor location (from anal verge):
    [Low(0–5.0 cm) Mid (5.1–10.0 cm) High (10.1–15.0 cm)]

*Relationship to anterior peritoneal reflection:* [Above At or straddles Below Not able to assess]

*Tumor Characteristics:*

Circumferential extent/location (clock face): [ ]
Tumor Length : [ ] cm
Mucinous: [No]

*Tumor Extent:*
Does [not ]extend beyond muscularis into perirectal fat. [ ]
There is [not ]spiculation of the periectal fat. [ ]
There is [not ]invasion of adjacent structures. [ ]
The distance of [tumor] to the mesorectal fascia is [ ] cm. [ ]

[For low rectal tumors only: Is the lower extent of the tumor at or below the upper border of the puborectalis sling? If YES, for the most penetrating component of the tumor below the upper border of the puborectalis sling, note:

- Possible confinement to the submucosa; no definite involvement of internal sphincter (suspected T1)
- Confined to the internal sphincter; no involvement of intersphincteric fat or external sphincter (early T2)
- Through the internal sphincter and intersphincteric fat; possible or definite involvement of the external sphincter (advanced T2)
- Through the external sphincter and into surrounding soft tissue; no organ involvement (T3)
- Through external sphincter and possible involvement of the adjacent organs (i.e., prostate, vagina) (T3/T4)
- Through external sphincter and definite involvement of adjacent organs (i.e., prostate, vagina) (T4)]

*Lymph Nodes:*
There are [no] perirectal lymph nodes [greater than 5mm]in the mesorectal fat. [The distance of the closest lymph node to the mesorectal fascia is [ ] cm.] [ ]
There are [no] extra-mesorectal nodes lymph nodes in the visualized pelvis. [ ]
There are [no] lymph nodes that are suspicious based on [heterogeneous] [speculated] morphology. [ ]
There is [no] evident vascular invasion. [ ]

*Impression:*
[]

Figure 12.16 Structured report template for rectal cancer staging at our institution.

can also be used reliably to assist in the detection of rectal cancers (42) (Figure 12.18). It is usually not practical and typically unreliable to differentiate between T1 (isolated to mucosa and submucosa) and T2 (involves muscularis propria) rectal tumors by MRI (Figure 12.19). The real utility of MRI is differentiating T2 from T3 and T3 from T4 tumors. T3 rectal tumors involve extension of the tumor beyond the muscularis propria and into the surrounding perirectal soft tissues. The low rectum is surrounded by high signal intensity mesorectal fat encased by the MRF, which is represented as a thin hypointense line on T2-weighted images (Figure 12.20). T3 involvement represents invasion into this surrounding fat. Invasion has been described as "broad based bulging or nodular configuration in continuity with the intramural portion of the tumor" (50) (Figure 12.21). Tumor extension may be confused with a similarly appearing benign desmoplastic reaction to underlying tumor, although differentiation may not be possible on MRI (40) (Figure 12.22). T3 involvement should also not

be confused with small penetrating vessels disrupting the muscularis propria (50). T3 tumors are further subdivided by their depth of invasion (mm) past the muscularis propria and whether the tumor involves the MRF. The MRF is the potential surgical resection plane, so involvement with the MRF (considered tumor within 1 mm) needs to be closely evaluated. MRF involvement requires therapy to downstage the lesion prior to surgery.

In the more superior rectum toward the sigmoid colon, the peritoneum begins to cover the anterior portion of the rectum at the anterior peritoneal reflection. Superior to this point, the rectum becomes gradually enveloped until it is completely encircled by the peritoneum. It is important to identify the peritoneal reflection in mid and high rectal tumors, which is depicted as a thin hypointense line on sagittal T2-weighted images connecting the superior aspect of the bladder to the anterior rectum (Figure 12.15b and c). Tumoral involvement into the peritoneum upstages the lesion to T4. T4 rectal tumors are further classified as T4a,

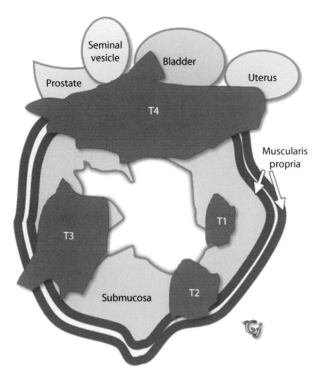

Figure 12.17 Tumor staging in rectal cancer. Stage T1 tumors are confined to the submucosa; stage T2 tumors involve the muscularis propria (arrows), which consist of inner circular and outer longitudinal muscle layers; stage T3 tumors extend beyond the muscularis propria; and stage T4 tumors involve adjacent organs and/or the peritoneum. (Republished image with permission from the RSNA. Kaur H et al. *Radiographics*. 2012;32:389–409.)

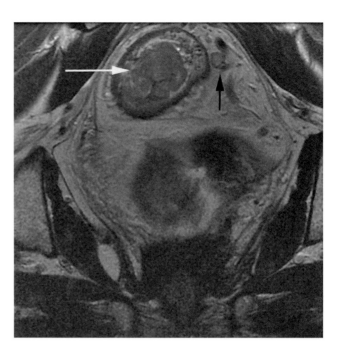

Figure 12.19 MRI. Oblique coronal T2 image of the pelvis demonstrates a rectal tumor (white arrow) that appears confined to the submucosa and muscularis propria (T1/T2). Note the submucosa is relatively hyperintense, and the muscularis propria is hypointense. Adjacent prominent lymph node (black arrow).

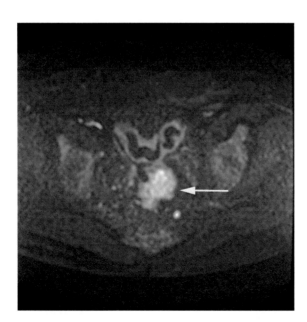

Figure 12.18 MRI. Axial diffusion-weighted image (DWI) of the pelvis depicts a hyperintense rectal tumor. DWI can be utilized for tumoral localization.

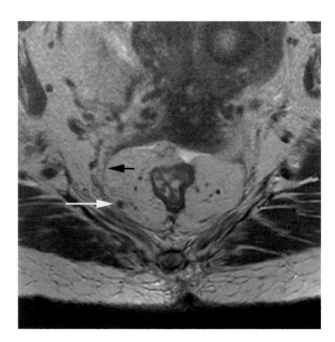

Figure 12.20 MRI. Oblique axial T2 image of the pelvis demonstrates a single prominent lymph node (white arrow) within 1 mm of the MRF, deemed MRF involvement. MRF (black arrow) is depicted as a thin hypointense line on T2-weighted MRI.

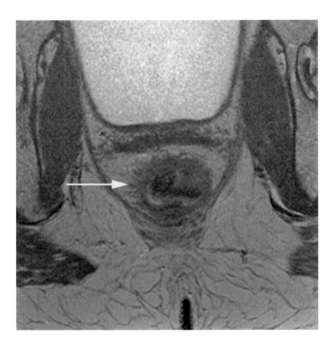

Figure 12.21 MRI. Oblique axial T2 image of the pelvis shows spiculated extension (white arrow) of the underlying tumor into the adjacent mesorectal fat indicating T3 involvement.

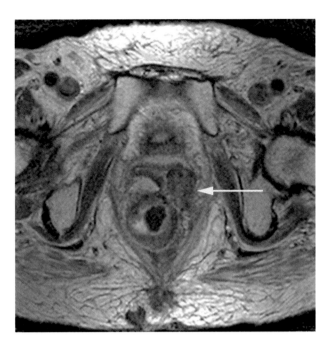

Figure 12.23 MRI. True axial T2 images of the pelvis show lobulated extension (white arrow) of the rectal tumor to involve the vagina, indicating T4 disease.

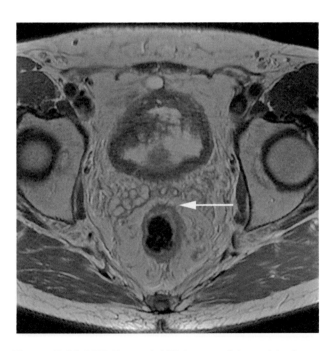

Figure 12.22 MRI. True axial T2 image of the pelvis shows hypointense spiculations (white arrow) extending into the surrounding mesorectal fat from the anterior rectum to suggest T3 invasion or benign desmoplastic reaction. The two processes are not reliably distinguishable by MRI.

involving the surface of the visceral peritoneum, or T4b, involving adjacent organs or structures (Figure 12.23).

Another important factor in initial rectal cancer staging is the evaluation of regional pelvic lymph nodes including mesorectal and internal iliac nodes. MRI has comparable ability in detecting lymph node involvement as TRUS (51), but the ability of MRI to differentiate benign from malignant nodes has been progressing. Location and number of nodes are important to consider in preoperative planning. Nodes located within the mesorectal fascia will be removed during transmesorectal excision, but those outside or involved with the MRF (defined as a node within 1 mm of the MRF) may indicate further treatment prior to surgery (Figure 12.20). An increasing number of involved nodes also has portended a poor prognosis and may also require neoadjuvant treatment. The ability to determine which if any of these nodes represents malignant involvement will further guide preoperative planning. Certainly the size and location of local nodes have some prognostic abilities. Lymph nodes greater than 5–8 mm tend to purport malignancy (37). The most frequently encountered nodes in rectal cancer are those in the surrounding mesorectal fat with the majority of malignant nodes within 5 cm of the tumor (52) and typically located in the lateral and dorsal mesorectum at or above the level of the tumor (53).

Morphologic nodal characterization with MRI is also a factor in determining malignant from benign nodes. Irregular border morphology and mixed signal intensity increase accuracy in diagnosing malignant nodes (52). Diffusion-weighted imaging (DWI) has also shown some utility in detecting pelvic lymph nodes, but limited utility in determining their involvement with tumor (54,55). Recent advances in lymph node–specific contrast agents such as ultrasmall superparamagnetic iron oxide, an iron-based nanoparticle, and gadofosveset, a gadolinium chelate that binds albumin, have shown promise in their ability to detect malignant from nonmalignant nodes and appear to be viable methods of doing such (56,57).

Although not part of the TNM staging criteria, extramural vascular invasion is a significant finding that should be commented on during a rectal cancer staging examination. Vascular invasion has been shown to be a significant risk factor in local recurrence and disease relapse (58,59). MRI has proven reliable in identifying vascular tumoral involvement as defined by irregularity and expansion of adjacent vessels (59) warranting inclusion in rectal cancer staging workups.

MRI is an invaluable tool in the initial workup of known rectal cancer. High-resolution T2 images provide valuable information to accurately determine tumor involvement and stage similar to transrectal ultrasound. MRI, however, has the added benefit of a greater field of view to more accurately assess lymph node involvement and local metastatic disease to inguinal nodes or the pelvic osseous structures. While providing details of nodal involvement, studies have indicated a role for MRI in differentiating benign versus malignant nodes, which has the potential to be a tremendous advantage in predicting surgical success or recurrent disease. Continued advances in magnetic resonance technology should only further the utility MRI has in guiding surgical workup and increasing the surgeon's ability to provide tumor-free resection margins.

## HEPATIC METASTATIC COLORECTAL CANCER

Close to a quarter of all patients diagnosed with colon and rectal cancer present with metastatic disease (60), and the most common location for colorectal metastases is the liver (61). Surgical treatment of hepatic metastatic disease has proven to be a successful option in a small subset of patients, but accurate diagnosis of the size, number, and extent of disease is needed before potential surgical intervention or neoadjuvant treatment can occur. Hepatic metastases can be evaluated by a variety of imaging modalities including ultrasound, CT, MRI, and fluorodeoxyglucose-positron emission tomography (FDG-PET); but MRI has repeatedly been shown as the superior imaging modality for the evaluation of metastatic disease and specifically colorectal metastatic disease.

A meta-analysis comparing the variety of imaging modalities in diagnosing hepatic metastatic colorectal disease was compiled by Floriani et al. and demonstrated similar sensitivities and specificities of ultrasound and CT in the diagnosis on a per patient basis (62). Ultrasound does not utilize ionizing radiation but is limited by its small field of view and is significantly operator dependent. CT can be a valuable screening tool as it has the ability of a large field of view acquired in a relatively short time period, but the repeated doses of ionizing radiation raise concern. In the same study, the evaluation of FDG-PET was somewhat limited by small sample size, but when compared to CT, it also

demonstrated similar per patient sensitivities in diagnosing hepatic metastatic colorectal cancer (62). FDG-PET utilizes fluorinated deoxyglucose to identify areas of hypermetabolic activity, presumed areas of tumor activity (Figure 12.24). FDG-PET is not without its limitations, especially in the liver, as the baseline hypermetabolic activity in the liver limits evaluation for small areas of increased uptake. To that end, several studies have validated this result. In comparing CT and FDG-PET, CT was found more sensitive in detecting hepatic metastases smaller than 1.5 cm (63). Studies have also shown that neoadjuvant chemotherapy lowers the sensitivity of FDG-PET in the detection of hepatic metastatic disease (64). When compared to MRI, however, CT and FDG-PET have shown to be inferior. In a direct comparison with contrast-enhanced CT, MRI was shown to have increased sensitivity to lesions less than 1 cm (65). When compared directly against FDG-PET, MRI demonstrated greater sensitivity on a per lesion basis, and the same study concluded that MRI had the most data supporting its use in detecting hepatic colorectal cancer over all modalities (62).

Metastatic lesions on MRI are typically iso- to hypointense on T1-weighted images and iso- to hyperintense on T2-weighted images (66), and further lose signal as compared to hemangiomas and cysts on increasingly T2-weighted sequences (67) (Figure 12.25a and b). Specifically, colorectal metastases tend to show central hypointensity secondary to necrosis with a surrounding rim of viable, hyperintense tumor (68). Contrast-enhanced images with gadolinium-based contrast agents typically

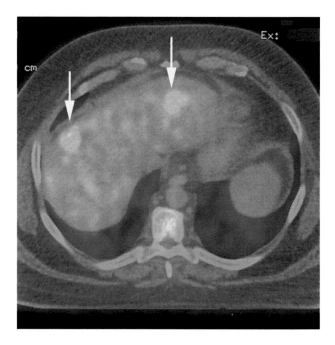

Figure 12.24 FDG-PET/CT. Axial image through the liver demonstrates two hypermetabolic foci in the liver (white arrows) indicating metastatic disease in this patient with colon cancer. Note the significant background activity of the liver, which could potentially mask a smaller lesion.

show relative hypoenhancement of metastatic colorectal lesions, which are more conspicuous on the portal venous phase (Figure 12.25c). In addition to conventional MRI sequences, more recent advances in diffusion-weighted imaging and hepatobiliary contrast agents such as gadoxetic acid (Gd-EOB-DTPA) for the evaluation of metastatic liver lesions have only further increased sensitivity (69,70). In fact a recent study demonstrated that higher sensitivities were generated when applying both diffusion and post-hepatobiliary contrast sequences (71). Hepatobiliary contrast agents are taken up by hepatocytes and excreted in the biliary system. Colorectal metastases or other non-hepatocyte-derived lesions will demonstrate relative hypoenhancement, allowing visualization.

The increased sensitivities MRI affords have to be balanced against the costs of the examination, which tend to be significantly higher than CT or ultrasound. Another factor to consider is the patient's ability to hold his or her breath for the acquisition (Figure 12.26). Although faster acquisition techniques have been generated, significant patient motion during the examination can severely degrade image quality and sensitivity. MRI is also contraindicated in patients with certain implantable devices such as pacemakers or defibrillators. In such cases, other imaging modalities must be pursued. Despite its limitations, current evidence supports MRI as the imaging modality most suited for the detection and quantification of colorectal liver metastases.

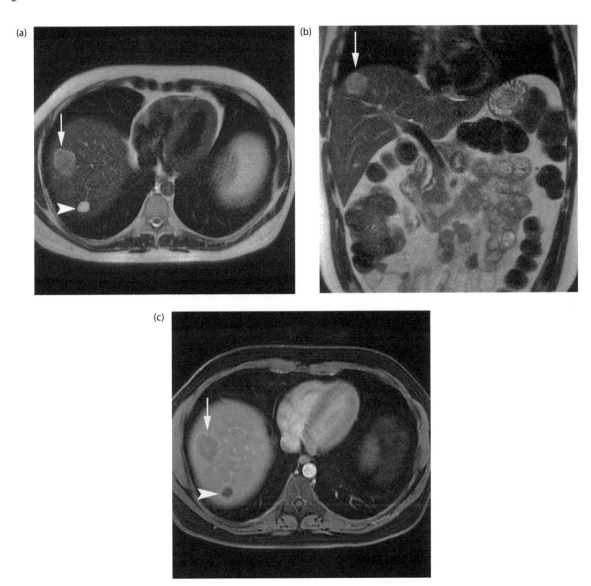

Figure 12.25 MRI. **(a)** Axial noncontrast T2 image through the liver demonstrates an intermediate-intensity liver lesion (white arrow) compatible with metastatic disease in contrast to an adjacent hyperintense cyst (arrowhead). Note the thin rim of T2 hyperintensity around the metastatic lesion (white arrow) to suggest viable tumor surrounding central necrosis. **(b)** Coronal noncontrast T2 image through the liver again shows the intermediate-intensity metastatic liver lesion (white arrow). **(c)** Axial postcontrast T1 fat-saturated image through the liver demonstrates the relative hypoenhancement of the metastatic colorectal lesion (white arrow). Also note the hypoenhancement of the adjacent cyst (arrowhead).

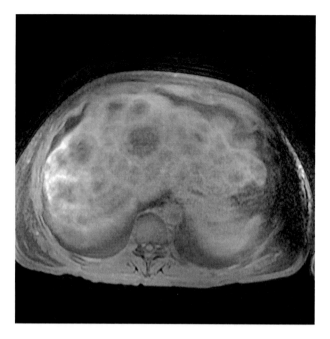

**Figure 12.26** MRI. Axial postcontrast T1 fat-saturated image through the liver demonstrates significant motion related to the patient's inability to hold the breath. Despite the motion blurring, several large hypoenhancing metastatic lesions are visible in this patient with colon cancer.

## REFERENCES

1. Sahani DV, Samir AE (eds). *Abdominal Imaging*. Maryland Heights, Missouri: Saunders, 2011, Chapter 51.
2. Ahn SH et al. *Radiology*. 2002;225:159–64.
3. Rockey DC et al. *Lancet*. 2005;365:305–11.
4. Johnson CD et al. *N Engl J Med*. 2008;359:1207–17.
5. Nobel Prize. Available from https://www.nobelprize.org/nobel_prizes/
6. Sahani DV, Samir AE (eds). *Abdominal Imaging*. Maryland Heights, Missouri: Saunders, 2011, Chapter 52.
7. Sahani DV, Samir AE (eds). *Abdominal Imaging*. Maryland Heights, Missouri: Saunders, 2011, Chapter 55.
8. Balthazar EJ. *AJR*. 1991;156:23–32.
9. Elsayes KM et al. *RadioGraphics*. 2010;30:1955–74.
10. Booya F et al. *Radiology*. 2006;241:787–95.
11. Baker ME et al. *AJR*. 2009;192:417–23.
12. Paulsen SR et al. *RadioGraphics*. 2006;26:641–62.
13. Del Gaizo AJ et al. *RadioGraphics*. 2013;33:1109–24.
14. Brenner DJ, Hall EJ. *N Engl J Med*. 2007;357:2277–84.
15. Kambadakone AR et al. *AJR*. 2011;196:W743–52.
16. Towbin AJ et al. *RadioGraphics*. 2013;33:1843–60.
17. Siddiki HA et al. *AJR*. 2009;193:113–21.
18. Masselli G et al. *Radiology*. 2016;279:420–31.
19. Flor N et al. *AJR*. 2016;207:15–24.
20. Zaidi E, Daly B. *AJR*. 2006;187:689–94.
21. Hulnick DH et al. *Radiology*. 1984;152:491–5.
22. Kircher MF et al. *AJR*. 2002;178:1313–8.
23. Siewert B et al. *AJR*. 2006;186:680–6.
24. Chintapalli KN et al. *Radiology*. 1999;210:429–35.
25. Sai VF et al. *Radiology*. 2012;263:383–90.
26. de Vries HS et al. *Surg Endosc*. 2014;28:2039–47.
27. Laine L et al. *Am J Gastroenterol*. 2012;107:1190–5.
28. Laing CJ et al. *RadioGraphics*. 2007;27:1055–70.
29. Lee SS et al. *Radiology*. 2011;259:739–48.
30. Rosch J et al. *Radiology*. 1971;99:27–36.
31. Bookstein JJ et al. *Radiology*. 1978;127:345–9.
32. Koo HJ et al. *AJR*. 2015;204:662–8.
33. Graca BM et al. *RadioGraphics*. 2010;20:235–52.
34. Artigas JM et al. *RadioGraphics*. 2013;33:1453–70.
35. Zink SI et al. *AJR*. 2008;191:1107–14.
36. Feuerstein JD et al. *AJR*. 2016;207:578–84.
37. Beets-Tan RG et al. *Eur Radiol*. 2013 Sep;23(9):2522–31.
38. Bipat S et al. *Radiology*. 2004;232(3):773–83.
39. Fernandez-Esparrach G et al. *GIE*. 2011;74(2):347–54.
40. Jhaveri KS, Hosseini-Nik H. *AJR*. 2015;205:W24–55.
41. Brown G et al. *Br J Radiol*. 2005;78(927):245–51.
42. Ichikawa T et al. *AJR*. 2006;187:181–4.
43. Figueiras RG et al. *AJR*. 2010;195:54–66.
44. Vliegen RF et al. *Radiographics*. 2005;234:179–88.
45. Alberda WJ et al. *Int J Colorectal Dis*. 2013;28(4):573–80.
46. Heijnen LA et al. *Eur Radiol*. 2014;24(2):371–9.
47. Sahni VA et al. *AJR*. 2015;205:584–8.
48. Younes M et al. *Cancer*. 1993;72(12):3588–92.
49. Hussain SM et al. *Radiology*. 1999;213(1):79–85.
50. Taylor FG et al. *AJR*. 2008;191:1827–35.
51. Bipat S et al. *Radiology*. 2004;232(2):773–83.
52. Koh DM et al. *Eur Radiol*. 2005;15(8):1650–57.
53. Engelen SM et al. *Eur J Surg Oncol*. 2008;34(7):776–81.
54. Heijnen LA et al. *Eur Radiol*. 2013;23(12):3354–60.
55. Cho EY et al. *Eur J Radiol*. 2013;82(11):e662–8.
56. Koh DM et al. *AJR*. 2010;194(6):W505–13.
57. Lambregts DM et al. *Abdom Imaging*. 2013;38(4):720–7.
58. Dresen RC et al. *Eur J Surg Oncol*. 2009;35(10):1071–7.
59. Smith NJ et al. *Br J Surg*. 2008;95(2):229–36.
60. van der Geest LG et al. *Clin Exp Metastasis*. 2015;32(5):457–65.
61. Riihimaki M et al. *Sci Rep [Internet]*. 2016 [cited January 12, 2017];6:Article 26975 [about 26 screens]. Available from: http://www.nature.com/articles/srep29765
62. Floriani I et al. *J Magn Reson Imaging*. 2010;31(1):19–31.
63. Ruers TJ et al. *J Clin Oncol*. 2002;20(2):388–95.
64. Lubezky N et al. *J Gastrointest Surg*. 2007;11(4):472–8.
65. Niekel MC et al. *Radiology*. 2010;257(3):674–84.
66. Saini S, Nelson RC. *Radiology*. 1995;197:575–7.
67. Namasivayam S et al. *Cancer Imaging*. 2007;7:2–9.
68. Sica GT et al. *Clin Liver Dis*. 2002;6(1):165–79.
69. Wu LM et al. *Eur J Cancer*. 2013;49(3):572–84.
70. Chen L et al. *PLOS ONE [Internet]*. 2012 [cited January 13, 2017];7(11):e48681 [about 10 screens]. Available from: http://journals.plos.org/plosone/article?id=10.1371/journal.pone.0048681
71. Vilgrain V et al. *Eur Radiol*. 2016;26(12):4595–615.

# 13

# Transanal endoscopy

AARON L. KLINGER AND BRIAN R. KANN

## CHALLENGING CASE

A 50-year-old man with a history of hypertension presents for screening colonoscopy. A 2 cm sessile polyp is found in the cecum and removed with a "hot" snare. He presents to the emergency department 2 days later with fevers to 101.5°F and abdominal pain with localized guarding over the right lower quadrant.

## CASE MANAGEMENT

You see and examine the patient. Blood is drawn for complete blood count (CBC), basic metabolic profile, and C-reactive protein (CRP). His white blood cell (WBC) count returns at 14 × 10³/mL, and CRP is 30 mg/dL. An upright chest x-ray does not show pneumoperitoneum, and a computed tomography (CT) scan with rectal contrast does not show extraluminal air or contrast extravasation. You admit the patient, start him on broad-spectrum antibiotics, and order bowel rest. Serial abdominal exams are performed to watch for generalized peritonitis. After 3 days, the patient's pain resolves and WBC normalizes. He is started on a clear liquid diet and advanced slowly. He is discharged home on hospital day 5.

## INTRODUCTION

Endoscopic evaluation of the lower gastrointestinal (GI) tract is a vital tool for the colorectal surgeon and should be viewed as an extension of the physical exam. Modalities include anoscopy, rigid proctoscopy, flexible sigmoidoscopy, and colonoscopy. Each procedure has its own benefits and limitations. It is important for a colorectal surgeon to be comfortable performing each technique and to know their indications. Knowledge of potential complications and their management is critical to successful patient management.

## BOWEL PREPARATION

### INTRODUCTION

Although significant debate continues regarding the benefit of preoperative bowel preparation for surgery, it is universally accepted that adequate bowel cleaning is crucial to proper colonoscopy. Despite this up to 25% of all colonoscopies are reported to have inadequate bowel preparation (1). If adequate mucosal examination cannot occur, a repeat procedure with additional costs and risks must occur. An ideal preparation must be safe, tolerable, and effective. Various preparations and methods of consumption exist, but consensus to the optimal regimen is lacking (2). The U.S. Multi-Society Task Force (USMSTF) on Colorectal Cancer (CRC) published its recommendations for precolonoscopy bowel cleaning in 2014. They concluded that the selection of a bowel-cleaning regimen should be determined based on a patient's history, other medications, and response to prior bowel preparations (3).

### POLYETHYLENE GLYCOL

Polyethylene glycol (PEG) is an inert osmotically active polymer commonly used for bowel preparation. It is generally mixed with an electrolyte lavage solution (ELS) to a volume of 4 L and functions as an electrolyte-balanced colonic lavage solution. "Low-volume" PEG regimens also exist, consisting of 2 L of PEG-ELS with an adjunct medication such as Bisacodyl or ascorbic acid.

### SODIUM PHOSPHATE

Sodium phosphate (NaP) formulations are hyperosmotic compounds that draw water into the GI tract to create bowel cleaning through a purgative action. Proponents of NaP refer to better patient tolerance compared to PEG without sacrificing bowel cleaning (4,5). Given its mechanism of action, NaP can result in significant fluid and electrolyte shifts. Patients must take a significant quantity of fluids orally if using this preparation to prevent dehydration. For this reason, NaP should not be used in elderly patients or those with congestive heart failure, decompensated cirrhosis, renal failure, or electrolyte disorders (6).

Reports of chronic renal failure or insufficiency from acute phosphate nephropathy led the U.S. Food and Drug Administration (FDA) to issue an alert regarding its use in 2006 (7). Last, NaP can cause mucosal lesions including aphthous ulcers and should be avoided in patients being evaluated specifically for inflammatory bowel disease (8). When used in a carefully selected patient, NaP remains a good option for precolonoscopy bowel cleansing. However, the limitations discussed previously have led manufacturers to withdraw many of the NaP products from the market (9).

## IRRITANT LAXATIVES (SODIUM PICOSULFATE)

Sodium picosulfate is a contact stimulant laxative that can either be used as a treatment for constipation or to prepare the large bowel before colonoscopy or surgery. Sodium picosulfate is a prodrug, and has no significant direct physiological effect on the intestine. Instead, it is metabolized by gut bacteria into the active compound 4,4'-dihydroxydiphenyl-(2-pyridiyl) methane, which increases peristalsis in the gut. Sodium picosulfate is typically prescribed in a combined formulation with magnesium citrate, which is an osmotic laxative. The use of sodium picosulfate can be associated with clinically significant hyponatremia and hypokalemia, and patients should be encouraged to drink large amounts of clear fluids as well as rehydrate to reestablish the electrolyte balance. In the United States, this drug combination is marketed as Prepopik (Ferring Pharmaceuticals, Parsippany, NJ).

## SINGLE VERSUS SPLIT DOSING

Whatever preparation formulation is chosen, there is good evidence to support using a split-dose protocol. A 2014 meta-analysis found good preparation in 85% of patients using a split dose compared to 63% in patients taking a single dose. They found the most important factor to be the "runway time"—the time between the last dose of preparation and the beginning of the colonoscopy. The benefit of split dose is lost if runway time exceeds 5 hours (2). Consistent with this finding, a 2012 single-blinded study evaluated split-day preparation with same-day preparation for afternoon colonoscopies. They found a same-day regimen (doses at 7:00 and 10:00 a.m.) to result in improved mucosal cleansing with greater patient satisfaction than a two-day regimen (10). As a result, the USMSTF's guidelines strongly recommend the use of split-dose cleansing for

elective colonoscopy with a same-day regimen as an acceptable alternative especially for afternoon endoscopy. They also emphasize the importance of patient education for increased compliance and quality of cleansing and recommend the use of both oral and written instructions as well as additional support measures to ensure correct preparation use (3).

## ANOSCOPY

### INDICATIONS

Anoscopy is used for examination of the anal canal and distal rectum following digital rectal exam (DRE). This procedure allows for evaluation of the anoderm, distal rectal mucosa, dentate line, and anal pathology, including internal/external hemorrhoids, fistulas, fissures, and anal masses. The device consists of a scope, often with a beveled end and an obturator. Light can be provided by a built-in light source, by a fiber-optic light cable, or from a separate light source. Disposable plastic anoscopes with built-in light sources are commercially available and are useful for bedside or emergency room examination.

### TECHNIQUE

The patient does not need any special preparation for anoscopic examination. The patient is placed in a prone jackknife or Sims' position. Following DRE, the anoscope is lubricated and slowly inserted with the examiner's thumb supporting the obturator while the patient bears down to assist in relaxation of the anal musculature. The obturator is then removed, and a circumferential examination is performed. Prior to turning the anoscope the obturator should be reinserted to avoid pinching the anoderm. As the anoscope is withdrawn, the patient is again asked to bear down to evaluate for any prolapsing hemorrhoids.

### COMPLICATIONS

Complications following anoscopy are rare. Bleeding may occur from irritation of hemorrhoids or from accidental tears to the anoderm.

## RIGID PROCTOSCOPY

### INDICATIONS

Rigid proctoscopy (to be referred to as simply "proctoscopy" for the remainder of this chapter) allows for visualization of the anus, rectum, and possibly sigmoid colon. Like the anoscope, it is made of a scope, generally 25 cm long, with an obturator, a light source, a viewing lens, and a bellows to allow for gentle air insufflation. Additional instruments such as suction, cotton-tipped swabs, and biopsy tools can be passed through the scope. Like anoscopes they come in a variety of adult and pediatric sizes and materials. Disposable scopes, made of clear plastic, may allow for additional visualization and do not need to be cleaned following use.

## TECHNIQUE

A full bowel preparation is not typically required for proctoscopy. Rather one or two enemas should be given within 1–2 hours of the procedure to clear stool for easy visualization and passage of the instrument. Enema use earlier than this period may allow stool from the more proximal bowel to migrate to the rectum. The procedure can generally be performed without anesthesia, although some patients may require sedation.

The patient is placed in a prone jackknife or Sims' position. Patients may have significant anxiety about this procedure, and it is important to explain that it will not hurt and that each step will be explained before being performed. Following DRE, a well-lubricated scope is inserted into the anal canal, aiming toward the umbilicus with the operator's thumb holding the obturator. Once past the sphincter muscles, the obturator is removed and the scope is repositioned to face the sacrum and is inserted into the rectum. Suctioning or swabbing to clear rectal contents is performed with the examiner's right hand while the left hand holds and advances the scope. If stool cannot be cleared with these techniques, the rectum can be cleared by inserting 50 mL of tap water, closing the lens, and providing insufflation.

At about 14 cm, the rectum turns anteriorly and the lumen may be difficult to follow. At this point the viewing lens can be closed and gentle insufflation can be provided to distend the bowel to allow further navigation. It is important to recognize that although most proctoscopes are 25 cm in length, it is not always possible to advance to this distance, and attempts to do so may cause the patient serious harm. In fact, a 1980 review of 1,000 proctoscopes performed at the University of Minnesota found the average depth of insertion to be 19.5 cm in males and 18.6 cm in females (11). If a fixed angle is encountered or the scope will not pass easily, advancement should stop. Blanching mucosa should be taken as a "danger sign." Attempts to force the scope further may result in pain or complications (12).

Although lesions encountered on insertion should be noted, full mucosal inspection should be done as the scope is withdrawn. All areas of the bowel wall should be examined, suctioning as needed, as the scope is withdrawn in a spiral motion. The endoscopist must be mindful of polyps, inflammation, tumors, or other abnormalities.

With the widespread availability of flexible sigmoidoscopy, the utility of proctoscopy has been questioned. Opponents note decreased rates of polyp detection, patient discomfort, ease of biopsy, and the ability of flexible scopes to be inserted further (13). Proctoscopy has proven itself invaluable in the localization of rectal tumors, however. A proctoscope has length markings on its outer surface and offers a more accurate estimate of lesion location than flexible endoscopy. In a recent study, the average difference between rigid and flexible measurements of tumors was found to be 3.1 cm in the upper rectum and 5 cm at the rectosigmoid junction. The addition of proctoscopy to flexible endoscopy changed the treatment options in up to 38% of rectal/rectosigmoid cancer patients (14).

## COMPLICATIONS

Serious complications of proctoscopy are rare. The most common complications are bleeding, especially at biopsy or polypectomy sites. Patients may have vasovagal reactions during the procedure. If a patient becomes faint or unresponsive, the scope should be removed and the patient should be taken out of the jackknife position, placed supine on the table, and oxygen should be provided. Perforation is very rare and should not happen if careful technique is utilized. In a review of 20 years of experience and over 300,000 proctoscopies at the Mayo Clinic, only four bowel injuries occurred and only one involved bowel perforation (15).

## FLEXIBLE SIGMOIDOSCOPY/ COLONOSCOPY

## HISTORY, INTRODUCTION, AND INDICATIONS

Documented attempts to use scopes to visualize the interior of body cavities have been made since the early 1800s. Early efforts were limited by lack of a reliable light source. Within just a few years of Edison's introduction of the electric light bulb, the technology was used for endoscopic purposes. The introduction of modern flexible endoscopy came with the advent of fiber optics in the 1960s and videoendoscopy in the 1980s (16).

Flexible lower endoscopy (flexible sigmoidoscopy and colonoscopy) is a commonly used procedure that can diagnose and treat conditions of the colon, rectum, and distal small intestine. It should be viewed as an extension of the colorectal physical examination and is an indispensable tool for the colorectal surgeon. These techniques allow for direct inspection of the mucosal surface, allowing the endoscopist to visualize and treat neoplasms, polyps, bleeding lesions, and inflammatory bowel disease. Successful colonoscopy is dependent on adequate sedation, bowel preparation, patient selection, and operator experience.

Flexible sigmoidoscopies are 35–65 cm in length (colonoscopes in comparison are 120–160 cm long). They are able to evaluate more bowel length than rigid sigmoidoscopy (although less than full colonoscopy), thereby increasing the chances of finding a lesion. In addition, given the flexible nature of the scope and smaller diameter, it is generally more comfortable for the patient. Disadvantages compared to rigid proctoscopy include the higher cost of the instruments, the need to clean after use, and the higher tendency for the instruments and their fiber optics to break. Unlike full colonoscopy, this technique can be performed without full bowel preparation and generally does not require sedation.

The indications for colonoscopy vary by condition and are often debated even among experts. Screening for CRC remains a primary use for the technique, and various appropriateness guidelines for screening colonoscopy have been published. In 2008, both the USMSTF on CRC and the American College of Gastroenterology (AGA) published their guidelines for CRC screening (17,18). Both suggest screening of *average-risk* individuals starting at age 50 to detect and prevent CRC. Although other screening tools exist, the AGA notes a 70%–90% reduction in CRC for patients undergoing colonoscopy and polypectomy compared to reference populations and the association of colonoscopy use with earlier and more favorable stages of CRC presentation. Furthermore, they refer to its wide availability, ability to examine the entire colon, and longer test interval than other screening options. For these reasons, colonoscopy remains the AGA's "preferred" screening strategy and should be the test offered to patients, saving other modalities for patients who decline colonoscopy (17).

## TECHNIQUE

### Sedation: Conscious sedation versus propofol: Comment on cost efficiency

While select colonoscopies can be performed without the use of sedation, most patients are given IV medication to reduce discomfort and facilitate the procedure (19). If sedation is to be used, it is important that the patient be provided with oxygen and has routine monitoring of blood pressure, heart and respiratory rate, pulse oximetry, and electrocardiogram, as well as postprocedural monitoring in the recovery area. There are four generally recognized stages of sedation, which range from minimal sedation to general anesthesia. Colonoscopy is generally performed under moderate sedation ("conscious sedation"), though some patients may require deep sedation or even general anesthesia.

Prior to the administration of any sedation, it is important to evaluate the patient for preexisting medical conditions or physical exam findings that may lead to compilations of sedation. The patient's American Society of Anesthesiologist (ASA) classification should be determined. Higher-risk patients (ASA class IV–V) should be evaluated by an anesthesia specialist prior to administration of sedatives. Women of childbearing age should be screened for pregnancy. If endoscopy is necessary during pregnancy, attempts should be made to postpone until the second trimester if possible, and an obstetrician should be consulted (20). Patients should fast for at least 2 hours following clear liquids to reduce the risk of aspiration (19).

Ideal drugs for endoscopic evaluation have rapid onset, short duration of action, do not alter hemodynamics, and have low side-effect profiles. The most commonly used medications for conscious sedation in the United States are benzodiazepines (midazolam and diazepam), which are generally given in conjunction with an opiate such as fentanyl (21). The most common alternative regimens consist of hypnotics such as propofol, which provides deep sedation. The use of propofol has increased steadily in recent years and has surpassed midazolam in some populations (22).

Advantages of propofol include reduced procedure time, reduced recovery time, and higher physician satisfaction. Furthermore, patients report greater satisfaction with its use compared to midazolam with fentanyl and are less likely to experience nausea or "hangover" symptoms (22). Unlike benzodiazepines and opioids, there are no reversal agents available for propofol, but it has a short (4–8 minute) duration of action (19). The major disadvantage of propofol is its narrow therapeutic index. The FDA therefore recommends it only be administered by a trained anesthesia specialist. A recent meta-analysis, however, found propofol to have a similar risk of cardiopulmonary adverse events compared to other sedatives. When used in simple endoscopic procedures, it is actually associated with a decrease in complications. In advanced endoscopic procedures, its use does not result in increased rates of complications compared to sedation with benzodiazepines/narcotics (23).

A major perceived disadvantage of propofol is an increased cost of its use compared to traditional sedatives. Both propofol and midazolam are inexpensive drugs, and propofol has been shown to reduce costs drastically by shortening recovery times (24). Due to concerns of increased risks of propofol use and the FDA's recommendations regarding its use, endoscopists are less likely to self-administer propofol than midazolam (19). The use of a trained anesthesia provider for endoscopy results in additional professional fees, which can be as high as $450 per procedure (25).

Despite FDA recommendations and endoscopist concerns, a growing body of literature supports the use of endoscopist-directed propofol (EDP) administration. A review of over 220,000 cases of EDP over 5 years found no instances of death and only one reported instance of intubation (26). The body of supporting data led the American Society for Gastrointestinal Endoscopy (ASGE), the American Gastroenterological Association, and the American College of Gastroenterology to release a joint statement endorsing EDP so long as the provider had been adequately trained in the drug's use (27).

### Maneuvers for difficult colonoscopy: Change position (supine/prone), abdominal pressure, etc.

Colonoscopy is a technically challenging procedure, and expertise requires adequate training, practice, patience, and knowledge of maneuvers. Technical challenges can occur due to redundant or floppy bowel, sharp angulation, or fixation from previous surgery.

It is important for an endoscopist to constantly use both hands during a procedure. While the left hand controls the direction of the tip with control knobs, the right hand works to both advance and withdraw the scope and provide torque. Rotation of the scope not only changes the viewing angle but also acts to help prevent or reduce loops.

Dithering refers to rapid back-and-forth jerking movements, where the endoscope is advanced and slowly withdrawn. This can result in pleating of the bowel over the scope rather than pushing it away and results in a shortened colon length. This technique can be especially useful in the descending and transverse colon and should be used even during portions of the procedure that are not difficult.

External pressure can be applied by an assistant or the endoscopist to the abdomen in attempts to splint areas of redundant bowel and help prevent or reduce loop formation. The presence of a formed loop can help guide pressure placement. In cases when no loop can be felt, pressure should generally be applied from the right upper quadrant toward the left lower quadrant. This maneuver can stabilize the redundant sigmoid colon, but care must be given to keep pressure gentle to avoid patient discomfort. Significant pressure may also contribute to gastroesophageal reflux and potentially aspiration.

When other maneuvers fail and the endoscope cannot be inserted further, repositioning the patient may assist with scope advancement. Colonoscopy generally starts with the patient in a left lateral decubitus position. Turning the patient to a supine position may assist with further navigation. During turns, the endoscopy team should move the patient together while the endoscopist maintains control of the endoscope and attempts to keep the scope in the middle of the bowel lumen. In some cases, especially with obese patients, turning the patient to a prone position can assist with advancement. Failure to be able to comfortably advance the scope despite the use of these maneuvers should be taken as an indication to abort the procedure.

## Need for prophylactic antibiotics

Cases of infectious endocarditis following colonoscopy have been reported, and given the high concentration of gram-positive bacteria in the colon, some argue that prophylaxis should be given to select high-risk patients including elderly patients, cancer patients, and immunocompromised patients (28). However, the most recent (2008) guidelines from the American College of Cardiology and American Heart Association do not recommend endocarditis prophylaxis for any GI tract procedures including colonoscopy. They acknowledge that transient bacteremia may occur but that there are few cases of infectious endocarditis following colonoscopy and that evidence that antibiotics can prevent endocarditis in these cases is lacking (29). Also, the risk of *Clostridium difficle* following antibiotic usage appears higher than the potential risk of bacteremia. The 2015 guidelines from the ASGE recommend against routine antibiotic prophylaxis as well. They do consider pre-endoscopy prophylaxis for patients with high-risk cardiac conditions such as new prosthetic heart valves or previous infectious

endocarditis and known GI tract infections that may include enterococci. The guidelines also recommend prophylaxis for active peritoneal dialysis patients, but they note that quality evidence for this recommendation is lacking (30).

## Patients on antithrombotic medications

An endoscopist should expect to encounter patients on antiplatelet or anticoagulation medications, especially as more antithrombotic medications become available and more patients are being treated with them. It is important to screen for use of these medications as well as the associated indication prior to scheduling a procedure. Consideration must be given to holding aspirin, clopidogrel bisulfate and other antiplatelet agents, and anticoagulants prior to colonoscopy, especially if a higher-risk therapeutic procedure (such as polypectomy or mucosal resection) is planned. It is important to recognize that each medication has its own duration of action, and therefore, "hold times" vary from drug to drug.

The 2016 ASGE guidelines (available at www.asge.org) include a table of commonly used antithrombotic agents, their durations of action, and reversal agents if available. Given the wide range of medications and indications, they do not provide a "one-size-fits-all" approach to holding antithrombotic medications. The endoscopist along with the patient's cardiologist or primary care provider must weigh the risk of endoscopy-induced bleeding to the patient's own cardiovascular risk. Generally speaking, the morbidity associated with thrombotic events outweighs that of bleeding. When possible, elective procedures should be delayed until temporarily antithrombotic drug courses have been completed.

In general, per ASGE guidelines, patients with low thromboembolic risk and high bleeding risk should have their medications held for the appropriate drug-specific interval. Heparin bridging therapy to be held in the immediate periprocedural period should be considered for those at high risk of bleeding and thrombotic events. Antithrombotic medications should be resumed as soon as possible after the procedure (30).

The most recent guidelines from the American College of Chest Physicians are similar to the ASGE guidelines. They suggest using heparin bridging therapy for patients at high risk of thromboembolism (to be held 4–6 hours before the procedure) and continuing aspirin or holding it at the time of surgery (as opposed to 7–10 days prior) for moderate to high cardiovascular risk patients (31) In contrast, low cardiovascular risk patients should have aspirin held 7–10 days prior to their procedure.

## TECHNICAL COMPLICATIONS

Although colonoscopy is very commonly performed and considered a low-risk procedure, it must be remembered that it is an invasive procedure and does carry an associated risk. The most commonly described serious complications of colonoscopy are bleeding, perforation, infectious complications, missed lesions, and cardiopulmonary events. A Centers for Disease Control and Prevention publication estimates the incidence of serious complication at 2.38 per 1,000 screening colonoscopies with rates in previous studies ranging from 0.79 to 8.4 per 1,000 procedures (32).

## HEMORRHAGE

Bleeding is the most common serious complication of colonoscopy with a reported incidence as high as 3%, though most recent publications report the incidence of serious bleeding at less than 3/1,000 (32,33). Hemorrhage usually comes from an intraluminal source, but it is also possible for bleeding to occur from mesenteric or splenic lacerations. Postpolypectomy bleeding occurs an average of 6 days after the procedure and can present up to 2 weeks later, though most bleeding is recognized and controlled at the time of the procedure. Risk factors for bleeding include polypectomy, which increases with the size of the polyp, and anticoagulation use (34).

Management of post-colonoscopy hemorrhage depends on the etiology of the bleeding source and knowledge of what was done at the time of the initial procedure. If postpolypectomy bleeding is suspected, repeat colonoscopy after a rapid prep allows for direct intervention if the bleeding site can be identified. Bleeding from a polypectomy site can be managed with endoclips, direct cautery, argon bean coagulation, and epinephrine injection. Unprepped colonoscopy in the setting of acute bleeding is often limited by lack of visualization due to a combination of stool, blood, and clots within the lumen of the colon, interfering with visualization. Alternatively, mesenteric arteriography with embolization of a bleeding source may be an effective means of dealing with post-polypectomy bleeding. Bleeding from an extramucosal source, such as the mesentery or spleen, usually requires direct operative intervention.

## PERFORATION

Perforation is a rare but serious complication of colonoscopy, with recent studies estimating the rate at far less than 1/1,000 procedures (34). In fact, the USMSTF on CRC set quality improvement targets for perforation of <1/1,000 for therapeutic examinations and <2/2,000 for screening procedures (33). Multiple mechanisms can cause perforation during colonoscopy. These include postpolypectomy and other procedural perforation, direct trauma from instrument passage (most commonly in the sigmoid colon), shearing injury caused by lateral bowel pressure from a bowing loop, and barotrauma from air insufflation (most commonly in the cecum).

Treatment of postcolonoscopic perforation depends on the patient's condition and presentation, time of perforation discovery, and the suspected nature of the perforation. In healthy patients with well-prepped bowel following polypectomy, it may be safe to admit the patient and treat nonoperatively. It should be mentioned, however, that patients treated operatively within 24 hours of perforation are less likely to develop peritonitis, require bowel resection or stomas, and have complications (35,36). Perforations from diagnostic endoscopy are more likely to be larger and thus less likely to be successfully treated with conservative measures.

Patients being treated conservatively should be admitted, started on antibiotics, have a nasogastric tube placed, and be put on bowel rest. Development of peritonitis is an indication for surgical exploration. Likewise, patients presenting late after colonoscopy are more likely to require operative intervention. Reports of successful repairs of perforations at the time of endoscopy using clips have been made as well (37,38). The most common signs and symptoms of perforation are abdominal pain, tachycardia, and leukocytosis (39). A CT scan with rectal contrast can help to confirm the diagnosis and may help guide operative intervention.

## POSTPOLYPECTOMY SYNDROME

Postpolypectomy syndrome (sometimes called postpoylpectomy coagulation syndrome or transmural burn syndrome) describes a variety of symptoms that can occur following colonoscopic polyp removal with electrocoagulation. This is more likely to occur following polypectomy in the thin-walled cecum and usually occurs following removal of sessile polyps >2 cm in diameter (40). Hypertension has also been shown to be an independent risk factor (41). Symptoms include abdominal pain (often with rebound and/or guarding), fever, and leukocytosis without frank perforation. Patients may present within hours of the procedure to as late as 5–6 days postprocedure.

Workup of suspected postpolypectomy syndrome should start with blood work and plain x-rays or a CT scan to rule out pneumoperitoneum. Leukocytosis and elevated CRP are suggestive of the syndrome. Patients can then be treated with broad-spectrum antibiotics and bowel rest and are followed with serial abdominal exams to assure the patient does not progress from localized to frank peritonitis (40,41).

## INFECTIOUS COMPLICATIONS

A rare but potentially serious complication of colonoscopy is the spread of transmittable diseases from improperly cleansed equipment or examiner exposure. Standard precautions should be taken with gowns, gloves, and face shields. Mechanical cleaning protocols, when followed correctly, should prevent the transmission of HIV and viral hepatitis (40). There have been no reported cases of endoscopy-transmitted HIV to date, and reports of transmission of viral hepatitis are limited to single digits. Reports of transmission of microorganisms such as *Pseudomonas aeruginosa* and *Salmonella* spp. by colonoscope have been made as well, including those with multidrug resistance. The true incidence of endoscopy-related infection is unknown but has been estimated to be approximately 1 in 1.8 million procedures (42). Despite the low incidence, it is important for the endoscopist to ensure that proper cleaning protocols have been followed prior to any endoscopy.

## POSTCOLONOSCOPY COLITIS (FROM DISINFECTANT)

Disinfectant colitis or glutaraldehyde-induced colitis is a condition first described in 1986 by Castelli (43). It is attributed to retention of a commonly used disinfectant, glutaraldehyde, in the colonoscopic channel. This condition typically presents with abdominal pain, tenesmus, and bloody diarrhea within 48 hours of colonoscopy, though milder cases can occur without bleeding. Laboratory workup can reveal leukocytosis and elevated CRP, and endoscopic features are similar to ischemic colitis. CT findings are also nonspecific and can include mural thickening or pericolonic fat stranding (44–46). Treatment is nonspecific and includes bowel rest; the disease course is self-limited. Incidence is estimated at 0.1%–4.7%, though given the difficulty in diagnosis and its self-limited nature, rates may actually be higher (47). Diagnosis remains one of exclusion, but it is important for the clinician to be aware of this potential complication and to consider it when other causes of pain or bleeding have been ruled out.

## INCOMPLETE COLONOSCOPY

A complete colonoscopy will not be possible in a certain number of patients. Reasons commonly include the presence of an obstructing mass, excess redundancy, poor preparation, medical instability, or lack of patient cooperation.

## MISCELLANEOUS COMPLICATIONS

Although the most common complications of colonoscopy are bleeding and perforation, a wide body of literature exists describing other rare but potential complications. Splenic injury following colonoscopy was first reported in 1974 and is becoming increasingly recognized (48). The injury is proposed to occur from excessive traction of the splenocolic ligament rather than from therapeutic maneuvers (40). Incidence is estimated at around 1 in 100,000 procedures, and it carries an overall mortality rate of about 5%, making prompt diagnosis and treatment vital. Traditionally treatment consisted of laparotomy with splenectomy. Although splenectomy remains a mainstay of treatment, there are recent trends toward embolization or conservative management (49).

Other rare complications include acute appendicitis, first reported in 1988 (50). Although rare with only about 30 reported incidences, one reported patient died despite appendectomy, and it is important to recognize appendicitis as a potential complication of lower endoscopy (51). Another rare but potentially serious complication is the incarceration of the colonoscope within an inguinal or ventral hernia. A "pulley" technique has been described where a large loop is intentionally created within the hernia sac, grasped manually, and withdrawn over the "pulley hand" limb by limb (52). Others report removal of the scope under x-ray guidance (53,54); however, an inability to remove the scope with gentle traction necessitates operative intervention (55).

### SUMMARY

Adequate training, knowledge, and experience as well as technical skill are vital to perform safe and effective endoscopy and to limit complications. It is important for the endoscopist to know the applications and limitation to the various modalities. Early recognition, workup, treatment, and understanding of potential complications are vital to minimize the risk of morbidity and mortality.

## REFERENCES

1. Harewood GC et al. *Gastrointest Endosc*. 2003;58(1): 76–9.
2. Bucci C et al. *Gastrointest Endosc*. 2014;80(4): 566–76.e2.
3. Johnson DA et al. *Gastrointest Endosc*. 2014;80(4): 543–62.
4. Curran MP, Plosker GL. *Drugs*. 2004;64(15):1697–714.
5. Cohen SM et al. *Dis Colon Rectum*. 1994;37(7): 689–96.
6. Parente F et al. *Dig Liver Dis*. 2009;41(2):87–95.
7. Markowitz GS et al. *J Am Soc Nephrol*. 2005; 16(11):3389–96.
8. Rejchrt S et al. *Gastrointest Endosc*. 2004;59(6): 651–4.
9. Marshal JB. *Clin Gastroenterol Hepatologu*. 2014;12: 1522–4.
10. Longcroft-Wheaton G, Bhandari P. *J Clin Gastroenterol*. 2012;46(1):57–61.
11. Nivatvongs S, Fryd DS. *N Engl J Med*. 1980;303(7): 380–2.
12. Ellis DJ, Bevan PG. *Br Med J*. 1980;281(6237):435–7.
13. Rao VS et al. *Colorectal Dis*. 2005;7(1):61–4.
14. Schoellhammer HF et al. *Am J Surg*. 2008;196(6): 904–8. discussion 908.
15. Beck DE. *Handbook of Colorectal Surgery*, 2nd Edition, Vol. xiv. New York, NY: Marcel Dekker, 2003.
16. Achord JL. The history of gastrointestinal endoscopy. In Ginsberg GG (ed). *Clinical Gastrointestinal Endoscopy*. St. Louis, MO: Elsevier Saunders, 2012, pp. 2–11.
17. Rex DK et al. *Am J Gastroenterol*. 2009;104(3): 739–50.
18. Levin B et al. *Gastroenterology*. 2008;134(5):1570–95.

19. Wiggins TF et al. *Clin Colon Rectal Surg.* 2010;23(1): 14–20.
20. Shergill AK et al. *Gastrointest Endosc.* 2012;76(1): 18–24.
21. Childers RE et al. *Gastrointest Endosc.* 2015;82(3): 503–11.
22. Schroeder C et al. *Dis Colon Rectum.* 2016;59(1): 62–9.
23. Wadhwa V et al. *Clin Gastroenterol Hepatol.* 2017;15(2):194–206.
24. Sipe BW et al. *Gastrointest Endosc.* 2002;55(7): 815–25.
25. Hassan C et al. *Endoscopy.* 2012;44(5):456–64.
26. Clarke AC et al. *Med J Aust.* 2002;176(4):158–61.
27. Lichtenstein DR et al. *Gastrointest Endosc.* 2008; 68(5):815–26.
28. Patane S. *J Cardiovasc Transl Res.* 2014;7(3):372–4.
29. Wilson W et al. *Circulation.* 2007;116(15):1736–54.
30. Committee ASOP et al. *Gastrointest Endosc.* 2015; 81(1):81–9.
31. Douketis JD et al. *Chest.* 2012;141(Suppl. 2): e326–50S.
32. Reumkens A et al. *Am J Gastroenterol.* 2016;111(8): 1092–101.
33. Rex DK et al. *Am J Gastroenterol.* 2002;97(6):1296–308.
34. Castro G et al. *Cancer.* 2013;119(Suppl. 15):2849–54.
35. Orsoni P et al. *Endoscopy.* 1997;29(3):160–4.
36. Castellvi J et al. *Int J Colorectal Dis.* 2011;26(9): 1183–90.
37. Kim JS et al. *Surg Endosc.* 2013;27(2):501–4.
38. Trecca A et al. *Tech Coloproctol.* 2008;12(4):315–21. discussion 322.
39. Avgerinos DV et al. *J Gastrointest Surg.* 2008;12(10): 1783–9.
40. Hicks TC. Transanal endoscopy. In Whitlow CB (ed). *Improved Outcomes in Colon and Rectal Surgery.* London, UK: Informa Healthcare, 2010, p. 132–9.
41. Cha JM et al. *Endoscopy.* 2013;45(3):202–7.
42. Kovaleva J. *Best Pract Res Clin Gastroenterol.* 2016; 30(5):689–704.
43. Castelli M et al. *Am J Gastroenterol.* 1986;81:887.
44. Yen HH, Chen YY. *Endoscopy.* 2006;38(Suppl. 2):E98.
45. Mohamad MZ et al. *Am J Emerg Med.* 2014;32(6): 685.e1-2.
46. Shih HY et al. *Kaohsiung J Med Sci.* 2011;27(12): 577–80.
47. Stein BL et al. *Can J Surg.* 2001;44(2):113–6.
48. Wherry DC et al. *Med Ann Dist Columbia.* 1974;43(4): 189–92.
49. Jehangir A et al. *Int J Surg.* 2016;33(Pt A):55–9.
50. Houghton A, Aston N. *Gastrointest Endosc.* 1988; 34(6):489.
51. Kuriyama M. *Clin J Gastroenterol.* 2014;7(1):32–5.
52. Koltun WA, Coller JA. *Dis Colon Rectum.* 1991;34(2): 191–3.
53. Kume K et al. *Endoscopy.* 2009;41(Suppl. 2):E172.
54. Fan CS, Soon MS. *Endoscopy.* 2007;39(Suppl. 1): E185.
55. Tas A et al. *Endoscopy.* 2015;47(Suppl. 1 UCTN): E125–6.

# 14

# Laparoscopy for colorectal disease

BRADLEY R. DAVIS AND KEVIN R. KASTEN

## CHALLENGING CASE

A 64-year-old woman with a history of arteriosclerotic peripheral vascular disease is undergoing a laparoscopic right colectomy for an early cancer. After the ileocolic artery and vein are divided with an energy-sealing device, pulsatile blood is noted from the proximal divided vessel.

## CASE MANAGEMENT

The proximal stump is grasped with a grasper, which controls the bleeding. A vessel loop is inserted and using a second grasper is placed around the vessel and tightened. This controls the bleeding.

## INTRODUCTION

Although laparoscopy has been in clinical use since the turn of the twentieth century, its use in general surgery was limited. That changed in the 1980s with the recognition that laparoscopic cholecystectomy could be performed with significant reduction in operative morbidity, hospital length of stay, and recovery. Now a host of complex surgeries are being performed preferentially using minimally invasive techniques with excellent outcomes.

Laparoscopic colon and rectal resections were demonstrated to be feasible in the mid-1990s (1,2), but the rate of adoption has been slower when compared to other minimally invasive procedures such as cholecystectomy (3). Laparoscopic colonic surgery is a significantly more challenging operation as it frequently involves multiple abdominal quadrants, identification and ligation of named vascular pedicles, mobilization and transection of the bowel, retrieval of the surgical specimen, and

performance of an anastomosis. The greater complexity of laparoscopic colectomy has been associated with longer operative times and a longer learning curve. For these reasons, despite its advantages, laparoscopic colectomy has taken many years to gain traction. In the early days of colorectal laparoscopy, it was estimated that only 3% of surgeons had performed more than 50 laparoscopic colectomies (2). The complexity of the procedure necessitated technological solutions that have evolved over the past 20 years so that surgeons are increasingly utilizing laparoscopy to treat colorectal disease. Some of the most recent estimates suggest about 40%–50% of colectomies are being performed laparoscopically, while about 5% are being performed with robotic assistance (4,5). While technical challenges have hampered its growth, other challenges remain including access to enough cases to overcome the learning curve, the perceived lack of benefit to the patient, as well as concerns regarding safety and oncologic outcomes. Some questions remain to be answered, but laparoscopy has now been shown to be equivalent in terms of oncologic outcomes in colon cancer, and the benefit to the patient has been clearly demonstrated. As more general surgery and colorectal trainees gain access to cases during their residencies, the penetration of minimally invasive techniques will continue to grow so that the day is approaching when the majority of colorectal resections will be done laparoscopically.

The Surgical Care and Outcomes Assessment Program evaluated the use of laparoscopy in 48 hospitals in the United States between 2005 and 2010. Of the 9,705 patients undergoing elective colorectal operations, 38% were performed laparoscopically (17.8% of the procedures were converted to open). The use of laparoscopic procedures increased from 23.3% in 2005 to 41.6% in 2010 (6). The authors found that hospital characteristics (urban location and less than 200 beds), diverticular disease, and right hemicolectomies were factors associated with the use of laparoscopy. They also found the greatest increase in the total number of colorectal operations among hospitals with the highest laparoscopy adoption rates.

In another recent study using the University Health System Consortium administrative database, which includes more than 300 academic hospitals, laparoscopic colorectal resection was attempted in 36,228 (42.2%) out of 85,712 patients, with 15.8% requiring conversion to open surgery. The authors concluded that there is a trend of increasing use of laparoscopy in colorectal surgery, across hospitals in the United States in recent years with acceptable conversion rates (7).

## ADVANTAGES

Laparoscopic surgery in general has many advantages compared to open surgery, including smaller incisions, which are expected to translate into decreased postoperative pain and offer a superior cosmetic result. More importantly, however, are a decreased risk of postoperative complications both long and short term, including ileus, surgical site infections, and adhesion formation, as well as incisional hernia formation. Postoperative pain has been evaluated in a number of prospective, randomized trials demonstrating a reduction in narcotic use following laparoscopic surgery (8–10). Further pain reduction can be seen with the use of multimodal pain management that has become common in enhanced recovery programs, including the use of transversus abdominis plane blocks (11) and multimodal drug therapy (12). Laparoscopy has been associated with a significant reduction in both incisional hernia and small bowel obstruction (SBO). In a review of 11 randomized controlled trials (RCTs) and 14 non-RCT comparative studies (6,540 patients), laparoscopy was associated with a significant reduction in the occurrence of SBO (relative risk [RR] 0.57; 95% confidence interval [CI], 0.42–0.76) and incisional hernia (RR 0.60; 95% CI, 0.50–0.72). No significant difference between laparoscopy and open surgery was found when the analysis was limited to studies with conversion rate: >15% demonstrating the importance of minimizing conversions. Length of follow-up did not substantially impact the results (13).

The incidence of both superficial and deep/organ space surgical site infections (SSIs) has decreased with the penetration of laparoscopy for colorectal disease (14). In a study looking at the National Surgical Quality Improvement Program, 10,979 patients undergoing colorectal surgery were analyzed (laparoscopy [LAP] 31.1%, open 68.9%). The SSI rate was 14% (9.5% LAP versus 16.1% open, $p < 0.001$). On multivariate analysis age, American Society of Anesthesiologists (ASA) stage $\geq 3$, smoking, diabetes, operative time >180 minutes, appendicitis or diverticulitis, and regional enteritis diseases were found to be significantly associated with high SSI while the LAP approach was associated with a reduced SSI rate (15). In a prospective study of SSIs in 1,011 patients undergoing elective colorectal resections, the overall rate of incisional SSI and organ/space SSI was 4.8% and 1.7%, respectively. Rates of incisional SSI in open and laparoscopic colorectal resection were 5.7% and

2.7%, respectively. Anastomotic leakage was the only factor that predicted organ/space SSI ($p < 0.01$). Independent risk factors of incisional SSI included blood transfusion ($p = 0.047$) anastomotic leakage ($p < 0.01$), and open colorectal resection ($p = 0.037$) (16). In another study of 3,701 patients, 2,518 (68%) underwent colon surgery and 1,183 (32%) rectal surgery. In colon surgery, the overall SSI rate was 16.4%, and the organ/space SSI rate was 7.9%, while in rectal surgery the rates were 21.6% and 11.5%, respectively ($p < 0.001$). Independent risk factors for organ/space SSI in colon surgery were male sex (odds ratio [OR] 1.57; 95% CI, 1.14–2.15) and ostomy creation (OR 2.65; 95% CI, 1.8–3.92), while laparoscopy (OR 0.5; 95% CI, 0.38–0.69) and oral antibiotics combined with IV antibiotic prophylaxis (OR 0.7; 95% CI, 0.51–0.97) were protective factors (17). Open surgery was shown to be a risk factor for superficial SSI after elective rectal surgery (18). Following elective rectal surgery, 8,880 patients were evaluated, and superficial SSIs were diagnosed in 861 (9.7%) patients. Multivariate analysis demonstrated the following risk factors: male gender, body mass index (BMI) >30, current smoking, history of chronic obstructive pulmonary disease (COPD), American Society of Anesthesiologists III/IV, abdominoperineal resection (APR), stoma formation, open surgery (versus laparoscopic), and operative time >217 minutes. The benefit of minimally invasive surgery with respect to SSIs has carried over to hand-assisted procedures as well (19). A limitation of many of the studies reviewed is the selection bias associated with selecting patients for a laparoscopic approach over an open procedure.

Postoperative ileus (POI) results in greater hospital length of stay and comes at a significant cost to the healthcare system (20). In a meta-analysis of 54 studies comprising 18,983 patients, the incidence of POI was 10.3%. A lower incidence of POI after laparoscopic resections was identified with an incidence of 6.4% (95% CI, 3.5%–11.5%) after laparoscopic resection and 10% (95% CI, 6.2%–15.8%) after open colorectal resection (21). Similar studies have demonstrated the protective effect of laparoscopy on POI following colorectal resections (22–24).

## DISADVANTAGES

While the advantages of laparoscopy are significant, they mostly favor patient outcomes at the expense of longer operative times and resource utilization in the operating room. In addition, there is a physical cost to the surgeon with as many as 74% experiencing musculoskeletal disorders attributable to performing minimally invasive surgery (25,26).

The conversion from laparoscopic to open surgery for colorectal disease is a predictable part of any practice. The proper patient selection and increasing expertise and experience, as well as improvements in equipment, will reduce the need for conversion and its overall impact.

Laparoscopy for colorectal disease is among the most complex minimally invasive procedures surgeons will perform. The challenge as in all laparoscopic procedures is the translation of a surgeon's expertise in open surgery to minimally invasive surgery. While good judgment and critical thinking in the operating room are common to both techniques, the skill sets and even the presentation of the anatomy are often quite different. Improvements in hand port technology have the potential to bridge the gap between open and minimally invasive procedures and afford the surgeon an opportunity to gradually acquire the necessary expertise.

There is a wide range of conversion rates published in the literature from as low as 3% to 30% (27,28). In early trials assessing the safety of laparoscopy in treatable colorectal cancer, all trial participants had to have completed a minimum of 20 laparoscopic colon resections for benign disease, and yet in the CLASICC trial there was a decrease in the conversion rate from 38% to 16% during the 6-year study, presumably reflecting an ongoing learning curve beyond 20 cases (29). While it is certainly possible that 20 cases will be adequate for some surgeons, the majority will require more—likely 50–70 cases—to fully master the technique (30). Much of this will depend on the choice of procedures— right-sided versus left-sided colectomies—the disease process, and the laparoscopic technique (31). In a more recent review of the published literature on learning curves for colorectal laparoscopy, it was found that the definition of proficiency was subjective, and the number of operations to achieve it ranged from 5 to 310 cases (32). It can be difficult for many surgeons in practice to achieve this volume of cases, and several options are available to facilitate the learning process. Simulators are still fairly crude but are being developed and improved upon constantly. Eventually a surgeon may be able to master a procedure through simulation prior to taking on a live case. While the numbers of laparoscopic cases being performed by general surgery residents is increasing, a recent review of graduating residents demonstrated an average case volume of just 20 laparoscopic colorectal resections, a number that when averaged over 5 years of training is probably inadequate to achieve competency (33,34). The number of cases performed by graduating colorectal surgery residents was 80 cases per resident, which reflects the increasing penetration of minimally invasive surgery techniques in colorectal practice (33).

Previous abdominal surgery does not preclude safe laparoscopy, but it is totally unpredictable. Open trocar insertion should be considered to avoid unintended bowel injury. The decision to proceed should be made early without a lot of time spent in laparoscopic adhesiolysis. With no ability to pack the abdomen, exposure is often obtained using gravity, with the patient at steep inclinations. Omental and small bowel adhesions will often prevent this, precluding safe visualization. As is true with all laparoscopic cases, feasibility should be decided as quickly as possible to prevent long operative times and unnecessary morbidity (35).

If named vessels are to be taken laparoscopically, the surgeon will need familiarity with a variety of commercially available instruments. It is important to be familiar with more than one device, as all of them can and will fail at some point. Staplers, vessel clips, sealant devices, as well as vessel loops are the standard tools used to achieve intracorporeal hemostasis. Early in a surgeon's experience, extracorporeal vessel ligation may be preferred.

While laparoscopy for patients with a BMI over 30 has been safely performed, increasing size will add to the challenge as is true with open surgery. Women tend to have much less intraabdominal adipose deposits, while obese men tend to have heavy, thick omentums with bulky mesenteries and large appendices epiploic. Therefore, laparoscopic colon resections in morbidly obese men tend to be more difficult and should be avoided early in a surgeon's experience. Obesity plays an important role in outcomes following laparoscopic surgery for colorectal disease. In a meta-analysis of 43 studies evaluating the impact of obesity, it was found that BMI was associated with significantly longer operative time ($p < 0.001$), greater blood loss ($p = 0.01$), and higher incidence of conversion to open surgery ($p < 0.001$). Moreover, BMI was a risk factor for overall complication rates ($p < 0.001$), especially for ileus ($p = 0.02$) and events of the urinary system ($p = 0.03$). Significant association was identified between higher BMI and risk of SSI ($p < 0.001$) and anastomotic leakage ($p = 0.02$). Higher BMI might also lead to a reduced number of harvest lymph nodes for patients with colorectal cancer ($p = 0.02$) (36).

While one study demonstrated that timely conversion to open surgery does not place a patient at increased risk of perioperative morbidity and mortality (37), most demonstrate that conversion results in worse outcomes compared to both laparoscopic and open procedures (38,39). In a retrospective study using the Premier Prospective database to evaluate predictors and outcomes of conversions for left-sided colectomies, 41,417 patients were evaluated; 63% of these cases were attempted laparoscopically with the incidence of conversion of 13.3%. Length of stay (LOS) in days was significantly lower for the Lap-Successful group (4.9 compared with Lap-Conversion 6.8 and Open-Planned 7.0), but Lap-Conversion and Open-Planned had similar LOS. Adjusted mean cost was higher for Lap-Conversion $20,165 compared to Open-Planned $18,797, but this difference was smaller than the cost savings for Lap-Successful $16,206 ± $219. Open-Planned had lower odds of anastomotic leak when compared to converted cases. Conversion risk factors included obesity, inflammatory bowel disease, and left hemicolectomy versus sigmoid colectomy. Colorectal specialists performing the procedure were associated with 38% decreased odds of conversion (40). With regard to long-term oncologic outcome, overall and disease-free survival in the case of converted patients undergoing laparoscopic colorectal cancer surgery seems to be worse than in those in whom the surgery was successfully completed minimally invasively. However, it remains difficult to draw a proper conclusion due to the heterogeneity of the current studies and reported outcomes as well as due to the inclusion of both colon and rectal cancer patients (41).

Converting from laparoscopy to open is usually accomplished through a midline laparotomy; however, for surgeons with experience using hand-assist techniques, alternatives to performing a midline laparotomy exist. For many left-sided and pelvic procedures, a Pfannenstiel incision can provide adequate to excellent exposure when used in combination with hand-assisted laparoscopic techniques. However, the surgeon should be certain that the lower transverse incision will adequately accomplish what needs to be addressed.

## TREATABLE CONDITIONS

## COLON CANCER

The impact of laparoscopy on long-term oncological outcome was a subject of controversy for many years and was a hurdle that had to be crossed for laparoscopy to become widely accepted. Early reports of trocar site cancer recurrence and concerns regarding lower number of lymph nodes retrieved (42,43) led to a self-imposed moratorium on laparoscopy for curable cancer, and the procedure lost some of its momentum further delaying widespread utilization. In fact, some series reported port site metastases and peritoneal dissemination in 10%–20% of patients (44,45). Many of the benign conditions (e.g., diverticular disease) tended to be more difficult to do laparoscopically, and surgeons were cautious to remove polyps as several of them contained adenocarcinoma on final pathological analysis. The relationship between different factors related to the laparoscopic technique (pneumoperitoneum) to the tumor (manipulation, degree of differentiation, and stage) and the host (immune and inflammatory factors) were investigated in several experimental studies (46,47). The "chimney effect," referring to leakage of carbon dioxide from trocars and aerosolizing of tumor cells, has been proposed as a causative factor (48). Based on these results, a series of recommendations were made to avoid port site metastasis (49,50). These included avoiding manipulation of the tumor to prevent exfoliation of malignant cells, using povidone-iodine solutions, emptying the $CO_2$ through the trocars, using a device to protect the wall incision, and closing all trocar holes.

To assess the outcomes of laparoscopy for colon cancer, a randomized multicenter trial was established to assess if laparoscopy was equivalent in terms of oncologic outcomes when compared to traditional open techniques (51). The results of the COST trial were published in 2004. The trial enrolled 872 patients with curable colon cancer and randomized them to open versus laparoscopic resection. The median follow-up was 4.4 years. There was no difference in oncological outcomes, and patients in the laparoscopic arm enjoyed a faster return of bowel function and earlier discharge. Surgeons who participated in the trial were selected based on proven expertise as decided by a review of a videotaped laparoscopic colectomy. Despite this proven ability, the conversion rate from laparoscopy

to open surgery was 21%. There have been several other well-designed prospective randomized multicenter trials that have demonstrated no differences in the incidence of metastasis in the surgical wound as well as in oncological outcomes when the laparoscopic approach was compared to open surgery (52–55).

While some studies have suggested better oncologic outcomes favoring laparoscopy, particularly in patients stage III colon cancer (51,56), the results have not been confirmed in all studies, but without question the use of laparoscopy for the management of colon cancer is currently accepted worldwide (57).

As a direct result of this data, the American Society of Colon and Rectal Surgeons as well as the Society of American Gastrointestinal and Endoscopic Surgeons have formulated a position statement in support of laparoscopy for curable colon cancer with the caveat that surgeons should have performed a minimum of 20 laparoscopic colectomies for benign disease or metastatic cancer before a curable cancer resection can be performed. Individual surgeons need to be certain that they can perform an adequate lymphadenectomy with negative margins and create an anastomosis before they take on curable cancer resections laparoscopically.

## RECTAL CANCER

With respect to rectal cancer, only one of these early trials reported on the outcomes, and the incidence of positive radial margin was higher in the laparoscopic arm with much higher conversion rates noted (52). More recent trials have assessed the safety and outcomes of patients undergoing a laparoscopic approach to rectal cancer, and the outcomes have been mixed. The need to perform a total mesorectal excision in a deep and narrow pelvis increases the technical complexity of this procedure and the risk of oncological compromise.

In a recent single-center randomized trial, Lujan et al. (58) compared surgical outcomes after laparoscopy and open surgery in patients with mid and low rectal cancers. Blood loss was significantly greater for open surgery ($p < 0.001$), and operating time was significantly greater for laparoscopic surgery ($p = 0.020$), while return to diet and hospital stay were longer for open surgery. Complication rates and involvement of circumferential and radial margins were similar for both procedures, but the number of isolated lymph nodes was greater in the laparoscopic group (mean 13.63 versus 11.57; $p = 0.026$). There were no differences in local recurrence or disease-free or overall survival.

In the COLOR II trial, 1,044 patients were randomized to undergo laparoscopic or open rectal resections for adenocarcinoma (within 15 cm from the anal verge—699 in the laparoscopic surgery group and 345 in the open surgery group) (59). At 3 years, the locoregional recurrence rate was 5% in the two groups (90% CI, −2.6 to 2.6). Disease-free survival rates were 74.8% in the laparoscopic surgery group and 70.8% in the open surgery group (95% CI, −1.9

to 9.9). Overall survival rates were 86.7% in the laparoscopic surgery group and 83.6% in the open surgery group (95% CI, −1.6 to 7.8). As with many of these trials, surgeons had to demonstrate expertise in laparoscopic total mesorectal excision through submission of unedited video prior to participation in the study. Conversion to open surgery was 16%. In the laparoscopic surgery group, the operating time was 52 minutes longer, bowel function returned 1 day earlier ($p < 0.0001$), and the hospital stay was 1 day shorter than in the open surgery group ($p = 0.036$) (60). There were no significant differences in the rates of anastomotic leaking, complication, or death. There were no significant differences between the groups with respect to macroscopic completeness of the mesorectum, involved circumferential resection margins, or distal resection margins (median, 3 cm in the two groups).

The ACOSOG Z6051 trial randomized patients with rectal cancer within 12 cm of the anal verge to undergo either open ($n = 222$) or laparoscopic ($n = 240$) total mesorectal excision. The trial was a noninferiority design, and the primary outcome was a composite of circumferential radial margin greater than 1 mm, distal margin without tumor, and completeness of total mesorectal excision (61).

Conversion to open resection occurred in 11.3% of patients. Operative time was significantly longer for laparoscopic resection (mean, 266.2 versus 220.6 minutes; $p < 0.001$). Length of stay (7.3 versus 7 days), readmission within 30 days (3.3% versus 4.1%), and severe complications (22.5% versus 22.1%) did not differ significantly.

Successful resection occurred in 81.7% of laparoscopic resection cases and 86.9% of open resection cases and did not support noninferiority. Quality of the total mesorectal excision specimen in 462 operated and analyzed surgeries was complete (77%) and nearly complete (16.5%) in 93.5% of the cases. Negative circumferential radial margin was observed in 90% of the overall group (87.9% laparoscopic resection and 92.3% open resection; $p = 0.11$). The distal margin result was negative in more than 98% of patients irrespective of type of surgery ($p = 0.91$).

The ALaCaRT trial randomized patients with T1–T3 rectal cancer within 15 cm of the anal verge to either open ($n = 237$) or laparoscopic ($n = 238$) total mesorectal excision (TME) in a European multicenter trial with a similar composite outcome measure and noninferiority design. Conversion to open surgery occurred in 9% of patients. Operative times were longer in the laparoscopy group, while length of hospital stay (8 days) and complication rates were not different among the groups. A successful resection was achieved in 194 patients (82%) in the laparoscopic surgery group and 208 patients (89%) in the open surgery group, which once again did not support noninferiority. The circumferential resection margin was clear in 222 patients (93%) in the laparoscopic surgery group and in 228 patients (97%) in the open surgery group ($p = 0.06$), the distal margin was clear in 236 patients (99%) in the laparoscopic surgery group and in 234 patients (99%) in the open surgery group ($p = 0.67$), and total mesorectal excision was complete in

206 patients (87%) in the laparoscopic surgery group and 216 patients (92%) in the open surgery group ($p = 0.06$).

Several systematic reviews and meta-analyses have recently confirmed the short-term benefits and oncological safety of the minimally invasive approach for rectal cancer surgery (62,63). While patients with rectal cancer benefit from laparoscopic approaches, surgeons must be very mindful of the results of the randomized trials and how patients are informed of the possibility that an open technique may be a better option. Individual surgeons will need to track their results, and it is likely that minimally invasive approaches to rectal cancer should be reserved for higher volume centers with access to more cases to achieve proficiency in these techniques.

## INFLAMMATORY BOWEL DISEASE

### Ulcerative colitis

Pooled data from 1975 to 2007 demonstrate overall morbidity and mortality of 40.1% and 1.8%, respectively, following open surgery for ulcerative colitis (UC) (64). Studies report 10%–45% of UC patients ultimately require surgery, even as that number declines due to a paradigm shift in medical treatment using biologic agents (65–67). These agents are keeping more patients out of the operating room; however, a significant volume of higher acuity patients still require surgical resection (68). Despite contradictory data regarding the effect of biologics on surgical complications, providers continue to strive for reduction in risk while maximizing quality of life (69). Minimally invasive surgery helps in risk reduction.

Specific patient populations have been shown to benefit from laparoscopic surgery for UC. While obesity is independently associated with conversion to open procedure, no differences were seen between laparoscopic and open procedures in overweight or obese patients compared with normal BMI patients (70). When comparing abdominal adhesions following laparoscopic and open ileal pouch-anal anastomosis (IPAA), the intraabdominal adhesion score was significantly lower in the laparoscopic group (median score 0 versus 4). Additionally, the adnexal adhesions score was significantly lower at 5.2 versus 20. These findings were independent of two- or three-stage procedures (71). With a median age of IPAA near 27 years and 65% of female patients experiencing infertility when undergoing an open procedure due to adhesions of the fallopian tubes (71), laparoscopy may benefit females interested in future childrearing. Studies of laparoscopic IPAA show significantly reduced infertility rates (27%–45%) that are comparable to UC patients undergoing laparoscopic appendectomy (65,72). Reduced adhesions following laparoscopic surgery for UC also benefits subsequent procedures. Operative time is reduced in subsequent procedures due to less time required for adhesiolysis, and there are lower rates of bowel obstruction (71). A conversion rate of 5% during second- and third-stage procedures is likely due to significantly fewer abdominal and interloop adhesions, even in patients with severe colitis (64,73,74). This is important to remember as surgeons become more aggressive in performing urgent minimally invasive colectomy for severe colitis. Newer published indices are being increasingly used by gastroenterologists and surgeons to determine patients at increased risk for surgical intervention. The simplest index is the Oxford Index that shows an 85% likelihood of requiring colectomy during that admission if the patient has stool frequency >8/day or stool frequency of 3–8/day with C-reactive protein (CRP) >45 mg/L on hospital day 3 (75). Such indices support decision-making algorithms that improve laparoscopic surgical outcomes for severe colitis.

When evaluating laparoscopic total abdominal colectomy (TAC) (straight lap, hand assisted laparoscopic surgery [HALS], single incision laparoscopic surgery [SILS]) for severe colitis, a 40% overall complication rate, 7.5% reoperation rate, 17.2% readmission rate, and 0.5% mortality rate were demonstrated. The most common complications were stump leak (15%), bowel obstruction (10%), and wound infection (9%), with no differences between types of laparoscopic approach (64). Studies also show significantly lower rates of infectious complications following laparoscopic procedures in this patient population (73). At Washington University, the use of laparoscopy for stage 1 total abdominal colectomy yielded less narcotic usage, faster return of bowel function, shorter postoperative length of stay, and no difference in complication rates. Further, when the first stage was done laparoscopically, patients received completion proctectomy and IPAA an average of 49 days earlier than patients with open abdominal colectomy. Subsequent ileostomy closure occurred a mean of 17 days earlier. Laparoscopic approach was the only factor independently associated with decreased elapsed time to completion of all surgical procedures (74).

A range of studies, including two RCTs, showed equivalence of laparoscopic and open IPAA in quality of life, mortality, morbidity, return of bowel function (ROBF), and postoperative LOS (76). In contrast, a Cochrane Review demonstrated shorter ROBF, shorter LOS, better cosmesis, longer operative time, higher operative cost, and lower total hospital cost for laparoscopic versus open IPAA (76,77). From a long-term standpoint, studies show similar outcomes between open and laparoscopic procedures, aside from cosmesis and body image scores. Further, long-term IPAA function at 20 years (regardless of surgical approach) demonstrates a mean of six bowel movements per day with one at night. Continence is maintained in greater than 70% of patients, with more than 80% able to defer defecation for 30 minutes. Overall pouch failure is 4.7%, with rates decreasing since 2000. And male sexual dysfunction rates are 2%–3%, with lower rates achieved when dissection is close to the rectal wall. Interestingly, up to 40% of women complain of sexual dysfunction following TAC/IPAA. Overall costs are no different between approaches (78).

Published practice parameters from the American Society of Colon and Rectal Surgeons do not favor one surgical procedure over another for management of UC, nor do they favor an open versus laparoscopic approach (79). Data on laparoscopic TAC and IPAA support a minimally invasive approach as safe and effective, with fewer complications and higher quality of life. Surgeons are encouraged to discuss all options, utilizing decision aids where available (66). Tailoring an approach based on patient condition, expectations for quality of life, and surgeon comfort with procedure are tantamount to success.

## Crohn disease

Despite advances in medical management, 15%–20% of patients undergo surgical resection within the first year of diagnosis, increasing to 65% within 10 years of diagnosis. A multidisciplinary approach with gastroenterology is necessary as 40%–50% of operative patients require repeat procedure within 10 years (80). Unlike UC, disease pathophysiology helps determine the role for laparoscopic intervention in Crohn disease (CD). While most patient populations benefit from a minimally invasive procedure, rates of complications and conversion to open surgery are predicated on uncomplicated versus complicated disease. For uncomplicated disease and nonrecurrent strictures, a minimally invasive approach is recommended with resultant decreased length of stay, decreased costs, lower complication rates, conversion rates below 10%, and long-term recurrence rates similar to open procedures (80). For complicated and recurrent Crohn disease, intraoperative or CT findings of abscess or fistula are independently associated with conversion and septic complications (80–82). Interestingly, prior open procedure is not associated with higher rates of conversion, although adhesive disease is the most common indication for conversion. Further, iterative procedures in complicated Crohn patients are not associated with higher rates of complications (80,82–84). As such, minimally invasive surgery for both uncomplicated and complicated Crohn disease in most cases is a reasonable option, understanding that some patients are at higher risk for conversion to an open procedure.

More than 95% of fistulizing Crohn disease patients require surgery, with 27% undergoing two procedures and 55% requiring more than two procedures (85). These operations are technically demanding when performed laparoscopically, but the patient benefit is clear. Despite rates of conversion nearing 40%, the postoperative complication rate is significantly reduced (12% versus 43%). This includes lower rates of SSI, anastomotic leak, and intraabdominal bleeding. Decreased complication rates result in shorter postoperative length of stay. Measurement of serum CRP and procalcitonin in these patients indicates significantly reduced postoperative stress response in laparoscopic patients versus their open counterparts (85). Further, multiple studies support minimally invasive procedures for Crohn disease due to lower rates of pulmonary dysfunction, shorter postoperative length of stay, lower complication rates, and similar long-term results compared with open procedures (86).

Most surgical interventions for Crohn disease involve terminal ileal disease and small bowel strictures. However, a certain number of patients will require surgery for Crohn disease or indeterminate colitis. In the 5%–10% of Crohn patients requiring an urgent or emergent colectomy, laparoscopy may be considered. Total abdominal colectomy with end ileostomy is advised in these cases due to safety and speed of procedure, combined with knowledge that only 50% of severe colitis cases can be defined as either Crohn disease or UC. In fact, some authors recommend saving the distal sigmoid and bringing it out as a mucous fistula for possible anastomosis in the future if proctectomy is not required (87). Laparoscopy in most cases for Crohn disease is safe, producing fewer complications, shorter postoperative length of stay, and lower costs. Based on significant literature on the subject, the use of minimally invasive procedures for inflammatory bowel disease patients should be the preferred approach, understanding that higher rates of conversion are expected but not detrimental to the patient.

## Diverticulitis

Surgical treatment of diverticulitis remains controversial. Recent studies indicate <5% of patients present with recurrent episodes worse than their sentinel presentations, most patients requiring abscess drainage do not require resection, and more than 90% of patients who develop diverticulitis will resolve with conservative treatment (88,89). A review of recent literature is important to provide patients with the best options for management of this disease process without undue risk of a surgical procedure. When resection is deemed necessary (stricture, inability to exclude malignancy, or ongoing sepsis), minimally invasive colectomy is encouraged for elective resection, emergent resection, elective closure of an end colostomy, and urgent or emergent washout of purulent peritonitis. In fact, more studies continue to demonstrate lower overall, minor, and major morbidity when laparoscopy is used (90). Additionally, reports indicate staying close to the colon wall for benign disease results in fewer complications with resection onto the upper rectum necessary to reduce recurrence rates (88). Understanding where and when to utilize each technique reduces complications while providing the best patient care.

### ELECTIVE RESECTION FOR DIVERTICULITIS

In the past decade, a few RCTs evaluating laparoscopy for diverticulitis were completed. The SIGMA trial was a multicenter, double-blind, parallel-arm study that blinded patients and staff for 5 days; allowed discharge decision-making by blinded, independent physicians; and sought to determine if laparoscopy produced fewer postoperative complications (91). For study inclusion, patients had confirmed diagnosis of diverticulitis via imaging (CT or barium enema) and colonoscopy, diagnosis of two recurrent attacks, or prior attack with complication (i.e., abscess, fistula, stricture, or bleeding requiring blood transfusion). From 2002 to 2006, 104 patients were randomized to each

group with results demonstrating a 15.4% (25% versus 9.6%) absolute reduction in major complications in the laparoscopic group. Interestingly, there was a 10% leak rate in open cases and 6% rate in laparoscopic cases. There was a 19.2% conversion rate (9.6% to hand-assist, 9.6% to open), with half of converted procedures due to adhesions and 15% due to obesity. While operative time was significantly longer in the laparoscopic group, there was less blood loss, no difference in return of bowel function, and a shorter length of stay (5 versus 7 days). No differences in mortality were seen between groups. Less reported pain in the laparoscopic group produced higher quality of life scores. In a 6-month follow-up analysis, there was no difference in late complications or recurrence between laparoscopic and open groups (92). Subsequent financial analysis of a large subset of SIGMA patients demonstrated a significantly higher operative cost in laparoscopic colectomy, which was negated by lower hospitalization, blood product, and emergency room visit expenditures (93). The cost of 1% reduction in complication rate attributable to laparoscopic colectomy was only 31 euros ($39), making minimally invasive colectomy for diverticulitis a bargain.

A subsequent study in 2010 with similar design showed no difference in complication rates between laparoscopic (13.5%) and open (9%) groups, longer operative time, reduced perception of pain with less morphine narcotic usage, and shorter length of stay (36 hours) in the laparoscopy group (94). Follow-up evaluation of long-term outcomes and quality of life was published in 2011 with a median follow-up of 30 months (95). Only one patient in each group developed recurrent diverticulitis treated with antibiotics. Incisional hernias were demonstrated in 9.8% of open cases and 12.9% of laparoscopic cases, and were not significantly different. Of note, four of the seven laparoscopy group patients with hernias had their first case converted to open. Quality of life scores were the same between groups, except for higher satisfaction with cosmesis in the laparoscopic group. Total calculated costs were similar between groups. The authors cautioned that converted patients experienced worsened outcomes, so choose patients carefully and attempt conversion to hand-assist instead of open whenever possible.

### EMERGENT OR URGENT PROCEDURES FOR DIVERTICULITIS

In 2016, results from the DILALA randomized trial comparing laparoscopic lavage (LL) to open Hartmann procedure (OHP) for perforated diverticulitis were published (96). Patients were randomized following confirmed Hinchey III classification by diagnostic laparoscopy. LL involved 3 L or more of body-temperature saline solution instilled and aspirated from all four abdominal quadrants until clear. A drain was left in the pelvis for at least 24 hours, with postoperative management comparable to those undergoing OHP procedure. A higher 30-day mortality was seen in the LL group (7.7% versus 0%); however, 90-day mortality was similar (7.7% versus 11.4%). Higher readmission occurred in the OHP group (0% versus 5.7%), although no differences were shown in number (52% lavage versus 40% OHP) or severity of complications. Additionally, no difference was demonstrated in the rate of 30-day reoperation, suggesting lavage was adequate for controlling the Hinchey III process. Length of stay was 6 days in the LL group, significantly shorter than 9 days in the OHP group.

Another prospective RCT published in 2015, the SCANDIV trial evaluated LL versus laparoscopic or open resection with or without primary anastomosis (97). A total of 101 LL and 98 colonic resection patients were compared with rates of 90-day severe postoperative outcomes as the primary endpoint. This endpoint was met in 30.7% of LL patients and 26% of resection cases, which was not statistically different. Mortality at 90 days was similar between groups (13.9% LL versus 11.5% resection). In this study, reoperation rate was significantly higher in the LL group (20.3%) compared to the resection group (5.7%). Also of note, four sigmoid cancers were missed on LL, indicating a strong need for follow-up colonoscopy in all patients not undergoing resection at time of presentation. In a meta-analysis of the DILALA, SCANDIV, and LADIES trials, the main conclusion was LL produced a significantly lower 12-month reoperation rate (OR 0.32), at a cost of increased 90-day morbidity (OR 1.7) attributable mostly to a higher rate of intraabdominal abscess formation (OR 3.5) (98). Of note, LL failed in 17% of patients, but no differences in mortality or morbidity were noted in patients when LL failed and required resection.

For patients undergoing Hartmann procedure for perforated diverticulitis, laparoscopy is a viable alternative to open. In a cost-effectiveness study from 2013 utilizing propensity-matched cohorts in the NSQIP data set, no differences in 30-day morbidity or mortality were seen between laparoscopic and open Hartmann procedure. Statistical modeling was used to account for inherent selection bias in patients undergoing laparoscopic Hartmann procedure for emergent condition, which may explain why operative times between groups were no different (99). While effective in the right hands, remember that, "In all cases, the adoption of laparoscopic lavage in emergent settings, abdominal exploration for generalized peritonitis, pelvic dissection in inflammatory conditions and possible suture of a diseased colon require the surgeon have a minimum of colorectal and minimally invasive skills" (100). When utilized, minimally invasive techniques for elective and emergent management of diverticulitis greatly benefit the patient.

## STOMA CREATION

The creation of a stoma can be easily accomplished using laparoscopic techniques and is an excellent way for surgeons to gain experience in laparoscopic colorectal surgery. Several studies have shown that laparoscopic stoma creation is a viable alternative to an open approach, with benefit in both morbidity and mortality (101,102). There is also evidence to support the use of single-incision laparoscopy for

the creation of stomas, which has the added value of no additional incisions beyond the stoma (103).

## RECTAL PROLAPSE

Abdominal approaches to rectal prolapse are associated with fewer recurrences when compared to the perineal approach. Operative approaches include resection rectopexy, suture rectopexy, or mesh rectopexy from either a ventral or posterior approach. All of the abdominal approaches have been described using laparoscopic techniques with comparable results in terms of recurrence and function when compared to open surgery (104), but with fewer postoperative complications and shorter hospital stay than open rectopexy (105). A review of 321 prolapse operations (laparoscopic rectopexy 126 patients, open rectopexy in 46, and resection rectopexy in 21 patients) with a median follow-up of 5 years demonstrated a 4% recurrence following laparoscopy. There was no significant difference between groups in terms of recurrence and postoperative complications (106). In contrast to the posterior approaches, the ventral mesh rectopexy (VMR) avoids posterolateral rectal mobilization and thereby minimizes the risk of postoperative constipation. Because of a low overall recurrence rate, good functional results, and low mesh-related morbidity in the short to medium term, VMR has been popularized in the past decade. Laparoscopic-assisted VMR is now being progressively performed, and several articles and guidelines propose the procedure as the treatment of choice for rectal prolapse (107).

## TECHNICAL CONSIDERATIONS IN MINIMALLY INVASIVE COLECTOMY

Minimally invasive surgery provides a technically equivalent outcome to open colorectal surgery, but with significant reductions in complication rate, pain, hospital length of stay, and adhesion formation. Myriad approaches include straight laparoscopic colectomy (SLC), hand-assisted laparoscopic surgery (HALS), and single-site laparoscopic surgery (SILS), each geared toward utilizing surgeon strengths to maximize patient outcomes. Being comfortable with these approaches enables surgeons to tailor surgical intervention to individual patients.

Maximizing success in minimally invasive colectomy begins with port placement and incision planning. It is possible to utilize 5 mm trocars for all minimally invasive procedures until confirmation that intracorporeal stapling will occur. A 5 mm trocar is placed circumumbilical for all colectomies, allowing for SLC, HALS, SILS, or a hybrid procedure following diagnostic laparoscopy. Trocars are placed based on target anatomy and likelihood of a hand port being used. In selected cases, a hand port through a Pfannenstiel incision 2 cm above the top of the pubic symphysis can be placed early in the procedure. Using this incision requires understanding that converting to open surgery via midline laparotomy carries significant risk of wound infection and incisional hernia formation. If doubts exist regarding the ability to complete a HALS procedure via Pfannenstiel incision, a midline incision is utilized. The importance of trocar placement cannot be overstated as poor triangulation, awkward surgeon stance, and poor visualization from inadequate traction lead to worsening technical outcomes and higher rates of conversion.

One of the earliest opportunities for injury occurs during trocar insertion into the abdomen. The initial trocar insertion will provide the greatest opportunity for a bad outcome, and as such, several different techniques have been described (108). These include an open technique, a blind technique using the Veress needle, and an optical technique using specialized trocars that allow visualization of the layers of the abdominal wall using the laparoscope. Mastery of one these techniques is essential for safe access to the abdomen, and knowledge of more than one is essential to keep the operating surgeon and the patient out of trouble; however, no one technique has been shown to be superior with potential pros and cons of each (109,110). A recent review including 28 RCTs with 4,860 individuals undergoing laparoscopy demonstrated no advantage using any single technique in terms of preventing major vascular or visceral complications. Using an open-entry technique compared to a Veress needle demonstrated a reduction in the incidence of failed entry (OR 0.12; 95% CI, 0.02–0.92). There were three advantages with direct-trocar entry when compared with Veress needle entry, in terms of lower rates of failed entry (OR 0.21; 95% CI, 0.14–0.31), extraperitoneal insufflation (OR 0.18; 95% CI, 0.13–0.26), and omental injury (OR 0.28; 95% CI, 0.14–0.55). Advocates of the open technique regard this as the safest and most effective means to place the initial trocar (111), although there are some limitations. It is very difficult to keep the skin incisions smaller than 1 cm, and larger trocars (11 or 12 mm) are generally needed to prevent loss of pneumoperitoneum during the case. It is not always desirable or necessary to have a 12 mm trocar, particularly in the midline, and placing a trocar using an open technique off midline is difficult in all but the thinnest patients. Additionally, while acute and chronic herniation can occur through trocars as small as 5 mm (112), it is generally acceptable to close the fascial defect of trocars larger than 12 mm (113,114) resulting in longer overall times using an open technique. Complications associated with the open technique include enterotomy and vascular and solid organ injury, as well as acute and chronic herniation, which in the immediate postoperative period can result in a bowel obstruction and need for emergent repair. In the obese patient, it can be very difficult to visualize the fascia through a small skin incision, and if necessary, it should be enlarged to ensure an adequate closure. It is probably best to avoid this technique altogether in the significantly obese patient, as the abdominal wall thickness will preclude adequate fascial visualization without a generous skin incision.

Understanding limitations reduces risk of conversion to open technique and the resultant worsened patient outcomes. Patient selection is of utmost importance. Factors associated with risk of conversion include BMI, surgical expertise, intraabdominal adhesions, stricture or fistula, and severity of diverticulitis/inflammation on pathologic examination (88). Review all available diagnostic films and endoscopy reports. Consider preoperative (or intraoperative) ureteral stent placement for help with identifying anatomy and reducing injury rates (88,115).

# STRAIGHT LAPAROSCOPIC COLECTOMY (SLC)

Following diagnostic laparoscopy, further 5 mm ports are placed and triangulated toward patient pathology. Fogging of the laparoscopic lens, splatter of irrigation fluid, blood, and bodily fluids are among those factors that affect a surgeon's ability to maintain a clear operating field, which is exacerbated by the use of a 5 mm camera. Aerosolization of fat and other debris will quickly diminish the optics and preclude safe visualization. Condensation on the lens due to temperature discrepancies will also degrade the optics and is perhaps the most common reason a surgeon will remove the laparoscope during surgery. Several commercial products exist to help mitigate the detrimental effects of smoke and condensation on the tip of the laparoscope, and a thorough evaluation of these technologies is appropriate for all surgeons considering laparoscopy as part of their colorectal practice. The most commonly used product is the fog reduction/elimination device (FRED, US Surgical, North Haven, Connecticut), which consists of less than 15% isopropyl alcohol, 2% surfactant, and more than 85% water (116). Advantages include ease of use, widespread availability, and low cost; the main disadvantage is the need to remove the laparoscope and the cooling that occurs upon removal of the laparoscope, leading to further condensation and worsening view. A newer product is the Clearify (Medtronic Minneapolis, Minnesota), a compact device that both heats the tip of the laparoscope and applies defogging solution at the same time. While it is still necessary to remove the laparoscope to utilize this device, the warming that occurs greatly eliminates the need for repeat cleanings. Another effective strategy to maintain the laparoscopic image is the use of heated insufflation tubing, which can also be used to humidify the gas as it enters the abdomen. This has also been shown to reduce postoperative hypothermia in clinical trials (117). The suction-irrigator can be used effectively in short bursts to keep the operative field free of smoke, especially when working in the narrow confines of the pelvis. On rare occasions when pulsatile bleeding strikes the camera, the operative field will be totally obscured, creating a situation that is particularly unnerving. It is important to determine the significance of the bleeding and to deal with it as quickly as possible. Often the camera operator is the least experienced surgeon or student involved in the case, and the senior surgeon must quickly take control of the situation. Blood in the trocar will frustrate any attempts at good visualization, and if it cannot be cleared quickly, then an alternate trocar should be chosen for the camera as long as it provides good exposure to the bleeding vessel. Alternatively, a 5 mm trocar can be upsized to accommodate a 10 mm laparoscope, which will be less temperamental in the face of blood and debris. Once the operative view has been restored, an assessment of the bleeding can be made and dealt with appropriately.

While segmental colectomy of the right or left can be completed with only two working trocars, the addition of a third trocar in the contralateral abdomen greatly enhances overall visualization and dissection. For intracorporeal anastomosis following right colectomy, an isoperistaltic anastomosis with stapling achieved through a left upper quadrant 12 mm trocar is an effective way to restore intestinal continuity. The common channel can be closed with either a 9″ 2.0 V-lock absorbable suture or a staple load fired transversely. A recent meta-analysis including 484 patients undergoing laparoscopic right colectomy, 272 with intracorporeal anastomosis and 212 with extracorporeal anastomosis, reported the best outcomes associated with intracorporeal anastomosis, especially in terms of return of bowel function, length of hospital stay, and cosmetic results. However, the meta-analysis did not show a significant difference between the two techniques for anastomotic leaks or overall short-term morbidity (118). In another review of this topic, 12 nonrandomized comparative studies were included in the analysis with a total number of 1,492 patients. No significant change in mortality was found, while short-term morbidity decreased significantly in favor of intracorporeal anastomosis (OR 0.68, 95% CI, 0.49–0.93). Length of stay was also decreased significantly. Subgroup analysis for papers published after 2012 resulted in an even larger decrease in short-term morbidity and decrease in length of stay (119).

Left colectomy is achieved in one of two ways. The first involves distal transection via an enlarged Pfannenstiel incision with anastomosis achieved under direct visualization using a circular stapler. The alternative involves intracorporeal transection through a right lower quadrant 12 mm trocar with specimen extraction via smaller Pfannenstiel incision and placement of stapling anvil. After reduction of conduit back into the abdomen, the anastomosis is completed under direct laparoscopic visualization.

## HAND-ASSISTED LAPAROSCOPIC SURGERY

Perhaps the most underrated minimally invasive approach to colectomy, HALS consistently provides the benefits of open surgery (tactile feedback, speed of dissection and decreased operative time, and shorter learning curve for most surgeons) with the beneficial outcomes of a laparoscopic approach (reduced pain, reduced hospital length of stay, and lower complication rate). HALS can be beneficial

in morbidly obese patients with voluminous mesenteric fat obscuring visualization, extensive intraabdominal adhesions from prior surgery, or when operative time is at a premium due to patient status. For cases when HALS is expected from the outset, a hand port can be placed in a variety of places depending on the anatomy—midline for a right colectomy and a Pfannenstiel incision for totals, lefts, and ileal pouch surgery.

After insufflation, it is of utmost importance to move all nonpathologic bowel out of the operative field. Take advantage of the hand port and insert lap pads as necessary to facilitate packing the bowel. Be sure to utilize patient bed positioning to assist in bowel positioning, but also for surgeon comfort while performing HALS. Do not hesitate to use both left and right hands during different portions of the operation. Patients can be placed on split-leg tables to facilitate operating from between the legs without fear of nerve injury. The ability to work from all sides during a HALS procedure ensures a technically precise dissection with limited surgeon strain. Finally, once mobilization has been completed, the surgeon should utilize the hand port incision for extraction and anastomotic creation. After appropriate mobilization, each anastomosis can be performed via this incision, so there is little reason to struggle with a laparoscopic anastomosis.

## SINGLE-SITE LAPAROSCOPIC SURGERY

This technique has gained only limited traction in the performance of colorectal surgery with most studies demonstrating parity to traditional multiport laparoscopy (120). Studies indicate the main benefit of SILS as cosmesis from a small incision hidden in the umbilicus. In a meta-analysis of studies using SILS, there was no significant reduction in length of hospital stay with SILS. Most patients selected for colonic SILS had a low BMI, nonbulky tumors, and were operated on by experienced laparoscopic surgeons (121). When utilized, several products are available for the SILS port, which can be used with a 5 mm 30° laparoscope and curved instruments to prevent collision and maximize tension for dissection.

## REFERENCES

1. Scott HJ, Spencer J. *Surg Laparosc Endosc.* 1995; 5(5):382–6.
2. Jacobs M et al. *Surg Laparosc Endosc.* 1991; 1(3):144–50.
3. Moloo H et al. *Can J Surg.* 2009;52(6):455–62.
4. Davis BR et al. *JSLS.* 2014;18(2):211–24.
5. Keller DS et al. *Surg Endosc.* 2017;31:1855–62.
6. Kwon S et al. *J Am Coll Surg.* 2012;214(6):909–18.e1.
7. Simorov A et al. *Ann Surg.* 2012;256(3):462–8.
8. Milsom JW et al. *J Am Coll Surg.* 1998;187(1):46–54; discussion 5.
9. Stage JG et al. *Br J Surg.* 1997;84(3):391–6.
10. Morneau M et al. *Can J Surg.* 2013;56(5):297–310.
11. Oh TK et al. *Surg Endosc.* 2017;7:903–8.

12. Helander EM et al. *J Laparoendosc Adv Surg Tech Part A.* 2017;27(9):903–8.
13. Pecorelli N et al. *Surg Endosc.* 2017;31(1):85–99.
14. Hennessey DB et al. *Int J Colorectal Dis.* 2016;31(2): 267–71.
15. Kiran RP et al. *J Am Coll Surg.* 2010;211(2):232–8.
16. Poon JT et al. *Ann Surg.* 2009;249(1):77–81.
17. Gomila A et al. *Antimicrob Resist Infect Control.* 2017;6:40.
18. Sutton E et al. *J Surg Res.* 2017;207:205–14.
19. Zhang X et al. *Medicine.* 2017;96(33):e7794.
20. Iyer S et al. *J Managed Care Pharmacy.* 2009;15(6): 485–94.
21. Wolthuis AM et al. *Colorectal Dis.* 2016;18(1):01–9.
22. Vather R et al. *Surgery.* 2015;157(4):764–73.
23. Wolthuis AM et al. *Int J Colorectal Dis.* 2017;32(6): 883–90.
24. Sugawara K et al. *J Gastrointest Surg.* 2018;22: 508–15.
25. Alleblas CCJ et al. *Ann Surg.* 2017;266(6):905–20.
26. Dalager T et al. *Surg Endosc.* 2017;31(2):516–26.
27. Luglio G et al. *Ann Med Surg (2012).* 2015;4(2):89–94.
28. Zelhart M, Kaiser AM. *Surg Endosc.* 2018;32(1): 24–38.
29. Lee JK et al. *Ann Surg Innovation and Research.* 2012;6(1):5.
30. Dincler S et al. *Dis Colon Rectum.* 2003;46(10):1371–8; discussion 8-9.
31. Tekkis PP et al. *Ann Surg.* 2005;242(1):83–91.
32. Barrie J et al. *Annals Surg Oncology.* 2014;21(3): 829–40.
33. Shanker BA et al. *JSLS.* 2016;20(3).
34. Malangoni MA et al. *J Surg Education.* 2013;70(6): 783–8.
35. Feigel A, Sylla P. *Clin Colon Rectal Surg.* 2016;29(2): 168–80.
36. He Y et al. *Dis Colon Rectum.* 2017;60(4):433–45.
37. Casillas S et al. *Dis Colon Rectum.* 2004;47(10): 1680–5.
38. Clancy C et al. *Colorectal Dis.* 2015;17(6):482–90.
39. Gouvas N et al. *J Laparoendosc Adv Surg Tech A.* 2018;28:117–26.
40. Etter K et al. *JSLS.* 2017;21(3).
41. Allaix ME et al. *World J Gastroenterol.* 2016;22(37): 8304–13.
42. Martinez J et al. A review. *Int Surg.* 1995;80(4): 315–21.
43. Berends FJ et al. *Lancet.* 1994;344(8914):58.
44. Lacy AM et al. *Surg Endosc.* 1998;12(8):1039–42.
45. Vukasin P et al. *Dis Colon Rectum.* 1996;39(10 Suppl): S20–3.
46. Bouvy ND et al. *Ann Surg.* 1996;224(6):694–700; discussion 1.
47. Watson DI et al. *Arch Surg.* 1997;132(2):166–8; discussion 9.
48. Whelan RL, Lee SW. *J Laparoendosc Adv Surg Tech A.* 1999;9(1):1–16.
49. Franklin ME, Jr. et al. *Dis Colon Rectum.* 1996;39(10 Suppl):S35–46.
50. Lacy AM et al. *Surg Endosc.* 1995;9(10):1101–5.
51. Clinical Outcomes of Surgical Therapy Study Group. *N Engl J Med.* 2004;350(20):2050–9.
52. Guillou PJ et al. *Lancet.* 2005;365(9472):1718–26.
53. Buunen M et al. *Lancet Oncol.* 2009;10(1):44–52.
54. Hazebroek EJ *Surg Endosc.* 2002;16(6):949–53.
55. Nakamura T et al. *Hepato-Gastroenterology.* 2006; 53(69):351–3.
56. Lacy AM et al. *Lancet.* 2002;359(9325):2224–9.
57. Bencini L et al. *World J Gastroenterol.* 2014;20(7): 1777–89.
58. Lujan J et al. *Br J Surg.* 2009;96(9):982–9.
59. Bonjer HJ et al. *N Engl J Med.* 2015;372(14):1324–32.
60. van der Pas MH et al. *Lancet Oncol.* 2013;14(3): 210–8.
61. Fleshman J et al. *JAMA.* 2015;314(13):1346–55.
62. Arezzo A et al. *Surg Endosc.* 2015;29(2):334–48.
63. Chen K et al. *Int J Surg.* 2017;39:1–10.
64. Gu J et al. *Colorectal Dis.* 2013;15(9):1123–9.
65. Bartels SA et al. *Ann Surg.* 2012;256(6):1045–8.
66. Cohan JN et al. *Dis Colon Rectum.* 2016;59(6):520–8.
67. Mao EJ et al. *Aliment Pharmacol Ther.* 2017;45(1): 3–13.
68. Abelson J et al. *J Am Coll Surg.* 2016;223(4):S31–2.
69. Coquet-Reinier B et al. *Surg Endosc.* 2010;24(8): 1866–71.
70. Krane MK et al. *J Am Coll Surg.* 2013;216(5):986–96.
71. Hull TL et al. *Br J Surg.* 2012;99(2):270–5.
72. Beyer-Berjot L et al. *Ann Surg.* 2013;258(2):275–82.
73. Bartels SA et al. *Br J Surg.* 2013;100(6):726–733.
74. Chung TP et al. *Dis Colon Rectum.* 2009;52(1):4–10.
75. Hindryckx P et al. *Nat Rev Gastroenterol Hepatol.* 2016;13(11):654–64.
76. Hata K et al. *Surg Today.* 2015;45(8):933–8.
77. Ahmed Ali U et al. *Cochrane Database Syst Rev.* 2009(1):CD006267.
78. Buskens CJ et al. *Best Pract Res Clin Gastroenterol.* 2014;28(1):19–27.
79. Ross H et al. *Dis Colon Rectum.* 2014;57(1):5–22.
80. Tavernier M et al. *J Visc Surg.* 2013;150(6):389–93.
81. Mino JS et al. *J Gastrointest Surg.* 2015;19(6): 1007–14.
82. Shigeta K et al. *Surg Today.* 2016;46(8):970–8.
83. Aytac E et al. *Surg Endosc.* 2012;26(12):3552–6.
84. Brouquet A et al. *Surg Endosc.* 2010;24(4):879–87.
85. Ren J et al. *J Surg Res.* 2016;200(1):110–6.
86. Neumann PA et al. *Int J Colorectal Dis.* 2013;28(5): 599–610.
87. Maggiori L, Panis Y. *Best Pract Res Clin Gastroenterol.* 2014;28(1):183–94.
88. Collins D, Winter DC. *Best Pract Res Clin Gastroenterol.* 2014;28(1):175–82.
89. Hall JF et al. *Dis Colon Rectum.* 2011;54(3):283–8.
90. Cirocchi R et al. *Colorectal Dis.* 2012;14(6):671–83.
91. Klarenbeek BR et al. *Ann Surg.* 2009;249(1):39–44.

92. Klarenbeek BR et al. *Surg Endosc.* 2011;25(4):1121–6.
93. Klarenbeek BR et al. *Surg Endosc.* 2011;25(3):776–83.
94. Gervaz P et al. *Ann Surg.* 2010;252(1):3–8.
95. Gervaz P et al. *Surg Endosc.* 2011;25(10):3373–8.
96. Angenete E et al. *Ann Surg.* 2016;263(1):117–22.
97. Schultz JK et al. *JAMA.* 2015;314(13):1364–75.
98. Ceresoli M et al. *World J Emerg Surg.* 2016;11(1):42.
99. Turley RS et al. *Dis Colon Rectum.* 2013;56(1):72–82.
100. Daher R et al. *World J Gastrointest Surg.* 2016;8(2): 134–42.
101. Oliveira L et al. *Surg Endosc.* 1997;11(1):19–23.
102. Liu J et al. *Tech Coloproctol.* 2005;9(1):9–14.
103. Miyoshi N et al. *World J Gastrointest Endosc.* 2016; 8(15):541–5.
104. Cadeddu F et al. *Tech Coloproctol.* 2012;16(1):37–53.
105. Tou S et al. *Cochrane Database Syst Rev.* 2015(11): CD001758.
106. Byrne CM et al. *Dis Colon Rectum.* 2008;51(11): 1597–604.
107. van Iersel JJ et al. *World J Gastroenterol.* 2016;22(21): 4977–87.
108. Varma R, Gupta JK. *Surg Endosc.* 2008;22(12): 2686–97.
109. Ahmad G et al. *Cochrane Database Syst Rev.* 2012;2: CD006583.
110. Deffieux X et al. *Eur J Obstet, Gynecol Reprod Biol.* 2011;158(2):159–66.
111. McKernan JB, Champion JK. *Endosc Surg Allied Technol.* 1995;3(1):35–8.
112. Moreaux G et al. *J Minim Invasive Gynecol.* 2009; 16(5):643–5.
113. Chiong E et al. *Urology.* 2010;75(3):574–80.
114. Yamamoto M et al. *JSLS.* 2011;15(1):122–6.
115. Coakley K et al. *American Society of Colon and Rectal Surgeons Annual Scientific Meeting;* June 10–14, 2017; Seattle, WA.
116. Material Safety Data Sheet: FRED Anti-Fog Solution. *North Haven CUSS. Material Safety Data Sheet: FRED Anti-Fog Solution. North Haven,* CT: United States Surgical 2004. [Available from: http://www. autosuture.com/imageServer.aspx?contentID=6591 &contenttype=application/pdf.]
117. Ott DE et al. *JSLS.* 1998;2(4):321–9.
118. Carnuccio P et al. *Tech Coloproctol.* 2014;18(1): 5–12.
119. van Oostendorp S et al. *Surg Endosc.* 2017;31(1): 64–77.
120. Gibor U et al. *J Laparoendosc Adv Surg Tech Part A.* 2018;28(1):65–70.
121. Fung AK, Aly EH. *Br J Surg.* 2012;99(10):1353–64.

# 15

# Medical legal issues

TERRY C. HICKS AND DAVID E. BECK

---

## CHALLENGING CASE

A 60-year-old woman with a strongly positive family history of colorectal cancer undergoes a colonoscopy. She has a 1.5 cm pedunculated polyp snared from the transverse colon. Five days after the procedure, she presents to the emergency room with a lower gastrointestinal (GI) bleed. She is hemodynamically stable, and you admit her for observation. She remains stable and is discharged 2 days later with no further bleeding episodes. The hospital risk manager calls you to discuss this case.

## CASE MANAGEMENT

When you meet with the risk manager, you inform her that you had seen the patient in your office prior to the procedure. During this office visit, you had discussed with the patient her risk factors, indications for the procedure, details of the procedure, and potential risks. This conservation was documented in your office note, and the patient signed a consent for the procedure. The procedure was performed in the usual fashion. Postpolypectomy is a recognized complication of the procedure. You feel that you have a good relationship with the patient, and the records are well documented. Although any untoward outcome could lead to litigation, the risk manager agrees that you have taken the appropriate actions to minimize your risk.

Despite efforts at tort reform in the United States, medical liability remains a serious issue. This chapter briefly reviews important aspects of the U.S. medical liability situation and then addresses some risk-prevention techniques for colorectal surgeons. This includes a general overview of the legal process pertaining to medical malpractice issues and tips to help prevent and defend such cases. It is intended to provide practical information that can be used by medical care providers.

## CURRENT STATUS OF MEDICAL LIABILITY AND INSURANCE

The cost of medical malpractice insurance began to rise in the early 2000s after a period of essentially flat process. Rate increases were precipitated in part by the growing size of claims, particularly in urban areas. Among other factors driving up prices was a reduced supply of available coverage as several major insurers exited the medical malpractice business because of the difficulty of making a profit (1). The number of claims filed has dropped over the last few years, and the cost of claims has moderated. Malpractice payouts in 2016 were over $3.8 billion (2). However, medical malpractice costs have outpaced other tort areas. Regardless of whether a case is won, going to court is expensive.

A study from the *New England Journal of Medicine* (3) found that 7.4% of all physicians could expect a medical malpractice claim to be filed against them in any given year, but only 1.6% of physicians would be subject to a claim that would lead to a payment.

Many states have considered tort reform, but limits on noneconomic damages have been found unconstitutional in some states. States with tort limits have seen reductions in suits filed (1). Despite these efforts, the cost of liability insurance is leading some doctors to retire prematurely, relocate their practices to nonlitigious areas, practice without insurance, or drop risky procedures.

The evidence is clear that there remain serious medical malpractice issues in the United States, and multiple grassroots efforts continue to address this on a local as well as on a national level. The current environment endangers care in rural areas and among low-income, inner-city populations.

Based on comprehensive jury verdict research, there is little doubt that soaring jury verdicts are serious, ongoing problems. At present, half of the jury awards in medical liability cases exceed $1 million, and the average award is $4.7 million (4). The number of mega-awards has skyrocketed, especially in states with no limits on noneconomic damages. For the past several years, juries have awarded lottery-size verdicts of $80 million, $90 million, or even $100 million (5).

Many physicians feel the medical liability crisis is very straightforward. They note that medical liability costs are soaring faster than the rate of overall health-care costs and the rate of inflation, leading directly to increasing insurance premiums for doctors. In short, their position is that the litigation system generates too many lottery-size verdicts and encourages too many meritless cases. As a result, insurance companies are fleeing the market, making it more difficult for doctors to obtain liability coverage at any price. The U.S. Department of Health and Human Services concluded: "The excess of a litigation system raises the cost of health-care for everyone, threatens Americans access to care, and impedes efforts to improve the quality of care" (6).

Other major impacts of the malpractice crisis are the practice of defensive medicine and a negative impact on the young physicians in training. In a patient American Medical Association survey, 48% of the students in their third and fourth years of medical school indicated the liability situation was a factor in their specialty choice.

It is of interest to note that overall, 75% of medical liability claims in 2004 were closed without payment to the plaintiff, and of the 7% of the claims that went to a jury verdict, the defendant won 83% of the time. Unfortunately, physicians that win at trial still have large fees to pay for their defenses. The average cost is $93,559 per case where the defendant prevailed at trial. In all cases where the claim was dropped or dismissed, the cost of the defendants averaged $18,774 (7).

Until medical liability issues are resolved, physicians will be forced to continue to deal with the present medical legal climate, and it is our hope that the following information will provide some guidelines to lower their exposure to medical legal risks by utilizing proactive risk management steps.

In today's litigious society, physicians who practice good medicine, exercise effective communications skills, establish rapport with the patient, and accurately document care have the best chance of averting malpractice claims. Even when physicians do all of these, however, a bad outcome may still result in the patient's filing of a claim for malpractice (8). Research appears to support the position that a patient who perceives the physician as having good interpersonal skills and communication is less likely to sue (9). There are ways to conduct a medical practice that deter patients from making claims and, even after one is made, can enhance the chances of winning the case.

## PHYSICIAN–PATIENT RELATIONSHIP

Medicine has changed dramatically in the last few decades because of extraordinary technologic advances that have resulted in specialization, such as colorectal surgery. This

fragmentation often decreases the opportunity to communicate effectively with patients, who have also become much more demanding consumers, increasingly aware of their "rights" through media and lawyer advertising. Health insurers contribute to the problem, not only by creating incentives that discourage referrals to a specialist but also by placing restrictions on the specialist, once referral is made, that can impede opportunities to establish rapport with the patient. Under such circumstances, it is important to make the most of each opportunity to listen to the patient, remember and use the patient's name, explain procedures in lay terms (avoid medical terminology), and take the time necessary to answer any and all questions. Remember that listening to a patient's questions and complaints will be much less time consuming than defending a malpractice claim.

Still one of the best books for improving communication and relationships is Dale Carnegie's *How to Win Friends and Influence People* (10). For a more practical guide with a medical orientation, one should read *Malpractice Prevention and Liability Control for Hospitals,* by Orlikoff and Vanagunas (11).

The frequency of medical malpractice claims has been on the rise since the early 1970s (12). As long as the contingency fee system exists and there is not a loser pay provision, the rise in suits against physicians will likely continue. Accordingly, it is incumbent on the well-educated and well-trained specialist to be aware of areas of treatment in colorectal disease that present an increased risk of malpractice claims.

## HIGH–RISK AREAS IN COLORECTAL TREATMENT

The following circumstances associated with increased risk for malpractice claims in colorectal disease have been identified (13):

1. Delay in diagnosis of colon and rectal cancer and appendicitis
2. Iatrogenic colon injury (e.g., colon perforation)
3. Iatrogenic medical complications during diagnosis or treatment
4. Sphincter injury with fecal incontinence resulting from anorectal surgery
5. Lack of informed consent

The colorectal physician who is aware of these potential high-risk conditions can use risk-prevention strategies to avoid litigation.

## INFORMED CONSENT

Physicians should be mindful that consent and informed consent are quite different concepts. Consent implies permission. Informed consent is assent given based on information provided or knowledge of the procedure and its inherent risks, benefits, and alternatives.

Courts have long recognized that "Every human being of adult years and sound mind has a right to determine what shall be done with his own body" (14). The law of informed consent may vary to some degree from state to state, but regardless of the law of the state, each patient should be allowed an exchange of information with the physician before a procedure is done. Informed consent is not satisfied by merely having the patient sign a form. It is satisfied when consent was obtained after full disclosure of the risks, benefits, and alternatives of the procedure.

Many states use the "reasonable practitioner standard" to judge whether informed consent was obtained. This standard focuses on what a reasonable physician would disclose. The physician's duty is not to disclose all risks but primarily those that are significant or material. A risk is material depending on its likelihood of occurrence or the degree of harm it presents. The focus is on whether a reasonable person in the patient's position probably would attach significance to the specific risk. This is the "reasonable patient standard" that some state courts apply.

Moreover, to prevail on a claim for lack of informed consent, in most states the patient must still prove causation (i.e., that he or she would not have consented to the procedure if informed of the risk). As a practical matter, it is difficult for a patient to persuade a judge or jury that even though the surgery was needed to relieve pain or disease, he or she would not have consented if told of the risk of, for example, perforation of the colon. This is particularly true when a patient is told of much more severe risks such as death or paraplegia and agrees to the surgery. In that regard, the question to be answered by the judge or jury on an issue of informed consent is whether a reasonable patient in the plaintiff's positions would have consented to the treatment or procedure even if the material information and risks were disclosed.

The following points should always be discussed with the patient:

- The general nature of the proposed treatment or procedure
- The likely prospects for success of the treatment (but no guarantee)
- The risks of failing to undergo the treatment
- The alternative methods of treatment, if any, and their inherent risks

Suffice it to say that good rapport with the patient coupled with accurate and complete charting are the best tools to deter suits based on informed consent and to provide a heavy shield in defending them.

## DOCUMENTATION

The importance of good communication and rapport with patients (i.e., treating patients as you would like to be treated)

cannot be overemphasized in deterring lawsuits; however, complete and accurate documentation of patient care is invaluable to a defense of claims. In addition, good documentation may well nip in the bud a potential claim when the plaintiff's attorney who is considering filing suit reviews the record and care is fully documented. Plaintiff attorneys are more likely to bring suit when the case is poorly documented, because they can more easily argue that what happened in the care of the patient was sinister and improper. Where documentation is clear and accurate, the plaintiff's attorney may be deterred from filing suit, because what happened is easily proved from the record. Thus, judgment becomes the issue when documentation is accurate, and judgment used by physicians in most cases is easier to successfully defend than a vague, evasive, and poorly documented chart.

The following are some time-honored rules for charting that help defend against malpractice claims.

## CHARTING

1. Thorough and accurate charting is your primary shield to liability.
2. If an event in which you are involved gives rise to litigation, chances are your testimony will not be taken for 1 or 2 years after the event. Accordingly, your chart will provide the content and guidelines for your testimony.
3. *Most important*: If it is not charted, it was not done, nor was it observed, administered, or reported. In *Smith v. State through Dept of HHR* (15), the court stated:

   The experts concluded that decedent's condition required continued monitoring and that charting should have been done on a regular basis. The experts also agreed that the lack of documentation indicated that no one was properly observing the decedent, based on the standard maximum *"not charted, not done."*

   The evidence indicates that the decedent was not adequately monitored in this case. The nurses did not specifically recall the patient, and thus the *best evidence of their actions would have been the documentation of the chart* (emphasis added).

4. General guidelines
   a. If you are the treating or primary physician, make a daily entry on the chart.
   b. Chart at the earliest possible time.
   c. If the situation prevents you from charting until later, state why and that the recorded times are best estimates and not fully accurate.
   d. Always record the time (designate a.m. or p.m.) and the date of every entry.
   e. Chart all consultations.
   f. Never black out or white out any entry on a chart. Should you make a mistake in charting, place a single line through the erroneous entry and label the entry "error in charting." However, if a hospital policy exists that governs errors in charting, follow it. An

addendum is acceptable if placed properly in sequence with the date and time it is made. An addendum squeezed between progress notes is inappropriate.

g. Write legibly.
h. Spell correctly.
i. Chart professionally; do not impugn or insult the patient.
j. *Never* alter the medical records.
k. Do not insult, impugn, or criticize colleagues, coworkers, or support staff.
l. *Always* designate the dose, site, route, and time of medication.
m. Sign your entries on the chart.
n. Do not chart an incident report in your notes.
o. Chart objectively, not subjectively; do not use ambiguous terms (examples follow).

| Subjective | Objective |
| --- | --- |
| Patient doing well | Patient denies any complaints. |
| | Awake, alert, and oriented. |
| | Vital signs stable: BP, 100/70: P, 72; R, 18 |
| | Respirations regular and unlabored |
| | Breath sounds clear and equal bilaterally on auscultation. No rales or rhonchi noted |
| Breath sounds within normal limits (WNL) | Pedal pulses noted bilaterally. |
| Circulation check WNL | Nail beds blanch quickly and toes warm to touch |
| | Patient denies any pain or tingling |

p. Document use of all restraints and safeguards, and patient positioning (extremely important in surgery).
q. Document all patient noncompliance.
r. Document all patient education and discharge instructions, and patient responses.
s. Always document patient status on transfer or discharge.
t. Record the patient's name on each page of the medical chart.
u. Use accepted medical abbreviations.
v. Do not chart in advance.
5. Guidelines for charting in the ambulatory setting
a. Always chart the return visit date and that the date was provided to the patient.
b. Always chart all cancelled and missed appointments.
c. Document all telephone conservations and their content.
d. Chart all prescriptions and refills, as well as patient teaching regarding prescriptions.
e. Chart all follow-up and discharge instructions. If possible, have the patient or his or her representative cosign these instructions.

## ELECTRONIC HEALTH RECORD

The federal government has encouraged adoption of electronic health records (EHRs), which have four major functions: documentation of clinical findings, recording of test and imaging results, computerized provider order entry, and clinical decision support. Basic EHRs include access to clinical information, provider notes, and order entry for medications. Comprehensive EHRs include these functionalities as well as more extensive order entry (labs and tests) and clinical decision support. The legal implications of EHRs extend beyond changes in medical liability and include liability related to privacy, disputes over ownership of health data, and heightened vulnerability to Medicare or Medicaid fraud (16). Additional advantages and limitations of the electronic medical record are discussed in depth in Chapter 7. This section highlights aspects related to medical legal liability. Implementation of electronic medical records can be divided into three phases: initial implementation, mature systems in place, and widespread use.

During initial implementation, transition from paper to electronic records may create documentation gaps. Inadequate training on EHR systems may create new error pathways such as incorrect or missing data or gaps in communication. System failure or bugs in the system could adversely affect clinical care. As the system matures in place, e-mail advice multiplies the number of patient interactions and provides the potential to offer advice with inadequate investigation or examination of the patient. Increased documentation creates more discoverable evidence for plaintiffs, including metadata. Copy and pasting of history, physicals, and notes risks missing new information and perpetuates previous mistakes. Failure to respond to patient e-mails in a timely fashion could constitute negligence. Information overload could cause clinicians to miss important information. Departure from clinical decision support guidelines could bolster a plaintiff's case.

Despite these potential limitations, successful implementation of EHR systems may reduce errors in care and adverse events. Better documentation may improve the ability to defend against malpractice when care was appropriate. Compliance with clinical decision support care guidelines provides evidence that the legal standard of care was met, Finally, better messaging may improve patient satisfaction and communication, reduce adverse events, and reduce claims or a propensity to sue.

As EHRs become widespread, better access to clinical information could lead to legal duties to act on information. Widespread use of clinical decision support may solidify standards of care that might otherwise be subject to debate. Rise of health information exchanges may increase a clinician's duty to search for information generated by other providers. Finally, failure to adopt and use electronic technologies may itself constitute a deviation from the standard of care. These potential liabilities are balanced by the situation where adherence to clinical decision support recommendations may protect providers from liability. The rise of health information exchanges may facilitate sharing of information, leading to better care and fewer claims.

In summary, EHRs have the potential to improve care and may increase or decrease medical liability. Clinicians must understand their systems and use them to their full potential.

## ANATOMY OF A MALPRACTICE SUIT

## INITIAL PHASE

Once a patient initiates a claim for medical malpractice, the physician should immediately place a call to the risk manager or the malpractice insurance carrier. An attorney will usually be selected, and the physician should insist that the appointed counsel be experienced and have a well-established reputation in the handling of malpractice cases.

Physicians should work closely with the defense attorney to review and analyze the allegations of the suit, with particular focus on the strengths and weakness of the case. This team effort can often substantially enhance the strength of the defense by educating the attorney on the medical aspects of the case.

## PRETRIAL DISCOVERY

During this stage, each side will discover the facts and opinions in the case. Written questions, or interrogatories, can usually be propounded to obtain written responses. Depositions usually follow the written discovery and are important to the overall outcome of the case. Before testifying by deposition or otherwise, it is advisable that the physician be thoroughly familiar with the facts, including previous and subsequent medical care of the patient and the allegations against the physician. This requires careful review of medical records, other depositions, and all medical data related to the case. A conference should be held with the attorney before the physician's deposition. They physician should allow ample time to confer with the defense attorney before testifying. Remember that the judicial system is adversarial, and the purpose of the deposition is not to convince the plaintiff's attorney to understand the case is frivolous. The physician is there to answer the questions and defend the care administered, not to educate the plaintiff's attorney.

The deposition is simply the physician's testimony, given under oath, before a court reporter, in an informal setting. Attorneys for both defendant and plaintiff are present. Any party to the lawsuit may be present, but often the physician is the only party present. The testimony is taken down in question-and-answer form. Under the laws of discovery, the plaintiff's attorney has the right to ask the defendant physician proper questions. The physician is present simply to discharge a legal obligation to answer proper questions.

The physician's deposition is most important. A good effort is essential for an effective presentation. Close cooperation with the defense attorney in preparation is fundamental. Above all, a physician must be his or her own person.

Thorough preparation will assist physicians in giving a deposition with which they will be perfectly comfortable when they see the printed transcript, that is, one that will be easily defended, should any part of it later be challenged.

The following suggestions for giving testimony in depositions can be helpful to the physician:

1. Tell the truth; you must testify accurately.
2. Do not guess or speculate. If you do not know the answer to a question, say so.
3. If you are not certain of what the attorney is asking, ask that the questions be clarified or repeated. Do not attempt to rephrase the question for the interrogator (e.g., "If you mean such and such").
4. Keep your answers short and concise. Do not volunteer information. Answer only the question posed.
5. Be courteous. Avoid jokes and sarcasm.
6. Think about each question that is posed. Listen to each work. Formulate an answer, and then give the answer. Do not permit yourself to become hurried.
7. Do not argue with opposing counsel. If an argument is necessary, your attorney will do it for you.
8. If you realize that you have given an incorrect answer to a previous question, stop at that moment and say so, and then correct your answer.
9. Be aware of questions that involve distances and time. If you make an estimate, make sure everyone knows it is an estimate.
10. Do not lose your temper, no matter how hard pressed. This may be a deliberate ploy; do not fall for it.
11. Do not anticipate questions. Be sure to let the attorney completely finish the question before you begin to respond.
12. Do not exaggerate or brag.

## DEPOSITION PITFALLS

*Testing your memory of the case.* You have the right to refer to the chart or hospital records whenever you wish. Your memory is usually a composite of events you recall as jogged by your records. Watch for generalities, ploys, and tricky questions by the plaintiff's attorney during the deposition.

*Generalities.* Often the plaintiff's attorney will begin with general questions, such as, "Doctor, how do you treat a patient when you suspect he has X disease?" In all likelihood, the lawsuit to which you are a party involves X disease or involves the plaintiff's attorney trying to make it X disease. You really cannot answer this question, and you should say just that. X disease probably occurs in various forms, and you have been given no particular information—no patient complaints, no patient history, no findings on physical examination, no results of laboratory studies, no clinical impression—all factors you must know to diagnose and treat intelligently. The question is simply too general.

A similar question might be, "Doctor, what are the standards for making a diagnosis of X disease?" Again, you should advise that this question is too broad and defies rational response because no details have been given. You, as a physician, do not immediately diagnose X disease or any other disease. You evaluate all the data in light of your formal training and clinical experience in considering or making a diagnosis. Patient signs and symptoms are innumerable. You must have specifics. For example, in one doubtful clinical presentation, you may have to order a particular set of laboratory studies; in another, the evidence of a certain disease process may be more definitive and clear-cut from the history and clinical examination.

A proper question is, "Doctor, what are the characteristics of X disease?" Particularly if your case involves X disease, you should know its characteristics, but you should also point out that they are general characteristics and most certainly will vary in specific instances.

The point is, you must avoid generalities. You must demand specifics. Try to make the questioner stick to the specific case.

## PLOYS

Question: "Doctor, you have no memory of events independent of your records, do you?"

Ploy: "Doctor, if an event is not noted in your records or in the hospital records, is it fair to say that event did not occur?"

Appropriate response: "That is incorrect. It is impossible for a physician to note everything that occurs. My records are for my own use, to jog my memory. Thus, I note pertinent highlights, which when later reviewed give me the complete picture at the time in question."

Remember that physicians treat patients, not charts. You may properly testify to the following:

1. What you actually recall
2. What you recall with the assistance of your records
3. What is recorded
4. What your routine or standard procedure is, even when such is not recalled and not recorded

*Tricky questions.* Many plaintiff attorneys will use questions cleverly phrased to evoke a response that can later be used against the physician.

*Possibilities.* Questions phrased in terms of possibility invite speculation and are improper. The criterion is reasonable medical probability.

Question: "Doctor, isn't such and such possible?" or "Couldn't such and such have happened?"

Appropriate response: "Most improbable."

*Doing things differently.* Almost all malpractice cases involve the "retro spectroscope" or Monday morning quarterbacking to suggest the physician knew things beforehand that were only learned later or that the physician has 100% control over the healing process.

Question: "Doctor, is there anything you would do differently now if you had Mrs. White's case to treat again?"

Appropriate response: "My recommendations to Mrs. White were based on her complaints, her history, and findings at the time and on my clinical impression at that time. The course I recommended was appropriate on the basis of those factors."

Question: "Doctor, you did not intend for Mrs. White to have this complication, did you?"

Appropriate response: "Of course, no harm to Mrs. White was intended. At the time of my recommendations, there were good prospects for a good result. The procedure (or regimen) does have known complications, and that is why the risks were explained to her beforehand."

Many other factors are involved in preparing for and successfully testifying by deposition or at trial (17). Suffice it to say that effective and sincere testimony is critical to a successful defense in malpractice cases. Ineffective testimony can render a defensible case indefensible. Many tricks and ploys may be used by the plaintiff attorney, and the physician who is prepared with a basic understanding of how to answer such questions can substantially enhance the defense.

## TRIAL

After pretrial discovery, the physician should have a clear understanding of the evidence and witnesses, the experts in particular, to be used against him or her at trial. Working with the defense attorney to rebut this evidence and to assist with selection of expert witnesses to testify for the defense is strongly advised and helps the physician to prepare the defense.

At the trial, the physician is carefully observed at all times by the judge and jury, and the physician's trial testimony, mannerisms, and behavior are critical to a favorable verdict. A well-trained and educated physician who portrays a sincere, conscientious, and caring attitude about the patient's well-being greatly increases the chances of a favorable jury verdict, even where severe complications have occurred and there may be questions of the appropriateness of the course of treatment chosen.

## CONCLUSION

The defense of medical malpractice claims is similar to the defense of criminal cases. The physician stands accused, and his or her reputation is usually an issue of great importance. The emotional costs to the physician are sometimes staggering. The physician should recognize that until additional tort reform is enacted, these cases will likely continue to increase and should be dealt with as a regrettable aspect of the practice (18). Under these circumstances, it is best to accept the reality of the medicolegal arena and use the best means available to aggressively defend and win the malpractice case (19).

## REFERENCES

1. Medical malpractice payout analysis. http://www. diederichhealthcare.com/the-standard/2017-medical-malpractice-payout-analysis/ Accessed October 26, 2017.
2. Medical malpractice update. https://www.iii.org/issue-update/medical-malpractice Accessed October 26, 2017.
3. Jena AB et al. *N Engl J Med*. 2011;365:629–63.
4. Manhattan Institute Malpractice maladies. https://www.manhattan-institute.org/pdf/TLI-IL.pdf. Accessed July 23, 2017.
5. Gay CF, Hicks TC. Medical legal issues. In: Whitlow CB, Beck DE, Margolin DA, Hicks TC, Timmcke AE. (eds) *Improved Outcomes in Colon and Rectal Surgery*. London, UK: Informa Healthcare, 2010:148–53.
6. Addressing the New Health Care Crisis. https://aspe. hhs.gov/basic-report/addressing-new-health-care-crisis-reforming-medical-litigation-system-improve-quality-health-care. Accessed, July 23, 2018.
7. American Medical Association Medical liability reform June 2006. https://www.ama-assn.org/sites/default/files/media-browser/premium/arc/mlr-now. pdf. Accessed July 23, 2018.
8. Entman SS et al. *JAMA* 1994:272:1588–91.
9. Hickson GB et al. *JAMA* 1992:267:1359–63.
10. Carnegie D. *How to Win Friends and Influence People*. New York, NY: Simon and Schuster, 1936.
11. Orlikoff J., Vanagunas A. *Malpractice Prevention and Liability Control for Hospitals*. Chicago, IL: American Hospital Association, 1988.
12. Danzon PM. *Law Contemp Probl* 1986;49:57–84.
13. Kern K. *Dis Colon Rectum* 1993;36:531–9.
14. *Schloendorff v. Society of New York Hospital*, 2112 NY125, 105 NE 92,93;1914.
15. *Smith v. State*, through Dept of HHR, 517 SO2d 1072 App 3d Cir;1987.
16. Mangalmurti SS et al. *NEJM* 2010:363:2060–7.
17. Taraska JM. *The Physician as Witness. In Legal Guide for Physicians*. New York, NY: Matthew Bender, 1994, pp 1–56.
18. Taraska JM. Tort reform. In *Legal Guide for Physicians*. New York, NY: Matthew Bender, 1994, pp 1–64.
19. Gay CE. Medicolegal issues. In: Hicks TC, Beck DE, Opelka FG, Timmcke AE. (eds). *Complications of Colon and Rectal Surgery*. Baltimore, MD: Williams and Wilkins, 1996, 468–77.

# 16

# Miscellaneous conditions

ALEXANDER T. HAWKINS AND M. BENJAMIN HOPKINS

---

**CHALLENGING CASE**

A 28-year-old construction worker is referred to your office for evaluation of a 9-month history of anal itching. He has oscillating constipation and diarrhea. Physical exam reveals excoriations and macerated anoderm. Digital rectal exam is normal. Anoscopy is unremarkable.

---

**CASE MANAGEMENT**

Empiric treatment for pruritus ani was initiated with increased dietary fiber and meticulous anal hygiene with instructions to minimize anal trauma. Punch biopsy is deferred at this time. Differential diagnosis includes anal condyloma, Paget disease, HIV-associated anorectal lesions, and other sexually transmitted disease.

---

## PRURITUS ANI

Pruritus ani is a dermatologic condition with a wide range of etiologies and potential diagnoses. It is characterized by itching or burning at the perianal area. Despite the marked impact on a patient's quality of life, it remains an underdiagnosed condition. Most patients choose to self-medicate and do not seek medical care (1). The incidence of pruritus ani is estimated to range from 1% to 5% in the general population with men more affected than women by 4:1. It is most commonly diagnosed in the fourth through sixth decades of life (2–4). Because pruritus ani often has a multifactorial etiology and high chronicity, most patients report symptoms and self-medication for a number of years. Pruritus ani can be caused by a spectrum of conditions, the most common of which is perianal eczema. Due to the wide range of causes, the disease can be a challenging condition to treat for both the patient and clinician.

## CLINICAL PRESENTATION

Most patients report perianal itching and burning that is exacerbated during hot, humid weather or after exercise. On physical exam, the affected area can vary from mild erythema and excoriations to marked skin thickening, cracking, and lichenification (Figure 16.1). Excessive scratching or vigorous cleansing of the affected area in an attempt to alleviate symptoms can instead exacerbate the condition and lead to a downward spiral of the disease.

## ETIOLOGY AND DIAGNOSIS

Pruritus ani can be classified as either primary (idiopathic, accounting for 50%–90% of cases) or secondary (due to a separate condition) (5). The causes of secondary pruritus ani can be divided into several broad categories: dermatologic, infectious, systemic disease, neoplastic, and anorectal causes (2,4). We first discuss common etiologies of secondary pruritus ani, as these are important to rule out in evaluation.

Many dermatologic conditions may present as pruritus ani. The most common is perianal eczema, but the differential diagnosis is wide and includes psoriasis, seborrheic dermatitis, atopic dermatitis, contact dermatitis, lichen planus, lichen sclerosis, and local malignancies. Proper diagnosis requires a comprehensive history, complete skin examination, and full thickness skin biopsy, preferably containing both normal and abnormal skin. Recent data have called attention to the prevalence of systemic contact dermatitis in patients with pruritus ani, advocating for patch testing (6). In one study of 150 patients with perianal dermatoses and pruritus ani, 40% had a positive reaction, and 20% of tests revealed relevant allergens to be avoided (7). Treatment should be focused on the condition identified.

Infectious causes of pruritus ani are multiple and can be fungal, bacterial, viral, and parasitic in origin. Bacterial agents include ß-hemolytic streptococci, *Staphylococcus aureus*, and *Corynebacterium* (8). Perianal streptococcal dermatitis occurs in adult patients more often than reported. It is mainly caused by group B ß-hemolysing *Streptococcus*.

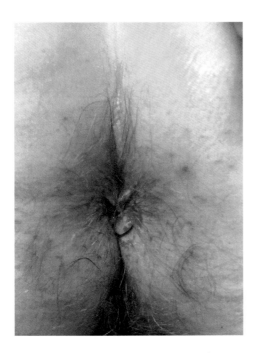

Figure 16.1 **(See color insert.)** Pruitis ani with excoriations.

Its diagnosis is important because it can cause serious systemic infections, especially in the elderly and in newborns. Antibiotics resolve the condition in a high proportion of patients (9). Though thought to be rare, data suggest that fungal infections may be more prevalent in patients than originally suspected (10,11). Fungal infections can account for 10%–43% of infectious causes of pruritus ani (8,10). The most common fungi identified is *Candida albicans* (12). Pinworms are a common cause of nocturnal and postdefecation symptoms, especially in children. HIV and sexually transmitted diseases are reviewed later in this chapter.

Though exact causation remains unknown, a number of systemic conditions are associated with pruritus ani including diabetes mellitus, liver disease, pellagra, renal failure, hyperthyroidism, and vitamin deficiencies (A and D) (2,4,8). Dermatologic neoplasms, including condyloma acuminata, Paget disease, and Bowen disease can present with pruritus ani. Biopsy is essential in securing these diagnoses. Condyloma acuminata and Paget disease are discussed later in this chapter. Bowen disease, also known as intraepithelial squamous cell carcinoma in situ of the anus, is rare but can often present with pruritus ani (13). Given the indolent natural history, treatment has shifted away from aggressive wide local excision to surveillance with targeted biopsies and destruction of discrete tissue (14).

A number of anorectal conditions can lead to pruritus ani, either on their own or via leakage and soiling. Hemorrhoids, skin tags, and chronic anal fissures all have been associated with pruritus ani. Anoscopy is usually sufficient to make the diagnosis, and treatment of the underlying condition often corrects the pruritus (15,16).

When a comprehensive investigation fails to identify associated disease conditions that cause secondary pruritus ani, the diagnosis of primary or idiopathic pruritus ani is

reached. Etiology can range from poor hygiene, to poorly absorbent or ventilated clothing, to excessive or improper cleaning, to dietary intolerances. Fecal soilage is a strong caustic substance leading to skin irritation. Causes of soilage can include incomplete wiping due to skin tags, loose or tenacious stool, and poor anal sensation or sphincter tone. A physiologic basis has been forwarded via the observation that patients with pruritus ani demonstrated a greater rise in rectal pressure associated with decreased anal pressure and longer duration of internal anal sphincter relaxation (17). Tight fitting and nonaerating underwear can exacerbate the problem. Foods such as caffeinated beverages, chocolate, tomatoes, and citrus fruit have been associated with pruritus ani (10,18,19). A dose response is seen in coffee consumption, possibly due to decreased internal sphincter tone similar to that found in relaxation of the lower esophageal sphincter in patients with gastroesophageal reflux disease.

## TREATMENT

Treatment of secondary causes of pruritus ani should focus on resolution of the underlying etiology. For patients with idiopathic pruritus ani, simple reassurance is the best initial treatment. Lifestyle changes should include improved cleanliness, changes in clothing, and diet modification with avoidance of the above-mentioned foods. Patients should cleanse themselves several times a day and avoid alcohol-based products and excessive wiping. Patients should be instructed to dry the areas with a hair dryer when possible. If the patient reports excessive moisture in the perianal region, sprinkling the area with baby powder and placing a dry cotton ball on the anal verge can help alleviate symptoms, as well as provide a reminder not to scratch the area. Hydrocortisone cream can be trialed but only for 2 weeks. Barrier creams, especially the zinc oxide–based types, can be helpful in protecting the skin.

For patients who fail conservative measures after 4–6 weeks, a more detailed examination for a secondary cause should be undertaken. If no secondary cause can be found, more extreme options are available. An intradermal application of 1% methylene blue solution has been associated with a positive effect on idiopathic pruritus ani with mild side effects related to sensory cutaneous innervation in all patients within the first 4 weeks following the procedure but with only a 20% 5-year success rate (20). Another study suggests that tacrolimus 0.1% ointment may be an effective treatment for idiopathic pruritus ani, resulting in a symptom reduction in 68% of the patients after 2 weeks of treatment (21). Long-term data are lacking.

## ANAL CONDYLOMA

Anal condyloma, or anal warts, present as growths in the perianal skin or anal mucosa. Human papillomavirus (HPV) is the causative pathogen in condyloma. The condition affects nearly 20 million sexually active adults with 5.5

million new cases occurring each year worldwide (22). The virus is spread by close contact with an infected individual, and autoinoculation to other body surfaces is possible. HPV-induced genital warts are the most common anorectal infection among homosexual men. In this population, intraanal lesions are especially common as are fistula in ano (23,24). Patients who are HIV positive or otherwise immunosuppressed are (1) more likely to develop anal condyloma, (2) less likely to respond to treatment, and (3) more likely to experience recurrence of anal condyloma. Patients can present with pain, pruritus, discomfort, bleeding, or even partial obstruction, depending on the location and size of the condyloma. Diagnosis is achieved through visual inspection and anoscopy. High-risk HPV types are more likely to progress to invasive squamous cell carcinoma of the anus. Oncogenic HPV infection is often associated with having a high lifetime number of either female sexual partners or male anal-sexual partners (25).

## TREATMENT

Treatment options include excision, destruction, and topical therapy. Excision of the condyloma allows for tissue diagnosis as well as typing of the causative papillomavirus (26). Due to the risk of malignant transformation, histopathological examination is recommended for all patients undergoing treatment. Excision usually is performed in the operating room using monitored anesthesia care, although treatment in an office setting is possible in the case of discrete lesions. Care must be taken to leave the underlying musculature, as well as normal skin and mucosa, intact. Complications of intraanal excision include strictures of the anal canal. Unfortunately, surgical excision has a high recurrence rate ranging from 9% to 46% (27,28).

Destructive techniques used in the treatment of condyloma include electrocautery, cryotherapy, and laser. Fulguration of condyloma using electrocautery is an effective tool in treating condyloma. It can be performed in the ambulatory setting with monitored anesthesia care. Deep burns, which can damage and scar both surrounding skin and the sphincter complex, must be avoided. Curettage of the fulgurated tissue with a sponge or curette is an effective adjunct. Cryotherapy is similar to electrocautery in that the condyloma and underlying tissue are destroyed with liquid nitrogen. Application causes tissue damage by formation of ice crystals, leading to disruption of cell membranes and cell death. Treatment success rates from randomized trials range from 44% to 75% (28). Laser therapy is another destructive technique useful in the elimination of condyloma. Clearance and recurrence rates after $CO_2$ laser treatment vary widely (29). Care must be taken to protect care providers from aerosolized viral particles that can cause respiratory papilloma (30).

There are a number of topical therapies available to treat anal condyloma. These therapies are most effective in patients with a low number of discrete warts. Trichloroacetic acid is a caustic agent used to chemically burn the wart. As such, it should be applied only to the wart itself. Patients need to return to the office every 7–10 days for reapplication. Clearance rates reported in randomized trials range from 56% to 81% (28). Podophyllin is a topical agent that can be applied either in the office or by the patient at home. Again, great care must be taken to apply the agent only to the condyloma. Podophyllin is a destructive agent that leads to necrosis. Pregnancy is an absolute contraindication for the use of topical podophyllin. Treatment success is as high as 50%, but recurrence is almost inevitable, requiring repeat administration. Complications of trichloroacetic acid and podophyllin can include skin necrosis, fistula in ano, and anal stenosis. Imiquimod is a newer agent that not only has destructive properties but also stimulates the innate and cell-mediated immune response to clear HPV-infected cells. A systematic review of randomized trials found imiquimod superior to placebo for achieving complete and partial regression of anogenital warts but did not identify superiority for recurrence rates or new wart development (31). The cream is applied to the wart and left in place for 8 hours before being washed off. A single treatment course involves application three times a week for up to 16 weeks. Imiquimod appears to have decreased incidence of skin necrosis and fistula in ano compared to the other two topical agents. It should be noted that all topical agents have decreased efficacy in treating highly keratinized warts.

Giant condyloma acuminatum (Buschke-Löwenstein tumor) of the anorectal region is a highly aggressive tumor with the propensity for recurrence and malignant transformation but without metastatic potential. A high rate of recurrence is seen in patients with long duration of the disease. Salvage of patients with recurrences can be achieved successfully with radical surgery (32). There are case reports of primary rectal adenocarcinoma presenting as a giant perianal mass mimicking giant condyloma acuminatum, and this diagnosis should be considered when treating (33).

HIV-positive and immunosuppressed patients have a higher risk of developing invasive squamous cell carcinoma of the anus and should be screened yearly to detect precursor lesions. This is commonly performed with anal Pap testing using a liquid medium to capture epithelial cells for analysis (34). Patients with suspicious cytology can be referred for surgical evaluation. High-resolution anoscopy can be used to inspect for areas of high-grade dysplasia. The best management of high-grade anal dysplasia, which is the precursor to invasive squamous cell carcinoma, remains unclear. Patients with high-grade intraanal dysplasia who undergo ablation have recurrence rates in the range of 50%. This number is higher in HIV-positive patients; however, there is a very low risk of progression to anal cancer (35).

There are currently two HPV vaccines (bivalent and quadrivalent) on the market, which offer protection against high-risk oncogenic HPV types. Both are effective at prevention of HPV-associated dysplasia, but treatment of anogenital warts with any HPV vaccine formulation is not recommended. Either vaccine should be given prior to becoming sexually active, and both are approved for both boys and girls aged 9–26 years (36). The quadrivalent vaccine has been shown to be effective at reducing the rates of anal condyloma development and high-grade anal dysplasia, and it also may decrease the risk of anal cancer (37,38). HPV vaccination of MSM is likely to be a cost-effective intervention for the prevention of genital warts and anal cancer (39).

## PERIANAL PAGET DISEASE

Perianal Paget disease (cutaneous adenocarcinoma in situ) was first reported in literature in the late 1800s. Due to its rarity, current recommendations for management are limited. Despite the infrequent occurrence of this disease, Paget disease and other malignancies warrant a strong clinical suspicion when dealing with persistent and unusual perianal lesions. The perineum is the second most common location for extramammary Paget disease. Primary disease is described as the presence of intraepithelial Paget cells without an associated malignancy. Secondary perianal Paget disease has an associated malignancy from either epidermoid extension of an adenocarcinoma of the anus and rectum or a synchronous cancer of the bladder, thyroid, endometrium, and breast (40,41). Associations with melanomas and acute leukemias also are described (40,41).

## CLINICAL PRESENTATION

Patients typically present with nonspecific anorectal problems of pain, pruritus, and perianal bleeding or with a palpable mass. Physical exam findings can range from an erythematous, scaly plaque to a hypopigmented or hyperpigmented lesion. Often, the lesion is associated with perineal fungal infections, psoriasis, and pruritus ani, which can lead to a delay in diagnosis. A report from the Mayo Clinic found a median delay in diagnosis of 2 years from the initial onset of symptoms (42). Patients seen in the colorectal clinic with longstanding complaints and perianal disease should undergo a punch biopsy to rule out the diagnosis of perianal Paget disease.

## ETIOLOGY AND DIAGNOSIS

Apocrine glands, hair follicles, and sebaceous glands of the skin are the sites of origin of extramammary Paget disease (40,41). A punch biopsy in the office can confirm the diagnosis of a suspicious lesion. While perianal Paget disease can have a similar gross appearance to Bowen disease, histologic slides of perianal Paget disease show signet ring cells that demonstrate vacuolated and pale cytoplasm and acid-Schiff positive mucin stain (41).

Preoperative workup for perianal Paget disease should first focus on ruling out potential associated malignancies. There are no guideline recommendations due to the rarity of this disease; however, workup with colonoscopy, esophagogastroduodenoscopy, and computed tomography of the chest/abdomen/pelvis is prudent.

## TREATMENT

Previous management of perianal Paget disease included wide local excision combined with perianal mapping. Mapping involved sequential punch biopsies in a circular pattern from the anus while maintaining location within four quadrants; if a biopsy in the quadrant demonstrated disease, the resection margins were enlarged to accommodate the affected skin. There is debate between wide local excision and perianal mapping with wide local excision. Perez et al. found a high rate of local recurrence despite utilizing punch biopsies in 1 cm intervals beyond the visualized tumor followed by a wide local excision. This led the authors to question the necessity of mapping procedures (41). Isik et al. described local excisions for perianal Paget disease as 0.5–1 cm macroscopic margins; wide local excision was described as a macroscopic margin of more than 1 cm. They found no significant difference in the survival of patients with local excision and wide local excision for primary perianal Paget disease. Additionally, there were comparable survival rates in patients with primary perianal Paget disease despite positive surgical margins (40).

Local excision with sphincter preservation should be the goal with noninvasive disease. Patients with invasive perianal Paget disease extending from an associated cancer proximal to the dentate line should be considered for abdominal perineal resection (APR).

Other modalities used to treat perianal Paget disease include topical imiquimod, photodynamic therapy, radiation, or chemoradiation (40–42). The paucity of Paget disease cases makes the studies of adjuvant therapies difficult, and there is not enough data to support their use.

Follow-up in those with invasive disease should include annual imaging of the chest and abdomen as well as an anorectal and inguinal lymph node exam with proctoscopy/flexible sigmoidoscopy. Those with noninvasive disease should have a visual inspection and endoscopy yearly (41).

## ANORECTAL MELANOMA

## CLINICAL PRESENTATION

Anal melanomas typically present with features similar to benign anorectal disease: bleeding, mass, pruritus, pain, and tenesmus (43,44). Due to the association with other anorectal conditions, diagnosis can often be delayed. The average duration of time from symptoms to diagnosis is 4–6 months, and a benign anorectal condition was initially misdiagnosed in 46 of 79 patients in one case series (43,45). Further confusing the diagnosis is the fact that a large number of reported anal melanomas are amelanotic (43).

## ETIOLOGY AND DIAGNOSIS

Anorectal melanoma comprises only 2% of all melanomas and 4% of all anal cancers (43,44). It is most commonly seen in patients in their seventh decade of life. Patients seen in clinic with prolonged symptoms should have a punch biopsy performed in order to rule out the disease. Hillenbrand et al. found no difference in patient survival of pigmented versus nonpigmented lesions and highlighted the importance of keeping melanoma in the differential when no pigment is present (46).

Unfortunately, a large proportion of patients present with nodal and/or metastatic disease (43,44). Therefore, appropriate staging after diagnosis should include an inguinal node exam, colonoscopy, and computed tomography of the head, chest, abdomen, and pelvis (43).

## TREATMENT

There are limited data to support a consensus statement on the management of nonmetastatic anal melanoma. Initially, anal melanomas were treated with an APR. While an APR does give better local control, there is no clear improvement in patient survival (44,47). Multiple case series comparing APR to wide local excision have shown no difference in survival, which has led to newer recommendations of wide local excision for initial treatment. Disease-free survival has been shown to be largely determined by metastatic spread and not local control; therefore, APR is reserved for large or circumferential tumors with concern for eventual obstruction (43). Inguinal lymph node dissection has been performed with positive disease, but this is a morbid surgery with limited data on patient outcomes. Radiation for anal melanoma has been described with equivocal results to an APR, leaving this as a potential option (48). Treatment with systemic chemotherapy has not been shown to increase survival (43,49). Five-year survival remains low with reports ranging from 6% to 20% (43,44,47,49). A review of the Surveillance, Epidemiology, and End Results (SEER) Program database by Kiran et al. demonstrated that stage of the anal melanoma is the best predictor of prognosis and that patients with local and regional disease had equivalent outcomes despite local excision or APR (49).

As anal melanoma remains a lethal disease regardless of therapy, treatment plans should be individualized with each patient with a clear understanding of patient goals and potential complications.

## HUMAN IMMUNODEFICIENCY VIRUS

Patients infected with HIV may have no outward symptoms save for chronic perianal complaints; therefore, "patients not known to be HIV-positive but who have multiple perianal disorders, should be questioned regarding their risk of HIV infection, because the initial diagnosis of this disease can be made by the colorectal surgeon" (50). HIV screening in high-risk patients is prudent and can make the initial HIV diagnosis in an otherwise asymptomatic patient.

Perianal ulcers have a multifactorial etiology, and treatment involves identification of the causative agent and appropriate medical management. Etiologies of anal ulcer in the HIV patient include herpes virus, syphilis, cytomegalovirus, and *Cryptococcus* (51,52). Surgical management is reserved for chronic, nonhealing ulcers despite medical management of the underlying disease and includes local debridement and unroofing of ulcerative cavities. Complications of surgery include prolonged drainage and poor wound healing. Incontinence and superinfections are risks that need to be discussed preoperatively, but these risks are unlikely.

With the advent of highly active antiretroviral therapy (HAART), patients with well-controlled HIV develop the same anorectal disorders seen in non-HIV-infected patients. Abramowitz et al. screened 473 HIV patients on HAART and found condyloma, hemorrhoids, and anal fissures to be the most common anorectal disorders in the HIV population followed by dermatologic disorders, anorectal infections, and incontinence (53). Their screening included a visual inspection of the perineum, digital rectal exam, and anoscopy, which revealed a 44% prevalence of anal condyloma in the 473 patients screened between 2003 and 2004. Of those infected with HIV, men who had sex with men were found to have the highest incidence of anal condylomas. Interestingly, they found no increased risk of hemorrhoidal disease or anal fissures in patents with HIV disease in relation to sexual practices (53).

Due to a depressed immune system, HIV-positive individuals are at increased risk of wound complications following surgery. Of those affected, more severe HIV disease leads to higher morbidity and mortality from minor surgical procedures including hemorrhoidectomy, lateral internal anal sphincterotomy, and transrectal biopsies as well as major surgical cases. Due to the high complication rates, surgical treatment of benign anorectal diseases should be approached carefully, and previous recommendations called for a CD4 count higher than 200 (54). With improved drug regimens to treat HIV (HAART), Barrett et al. described their experience in operating on the HIV population from 1989 to 1996 and reported on 260 patients receiving treatment for their perianal disease (50). They described anorectal and abdominal surgery in an HIV patient population with a median CD4 count of 175 and with 34% meeting criteria for the Centers for Disease Control and Prevention's definition of acquired immune deficiency syndrome (AIDS). Their study showed minimal complications from major and minor surgery with 2% preoperative complications. The main complication was slow wound healing, and they showed 44% of patients were completely resolved at 13 weeks. Surgical management was not limited in patients with CD4 counts less than 200, despite concerns for poor wound healing, and their patients experienced significant symptom relief. Their conclusion was that aggressive therapy was warranted regardless of the high recurrence of pathology and prolonged wound healing.

Human immunodeficiency disease complicates benign anorectal disease. While complication rates following surgery are low in the HAART era, discussions with patients regarding surgical risks and prolonged wound healing need to be emphasized. There is a high rate of recurrence with anal condyloma in the HIV population, and continued surveillance is recommended after treatment to evaluate both for recurrent disease and for squamous cell carcinoma (50,53).

## COMMON ANORECTAL SEXUALLY TRANSMITTED DISEASES

Anorectal sexually transmitted diseases (STDs) typically present with perianal skin changes, pruritus, pain, and bleeding. However, many also can be asymptomatic. A study of men having sex with men found that 85% of rectal infections were asymptomatic, supporting the need for routine screening (55). Coinfections also can be present at time of STD diagnosis and must be taken into consideration and tested (56). One needs to have a high index of suspicion and ensure testing in concerning patients or in those who are not improving with conservative management.

Herpes simplex virus (HSV) is transmitted via direct skin contact and results in small, painful vesicles about the perianal skin. Lesions typically last for 2 weeks and remain contagious even in the asymptomatic stage. Vesicles can become secondarily infected and are noted to have erythematous edges. Proctitis can occur and is diagnosed with endoscopic evaluation demonstrating an inflamed and friable mucosa. Swabs taken from the ulcerations are sent for viral culture and polymerase chain reaction (PCR). Treatment involves medical management (valacyclovir) and local debridement for superimposed infections. Additional management includes local analgesic creams for symptomatic relief and good hygiene to prevent secondary infections of the affected area. Patients must be counseled that viral shedding and transference can occur at any stage in the disease progression, even when the patient is asymptomatic.

Chlamydia trachomatis infections can lead to proctitis, with symptoms of rectal urgency, bleeding, and pain. If the infection progresses proximally, bloody diarrhea can occur. Endoscopic evaluation demonstrates diffuse inflammation and ulcerations. PCR and cultures reveal the diagnosis. Treatment includes antibiotics such as doxycycline and azithromycin.

Neisseria gonorrhea is a gram-negative diplococcus that infects the mucous membranes via direct contact. This infection can lead to proctitis, urethritis, cervicitis, pharyngitis, and conjunctivitis. In men, transmission occurs via anal receptive intercourse. Women may become infected by similar means or from autoinoculation secondary to a vaginal infection. After an incubation period ranging from 3 days to 2 weeks, proctitis or cryptitis may occur.

Symptoms can include pruritus ani, bloody discharge, and pain. Disseminated gonorrhea occurs if the disease is not treated; pericarditis, meningitis, and arthritis are manifestations of disseminated disease. A thick, purulent discharge can be expressed from the anal crypts and is highly suspicious for gonococcal proctitis. This discharge should be collected on Thayer-Martin plates for identification via culture. Management includes systemic antibiotics with amoxicillin, fluoroquinolones, or ceftriaxone. Current treatment of gonorrhea also includes treatment of a presumed Chlamydia infection with doxycycline and azithromycin.

Another common sexually transmitted disease is syphilis, caused by the spirochete, Treponema pallidum. Anorectal disease presents much like other sites of inoculation: a chancre represents the first stage of the disease. These ulcerative lesions may be associated with pain and inguinal adenopathy. Rectal symptoms may include discharge or bleeding. If untreated, the first stage of syphilis resolves within 2–4 weeks with subsequent progression to secondary syphilis. A macular rash on the torso and extremities denotes secondary syphilis. Condyloma may be present during this time as well as mucosal ulcerations. Without treatment, this condition will spontaneously resolve within a few weeks. Tertiary syphilis with its neurologic and vascular sequelae will eventually develop if left untreated. Serologic testing with Venereal Disease Research Laboratory (VDRL) and rapid plasma reagin (RPR) will provide the diagnosis. The treatment of choice remains penicillin G and doxycycline.

## REFERENCES

1. Nelson RL et al. *Dis Colon Rectum.* 1995;38(4):341–4.
2. Hanno R, Murphy P. *Dermatol Clin.* 1987;5(4):811–6.
3. Mazier WP. *Surg Clin North Am.* 1994;74(6):1277–92.
4. Zuccati G et al. *Dermatol Ther.* 2005;18(4):355–62.
5. Metcalf A. *Postgrad Med.* 1995;98(5):81–4, 87–9, 92–4.
6. Silvestri DL, Barmettler S. *Dermatitis.* 2011;22(1): 50–5.
7. Abu-Asi MJ et al. *Contact Dermatitis.* 2016;74(5): 298–300.
8. Siddiqi S et al. *Ann R Coll Surg Engl.* 2008;90(6): 457–63.
9. Kahlke V et al. *Colorectal Dis.* 2013;15(5):602–7.
10. Kranke B et al. *Wien Klin Wochenschr.* 2006;118(3–4): 90–4.
11. Markell KW, Billingham RP. *Surg Clin North Am.* 2010;90(1):125–35, Table of Contents.
12. Dodi G et al. *Br J Surg.* 1985;72(12):967–9.
13. Marchesa P et al. *Dis Colon Rectum.* 1997;40(11): 1286–93.
14. Halverson AL. *Semin Colon Rectal Surg.* 2003;14(4): 222–5.
15. Bowyer A, McColl I. *Proc R Soc Med.* 1970;63(Suppl): 96–8.
16. Murie JA et al. *Br J Surg.* 1981;68(4):247–9.
17. Farouk R et al. *Br J Surg.* 1994;81(4):603–6.

18. Daniel GL et al. *Dis Colon Rectum.* 1994;37(7):670–4.
19. Friend WG. *Dis Colon Rectum.* 1977;20(1):40–2.
20. Samalavicius NE et al. *Tech Coloproctol.* 2012;16(4): 295–9.
21. Suys E. *J Am Acad Dermatol.* 2012;66(2):327–8.
22. Sauder DN et al. *Sex Transm Dis.* 2003;30(2):124–8.
23. Nadal SR et al. *Int J Colorectal Dis.* 2010;25(5):663–4.
24. Silvera RJ et al. *Dis Colon Rectum.* 2014;57(6):752–61.
25. Giuliano AR et al. *Lancet.* 2011;377(9769):932–40.
26. Wexner SD. *Dis Colon Rectum.* 1990;33(12):1048–62.
27. Gollock JM et al. *Br J Vener Dis.* 1982;58(6):400–1.
28. Lacey CJ et al. *J Eur Acad Dermatol Venereol.* 2013; 27(3):e263–70.
29. Carrozza PM et al. *Dermatology.* 2002;205(3):255–9.
30. Ilmarinen T et al. *Eur Arch Otorhinolaryngol.* 2012; 269(11):2367–71.
31. Grillo-Ardila CF et al. *Cochrane Database Syst Rev.* 2013; Issue 2. Art. No.: CD010389. DOI:10.1002/14651858.CD010389
32. Chu QD et al. *Dis Colon Rectum.* 1994;37(9):950–7.
33. Long CA et al. *Am Surg.* 2013;79(6):2E228–30.
34. Palefsky JM et al. *J Acquir Immune Defic Syndr Hum Retrovirol.* 1998;17(4):320–6.
35. Goldstone SE et al. *Dis Colon Rectum.* 2014;57(3): 316–23.
36. Workowski KA et al. *MMWR Recomm Rep.* 2010; 59(RR-12):1–110.
37. Palefsky JM et al. *N Engl J Med.* 2011;365(17): 1576–85.
38. Swedish KA, Goldstone SE. *PLOS ONE.* 2014;9(4): e93393.
39. Kim JJ. *Lancet Infect Dis.* 2010;10(12):845–52.
40. Isik O et al. *Int J Colorectal Dis.* 2016;31(1):29–34.
41. Perez DR et al. *Dis Colon Rectum.* 2014;57(6): 747–51.
42. Padrnos L et al. *Rare Tumors.* 2016;8(4):6804.
43. Meguerditchian AN et al. *Dis Colon Rectum.* 2011; 54(5):638–44.
44. Homsi J, Garrett C. *Dis Colon Rectum.* 2007;50(7): 1004–10.
45. Zhang S et al. *J Cancer Res Clin Oncol.* 2010;136(9): 1401–5.
46. Hillenbrand A et al. *Colorectal Dis.* 2008;10(6):612–5.
47. Matsuda A et al. *Ann Surg.* 2015;261(4):670–7.
48. Ballo MT et al. *J Clin Oncol.* 2002;20(23):4555–8.
49. Kiran RP et al. *Dis Colon Rectum.* 2010;53(4):402–8.
50. Barrett WL et al. *Dis Colon Rectum.* 1998;41(5):606–11; discussion 611–2.
51. Cohen SM et al. *Int J Colorectal Dis.* 1994;9(4): 169–73.
52. Viamonte M et al. *Dis Colon Rectum.* 1993;36(9): 801–5.
53. Abramowitz L et al. *Dis Colon Rectum.* 2009;52(6): 1130–6.
54. SDW. *Perspect Colon Rectal Surg.* 1989;2:19–54.
55. Kent CK et al. *Clin Infect Dis.* 2005;41(1):67–74.
56. Assi R et al. *World J Gastroenterol.* 2014;20(41): 15262–8.

# 17

# Outcomes and quality

SHAUN R. BROWN AND KURT G. DAVIS

## CHALLENGING CASE

A 56-year-old man living in a rural community presents to his primary care physician for what he believes are symptomatic hemorrhoids. On physical exam he is found to have a low rectal mass. Further workup, to include colonoscopy with biopsies, confirms the diagnosis of rectal cancer. The patient's primary care physician refers the patient to the local oncologist who orders a staging workup. The patient has no evidence of metastatic disease on preoperative computed tomography (CT) imaging, and pelvic magnetic resonance imaging (MRI) demonstrates a T2N1MO lesion, 5 cm from the anal verge. The patient's community has a regional hospital with a three-person general surgery group. After consultation with the local surgeon, the patient is offered an abdominoperineal resection to treat his rectal cancer. The patient is unsure of this recommendation and seeks a second opinion.

## CASE MANAGEMENT

The man is seen by a colorectal surgeon who reviews the patient's workup and presents the patient to a Multidisciplinary Tumor Board. The consensus was for the patient to receive long-course chemoradiotherapy followed by a sphincter saving resection.

## INTRODUCTION

The landmark paper published by the Institute of Medicine in 2000 titled, "To Err Is Human, Building a Safer Health System," shined a spotlight on the epidemic of medical mistakes, bringing quality and safety concerns to the forefront for many American hospitals (1). The report estimated that 44,000–98,000 deaths occur annually in the United States due to medical errors. A second report published in 2001, titled "Crossing the Quality Chasm: A New Health System for the 21st Century," attempted to provide guidance on how to achieve the goals of improving the quality of health care delivered (2). As a consequence of these reports, awareness and attention increased, resulting in an explosion of research aimed at improving quality and outcome measures. In this chapter, we explore the concept of quality, and the various methods of quality improvement with special emphasis on quality improvement related to the specialty of colon and rectal surgery.

## HISTORY OF QUALITY ASSESSMENT AND IMPROVEMENT

*—where all the women are strong, all the men are good-looking, and all the children are above average …*

Garrison Keillor

Like the children in the fictitious hometown of Garrison Keillor, surgeons certainly all consider themselves above average. A certain amount of hubris is required to perform complex operations on patients with multiple, often complex medical comorbidities and with significant consequences for complications that can be labeled as a mistake whether or not an error actually occurred. It is inherent in what we, as surgeons, do daily both in and out of the operating room to have the training, experience, and confidence to perform technically challenging operations and make difficult decisions for our patients. Despite the difficulty in defining, measuring, and codifying medical and surgical quality, surgeons take great pride and are committed to improving the care that is delivered to their patients.

The search for quality has likely always been an aim for physicians. Hippocrates is attributed with saying, "Make a habit of two things: to help; or at least to do no harm (3)." This is nothing else if not a call for physicians to pursue quality. That is what surgeons are attempting to do—to help the patient. Yet all surgeons know that harm does sometimes befall our patients. How do we look at our own results—or those of our colleagues or peers and determine if quality surgery is being practiced?

A surgeon, Ernest Amory Codman was one of the pioneers of medical quality. Although also an innovative technical surgeon whose eponymous exercises and tumor are still in use, he is most widely hailed today as the forefather of outcomes and quality measurement. While it seems self-evident, he was the first physician to look at results from the patient's perspective, using the end result.

Codman used end-result cards to keep track of information on every patient that he operated on and sought to track the long-term outcomes from his surgeries. He sought to determine if the treatment that was administered had been successful, and if it had not, then the reason for the failure was sought. He felt that this should be practiced by all hospitals and surgeons, and he aimed to make this information available to the public, so that it could be used to assist them in their decisions on where to receive medical care. He felt that by tracking outcomes we, as physicians, could learn from our patients and advance the field of medicine. His ideas were not well received in his time, yet he leaves behind a broad legacy (4).

One facet that he left is the practice of regular morbidity and mortality conferences. He sought to determine if there was an unsuccessful outcome, "was it the fault of the surgeon, the disease, or the patient," and could we prevent similar failures in the future (5)? He was indeed prescient in that before the explosion of information and the development of the Internet, he knew that in order for hospitals to implement these tasks, that they would be "difficult, time-consuming, and troublesome, and would lead … to much onerous committee work" by members of the staff (5). Another legacy of Ernest Codman remains within the Joint Commission. He developed and then chaired the Committee on the Standardization of Hospitals that became the Joint Commission on Accreditation of Hospital Organizations, now simply the Joint Commission, which continues to be a continuous aspect of modern medical care.

It is obvious that the ideas of Codman were revolutionary, but it remains to be seen if adopting his ideas, which is certainly done today, has actually led to improved quality or better outcomes. In addition, while Codman focused on outcomes, is outcomes research the only marker of quality, or is it the only marker that should be studied?

## THE DONABEDIAN MODEL OF QUALITY OF CARE

One of the more common models of quality medical care in use today was developed by the physician Avedis Donabedian in 1966 (6). In this model, information regarding quality of medical care can be taken from three separate categories: structure, process, and outcomes. The structure is devoted to the context in which medical care is delivered, the process is the actual medical care that is delivered, and the outcomes are the effects that are actually seen by the patients.

## STRUCTURE

The structure as it relates to the Donabedian model is the setting where the medical care is delivered. This includes the physical building, the equipment, as well as the human resources including the qualifications and the training of these individuals.

The structure is relatively easy to observe and measure. Examples of structure as it relates to colon and rectal surgery could include how many surgeons at an institution have additional training in colon and rectal surgery or have attained certification by the American Board of Colon and Rectal Surgeons (ABCRS). In addition, whether a facility employs a coordinator for the cancer program or a multidisciplinary approach is used for all patients with defecatory disorders, the majority of the early focus on quality in colorectal surgery revolved around structural measures. For colorectal cancer surgery, hospital and surgeon volume are associated with a reduction in operative morbidity and an improvement in 5-year survival (7,8). Additionally, there is a similar relationship between complications and volume in complex inflammatory bowel disease surgery (9).

While the structure is relatively easy to measure, it is more difficult to extrapolate these measurements or attribute any outcome measures based on the structure. Do improved outcomes result from a program coordinator, more training, a multidisciplinary approach, or the presence of a water feature in the lobby of the hospital? These are all elements of the structure of health care, but extrapolating these to quality measurements can be arbitrary.

## PROCESS

The process in the Donabedian model is the combination of all of the actions that comprise the medical care that is delivered to the patient. It is the collection of everything that is done in the administration of health care. This includes any preventative services, diagnostic tests, or treatments that are rendered. Process measures focus on the details of the health care delivered—prophylactic antibiotics, preoperative bowel preparation, and deep vein thrombosis prophylaxis—and are relatively easy to monitor for compliance. Unfortunately, excellent compliance with surgical process measures has largely failed to demonstrate an improvement in outcomes. An example of this is the Surgical Care Improvement Project (SCIP). The SCIP initiative was formalized in 2006 and met with widespread endorsement, and it resulted in mandatory implementation. While there was significant improvement in the surgical care process (compliance with preoperative antibiotics), this failed to translate into an improvement in outcomes (10,11).

Process measures are generally evaluated by examining the medical records or by directly interviewing health professionals or the patients. Some examples of process as it relates to colon and rectal surgery are the percentage of patients who undergo screening colonoscopy, the percentage of colectomies that are performed laparoscopically, or the understanding of postoperative instructions in patients undergoing surgical hemorrhoidectomy. Again, while it is possible to examine numerous aspects of the process of medical care, it remains arbitrary to attribute these to quality.

## OUTCOMES

The outcomes, as in the time of Codman, are the effects of the process of health-care delivery on the patients and patient populations. Encompassed within this are not only direct outcomes, but also patient satisfaction. So outcome measures of colon and rectal surgery will include not only anastomotic leak rate or permanent ostomy rates but also patient quality of life measurements.

Outcome measures garner a significant amount of attention from researchers and hospital administration in regard to quality. The majority of data collected in regard to outcome measures is collected from administrative data and clinical registries (12). Administrative data are collected retrospectively and derived from hospital billing information, whereas clinical registries collect clinical variables with high fidelity utilizing dedicated personnel to extract and audit the data from patient charts. An excellent example of a surgical registry is the American College of Surgeons National Surgical Quality Improvement Program (NSQIP). The ACS NSQIP database includes numerous data points, including demographic information, intraoperative data, and postoperative complications, to name a few. In 2015 alone, the NSQIP Participant Use Data File (PUF) included 885,502 cases from 603 hospitals (13). Colorectal surgery is one of the key areas of focus of the NSQIP database, with a separate targeted database for colorectal surgery. Again in 2015, the targeted colectomy PUF included 31,307 cases, from 239 hospitals (13). This high-volume data collected from a diverse collection of hospitals across the United States provides significant power for research related to outcome measures. One of the pitfalls identified with clinical registries is that physician-surrogates who rely on the medical records typically enter the data. This may limit the quality of the data entered, omitting critical information known only to the surgeon. In an attempt to overcome these shortcomings, the Vermont Colorectal Cancer Project was established. Published in 2002, the purpose of this study was to assess the feasibility of performing a quality study of the surgical management of colorectal cancer in Vermont using a surgeon-initiated, prospective database (14). The motivation for this study was, in the authors' opinion, that the surgeon is in the best position to provide reliable and accurate data regarding tumor characteristics, surgical technique,

and the nature of complications. The results demonstrated that overall compliance was high, and surgeons are willing to report their outcomes, and generally work together on a quality improvement project under peer review protection (14). The New England Colorectal Cancer Quality Project confirmed these findings, on a broader geographical scale, demonstrating a willingness of surgeons to participate and report their data to a multi-institutional quality database (15). The authors concluded that surgeon data entry can supplement the data entered by physician surrogates and can extend the achievements in quality seen in NSQIP (15).

It should be emphasized that the Donabedian method was developed to assess the quality that is in clinical practice, but it suffers from the lack of a definition of quality, and all three of the domains have both advantages and disadvantages that require researchers to draw conclusions regarding causality. Donabedian points out that while at one time, the idea of measuring quality was ridiculed, now perhaps the pendulum has swung too much in the opposite direction. Those who wish to measure medical quality, especially those who are not clinicians, "demand measures that are easy, precise, and complete—as if a sack of potatoes was being weighed" (16). This is clearly not realistic, and it is imperative that surgeons remain at the forefront of how quality is defined and measured.

## QUALITY AND OUTCOME MEASURES SPECIFIC TO COLORECTAL SURGERY

The practice of colorectal surgery, while considered a surgical subspecialty, encompasses a broad range of pathology, from infectious processes to cancer. Several quality improvement measures specific to colorectal surgery have previously been addressed in this chapter. However, two areas of interest in regard to both quality and outcomes that have garnered significant attention are the management of rectal cancer and the performance of colonoscopy.

Rectal cancer surgery is more technically difficult compared to colon cancer surgery, due to the constrained working space of the pelvis and the resulting challenge of achieving adequate resection margins with close proximity to vital structures. In the United States, the majority of rectal cancer surgeries are performed by general surgeons who may or may not have had additional training or possess an interest in colorectal surgery. There is significant room for improvement in the outcomes of rectal cancer surgery, as evident by the variations in quality of resection, such as positive distal or circumferential radial margins, local recurrence, use of neoadjuvant/adjuvant chemoradiotherapy, and permanent stoma creation (7,17,18). The fundamentals of rectal cancer management have evolved over the past 30 years with the introduction of total mesorectal excision (TME), chemoradiotherapy (CRT), and multidisciplinary team (MDT) approach to care (19). Throughout this evolution, five main principles have been identified, and when

Table 17.1 Five principles of rectal cancer management

| Principles of rectal cancer management | |
| --- | --- |
| 1 | Total mesorectal excision and associated surgical principles |
| 2 | Pathologic assessment of surgical quality and accurate staging |
| 3 | Preoperative imaging to identify those patients at risk for local recurrence |
| 4 | Implementation of updated neoadjuvant/ adjuvant chemotherapy and radiotherapy |
| 5 | Multidisciplinary team (MDT) approach to every individual patient |

combined, have led to a significant reduction in the rates of local recurrence, increased disease-free and overall survival, and a reduction in permanent stoma rates (19). These five principles are depicted in Table 17.1.

Implementation of these principles requires a hospital system, with specialized surgeons, pathologists, oncologists, radiation oncologists, radiologists, and associated support staff available to deliver higher-quality care. These five principles related to quality are the basis for the formation of Rectal Cancer Centers of Excellence (ReCCoEs). Several European countries have established ReCCoEs, which has resulted in a significant improvement in short- and long-term outcomes in rectal cancer (20,21).

The Rectal Cancer Coordinating Committee (RCCC) of the American Society of Colorectal Surgery (ASCRS) was established to coalesce knowledge and activity regarding ongoing North American rectal cancer initiatives (22). A primary goal of the RCCC is to develop a surgical skills education module for TME. This committee, along with the OSTRiCH Consortium (Optimizing the Surgical Treatment of Rectal Cancer) and the American College of Surgeons Commission on Cancer, is working to define and establish Centers of Excellence for rectal cancer care.

The OSTRiCH Consortium is a group of health-care institutions that have come together with the ultimate goal of providing access to high-quality rectal cancer care for all Americans (23). The Consortium plans to achieve this goal through the establishment of new Rectal Cancer Centers throughout the United States with a highly trained multidisciplinary team focused on providing care based on the five core principles of evidence-based rectal cancer care.

## COLONOSCOPY

There are approximately 3.3 million screening colonoscopies performed in the United States annually. Optimal effectiveness and quality of colonoscopy depend on several factors, including preprocedure bowel preparation, meticulous inspection and appropriate withdrawal times, adenoma detection rate (ADR), technical expertise to

minimize complications, and finally appropriate postprocedure recommendations (24). The appropriate goal for an individual metric such as withdrawal time remains controversial. While it is easy to measure, the relationship of withdrawal time to other metrics such as ADR or the incidence of interval cancers is problematic. Will the identification of 2–3 mm adenomas in a patient who will undergo regular surveillance lead to improved care or just add cost to the procedure? As in other areas of medicine, improving some of these process measures has yet to translate into improved outcomes.

A quality indicator is often reported as a ratio between the incidence of correct performance and the opportunity for correct performance (25). As previously stated, quality indicators can be divided into three categories: structural measures, process measures, and outcome measures. Specific to colonoscopy, structural measures assess the health-care structure, process measures assess the performance of the procedure (ADR, cecal intubation rate, and withdrawal time), and outcome measures assess the results of care (prevention of cancer through screening and reduction in colonoscopic complications) (26). The American Society of Gastroenterology has defined specific quality indicators and performance targets based on preprocedure, intraprocedure, and postprocedure metrics (Table 17.2) (26). For the first time, in 2015, the ASGE task force recommended three priority indicators that every colonoscopy practice should track. The priority indicators are as follows:

1. Frequency with which adenomas are detected in asymptomatic average-risk individuals
2. Frequency with which colonoscopies follow recommended postpolypectomy and postcancer resection surveillance intervals and 10-year intervals between screening colonoscopies in average-risk patients who have negative examination results and adequate bowel cleansing
3. Frequency with which visualization of the cecum by notation of landmarks and photo documentation of landmarks is documented in every procedure

The advantage of these priority indicators is that they are all actionable metrics that readily measure quality and can be acted upon accordingly (26).

## PUTTING IT TOGETHER

The focus and resources allocated to researching and implementing quality and outcome measures have expanded exponentially since the start of the twenty-first century. The terms "quality," "value," and "outcomes" have become part of the common vernacular permeating throughout our health-care systems, yet they remain poorly defined. This evolution has contributed to the expansion of sophisticated data systems and the creation of task forces dedicated to

Table 17.2 Summary of proposed quality indicators for colonoscopy

| Quality indicator | Grade of recommendation | Measure type | Performance target (%) |
|---|---|---|---|
| **Preprocedure** | | | |
| 1. Frequency with which colonoscopy is performed for an indication that is included in a published standard list of appropriate indications, and the indication is documented | 1C+ | Process | >80 |
| 2. Frequency with which informed consent is obtained, including specific discussions of risks associated with colonoscopy, and fully documented | 1C | Process | >98 |
| 3. Frequency with which colonoscopies follow recommended postpolypectomy and postcancer resection surveillance intervals and 10-year intervals between screening colonoscopies in average-risk patients who have negative examination results and adequate bowel cleansing (priority indicator) | 1A | Process | ≥90 |
| 4. Frequency with which ulcerative colitis and Crohn colitis surveillance is recommended within proper intervals | 2C | Process | ≥90 |
| **Intraprocedure** | | | |
| 5. Frequency with which the procedure note documents the quality of preparation | 3 | Process | >98 |
| 6. Frequency with which bowel preparation is adequate to allow the use of recommended surveillance or screening intervals | 3 | Process | ≥85 of outpatient examinations |
| 7. Frequency with which visualization of the cecum by notation of landmarks and photodocumentation of landmarks is documented in every procedure (priority indicator) | 1C | Process | – |
|     Cecal intubation rate with photography (all examinations) | – | – | ≥90 |
|     Cecal intubation rate with photography (screening) | – | – | ≥95 |
| 8. Frequency with which adenomas are detected in asymptomatic average-risk individuals (screening) (priority indicator) | 1C | Outcome | – |
|     Adenoma detection rate for male/female population | – | – | ≥25 |
|     Adenoma detection rate for male patients | – | – | ≥30 |
|     Adenoma detection rate for female patients | – | – | ≥20 |
| 9a. Frequency with which withdrawal time is measured | 2C | Process | >98 |
| 9b. Average withdrawal time in negative-result screening colonoscopies | 2C | Process | ≥6 minutes |
| 10. Frequency with which biopsy specimens are obtained when colonoscopy is performed for an indication of chronic diarrhea | 2C | Process | >98 |
| 11. Frequency of recommended tissue sampling when colonoscopy is performed for surveillance in ulcerative colitis and Crohn colitis | 1C | Process | >98 |
| 12. Frequency with which endoscopic removal of pedunculated polyps and sessile polyps <2 cm is attempted before surgical referral | 3 | Outcome | >98 |
| **Postprocedure** | | | |
| 13. Incidence of perforation by procedure type (all indications versus colorectal cancer screening/polyp surveillance) and postpolypectomy bleeding | 1C | Outcome | – |

*(Continued)*

Table 17.2 (Continued) Summary of proposed quality indicators for colonoscopy

| Quality indicator | Grade of recommendation | Measure type | Performance target (%) |
|---|---|---|---|
| Incidence of perforation—all examinations | – | – | <1:500 |
| Incidence of perforation—screening | – | – | <1:1,000 |
| Incidence of postpolypectomy bleeding | – | – | <1 |
| 14. Frequency with which postpolypectomy bleeding is managed without surgery | 1C | Outcome | ≥90 |
| 15. Frequency with which appropriate recommendation for timing of repeat colonoscopy is documented and provided to the patient after histologic findings are reviewed | 1A | Process | ≥90 |

improving both quality and outcomes. There is no question that colorectal surgeons are committed to improving the health care delivered to our patients, and that we must maintain a voice in the constant search for quality.

# REFERENCES

1. Medicine IO. *To Err Is Human: Building a Safer Health System.* Washington, DC: National Academy Press, 2000. https://doi.org/10.17226/9728
2. Richardson WC et al. nationalacademies.org, 2001.
3. Grammaticos PC, Diamantis A. *Hell J Nucl Med* 2008; 11:2–4.
4. Brand RA. Biographical sketch: Ernest Amory Codman, MD (1869–1940). *Clin Orthop Relat Res* 2013;471(6):1775–7.
5. Codman EA. Boston, MA: Thomas Todd Co.; 1918.
6. Donabedian A. *The Milbank memorial fund quarterly,* 1966.
7. Gietelink L et al. *Ann Surg* 2016;263:745–50.
8. Liu CJ et al. *Cancer* 2015;121:2782–90.
9. Kennedy ED et al. *Dis Colon Rectum* 2006;49:958–65.
10. Stulberg JJ et al. *JAMA* 2010;303:2479–85.
11. Munday GS et al. *Am J Surg* 2014;l208:835–40.
12. Lawson EH et al. *Ann Surg* 2012;256:973–81.
13. American College of Surgeons National Surgical Quality Improvement Project: ACS NSQIP. (2017). https://www.facs.org/quality-programs/acs-nsqip. Accessed July 23, 2018.
14. Hyman N, Labow SB. *Arch Surg* 2002;137:413–6.
15. Hyman NH et al. *J Am Coll Surg* 2006;202:36–44.
16. Donabedian A. *JAMA* 1988;260:1743–8.
17. Wexner SD, Rotholtz NA. *Dis Colon Rectum* 2000; 43:1606–27.
18. Archampong D et al. *Cochrane Database Syst Rev* 2012;(3):CD005391.
19. Abbas MA et al. *Dis Colon Rectum* 2014.
20. Dahlberg M et al. *Br J Surg* 1999.
21. Khani MH, Smedh K. *Colorectal Dis* 2010;12:874–879.
22. Rectal Cancer Coordinating Committee. May 2017. https://www.fascrs.org/rectal-cancer-coordinating-committee
23. OSTRiCh consortium: Optimizing the Surgical Treatment of Rectal Cancer. May 2017. http://www.ostrichconsortium.org/about.htm#.WvG75dMvwWo
24. Rex D et al. *Am J Gastroenterol* 2015.
25. Harewood GC et al. *Gastrointest Endosc* 2003;58:76–9.
26. Rex D et al. *Am J Gastroenterol* 2015;110:72–90.

# 18

# Hemorrhoidal surgery

JEFFERY MINO AND MASSARAT ZUTSHI

## INTRODUCTION

Hemorrhoids are a normal part of the anal canal and are symptomatic when they protrude into the anal canal causing bleeding with bowel movements or prolapse. Few diseases are more chronicled in human history than symptomatic hemorrhoidal disease (1,2). Citations of hemorrhoidal disease have been noted in historic texts dating back to Babylonian, Egyptian, Greek, and Hebrew cultures (1,2). A multitude of treatment regimens have been offered including anal dilation, various topical liniments, and even the often feared red hot poker (3,4). Although few people have died of hemorrhoidal disease, some patients wish they had, particularly after therapy, and this fact led to the beatification of St. Fiachre, the patron saint of gardeners and hemorrhoidal sufferers (5). This chapter guides the practitioner to a more humane approach to hemorrhoidal disease with an emphasis on short- and long-term outcomes.

## ANATOMY AND PHYSIOLOGY

The understanding of the anatomy of hemorrhoidal disease has not changed substantially since 1975 when Thomson published his master's thesis based on anatomic and radiologic studies and first used the term "vascular cushions" (6). The hemorrhoidal cushions are located in the upper anal canal and exist within the submucosal layer, which clusters into columns in the anal canal rather than forming a continuous circumferential ring. These cushions are a normal component of anorectal anatomy and contribute up to 20%–30% of the resting tone of the anus, as well as allowing the anal canal to dilate during defecation without tearing. They are composed of sinusoidal blood plexuses, smooth muscle from the internal sphincter, and conjoined longitudinal muscle, connective tissue, and elastic tissue (Figure 18.1). Because they lack a defined muscular wall, they are predisposed to bleeding, and may prolapse as the elastic connective tissue holding them in suspension wears down from age and trauma during defecation.

While they have classically been described as forming three pillars in the right anterior, right posterior, and left lateral positions within the anal ring, in truth there are often secondary hemorrhoidal complexes, which can lead to pathologic hemorrhoidal disease at any position. Blood supply is derived from the paired vessels of the superior rectal arteries as branches of the inferior mesenteric artery, the middle rectal arteries as branches of the internal iliac arteries, and the inferior rectal arteries as branches of the internal pudendal arteries (themselves branches of the internal iliac arteries). Venous drainage corresponds to the arterial

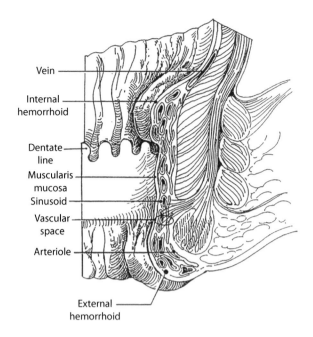

Figure 18.1 Hemorrhoidal anatomy.

supply, with the superior rectal veins draining the region above the dentate line into the portal system, while the inferior veins drain into the systemic system below the dentate line. Consequently, hemorrhoids are divided into two groups, internal and external, separated by their relation to the dentate line. External hemorrhoids are located distally and covered by the anoderm, a modified squamous epithelium. Internal hemorrhoids are located proximally and covered by columnar or transitional epithelium. This distinction has clinical importance, as the relative lack of sensation in the internal hemorrhoids allows for significantly more invasive and thus definitive management options compared to external hemorrhoids.

Internal hemorrhoids are commonly classified into one of four grades based on the level of prolapse. Grade I internal hemorrhoids protrude into the lumen, grade II protrude spontaneously with bowel movements and regress spontaneously once straining ceases, grade III protrude spontaneously with bowel movements and must be manually reduced, and grade IV are permanently prolapsed and irreducible. Mixed hemorrhoids include a component of both internal and external cushions. While the grade of internal hemorrhoids correlates well with appropriate medical and operative management, ultimately the therapeutic decisions should be based on symptoms and overall patient health rather than grade alone. The presence or absence of an external component must be factored in as well (7).

## ETIOLOGY

There are a number of potential clinical causes of symptomatic hemorrhoidal disease. Ultimately, they converge in the physiologic condition of disruption of the connective tissue within these cushions, producing bleeding with or without prolapse of the hemorrhoidal tissue (7). Dietary patterns including a low-fiber diet, behavioral factors including excessive straining or prolonged sitting on a commode, chronic constipation, and sphincter dysfunction can all result in symptomatic hemorrhoids. The prevailing explanation is that during straining, the hemorrhoids become engorged due to Valsalva pressure impairing venous return. Over time, as this process continues, the connective tissue that supports the muscular submucosa weakens, allowing the hemorrhoidal tissue to elongate, ultimately resulting in prolapse. Once the tissue prolapses far enough into or past the internal sphincter, its contracted resting tone further prevents blood return leading to a vicious cycle of further engorgement. The stretch of this tissue also results in thinning of the vascular walls, leading to transudative bleeding and/or rupture of the vessels, resulting in the classic symptoms associated with the disease. Haas et al. noted that the connective tissue can be shown to deteriorate by the third decade of life on microscopic examination (8). Additionally, neovascularization appears to play a role in enlarging hemorrhoids. Several studies have found evidence that terminal branches of the superior hemorrhoidal artery were larger with greater flow in patients with symptomatic hemorrhoids (9,10), greater microvascular density, higher markers of proliferation, and increased angiogenesis-related proteins such as vascular endothelial growth factor (11).

## CLINICAL PRESENTATION

When patients present with any of a varied number of anorectal pathologies, their presenting complaint is often, "I have hemorrhoids." The clinician should be wary of taking this statement at face value. A study by Ganchrow et al. reported on a series of 500 patients with anorectal complaints they associated with hemorrhoids, while only 35% of patients were found to have any hemorrhoidal disease at all (12). The most common complaints include bleeding and protrusion for internal hemorrhoids and pain and itching for external.

Pain is an unusual presentation for internal hemorrhoids due to their relative lack of sensory nerves corresponding to their location above the dentate line. Exceptions to this are thrombosed or strangulated internal hemorrhoids. Barring these, the clinician should thoroughly investigate other causes of the problem. Similarly, hemorrhoidal bleeding is typically fresh and thus bright red in nature. Dark blood or melena should raise suspicion of another etiology. The bleeding from hemorrhoids is most often seen on tissue paper after wiping or streaked in the toilet bowl. Occasionally larger volumes of blood can occur as hemorrhoids enlarge, particularly in advanced stages when a portion of the complex is fixed externally, allowing the blood to drip or spurt into the commode. Frequency will often increase over time as the hemorrhoids enlarge through their stages. Nonetheless, bleeding to a sufficient extent to cause clinical anemia is extremely rare, estimated at 0.5 per 100,000 per year (13). Thus, the index of suspicion should be high for another source of blood loss in patients who present with anemia.

Prolapse of the internal hemorrhoid is also quite common, hence the creation of the grading system. While the vast majority may reduce either spontaneously or with minimal manipulation, grade IV internal hemorrhoids are prolapsed all the time and cannot be manually reduced. These are at high risk of strangulation and definitive management should be offered expeditiously.

External hemorrhoids have a rich vascularization and innervation. Itching due to leakage of minute amounts of rectal content via capillary action and pain likely due to acute and chronic inflammation of the tissues as they chafe against one other during movement are the hallmarks of these entities, and bleeding is common as well from much the same etiology as internal hemorrhoids, thus leading to overlapping symptoms between the two. In addition, because these enlarge in size due to engorgement with blood, it is often difficult to tell on symptoms alone without clinical examination between an external hemorrhoid and a prolapsed internal one. A cause of severe pain is the classic thrombosed external hemorrhoid, which typically leads to a sudden onset, constant and unrelenting pain without palliating factors. If brought to attention before the clot has matured, it may be extracted and the hemorrhoid excised, typically within 72 hours. However, after this it is often better to treat conservatively, and allow the thrombosis to reabsorb over the next several weeks.

## CLINICAL EVALUATION

Prior to inspection of the anus, a focused physical examination should be performed, paying attention to the abdomen, groins, and perineal area (14). Patients should be examined first in the supine position and then either in the left lateral or prone jackknife position. Careful examination of the anus should then commence, with detailed explanation by the clinician for everything that they are doing. Visual inspection should commence with the spreading of the buttocks to evaluate for external hemorrhoids, and other conditions such as skin tags, condylomata, anal and perianal neoplasms, fissures, fistulae, and stigmata of Crohn disease. The patient should be asked to Valsalva, to inspect for engorgement of external hemorrhoids and also prolapse of internal ones. A digital rectal exam should then be performed with focus on any internal masses, tenderness at any specific point along the sphincter, the robustness of sphincter tone, and in a male, the contour and size of the prostate. Anoscopy should follow, paying specific attention to the left lateral, right anterior, and right posterior regions of the anal canal for documentation of size, friability, presence of bleeding or inflammation, ease of prolapse of any hemorrhoidal tissue, and reducibility of the prolapsed tissue. Following

this, a decision must be made regarding further evaluation. This should be done based on the age of the patient, family history, characteristics of bleeding, etc. In general, anyone over 50 years should undergo full colonoscopy even with "classic" findings, while a young patient with no family history likely needs no further testing. In a large series of classic "outlet" bleeding, colonoscopy revealed adenomas in less than 2% and no cancers in patients less than 50 years. When considering all age groups, 6.7% of patients had a significant lesion that would have otherwise been missed (15).

## MEDICAL AND NONSURGICAL MANAGEMENT

Excisional hemorrhoidectomy is becoming less common as we learn more about the disease and better nonoperative options have emerged. Dietary and lifestyle modifications, including increasing dietary fiber, increasing water intake, stool softeners, and limiting straining and the duration of time on the commode are all first-line interventions for symptomatic hemorrhoids. Sclerotherapy, infrared coagulation, and rubber band ligation are the most common nonsurgical modalities utilized for control of grade II hemorrhoids. These procedures are covered in Chapter 19.

## EXCISIONAL HEMORRHOIDECTOMY

Approximately 5%–10% of patients will require surgical management of their hemorrhoids (16). Patients with low-grade hemorrhoids that are nonetheless refractory to nonsurgical therapies, high-grade symptomatic hemorrhoids, and those with complications such as thrombosis or strangulation are candidates for surgical treatment. Excisional hemorrhoidectomy remains the gold standard treatment for grades II–IV or complicated hemorrhoids; however, techniques are continually developing to find an alternative approach with less postoperative pain that nonetheless maintains the low rate of recurrence and complications found with these procedures. Options for surgical resection include the Milligan-Morgan open hemorrhoidectomy, the Ferguson closed hemorrhoidectomy, stapled procedure for prolapsed hemorrhoids (PPH), Doppler-guided hemorrhoidal arterial ligation with or without mucopexy, and historically, the Whitehead hemorrhoidectomy.

## OPEN/MILLIGAN-MORGAN

The Milligan-Morgan open hemorrhoidectomy is popular in Europe and has stood the test of time and rigorous documentation. First described in 1937, it involves resection of the internal and external hemorrhoids and ligation of the arterial blood supply, leaving the excision sites open to granulate in by secondary intention. The procedure begins with digital rectal examination and then insertion of a Hill-Ferguson retractor through the anus. Lidocaine with epinephrine 1:200,000 is injected around the anus and within the hemorrhoids themselves to decrease bleeding during the case. The external and internal hemorrhoidal components are grasped with Allis clamps and retracted caudally. After the patient is adequately sedated, an elliptical or rhomboid incision is created, encompassing both components, beginning with the external, and the dissection is carried out. The mucosa and submucosa are elevated and then lifted off of the internal anal sphincter with either blunt or sharp dissection. The dissection should continue proximally until the feeding artery is reached. At this point, the base of the hemorrhoid should be clamped and the hemorrhoid excised. The vessel is then suture ligated. If multiple hemorrhoids are to be excised, intervening skin bridges must be left in place in order to minimize the risk of an anal stricture. The open wounds typically heal in approximately 4–8 weeks, leading to significant postoperative pain and discomfort. The procedure is summarized in Figure 18.2.

## CLOSED/FERGUSON

Due to the long recovery time of the Milligan-Morgan technique, the closed hemorrhoidectomy has enjoyed widespread adoption since its introduction in the 1950s by Dr. Lynn Ferguson, and it is currently the most common hemorrhoid surgery performed in the United States. Nearly identical to the open technique, the Ferguson procedure differs in that the suture used to ligate the vascular pedicle is then used to close the defect longitudinally in a running fashion (Figure 18.3). This reduces postoperative pain and discomfort as the underlying tissue is no longer exposed to the fecal stream. It is important in this procedure to take care to line up the anal verge precisely during reapproximation in order to avoid formation of an ectropion. Occasionally, it is necessary to undermine flaps of anoderm and perianal skin to allow excision of intermediate hemorrhoidal tissue, while preserving the bridges of anoderm between pedicles. This technical adjustment will avoid postoperative stricture.

## WHITEHEAD

The Whitehead procedure is a technique rarely practiced today due to its potential for significant adverse outcomes. Developed in the 1890s, it begins with a circumferential incision around the sphincter complex. The entirety of the hemorrhoid-bearing mucosa and submucosa is dissected from the internal sphincter and removed as specimen. Hemostasis is achieved with suture ligation or cautery, and the rectal mucosa is then mobilized and anastomosed down to the distal cut edge of the anoderm at the dentate line (Figure 18.4). This results in removal of all hemorrhoidal tissue. Typically, this procedure was performed only in

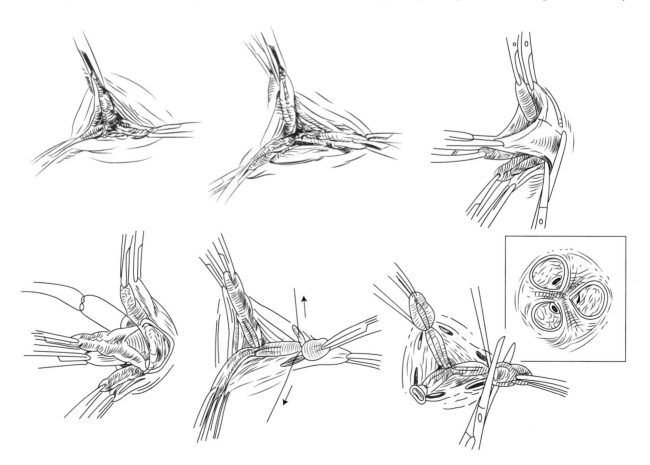

Figure 18.2 Open/Milligan-Morgan procedure.

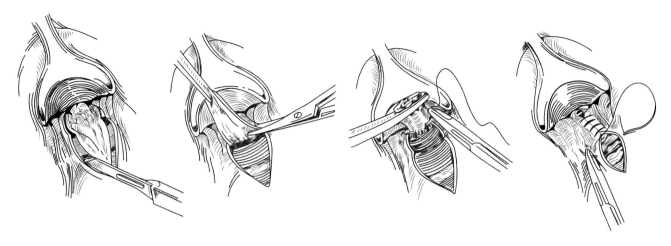

Figure 18.3 Closed/Ferguson.

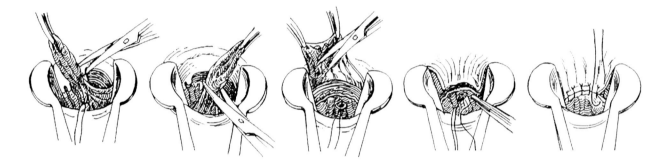

Figure 18.4 Whitehead.

patients with multiple, severe grade IV hemorrhoids, where they cannot be reduced, and it is not possible to distinguish and separate the three piles. If the procedure is performed incorrectly, complications are numerous and affect quality of life significantly. Ectropion can develop if the mucous-producing rectal mucosa is sutured down to the anal verge, rather than the dendate line, resulting in constant drainage, known as the Whitehead deformity. Anal stenosis is another potential complication of the Whitehead radical hemorrhoidectomy, as the rectal mucosa can be difficult to mobilize and is thus sutured with tension, resulting in poor healing, dehiscence, and subsequent stricture formation. Last, when stricture does not occur, incontinence may be significant, as the hemorrhoidal tissues account for as much as 20% of the resting tone of the anus and are especially important in the continence of flatus. As a result of these potential complications, the Whitehead procedure is rarely performed.

## STAPLED HEMORRHOIDECTOMY OR PROCEDURE FOR PROLAPSED HEMORRHOIDS

The stapled hemorrhoidopexy is a procedure first described in 1998 (17) as an alternative to the standard excisional hemorrhoidectomy. While not truly a primarily resectional procedure, it is also referred to as PPH. This technique is utilized for the treatment of grade III and some grade IV hemorrhoids and involves a 33 mm circular stapler with resection of a cuff of tissue above the hemorrhoids resulting in retraction and relocation of the tissue more proximally. The procedure starts with the insertion of an anoscope into the anal canal with reduction of the prolapsing hemorrhoids. Next a circumferential purse-string suture through the submucosa is applied 4 cm proximal to the dentate line above the apices of the hemorrhoids. The circular stapler is then inserted with the nondetachable anvil fully extended, and this is placed above the purse-string. This is then tightened around the shaft of the anvil, which is then retracted into the body of the stapler while holding gentle traction on the purse-string externally. As the stapler is closed, the prolapsing hemorrhoidal tissue is brought within the circle (Figure 18.5). Once tightened, the vagina should be inspected in females to ensure that the vaginal wall has not been caught within the anvil and the stapler. The stapler is then fired, excising a cuff of rectal mucosa and submucosa. This pulls the residual hemorrhoidal tissue up into the rectum while often cutting off the vascular pedicle of the hemorrhoids leading to atrophy of any remaining tissue. The staple line should be inspected for hemostasis as several small sites of bleeding are common. These should be controlled with figure-of-eight absorbable sutures.

Multiple randomized controlled trials have been conducted comparing stapled PPH to traditional excisional

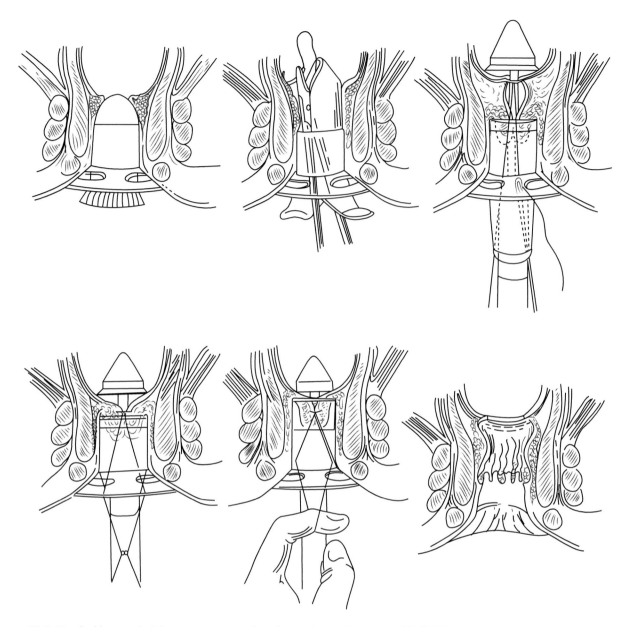

Figure 18.5 Stapled hemorrhoidectomy or procedure for prolapsed hemorrhoids (PPH).

hemorrhoidectomy. Overall findings include decreased operative times, less pain and analgesic use, earlier return to work, and similar symptom control (18–21). However, as more long-term data are accumulated, it appears clear that the stapled hemorrhoidopexy is a less durable procedure with increased recurrence after 1 year. A Cochrane analysis of 25 randomized controlled trials found a recurrence incidence of 5.7% (for PPH) versus 1% (for excisional hemorrhoidectomy) at 1 or more years (21). In addition to this, unique complications are attributable to this procedure, which while rare, can be devastating. These include rectal perforation or leak if the purse-string suture is taken full thickness, pelvic sepsis, incontinence if the purse-string is placed too low resulting in resection of the dentate line and/ or part of the sphincter complex, rectal obstruction, and anovaginal or anoprostatic fistulae if extraneous tissues are

caught within the staple line. Chronic debilitating rectal pain is a particularly difficult to resolve complication that has been reported. Because the recurrence rate is higher than with traditional excisional procedures, and because of the severity of these rare complications, the stapled procedure for prolapse using a hemorrhoidopexy has begun to fall out of favor.

## DOPPLER-GUIDED HEMORRHOIDAL ARTERIAL LIGATION

Transanal hemorrhoidal ligation using Doppler assistance is a relatively new technique first described by Morinaga in 1995 (22). This was further refined by Dal Monte with the inclusion of hemorrhoidopexy. It is an alternative to traditional hemorrhoidectomy in that it involves no excisional

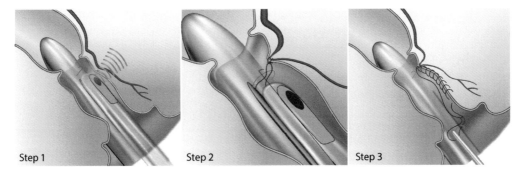

Figure 18.6 Doppler-guided hemorrhoidal arterial ligation.

component. It is based on the premise that the prolapsing tissue is a secondary result of its vascular inflow, and dealing with the latter will result in resolution of the former without need for resection. The preparation for the procedure is the same as for excisional hemorrhoidectomy, namely the use of preoperative enemas to clear the rectal vault. A specially designed anoscope that incorporates a Doppler transducer is inserted into the anus, and the Doppler is used to identify the hemorrhoidal vessels 2–3 cm above the dentate line. Once identified, the vascular pedicles are suture ligated with absorbable sutures leading to cessation of flow into the hemorrhoidal plexuses (Figure 18.6). The anoscope is moved around circumferentially, and all of the vessels leading to prolapsing tissue are similarly identified and ligated. Once done, the redundant, prolapsing hemorrhoids are then relocated proximally and pexied using a 2–0 Vicryl running suture starting in the distal anal canal and ending at least 5 mm above the dentate line (23), thereby repositing the hemorrhoid back into the anal canal. This is an effective procedure for grades II and III hemorrhoids, and while it may be safely used in grade IV, it appears to have a higher rate of recurrence. Postoperative complications and pain appear to be lower, as would be expected with a nonexcisional procedure. Bleeding requiring intervention is approximately 11% (24), and urinary retention, hematoma, and thrombosis have been described in the literature, although with low overall incidences. Prolapse recurrence rates are higher than either excisional hemorrhoidectomy or PPH at 10.3% at 1 year (25).

## USE OF ALTERNATIVE ENERGY SOURCES

Due to the extreme amount of pain classically associated with traditional hemorrhoidectomy procedures, alternative approaches and devices have been investigated, including the Harmonic Scalpel and LigaSure. These devices confine energy to minimal collateral damage and limited tissue charring, as thermal spread is confined within 2 millimeters of surrounding tissue (26). There have been multiple randomized controlled trials published in order to assess the efficacy of these (26–36). Most of these demonstrate a

reduction in postoperative pain and operating time using the LigaSure; however, there are inconsistent results regarding short-term benefits of the Harmonic Scalpel for postoperative pain. A multicenter, prospective, randomized study by Altomare et al. showed significantly less pain 12 hours after defecation, lower analgesic requirements, and faster return to work and normal activity, with no difference in early or late complications. However, this benefit was not significant after 2 weeks (35). Regardless, both energy devices are safe and effective; however, the added cost, conflicting short-term outcomes, and lack of long-term follow-up preclude recommendations for their routine use purely from a cost standpoint. Nonetheless, they may have benefit in reducing short-term pain.

## COMPARISON OF TECHNIQUES AND RESULTS

As one might imagine with the number of different procedures that are practiced for the treatment of symptomatic hemorrhoids, debate remains vigorous as to the best approach. Outcomes including postoperative pain, bleeding, time to complete healing, wound infection, and anal stenosis are the common results for which various procedures have been compared. Perhaps the most well-studied comparison is between the open and closed excisional hemorrhoidectomy techniques. Multiple studies have found that the Ferguson closed technique is superior to the Milligan-Morgan procedure in terms of time to postoperative healing, wound infection, and bleeding. This is intuitive, as healing by secondary intention will always take longer than primary closure, and bleeding is to be expected with passage of stool across an open wound. However, there appears to be no significant reduction in postoperative pain, and operative times are understandably longer (37). Rehman et al. in fact noted an increase in postoperative pain in the closed group compared with an open technique, while Arroyo et al. (2004) noted the opposite, with increased pain in the open hemorrhoidectomy group, but the difference was only significant during bowel movements (38,39). Regardless, nearly all studies agree that long-term results are similar with either procedure, with recurrence rates of approximately 1%.

Overall findings for stapled hemorrhoidopexy include multiple improved outcomes (39–42). Randomized controlled trials on stapled hemorrhoidopexy versus conventional excisional hemorrhoidectomy showed significantly lower operative times, less pain at first defecation, lower mean pain scores, less analgesia consumption, and an earlier return to work (20,40,41).

Complications of stapled hemorrhoidectomy are similar to those of closed hemorrhoidectomy, in addition to rare but potentially catastrophic complications including anastomotic leak with pelvic sepsis, anovaginal fistula, and Fournier gangrene (42,43). While PPH causes less postoperative pain compared with conventional excisional hemorrhoidectomy, some patients will experience chronic pain after the procedure. Unrelenting pain of unknown etiology after stapled hemorrhoidopexy is known as PPH syndrome (44); 15.1% of surgeons surveyed report experience with patients having unrelenting pain lasting for months. This has been postulated to be due to fibrosis around the staples or direct trauma to the pudendal or sacral nerve spindles. Even removal of the staples does not always result in relief. In addition, recurrence rates are higher with stapled hemorrhoidopexy at 5.7% versus 1% for excisional hemorrhoidectomy (21) for grades II and III disease and a surprisingly high rate of recurrence up to 50% for grade IV hemorrhoids (45,46).

Doppler-guided hemorrhoidal artery ligation is effective for grade II hemorrhoids, with a recurrence rate of 5.3%–6.7% at less than 1 year follow-up and a recurrence of 12% at greater than 1 year (47). Complications are few, with improved postoperative pain and return to work, and the procedure may be repeated without difficulty. However, when used for grade III hemorrhoids, recurrence rates are higher, up to 18%–31% (48,49). In a randomized controlled trial comparing ligation versus stapled hemorrhoidopexy, ligation was found to have a shorter operating time, lower mean pain scores, less postoperative discomfort, and less postoperative complications (49). Nonetheless, this improved pain profile appears to come at the cost of increased recurrence. Ultimately, excisional hemorrhoidectomy remains the gold standard in terms of durability of repair.

## POSTOPERATIVE PAIN AND BOWEL MANAGEMENT

Traditionally, hemorrhoid surgery has been very painful, and the postoperative pain was managed with opioids. The pain and the medication used to treat it often resulted in constipation or impaction, which added to patients' morbidity. Modern multimodality pain management has significantly improved the patient's experience (50,51). The editors currently use preoperative IV ibuprofen and acetaminophen and intraoperative liposomal bupivacaine. Additional discussion is provided in Chapters 3, 9, and 10.

To avoid postoperative constipation, patients should be encouraged to consume adequate fiber and enough polyethylene glycol to keep their stool soft. If an impaction occurs, disimpaction may require a general anesthetic.

## SPECIAL SITUATIONS

## THROMBOSED EXTERNAL HEMORRHOIDS

Acute thrombosis of an external hemorrhoid may be an exquisitely painful occurrence. While a precipitating event may be present, often these will occur at random, for no apparent reason that the patient can recall. Known risk factors include recent constipation and traumatic vaginal delivery (52,53). The patient will typically describe the acute onset of constant, sharp pain in the anal region, often accompanied by a tender, palpable nodule in the perianal region. The pain typically will increase over time through days 3–4, after which it will gradually subside as the inflammation decreases. In some situations, the thrombosis will result in pressure necrosis of the overlying skin, resulting in spontaneous evacuation of the clot and immediate improvement of symptoms.

Conservative treatments include stool softeners, increased fiber, increased fluid intake, Sitz baths, and nonsteroidal anti-inflammatory drugs (54–56). Topical calcium channel blockers have shown improvement of pain compared to traditional topical lidocaine (57). Nonetheless, none of these treatments have been shown to shorten the time to symptom resolution or reduce the frequency of recurrence compared to surgical excision. This is a simple bedside procedure within the purview of an office-based or emergency practitioner and offers low recurrence and complication rates with high levels of patient acceptance and satisfaction (58). It can typically be done under local anesthesia. An elliptical incision is made overlying the thrombosis, and the clot is enucleated. (Figure 18.7) Bleeding is usually minimal but can be addressed with pressure, silver nitrate, or suture ligation. The skin may then either be left open to close by secondary intention, or reapproximated with absorbable suture (59). A retrospective study by Greenspon et al. showed that surgical excision resulted in faster symptom resolution (3.9 versus 24 days) and lower recurrence rates (6.3% versus 25.4%) (60).

## STRANGULATED HEMORRHOIDS

Strangulated hemorrhoids are internal hemorrhoids that have become irreducibly incarcerated with compromised blood flow due to the constricting action of the anal sphincter. While internal hemorrhoids are classically nonpainful, strangulated ones will often present with an acute episode of pain. Urinary retention may also be present. Edema is

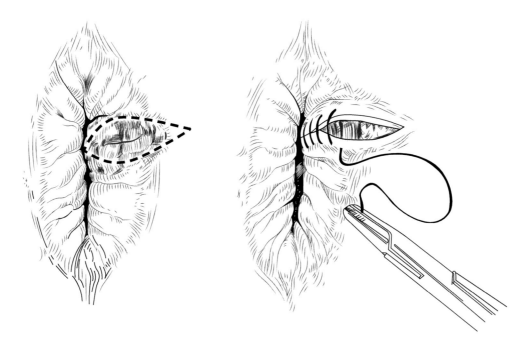

Figure 18.7 Excision of thrombosed external hemorrhoid.

often severe in these situations and is both a result of and contributing factor to further strangulation. This is considered a surgical emergency, as these hemorrhoids may progress to necrosis, gangrene, pelvic sepsis, and ultimately death. As such, a careful examination must be carried out. If the hemorrhoids are incarcerated but show no signs of necrosis, a manual reduction may be attempted (with the aid of an anal block of lidocaine with epinephrine). Often this can be augmented by the application of sugar over the hemorrhoids to draw out the edema or injection with hyaluronidase. Topical nitrates may also be used as an adjunct to relax the sphincter muscle. If successful, the patient may be observed for signs of systemic sepsis. However, if necrosis or other concerning signs of strangulation are present, the patient should be taken expeditiously to the operating room for an excisional hemorrhoidectomy.

## PORTAL HYPERTENSION

Unlike hemorrhoids, varices result from portal venous hypertension. These arise from the anastomoses between the portal and systemic venous circulation via the inferior and middle rectal veins. Differentiation from hemorrhoids is essential because excision of varices may result in venous bleeding that may be difficult or impossible to control. Anorectal varices are extremely common in patients with portal hypertension, found in up to 78% of individuals, although the vast majority are asymptomatic (61). A history of anal bleeding in a cirrhotic patient should arouse suspicion. Varices may be present in the rectum, anal canal, or anal verge (62). Doppler ultrasonography of the anorectum can confirm the diagnosis. Active bleeding from varices will usually require oversewing with a continuous suture

technique. Treatment is almost universally nonsurgical. Banding should be avoided as it may result in profuse bleeding at home after tissue necrosis. Sclerotherapy or photocoagulation are acceptable options for the treatment of bleeding varices, and a transjugular intrahepatic portosystemic shunt (TIPS) procedure, surgical shunt, or liver transplant should be considered to address the underlying etiology.

## PREGNANCY

Postpartum hemorrhoids that are refractory to conservative measures may require surgical management. Hemorrhoidectomy in this setting is safe, has a low prevalence of complications, and in many cases will minimize recovery time. Proper patient positioning (usually left lateral Sims) and good anesthetic techniques are important. As in other urgent hemorrhoidectomies, preservation of as much anoderm as possible is also critical.

## CROHN DISEASE

Unfortunately, patients with Crohn disease are just as if not more susceptible to hemorrhoids as the general population, due to their increased frequency of bowel movements and diarrhea. Patient selection is critical in this group if surgical excision is considered. A history of perianal Crohn disease is a relative contraindication due to the prolonged wound healing and increased risk of wound complications. Surgery should be reserved for patients with no history of perianal disease or in patients who have well-controlled disease off steroids. Resection in patients with active disease may result in proctectomy for surgical complications not manageable with conservative means (63).

## IMMUNOCOMPROMISED STATE

Any invasive intervention should generally be avoided if possible in patients with immunocompromised states. Similar to Crohn patients, sepsis and prolonged wound healing are the major concerns. Thus, conservative management is the mainstay of treatment. Injection sclerotherapy appears to be a safer alternative to band ligation or surgical excision (64,65); however, if a more invasive approach is required, antibiotic prophylaxis should be given due to the increased risk of bacteremia.

## REFERENCES

1. Holley CJ. *South Med J.* 1946;39:536–41.
2. Madoff R. *Presented at the Midwest Society of Colon and Rectal Surgeons' Meeting Brechenridge, CO.* 1991.
3. Dirckx JH. *Am J Dermatopathol.* 1985;7(4):341–6.
4. Maimonides M. *Treatise on Hemorrhoids.* Philadelphia, PA: JB Lippincott. 1969.
5. Rachochot J et al. *Am J Proctol.* 1971;22:175–9.
6. Thomson WH. *Br J Surg.* 1975;62(7):542–52.
7. Morgado PJ et al. *Dis Colon Rectum.* 1988;31(6): 474–80.
8. Haas PA et al. *Dis Colon Rectum.* 1984;27(7):442–50.
9. Aigner F et al. *J Gastrointest Surg.* 2006;10(7):1044–50.
10. Aigner F et al. *Int J Colorectal Dis.* 2009;24(1): 105–13.
11. Han W et al. *Zhonghua Wei Chang Wai Ke Za Zhi.* 2005;8(1):56–9.
12. Ganchrow MI et al. *Dis Colon Rectum.* 1971;14(2): 128–33.
13. Kluiber RM, Wolff BG. *Dis Colon Rectum.* 1994;37(10): 1006–7.
14. Steele SR et al. *The ASCRS Textbook of Colon and Rectal Surgery* 3rd Ed. Springer 2016.
15. Monson JR et al. *Dis Colon Rectum.* 2013;56(5): 535–50.
16. Bleday R et al. *Dis Colon Rectum.* 1992;35(5):477–81.
17. Longo A. *Proceedings of the 6th World Congress of Endoscopic Surgery*, Rome, Italy. 1998:777–84.
18. Shalaby R, Desoky A. *Br J Surg.* 2001;88(8):1049–53.
19. Pavlidis T et al. *Int J Colorectal Dis.* 2002;17(1):50–3.
20. Senagore AJ et al. *Dis Colon Rectum.* 2004;47(11):1824–36.
21. Tjandra JJ, Chan MK. *Dis Colon Rectum.* 2007;50(6): 878–92.
22. Morinaga K et al. *Am J Gastroenterol.* 1995;90(4): 610–3.
23. Infantino A. *Colorectal Dis.* 2010;12(12):1274.
24. Greenberg R et al. *Dis Colon Rectum.* 2006;49(4): 485–9.
25. LaBella GD et al. *Tech Coloproctol.* 2015;19(3):153–7.
26. Kennedy JS et al. *Surg Endosc.* 1998;12(6):876–8.
27. Khan S et al. *Dis Colon Rectum.* 2001;44(6):845–9.
28. Armstrong DN et al. *Dis Colon Rectum.* 2001;44(4): 558–64.
29. Tan JJ, Seow-Choen F. *Dis Colon Rectum.* 2001;44(5): 677–9.
30. Bessa SS. *Dis Colon Rectum.* 2008;51(6):940–4.
31. Wang JY et al. *World J Surg.* 2006;30(3):462–6.
32. Chung YC, Wu HJ. *Dis Colon Rectum.* 2003;46(1): 87–92.
33. Franklin EJ et al. *Dis Colon Rectum.* 2003;46(10): 1380–3.
34. Jayne DG et al. *Br J Sur.* 2002;89(4):428–32.
35. Altomare DF et al. *Dis Colon Rectum.* 2008;51(5): 514–9.
36. Palazzo FF et al. *Br J Sur.* 2002;89(2):154–7.
37. Arbman G et al. *Dis Colon Rectum.* 2000;43(1):31–4.
38. Rahman ASMT RA, Biswas SK. *Faridpur Med Coll J.* 2012;7:37–41.
39. Arroyo A et al. *Int J Colorectal Dis.* 2004;19(4):370–3.
40. Huang WS et al. *Int J Colorectal Dis.* 2007;22(8): 955–61.
41. Ammaturo C et al. *Il Giornale di chirurgia.* 2012;33(10): 346–51.
42. Molloy RG, Kingsmore D. *Lancet.* 2000;355(9206):810.
43. Wong LY et al. *Dis Colon Rectum.* 2003;46(1):116–7.
44. Yeo D, Tan KY. *World J Gastroenterol.* 2014;20(45): 16976–83.
45. Ortiz H et al. *Br J Surg.* 2002;89(11):1376–81.
46. Ortiz H et al. *Dis Colon Rectum.* 2005;48(4):809–15.
47. Avital S et al. *Tech Coloproctol.* 2012;16(4):291–4.
48. Avital S et al. *Tech Coloproctol.* 2012;16(1):61–5.
49. Avital S et al. *Tech Coloproctol.* 2011;15(3):267–71.
50. Haas E et al. *Am Surg.* 2012;78(5):574–81.
51. Beck DE et al. *Ochsner J.* 2015;15(4):408–12.
52. Oh C. *Mount Sinai J Med.* 1989;56(1):30–2.
53. Abramowitz L et al. *Dis Colon Rectum.* 2002;45(5): 650–5.
54. Stites T, Lund DP. *Semin Pediatr Surg.* 2007;16(1): 71–8.
55. Alonso-Coello P et al. *Am J Gastroenterol.* 2006; 101(1):181–8.
56. Mounsey AL, Henry SL. *J Fam Pract.* 2009;58(9):492–3.
57. Perrotti P et al. *Dis Colon Rectum.* 2001;44(3):405–9.
58. Jongen J et al. *Dis Colon Rectum.* 2003;46(9):1226–31.
59. Grosz CR. *Dis Colon Rectum.* 1990;33(3):249–50.
60. Greenspon J et al. *Dis Colon Rectum.* 2004;47(9): 1493–8.
61. Chawla Y, Dilawari JB. *Gut.* 1991;32(3):309–11.
62. Corman M. Complications of hemorrhoidal and fissure surgery. In Ferrari BT, Ray JE, Gathright JB (eds). *Complications of Colon and Rectal Surgery.* Philadelphia, PA: WB Saunders, 1985:91–100.
63. Jeffery PJ et al. *Lancet.* 1977;1(8021):1084–5.
64. Buchmann P, Seefeld U. *Int J Colorectal Dis.* 1989; 4(1):57–8.
65. Scaglia M et al. *Dis Colon Rectum.* 2001;44(3):401–4.

# 19

# Nonoperative therapy for hemorrhoidal disease

JOSEPH C. ADONGAY AND SCOTT A. BRILL

## CHALLENGING CASE

A 72-year-old woman taking Coumadin for atrial fibrillation is referred for treatment of bleeding hemorrhoids and resulting anemia with a hemoglobin of 9.2 g/dL. She reports daily painless bright red bleeding and prolapse usually requiring manual reduction with bowel movements. Recent colonoscopy reports nonbleeding diverticulosis of the sigmoid colon. Anoscopy reveals enlarged, friable, and prolapsing internal hemorrhoid in each of the three major positions. The patient reports soft, formed stools daily, and has been on a high-fiber diet for years as recommended for her diverticular disease.

## CASE MANAGEMENT

Given that this patient has already achieved optimal stool consistency, efforts to increase fiber consumption are unlikely to improve her symptoms. While management of anticoagulation complicates rubber band ligation (RBL), treatment with sclerotherapy or infrared coagulation (despite their safer bleeding profiles) is unlikely to succeed at treating prolapsing grade III hemorrhoids. Options for managing anticoagulation for RBL include (1) performing the procedure fully anticoagulated, (2) discontinuing Coumadin for 1 week prior with continued suspension for up to 2 weeks postprocedure, or (3) using regimens designed to minimize the period of thromboembolic risk while off therapy by beginning Coumadin suspension on the day of RBL and resuming regular dosing on post-RBL day 7. This schedule exploits the drug's therapeutic nadir to coincide with the period of greatest risk of hemorrhage (days 5–10), and in one published retrospective study achieved a bleeding risk comparable to that of nonanticoagulated patients. An option used by the editors is to do RBL with the patient anticoagulated, with the understanding that the risks of bleeding are less than the risks associated with stopping the anticoagulation. Finally, some would argue that the safest approach in such a patient is operative hemorrhoidectomy, as it can be performed with the shortest suspension of anticoagulation.

## INTRODUCTION

It is customary to begin discussions of hemorrhoid management by providing compelling data regarding the number of Americans who suffer from this entity or the money spent annually on over-the-counter and prescription remedies of questionable efficacy. Perhaps a more meaningful contemporary figure is that the term "hemorrhoids" was Google searched up to 120,000 times per week in 2013, and was the top trending U.S. health-care issue in the Google Zeitgeist 2012 data review. Hemorrhoidal disease remains as troublesome in our digital age as when Hippocrates wrote of it in his Treatises of 460 BC (1), and patients will go to great lengths to self-diagnose and treat rather than seek help from a knowledgeable physician for their embarrassing symptoms. Although surgical intervention is for some the most successful and durable intervention, excellent symptom control can be achieved for most with nonoperative management.

## ANATOMY AND PATHOPHYSIOLOGY

The understanding of hemorrhoids has not changed significantly since Thomson published his seminal paper in 1975. He described hemorrhoids as specialized arteriovenous sinusoids between the terminal branches of the hemorrhoidal arteries and veins forming cushions of connective tissue in the subepithelial space of the anal canal. Age and trauma may compromise the connective tissue matrix that supports these cushions leading to their prolapse. As the sinusoids lack a defined muscular wall, prolapse and trauma predispose to characteristic hemorrhoidal bleeding (2).

## CLINICAL EVALUATION

As patients and their referring providers will attribute anorectal symptoms of all sorts to "hemorrhoids," a careful history and physical examination must be obtained to distinguish hemorrhoid disease from other anorectal pathology.

The most frequent patient complaint is painless bright red bleeding that may be noted in scant amounts on the toilet tissue, dripping into the commode, or more significantly as pulsatile bleeding from the anus. Anemia attributable solely to hemorrhoidal bleeding is reportedly rare (0.5 patients/100,000 population) (3–5) but has been encountered not infrequently in the authors' practices.

Prolapsing hemorrhoids may cause irritation often described by patients as "burning," as well as pruritus, the sensation of incomplete fecal evacuation, and minor mucus seepage resulting in hygiene-related concerns. Patients can reliably describe the occurrence of prolapse, and if this reduces spontaneously (grade II), or requires manual reduction (grade III) (Table 19.1). Complaints of more intense pain should guide the clinician toward other likely diagnoses such as thrombosis, anal fissure, or abscess. In order to avoid unnecessary surgical treatment of hemorrhoids, it is important to correctly diagnose burning and itching secondary to prolapse as opposed to those symptoms being caused by perianal skin irritation from contact irritants and/or excoriation from overzealous hygiene practices.

Physical examination should include visual inspection of the anus, digital rectal examination, and anoscopy. Concomitant or alternative diagnoses such as fissure, fistula, abscess, or evidence of Crohn disease will frequently be discovered (6,7). For patients who present with hematochezia, there should exist a low threshold for evaluation with colonoscopy (8).

Table 19.1 Grading of symptomatic internal hemorrhoids

| Grade | Physical characteristics |
| --- | --- |
| I | Prominent vasculature; bleeding without prolapse |
| II | Prolapse with Valsalva; reduces spontaneously |
| III | Prolapse with Valsalva; requires manual reduction |
| IV | Prolapsed hemorrhoid that does not reduce |

## TREATMENT

## CONSERVATIVE MANAGEMENT

Constipation and straining may result in congestion, prolapse, and trauma to the hemorrhoids. Optimization of stool consistency should therefore be an early goal of conservative management. The average American consumes only 10–15 g of the 20–30 g that are recommended daily (9). Dietary consumption can be improved with patient education materials outlining fiber content of common fiber-rich foods. Efficacy of fiber consumption results from bulking and softening the stool by the passive absorption of water. Psyllium is a water-soluble natural source of pure fiber from the husks of psyllium plant seeds that is sold in powder form.

Patients who are unable to tolerate psyllium because of increased flatulence or bloating from its fermentation may prefer insoluble fibers such as FiberCon (polycarbophil) or Benefiber (wheat dextrin—United States, inulin—Canada) that pass through the gastrointestinal tract largely unfermented. Gradual increases in fiber consumption should be prescribed with adequate fluid (six to eight glasses of a noncaffeinated beverage daily) to avoid constipation (9). Behavioral modification should minimize stooling times to 3–5 minutes with minimal straining. A Cochrane review of seven investigations including 378 patients randomized to treatment with fiber supplement versus controls demonstrated a statistically significant benefit in the reduction of symptomatic prolapse (relative risk [RR] = 0.53) and bleeding (RR = 0.50) (10,11).

Little evidence exists supporting the use of stool softeners and laxatives in the treatment of symptomatic hemorrhoids, but such adjuncts may be useful to patients who are chronically constipated and for whom bulking agents and increased fluid alone are insufficient.

Warm sitz baths have been theorized to be beneficial in the treatment of symptomatic hemorrhoids due to an observed decrease in anal canal pressure. Their use, however, has not been subjected to a randomized trial (12,13). Their use is typically most beneficial in the acute setting.

Numerous topical agents are available for the treatment of hemorrhoids that combine varying concentrations of local anesthetics (pramoxine, lidocaine, and dibucaine), anti-inflammatories (hydrocortisone and 5-ASA), local vasoconstrictors (phenylephrine), and astringents (witch hazel). As some prescription preparations can be quite costly for patients, thoughtfulness on the prescriber's part is required given the limited proven efficacy of these compounds. Only 5-ASA has been subjected to a randomized clinical trial, which did show a decrease in hemorrhoid-associated pain and bleeding (14). The others do seem to offer relief from acute symptoms and have favorable safety profiles with local allergic reaction being the most common adverse effect. Topical steroids should not be advocated for long-term use due to a potential to cause chronic perianal dermatitis (15).

Flavonoids are a group of plant metabolites found in a variety of fruits and vegetables. They are thought to provide numerous health benefits through their antioxidant effects. Their proposed utility in hemorrhoid treatment includes modulation of venous tone and capillary resistance with resulting improvement of lymphatic drainage, venous acidosis, and inflammation of the microcirculation (16,17). Several studies have assessed oral micronized purified flavonoid fraction (MPFF) in treating hemorrhoid symptoms. Two placebo-controlled trials showed symptomatic improvement with flavonoid dosing, but results were inconsistent when combined with fiber. Ho and colleagues reported that MPFF with fiber led to faster relief of bleeding than either fiber and RBL or fiber alone (18). In contrast, Thanapongsathorn compared fiber with and without MPFF in a double-blind trial and found similar improvement in both groups at 14 days (19). Diosmiplex consists of diosmin, synthetically produced from the citrus flavonoid hesperidin, coupled with an alka4 complex. It has been commercially available as Vasculera in the Analpram Advanced kit (Ferndale Laboratories, Inc., Ferndale, Michigan) as 630 mg tablets with a recommended dose of one tablet three times daily for 4 days, followed by one twice daily for 9 days. It has a U.S. Food and Drug Administration GRAS (generally recognized as safe) designation for medical foods.

## SCLEROTHERAPY

Injection sclerotherapy, first described by John Morgan of Dublin in 1869 using iron persulfate, can be effective in the treatment of symptomatic grade I and II internal hemorrhoids (20). Currently used sclerosants include 5% phenol in oil, 5% quinine and urea, and 1%–3% sodium tetradecyl sulfate. Volumes of 1–3 mL of agent are injected using a 25-gauge spinal needle into the submucosa at the apex of each hemorrhoid. Treatment aims to obliterate the vascular component of the hemorrhoid leading to fibrosis and fixation with prevention of further prolapse. Repetitive sclerotherapy may lead to scarring and stricture and is therefore not recommended (21).

Complications stem from injection into unintended spaces. Bleeding can be exacerbated by superficial injection causing mucosal slough. Significant pain, infection, and abscess can occur with injection too deeply into or through the underlying muscle (22). Impotence, prostatic abscess, and urinary retention may result from deep anterior injection in the male patient (23,24). There have been numerous case reports of life-threatening retroperitoneal sepsis and necrotizing fasciitis after injection sclerotherapy (25–27).

Mann and colleagues in 1988 surveyed 100 patients after sclerotherapy for first-degree hemorrhoids and found 62% of patients had no bleeding at 24 hours, but only 41% remained symptom free after 28 days. Nonetheless, 88% felt their symptoms had improved with treatment (28). The same year, Senapati and Nicholls found no significant difference in bleeding in a randomized controlled trial comparing sclerotherapy to bulk laxatives (29).

Takano and colleagues published a review of sclerotherapy using aluminum potassium sulfate and tannic acid (ALTA), a recently developed agent in Japan. Treating internal hemorrhoids grades II through IV, they reported similar relief of symptoms compared to those treated with hemorrhoidectomy at 28 days postintervention. Recurrence rate after 1 year was 16% versus 2% in the excisional hemorrhoidectomy group (30,31). At present, this formulation is not approved for use in the United States.

## RUBBER BAND LIGATION

Ligation of the hemorrhoid mass has been the basis of hemorrhoidal treatments for centuries (1). The modern application of this principle utilizes a small rubber band to obliterate the hemorrhoid's feeding vessels leading to ulceration, sloughing, and fixation of the ulcer base to the underlying sphincter muscle. This was described by Blaisdell in 1958 and popularized by Barron in 1963, who initially used bands cut from pieces of a urinary catheter fired from a modified umbilical ligator (32,33). The technique's simplicity, effectiveness, and overall safety have made it the most widely used technique in the United States for treating first-, second-, and third-degree hemorrhoids (21).

After obtaining informed consent, the patient is positioned either on a proctoscopy table or in the left lateral Sims' position. Anoscopy allows for the hemorrhoid to be identified. Two types of ligators can be used: the McGown ligator draws the hemorrhoid bundle into its barrel using gentle pneumatic suction, whereas the Barron or McGivney ligator requires an atraumatic grasper for this (Figures 19.1 and 19.2). Both devices use a trigger release to deploy a small rubber band at the base of the hemorrhoid. Typically, two bands are preloaded onto the apparatus to prevent slippage or premature band rupture. As the McGown suction ligator can be used without an assistant, it has become the authors' and editors' preference. With increasing prevalence of

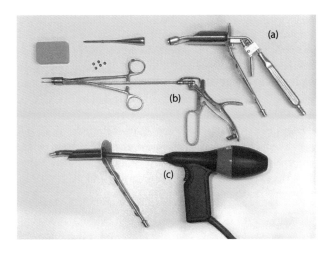

Figure 19.1 (a) McGown suction rubber band ligator; (b) Barron-McGivney rubber band ligator; (c) Infrared coagulator.

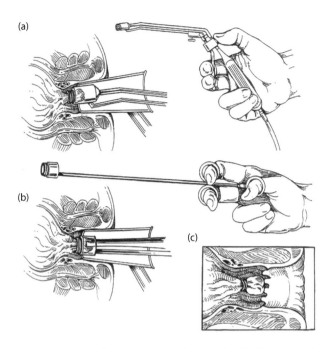

Figure 19.2 Banding an internal hemorrhoid. The internal hemorrhoid is teased into the barrel of the ligating gun with **(a)** a suction (McGown) ligator or **(b)** a McGivney ligator. **(c)** The apex of the banded hemorrhoid is well above the dentate line to minimize pain.

patient latex allergy, the authors and editors have switched to commercially available latex-free bands (George Percy McGown, Brooklyn, New York) without any noticeable increase in premature rupture or band slippage.

Proper placement of the bands is crucial to the procedure's success, and for this reason the authors have not endorsed the blind deployment of bands using disposable banding systems marketed for this sort of use. Inclusion of somatically innervated anoderm will result in excruciating pain. To prevent this, the bands should be applied at the apex of the hemorrhoid bundle, well proximal to the visualized dentate line. We favor the use of a lighted beveled anoscope to optimize visualization. If the patient expresses discomfort when either the grasper or suction is applied, the application should be aborted and a more proximal site selected. Some have suggested injection of local anesthetic either into the banded pedicle itself or the upper anal canal (5 mm above dentate line, 1.5 mL in four quadrants) (34,35). The authors have found that this is seldom necessary.

Disagreement exists as to how many hemorrhoids should be banded per session. Barron advocated ligation of one hemorrhoid at a time, with future sessions at 3-week intervals so as to minimize patient discomfort and to allow reassessment as to the need for additional bandings (33). Others have described no significant increase in patient discomfort with multiple bandings in a single session (36,37). Davis and colleagues reported their experience with combined colonoscopy under moderate sedation followed by immediate three-quadrant hemorrhoid ligation using a TriView (tri-slotted) anoscope and a Short-Shot multifire banding

apparatus. Although they comment on their need to excise thrombosed external hemorrhoids in 2.8% of patients treated thusly, they conclude that this approach is a safe, cost-effective, and well-tolerated method of treating hemorrhoids and excluding more serious colonic pathology at one setting (38). The editors' practice is to band the two largest bundles at the first treatment.

Complications are infrequent following RBL (<2%) and include vasovagal symptoms, pain, bleeding, external hemorrhoidal thrombosis, and rare cases of life-threatening pelvis sepsis (39,40). Allowing the patient to rest and recline for several minutes with a cold forehead compress is usually all that is required for vasovagal response. For mild pain immediately following band placement, injection of local anesthetic into the base of the banded tissue is often effective, as are the use of mild analgesics and warm sitz baths. More severe pain in the immediate postprocedure setting is best managed by removing the band with a hooked cutting probe after the site has been locally anesthetized.

A review of 10 papers describing 17 patients for whom RBL resulted in pelvic sepsis was made by McCloud and colleagues in 2006 (40). First reported in 1980, the complication is believed to be secondary to necrosis resulting in infection of the adjacent soft tissues (41,42). Although the absolute risk seems very small in immune-competent patients, common presenting factors that should alert the surgeon to this devastating possibility are worsening perineal or pelvic pain, urinary retention, and fever. These findings mandate urgent examination, often under anesthesia, computed tomography scan, empiric broad-spectrum antibiotics, and drainage of any identified abscess with debridement of necrotic tissue and possible fecal diversion. It has been the authors' practice to warn and reinforce this possibility to patients with written instructions upon leaving the office following each session of RBL.

Bleeding is a far more commonly described complication, and although most episodes are insignificant, cases resulting in hemodynamic instability and transfusion requirements do occur and are more common in patients receiving platelet inhibitors or systemic anticoagulation. Many surgeons have therefore avoided RBL in these patients, or at least insisted that such medications be suspended to reduce this risk. Few data exist regarding safe strategies for RBL in such patients. Part of the difficulty lies in the unpredictable time frame in which the banded hemorrhoid will slough and put the patient at greatest risk for hemorrhage. Although this usually occurs within 5 to 10 days, delayed bleeding is indeed encountered (43,44).

Some have recommended offering this procedure only after antiplatelets have been held for 7 days, followed by another 7–10 days thereafter before restarting (35,45).

If only one hemorrhoid is banded per session, this will result in a significant number of days off therapy and an increased risk of thromboembolic events. Nelson and colleagues described their preference of minimizing patients' time off these medications by offering RBL on the day of initial consultation, followed by immediate suspension of antiplatelet medications (aspirin or clopidogrel) for 10 days, and Coumadin for 7 days. This approach allows for recovery of platelet and coagulation capacity by the time the patient is theoretically at greatest risk of bleeding (5–10 days), and minimizes the total number of days they are at increased risk of thromboembolic events while these medications are suspended. They described 605 bands placed on 364 patients while on either anticoagulation or antiplatelet therapy, with a risk of significant bleeding of less than 1%. If clopidogrel was not included, this risk dropped to less than 0.5%. They point out that these rates of bleeding do not differ significantly from what has been reported in the literature for patients not taking antiplatelet or anticoagulation agents, but that patients taking clopidogrel showed a trend toward greater bleeding rates (46,47). This thoughtful approach appears to safely allow these medically challenging patients the benefits of RBL over less successful (sclerotherapy) or more invasive (hemorrhoidectomy) alternatives.

## INFRARED PHOTOCOAGULATION

Infrared photocoagulation (IRC) uses infrared radiation focused by a photoconductor to create protein coagulation at the base of the pedicle, causing scarring and fibrosis (Figures 19.1 and 19.3). Alteration of the optical wavelength of the coagulator and contact time controls the depth of tissue penetration to approximately 3 mm (24). A slotted anoscope is used to visualize the base of the targeted hemorrhoid. Three or four pulses of 1–1.5 seconds each are made around each hemorrhoid apex, producing a 3–4 mm$^2$ area of coagulation, which appears immediately as a whitish circular eschar. Proponents advocate treating one to three hemorrhoids per session. Treatment of additional hemorrhoids can be offered at 3- to 4-week intervals (21,39). However, governmental reimbursement currently applies a 90-day global to IRC. Additional treatments during this period will not be reimbursed.

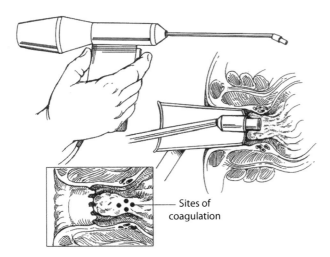

Sites of coagulation

Figure 19.3 The infrared photocoagulator creates a small thermal injury. Thus, several applications are required for each hemorrhoidal column.

Complications after IRC are infrequent. As with RBL, pain occurs if the energy is applied too near the somatically innervated anoderm; the discomfort, however, is typically of a shorter duration and lesser severity than misplaced hemorrhoidal bands. For this reason, IRC can be used to treat small distal internal hemorrhoids that are not suitable for RBL. Excessive application can result in bleeding. Rarely, ulceration can progress to fissure formation (39). IRC has been shown to be effective for the treatment of hemorrhoidal bleeding, but less so for alleviating significant prolapse (48). It is our practice to use IRC as a preferred alternative to sclerotherapy for hemorrhoids too small or distal for RBL.

## COMPARISON OF TECHNIQUES

In comparing RBL to sclerotherapy, RBL is associated with a more frequent occurrence of postprocedure pain from 30 minutes up to 72 hours. RBL is also associated with more episodes of bleeding in the immediate 24 hours postprocedure period (49). In a meta-analysis compiled in 1995, MacRae and associates showed that patients treated with RBL were less likely to need additional treatment versus patients treated with sclerotherapy ($p = 0.031$) or IRC ($p = 0.0014$) (50). However, a more recent randomized trial showed the number of sessions needed to reach symptomatic relief was equivalent between RBL and IRC (1.6 SD 0.9) (48). In the case of third-degree hemorrhoids, patients treated with RBL were more consistently symptom free versus those treated with IRC, with no difference noted between these therapies for treatment of first- and second-degree hemorrhoids (48,51).

### SUMMARY

The great majority of patients with hemorrhoidal disease may be treated nonoperatively, beginning with dietary modification intended to optimize stool consistency and ease of defecation, selective use of over-the-counter and prescription strength preparations for alleviation of mild acute symptoms, and escalation to office-based interventions to treat chronic symptoms such as bleeding and prolapse. Although treatment with sclerotherapy and infrared coagulation shows results comparable to treatment with RBL for stages I and II internal hemorrhoids, patients with more significant prolapse (grade III) achieve improved and more durable results with RBL. Management of platelet inhibitors and anticoagulation around these procedures requires some thoughtfulness and should be tailored to the procedure's bleeding risk (greatest with RBL), and the patient's unique thromboembolic risk while these agents are suspended. Although quite rare, the presenting symptoms and signs of pelvic sepsis following these procedures must be conveyed to the patient, and clinicians, once alerted to this possibility, must evaluate and intervene rapidly in order to salvage patients from this potentially fatal complication. Last, although some have claimed that nearly all hemorrhoidal disease can be treated non-operatively, good clinical judgment can often predict which patients will be better served by operative management. Such patients, as well as those whose symptoms are not well controlled after an appropriate trial of nonoperative intervention, should be offered excisional hemorrhoidectomy without further delay.

## REFERENCES

1. Parks AG. Guys Hosp Rep. 1955;104:135–56.
2. Thomson WHF. Br J Surg. 1975;62:542–52.
3. Nakama H et al. Am J Med. 1997;102:551–4.
4. Korkis AM, McDougall CJ. Dig Dis Sci. 1995;40:1520–3.
5. Kluiber RM, Wolff BG. Dis Colon Rectum. 1994;37:1006–7.
6. Madoff RD, Fleshman JW. Gastroenterology. 2004;126:1463–73.
7. Fazio VW, Tjandra JJ. Adv Surg. 1995;29:59–78.
8. Rivadeneira DE et al. Dis Colon Rectum. 2011;54:1059–64.
9. Villalba H, Abbas M. Perm J. 2007;11(2):74–6.
10. Alonso-Coello P et al. Cochrane Database Syst Rev. 2005;(4):CD004649.
11. Alonso-Coello P et al. Am J Gastroenterol. 2006;101:181–8.
12. Dodi G et al. Dis Colon Rectum. 1986;29:248–51.
13. Tejirian T, Abbas M. Dis Colon Rectum. 2005;48:2336–40.
14. Gionchetti P et al. Can J Gastroenterol. 1992;6(1):18–20.
15. Johanson JF. J Gastrointest Surg. 2002;6:290–4.
16. Desnoyers P. In: European Symposium on Venous Disease and its Treatment. Rome, Italy, April 1978. Gazette Medicale de France, 1987:17–21.
17. Klemn J. Gazette Medicale de France. 1976;83:3158–65.
18. Ho YH et al. Dis Colon Rectum. 2000;43:66–9.
19. Thanapongsathorn W, Bajrabukka T. Dis Colon Rectum. 1992;35:1085–8.
20. Morgan J. Medical Press and Circular. 1869;29–30.
21. Beck DE. Hemorrhoidal disease. In Beck DE, Wexner SD. (eds). Fundamentals of Anorectal Surgery, 2nd Edition. Bailliere Tindell, 1998, pp. 237–53.
22. Sim AJ et al. Surg Gynecol Obstet. 1983;157:534–6.
23. Bullock N. BMJ. 1997;314:419.
24. Hardy A et al. Dig Surg. 2005;22:26–33.
25. Ribbans WJ, Radcliffe AG. Dis Colon Rectum. 1985;28:188–9.
26. Kaman L et al. Dis Colon Rectum. 1999;42:419–20.
27. Barwell J et al. Dis Colon and Rectum. 1999;42(3):421–3.
28. Mann CV et al. J R Soc Med. 1988;81:146–8.
29. Senapati A, Nicholls RJ. Int J Colorectal Dis. 1998;3:124–6.
30. Takano M et al. Int J Colorectal Dis. 2006;21:44–51.
31. Takano M et al. 2010, May 15. Proceedings of the Annual Meeting of 2010. The American Society of Colon and Rectal Surgeons (ASCRS), Minneapolis, MN, 52–4.
32. Blaisdell PC. Surg Gynecol Obstet. 1958;106:485–8.
33. Barron J. Dis Colon Rectum. 1963;6:109–13.
34. Law WL, Chu KW. Dis Colon Rectum. 1999;42:363–6.
35. Gordon PH, Nivatongs S. Principles and Practice of Surgery for the Colon, Rectum and Anus, 3rd Edition. New York, NY: Informa Healthcare, 2007, p. 148.
36. Khubchandani IT. Dis Colon Rectum. 1983;26:705–8.
37. Lee HH et al. Dis Colon Rectum. 1994;37:37–41.
38. Davis KG et al. Dis Colon Rectum. 2007;50:1445.
39. Larach S et al. Nonoperative treatment of hemorrhoidal disease. In Hicks TC, Beck DE, Opelka FG, Timmcke AE. (eds). Complications of Colon and Rectal Surgery. Baltimore, MD: Williams and Wilkens, 1997, pp. 173–80.
40. McCloud JM et al. Colorectal Dis. 2006;8:748–55.
41. O'Hara VS. Dis Colon Rectum. 1980;23:570–1.
42. Russell TR, Donohue JH. Dis Colon Rectum. 1985;28:291–3.
43. Corman ML. Colon and Rectal Surgery, 6th Edition. Lippincott Williams and Wilkins, Philadelphia, PN, 2013, p. 288.
44. Patel S et al. World J Clin Cases. 2014;2(4):86–9.
45. Beattie GC et al. Ulster Med J. 2004;73:139–41.
46. Bat L et al. Dis Colon Rectum. 1993;36:287–90.
47. Iyer VS et al. Dis Colon Rectum. 2004;47:1367–70.
48. Poen AC et al. Eur J Gastroenterol Hepatol. 2000;12:535–9.
49. Marques CF et al. Tech Coloproctol. 2006;10:312–7.
50. MacRae HM, McLeod RS. Dis Colon Rectum. 1995;38:687–94.
51. Linares Santiago E et al. Rev Esp Enferm Dig. 2001;93:238–47.

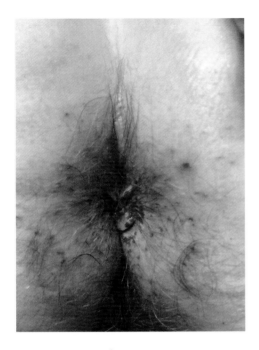

Figure 16.1 Pruitis ani with excoriations.

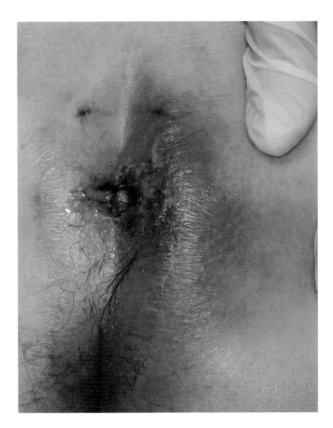

Figure 22.2 Acute pilonidal abscess. Note midline opening with abscess slightly to the right of midline.

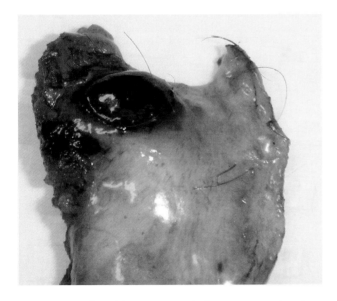

Figure 22.1 Pilonidal cyst opened after excision showing hair inside cavity.

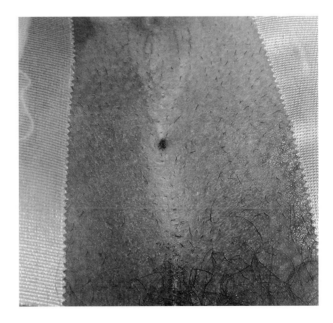

Figure 22.3 Chronic pilonidal disease showing midline pit.

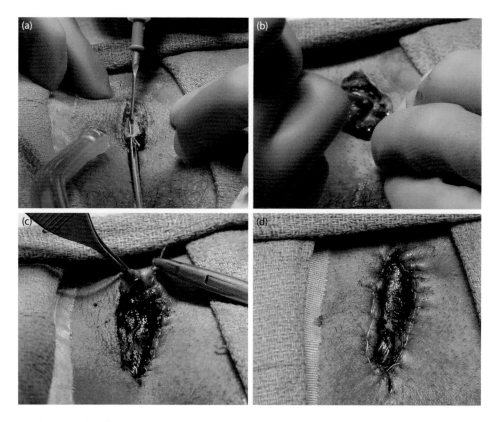

Figure 22.4 Marsupialization the diseased tissue is excised with electocautery **(a)**, and the cavity is debrided **(b)**. The edges of the wound are then sutured down to the base of the wound using absorbable suture **(c)**, resulting in a small open wound **(d)**.

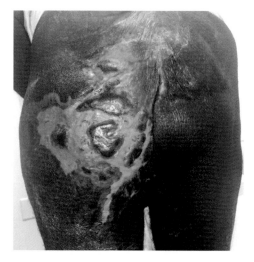

Figure 22.10 Chronically recurrent Hurley stage III HS in the setting of multiple incision and drainage and local excision procedures.

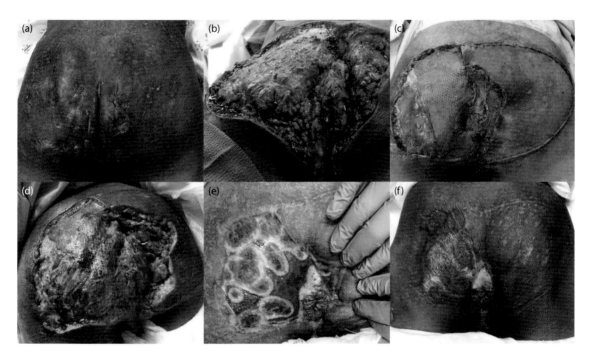

Figure 22.11 **(a)** Severe Hurley III perianal HS affecting the left > right. **(b)** Status/post wide radical excision with exposed external sphincter. **(c)** Immediate reconstruction via a right-sided V-Y advancement flap and split-thickness skin grafting. **(d)** Early loss of large portions of the skin graft due to fecal contamination and poor patient mobility. **(e)** Excellent reepithelialization from areas of viable graft at 6 weeks. **(f)** Complete healing without disease recurrence at 16 weeks.

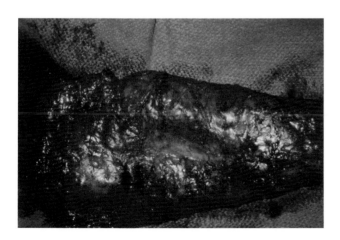

Figure 27.3 Total mesorectal excision specimen with a smooth, intact fascia propria. (Courtesy of the author.)

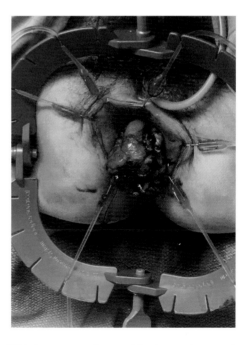

Figure 27.6 Intraoperative positioning and retraction for establishing a hand-sewn anastomosis following an intersphincteric proctectomy. (Courtesy of the author.)

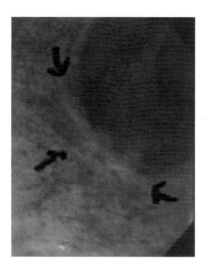

Figure 30.1 Endoscopic view of a complete clinical response with whitening of the mucosa within the area of the scar (original area of the primary tumor).

Baseline                                    12-weeks

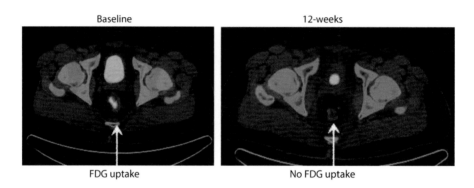

FDG uptake                                  No FDG uptake

Figure 30.4 PET/CT images performed at baseline (showing FDG uptake) and after 12 weeks from nCRT completion (showing no residual FDG uptake) consistent with a complete response to treatment.

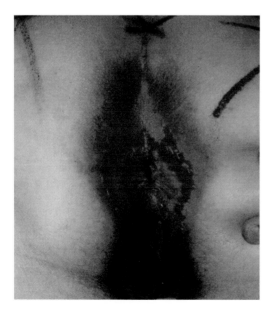

Figure 34.1 Radiation dermatitis.

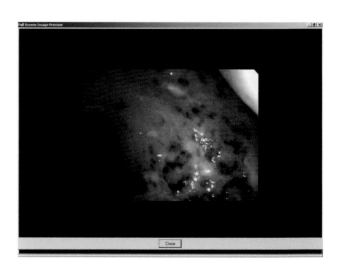

Figure 34.2 Radiation proctitis.

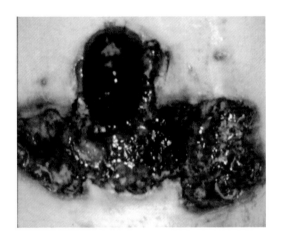

Figure 38.1 Pyodermia gangrenosum.

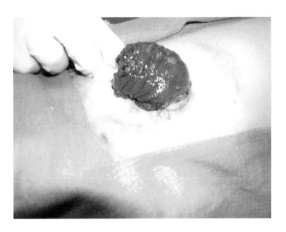

Figure 38.7 Stomal prolapse.

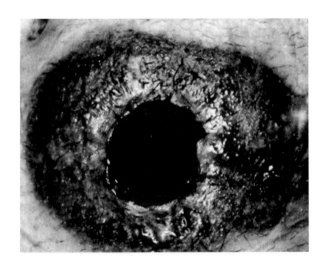

Figure 38.8 Parastomal varices.

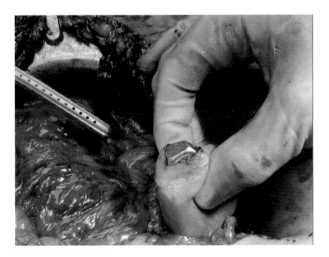

Figure 40.1 Shrapnel injury to the small bowel with a hex nut. Similar injuries were present to the small and large bowel.

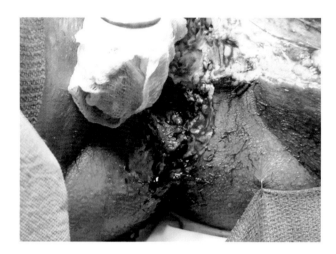

Figure 40.2 Perineal injury.

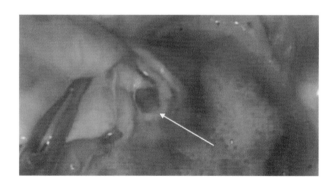

Figure 40.4 Rectal injury identified on laparoscopy (white arrow).

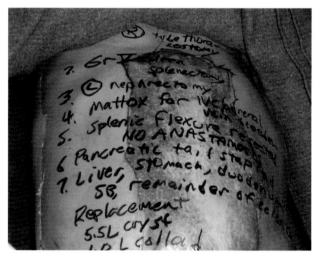

Figure 40.6 Damage control laparotomy in a combat environment.

# 20

# Surgery and nonoperative therapy of perirectal abscess and anal fistulas

MOHAMMED IYOOB MOHAMMED ILYAS AND CRAIG A. REICKERT

## CHALLENGING CASE

A 40-year-old male with poorly controlled HIV infection presents with incision and drainage of a perirectal abscess 2 cm right posterolateral to the anal verge. He is treated with a short course of oral antibiotics with resolution of the acute event. Several months later, he presents with purulent discharge from the drainage site as well as a second area in the posterior midline, 4 cm from the anal verge. Exam under anesthesia demonstrates a single primary fistula opening in the anal canal, in the posterior midline 3 cm proximal to the dentate line, which communicate with both secondary openings. Draining setons are placed, and biopsies from the fistula tracts show no evidence of Crohn disease or malignancy. Six weeks later, he presents in septic shock due to worsening perineal infection.

## CASE MANAGEMENT

The patient is initially managed with additional drainage and a diverting colostomy. After recovering, he is initiated on highly active antiretroviral therapy (HAART) with an excellent response in his CD4 count, and his viral load becomes undetectable. After magnetic resonance imaging (MRI) of the pelvis demonstrates no further infection in the pelvis, an anal fistula plug is placed to attempt to close the fistula; within a week, the plug has dislodged. An attempt at closing the fistula with an endorectal advancement flap several weeks later also fails. Further biopsies again show no evidence of Crohn disease or malignancy, and a second attempt at endorectal advancement flap closure performed 12 weeks later also fails. The patient

has decided not to pursue further surgery for the fistula and remain diverted via a colostomy with draining setons in place. Anorectal abscesses and fistulas can be incredibly frustrating, both for the patient and the managing physician. Meaningful outcomes data with large, prospective randomized trials regarding the management of these entities are extremely limited. This chapter addresses the surgical as well as non-operative management of these common problems, focusing on means of improving clinical outcomes.

## INTRODUCTION

A good understanding of the anatomy of the various perianal spaces in relation to the sphincters and the pelvic floor is essential in the clinical management of perianal abscess and fistulas. It also requires understanding the local anatomical factors along with the etiology, systemic, and local patient factors, and the various treatment options available.

## ANATOMICAL CONSIDERATIONS

Successful management of perianal abscesses and fistulas requires a good understanding of the anatomy of the anal canal, perianal region, and etiopathogenesis of abscesses and fistulas. The anal canal anatomically extends from the anal verge to the anorectal junction (cephalad extent of the pelvic diaphragm), measures about 2–4 cm, and is divided by the dentate line into the proximal endothelium lined (columns of Morgagni) part and distal part lined with squamous epithelium. Between the columns of Morgagni are unevenly distributed anal crypts, the ducts of which extend through the internal sphincter into the intersphincteric space or into the external sphincter (2–4).

There are six potential spaces around the anorectum (4) that can become sites of infection (Figure 20.1). The subcutaneous space is filled with fat and fibers of the corrugator cutis ani and is in communication with the central space and laterally with the ischiorectal space. The subcutaneous space is also considered to be part of the ischioanal space. The central space is considered the main perianal space which is in communication with others. It surrounds the anal canal and is bounded above by the termination of longitudinal muscles and below by the muscular loop of the external sphincter complex. The intersphincteric spaces are four upward longitudinal extensions from the central space below into and between the longitudinal intersphincteric muscles spaces. From lateral to medial, the first and the third of the four spaces open into the ischioanal space, the second space opens into the pelvirectal space, and the medial most space communicates with the submucosal space. Knowledge of these spaces, particularly of the central and intersphincteric spaces, helps in understanding the progression of perianal abscesses when not drained. The ischioanal or ischiorectal is a pyramidal space posterior to the urogenital diaphragm, with its medial wall formed

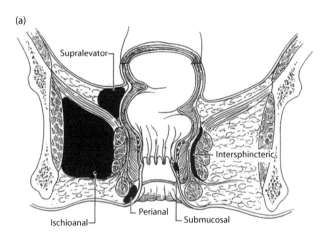

(a)

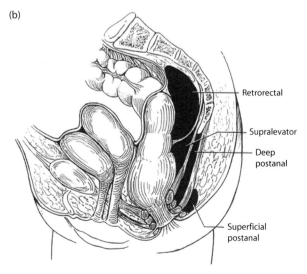

(b)

Figure 20.1 Anorectal spaces. **(a)** Coronal section. **(b)** Sagittal section.

by the external anal sphincter and levator muscle and the lateral wall formed by the obturator internus muscle. The two ischiorectal spaces communicate posteriorly behind the anus through the retrosphincteric space. The pelvirectal spaces are found between the levators and the pelvic peritoneum. The submucosal space lies between the anal mucosa and the internal sphincter muscle (4–9).

The cryptoglandular theory initially proposed by Eisenhammer and Parks has been generally espoused in the etiopathogenesis of perianal abscess. Stasis within the ducts of these glands leads to obstruction and formation of abscess formation in a majority (90%) of these cases (10). Chronic anal fissure has also been reported to be involved in the etiopathogenesis of anal fistula. The remaining 10% of the abscesses are secondary to other predisposing factors like inflammatory bowel disease, trauma, malignancy, radiation, tuberculosis, actinomycosis, and lymphogranuloma venereum. Perianal abscesses and fistulas are considered two phases of the same disease process (11). The first phase involves obstruction of the mucous anal gland leading to stasis and infection. Most glands are confined to the submucosa and when obstructed and infected will discharge into the anal canal with spontaneous healing. Nearly half of these glands do have extensions traversing the internal anal sphincter and may not discharge easily in the anal canal secondary to tonic contraction of the internal anal sphincter. Pus may then follow along with the path of least resistance between the internal and external anal sphincter or through the external sphincter into the ischioanal fossa (12).

A fistula is defined as an abnormal communication between two epithelial lined surfaces with 90% of cases associated with cryptoglandular etiology. Trauma, postoperative states, inflammatory bowel disease, anal fissure, and tuberculosis accounts for the rest. Anal fistulas are characterized as simple and complex. Simple fistulas are those that are superficial or low transsphincteric, have a single external opening, and have no associated abscess (Figure 20.2). Complex fistulas include those that are high intersphincteric, high transsphincteric, extra- and suprasphincteric fistulas, or have multiple external openings or are associated with abscesses, rectovaginal fistulas, or anorectal strictures. Fistulas involving more than 30% of the external sphincter or anteriorly located in females and fistulas associated with local irradiation or Crohn disease are also considered as complex fistulas.

The true incidence of the anorectal abscess is difficult to assess, as many such abscesses drain spontaneously or are drained in the physician's office or in the emergency room. The incidence of anorectal abscess in the United States falls between 68,000 and 96,000 per annum (1).

Intersphincteric fistulas account for nearly one-third of the cases and are known to branch out in the intersphincteric plane only without involving the external anal sphincter. Transsphincteric fistulas account for up to two-thirds of the fistulas with variable involvement of the external sphincter muscle. Transsphincteric fistulas may be associated with a blind tract leading to the ischiorectal

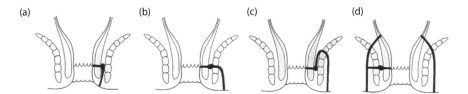

Figure 20.2 Classification of fistula-in-ano. **(a)** Intersphincteric. **(b)** Transsphincteric. **(c)** Suprasphincteric. **(d)** Extrasphincteric.

fossa or through the levator muscle into the pelvic cavity. Perforation of the blind tract during evaluation may lead to an extrasphincteric fistula. Suprasphincteric fistulas are uncommon and have tracts extending from above the puborectalis, through the levator plate, and into the ischiorectal fossa and skin. Suprasphincteric fistulas can be associated with an ischiorectal abscess. Extrasphincteric fistulas are outside of the external sphincter complex and are less common and extend from the perianal skin through the ischiorectal fossa and levator muscles into the rectum.

## DIAGNOSIS OF ABSCESSES

Physical examination (in the prone position preferably) is the most important diagnostic study when an anorectal abscess is suspected. Severe tenderness or fluctuance on the digital rectal exam are suggestive of intersphincteric abscess. Examination under anesthesia should be considered in cases of ambiguous clinical exam. Imaging is useful when a diagnosis could not be confirmed on physical exam or when supralevator abscesses are suspected. Triple contrast computed tomography imaging of the pelvis with 2.5 mm cuts is more helpful in an acute setting than magnetic resonance imaging (MRI) of the pelvis. Imaging is also useful to evaluate recurrent or incompletely drained abscesses or to evaluate complex abscesses. Endoanal ultrasound and transperineal sonography are other imaging modalities used to evaluate perianal and perirectal abscesses.

Fistulas resulting from the cryptoglandular disease often have a history of prior anorectal abscesses. Associated symptoms include bleeding secondary to granulation tissue from healing and irritation from the discharge. Pain is usually associated with chronic inflammation, but severe pain is associated more with Crohn disease and malignancy. Clinical evaluation of patients with perianal fistulas should include the history of prior anal procedures, history of incontinence, history of inflammatory bowel disease, radiation to the pelvis, and obstetric history. Physical examination in the office is more helpful with delineating superficial and transsphincteric fistulas and is expectedly less accurate with supralevator fistulas and intersphincteric fistulas.

Goodsall's rule has been estimated to have a positive predictive value in less than two-thirds of the cases and is more accurate in locating posterior compared with anterior fistulas (Figure 20.3). Patients with abdominal symptoms or findings suggestive of noncryptoglandular etiology should

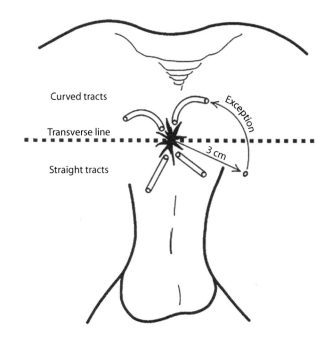

Figure 20.3 Goodsall's rule.

have a colonoscopy performed. MRI is helpful in delineating the anatomy of the fistula in relation to the sphincter complex and demonstrating pelvic sepsis, if any. It is operator independent and does not need any instrumentation of the anus. It is indicated when a complex fistula is suspected with multiple external openings, in those where an internal opening could not be identified, or in recurrences following a fistulotomy when cure is expected.

Endoanal ultrasound with hydrogen peroxide injection into the external opening can identify primary and secondary tracks. Endoanal ultrasound is more helpful with diagnosing transsphincteric fistula compared with inter- or suprasphincteric fistulas.

## MANAGEMENT OF ABSCESSES

Adequate drainage of abscesses remains the cornerstone of management of perianal and perirectal abscesses. Antibiotics are indicated when there is associated cellulitis or when patients are immunosuppressed but are not adequate treatment without incision and drainage and do not have any protective effect on subsequent fistula formation. Amoxicillin-clavulanic acid combination has been shown to offer the antibacterial spectrum necessary to cover the gram-negative enteric bacteria and gram-positive epidermal bacteria typically found in the perianal region (13). *Escherichia coli* and *Klebsiella pneumoniae* are the most common antibiotics isolated from perianal abscesses in patients without and with diabetes, respectively (14). The specificity of the microbiologic information from the anorectal abscesses has been shown to be low and is not a reliable predictor of fistula formation; thus, routine cultures are not performed during drainage of perianal abscesses. Studies also have shown no differences in progression to fistula formation with or without the use of antibiotics (13).

## DRAINAGE OF ABSCESSES

The extent of the incision and drainage depends on the type of abscess. Superficial perianal and ischiorectal abscesses can be drained in the surgeon's office or in the emergency room, with or without conscious sedation. Understanding the concept of the skeletal muscle rule helps deciding "inward" versus "outward" drainage of perianal/perirectal abscesses. As a rule, submucosal abscesses, intersphincteric abscesses, and supralevator abscesses from an intersphincteric fistula or from the pelvic disease are drained "inward" into the rectum. Supralevator abscess from an upwardly extending transsphincteric fistula, ischioanal abscess from a transsphincteric fistula, or ischioanal abscess from a supralevator abscess caused by an intersphincteric fistula penetrating the levator plate are drained "outward." The rule of thumb is that if the sepsis does not pass through the skeletal muscle (external anal sphincter and levator ani), the abscess should be drained inward, whereas if it traverses the muscle it should be drained outward (15). MRI can direct the surgeon to choose the correct direction of the drainage and is indicated in all supralevator abscesses. If the source of the abscess is intraabdominal, transrectal drainage is indicated. Also, abdominal drainage can be performed based on ease of access and directionality of the abscess cavity. Also, percutaneous drainage may prevent the creation of the fistulous track through the levator plate and is more successful than transrectal drainage.

Horseshoe abscesses or bilateral abscesses arise from the deep postanal space and require operative drainage for source control and to delineate the abscess. Hanley or modified Hanley procedure consists of open drainage of the postanal space through the anococcygeal ligament, posterior midline incision of the internal sphincter, and open drainage of the bilateral ischiorectal fossae. Modifications to this drainage include elliptical incisions on both ischiorectal space and internal sphincterotomy and drainage of deep space with or without placement of seton in the midline (16) (Figure 20.4).

Drainage catheters help minimize the perianal incisions with adequate drainage of large abscess cavities

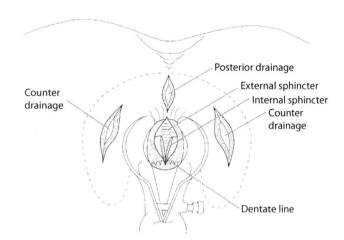

Figure 20.4 Hanley procedure.

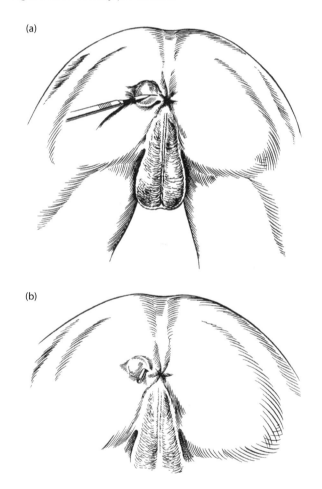

Figure 20.5 Catheter drainage of abscess.

(Figure 20.5a,b). The catheter can be secured to the skin to ensure adequate drainage of the abscess cavity until resolution of the abscess, and could also be used to perform a drain study to decipher the anatomy.

Drainage with primary fistulotomy in the acute setting is controversial. Historically it is performed along with the abscess drainage to obtain source control and increase the healing rate without the need for the subsequent procedure. A meta-analysis of six randomized control studies showed that fistula surgery during the initial incision and drainage of the abscesses reduced significantly the recurrence, persistent abscess/fistula, or repeat surgery. Incontinence at 1 year following drainage with fistula surgery was not statistically different (pooled relative risk [RR] 3.06, 95% confidence interval [CI] 0.7–13.45) (17). But, when the amount of sphincter involvement is confounded by the acute inflammation, placement of seton may be indicated to prevent unintended consequences of the excessive division of sphincter and its associated consequences (18,19).

Identification of the crypt of origin during the initial incision and drainage of the abscess could be performed by manual pressure over the abscess cavity, by careful insertion of the probe into the suspected duct by direct visualization, or injection of hydrogen peroxide via a catheter inserted into the external opening. If the offending duct is identified, the incidence of subsequent fistula could be lower than 30% as reported, confirming the role of primary fistulotomy during initial incision and drainage procedure (17,20). Microbiological origin of the abscess has not been shown to be helpful in the management of anorectal abscess of cryptoglandular origin (21–23).

Postoperative management should include local wound care with sitz baths, and packing of the abscess cavity should be avoided to facilitate drainage of the abscess cavity. Antibiotics are indicated when cellulitis persists or in patients who are immunosuppressed.

## MANAGEMENT OF FISTULA

The challenges associated with anal fistula management have been touted as the chief reason for the opening of St. Mark's Hospital in London, England. The goals of fistula management include elimination of sepsis, closure of the fistula tract, maintenance of continence, and prevention of recurrence (24).

Examination under anesthesia with the use of adjuncts (fistula probe or methylene blue or hydrogen peroxide injection) helps identify the internal opening and assess the sphincter involvement. The treatment modality depends on the amount of sphincter involvement.

The simple and most distal intersphincteric fistula can be managed with laying open the fistula tract to the anoderm. Multiple studies since 1987 have shown fistulotomy to be effective with recurrence rates ranging from 3% to 7% (21). Recurrence rates are lower (4%) for intersphincteric fistulas and higher for transsphincteric (7%) and suprasphincteric fistulas (33%) (25). Fistulotomy wounds typically heal by 4–6 weeks, and marsupialization of the wound edges leads to less bleeding and a decrease in the size of the wound, without increasing postoperative pain and sepsis. It has also been shown to result in faster healing with a shorter duration of wound discharge (26–28). Incontinence rates are higher with fistulotomy when it is associated with complex fistulas, female gender, prior fistula surgeries, and surgeon experience.

Setons have been in use since ancient times, when a caustic chemical seton from a plant extract known as ksharasutra was used to obliterate the tract. A variety of other materials have been used since, including different types of sutures, stainless steel wires, Pezzer catheters, self-locking cables, Penrose drains, vessel loops, and rubber bands (29–31). Grooved Lockhart-Mummery probes are used to probe fistula track and help with seton insertion. Fistula probes are modified with an eye near the tip of the probe through which the seton may be passed and withdrawn through the tract. Other modifications used for fistula probe insertion include using a railroad technique with the use of a plastic infusion line or use of a plastic infusion line and olive-tip malleable metaguide for seton placement (32–34). Setons are used when fistulotomy is not possible, as with higher fistulas, or not advisable, as with anterior fistulas in women or in Crohn disease. The use of a seton helps stimulate fibrosis around the track to make it obvious and helps identify the track for sphincter-sparing procedures like placement of a fistula plug, fibrin glue, or ligation of the intersphincteric tract (LIFT).

Seton could be used as a single-stage cutting seton, two-stage seton fistulotomy, or draining seton followed by a definitive procedure. The cutting seton is used purely to divide the muscle, while the staged technique is advocated when the muscle is too thick or to avoid the pain on the patient that a cutting seton would inflict while cutting through the anoderm. Cutting setons require maintaining tension by the use of leg strap and tourniquet, use of a synthetic cable tie, use of a hangman's tie using a polypropylene or nylon suture, or use of rubber band ligator to manage the tension. Use of cutting setons has a reported recurrence rate with variation based on the preservation or partial division of the internal anal sphincter. When the internal anal sphincter is preserved, the recurrence rate was 3%, and the incontinence rate was 5.6% versus 5% and 25.2% when the internal anal sphincter partially divided. A "snug" seton technique was also described where the seton is tied snugly around the sphincter muscles with minimal tension. A "two-thread" technique involves passing two No. 0 silk ties around the fistula track, tying one of the threads, and leaving the second untied initially and tying after 1 month when the first thread is removed. Another technique described is the use of a drainage seton along with a primary cutting seton. The use of multiple setons simultaneously has also been discussed with five 1-0 silk sutures, and at weekly intervals each suture is tightened progressively after taking out the previously tightened suture, which becomes lax (24,35). Multiple setons could also be used as modified cutting setons along with partial fistulotomy (staged seton), wherein the fistula tract is laid open to the dentate line. Use of the seton as a long term-draining seton for low transsphincteric and intersphincteric fistulas has been shown to be a good alternative to primary surgical treatment with similar healing rates and recurrence rates compared with primarily surgically treated patients, but incontinence has been shown to be rare (36). The major disadvantage is that the treatment takes a longer period compared with primary surgery (37). When draining setons are used, the second-stage surgery when performed is usually 6–8 weeks after, to allow for adequate healing of the cephalad portion of the sphincter.

## DRAINAGE TUBES IN FISTULAS

A tube loop seton drainage has been described with the use of a 16–18Ch Nelaton catheter for multiple recurring high-spreading extrasphincteric fistulas. It helps with irrigating the cavity and bidirectional drainage from the space. Use of an 8 mm Penrose drain with multiple holes with a Penrose drain fixed to the distal one-third point of the punctured Penrose drain has also been described for draining abscess cavities associated with high intersphincteric or trans-sphincteric fistulas. Similarly, Malecot catheters have been used to drain the abscess cavity as well.

There are conflicting data on the predisposition of certain perianal abscesses to fistula formation. Earlier reports were suggestive of perianal abscesses more predisposed to fistula formation than horseshoe abscess. Other studies showed eightfold higher fistula formation with ischiorectal abscess and threefold increase with intersphincteric abscesses compared with perianal abscesses (38).

## FIBRIN GLUE

Fibrin glue is a mixture of fibrinogen and thrombin and has been in use for over three decades in the management of anal fistulas. The fibrin sealant (Tissucol; Baxter Laboratory, Maurepas, France) contains Aprotinin as a fibrin stabilizer along with coagulation factor XIII and calcium chloride. It is injected using an appropriate-sized catheter from the external opening of the fistula, which is withdrawn slowly to leave a bleb of glue at the external opening. The patient is kept immobile on the operating table for a few minutes to ensure the glue solidifies. When injected into the fistula tract, it is expected to seal the tract, enhance wound healing, promote hemostasis and angiogenesis, and serve as a matrix for fibroblast ingrowth and formation of a collagen network over a period of 1–2 weeks. Fibrin installation is carried out after control of local sepsis and ensuring that the tract is relatively dry (39).

Fibrin glue instillation is easy to apply, associated with minimal discomfort, minimal postoperative analgesia, and early return to normal activity. Hjortrup et al. reported their initial modest success with fibrin instillation with a fistula

closure rate of 50% with one attempt, increasing to 72% with two or three attempts, and 26% failure rate even after multiple injections of fibrin (40). Since then multiple studies have reported conflicting success rates ranging from 10% to 78% (41–50). A figure-of-eight absorbable suture to prevent early expulsion of the glue into the rectum was placed by some investigators but did not show a significant difference in the success rate in a prospective controlled study.

Fibrin glue instillation is contraindicated in the presence of active inflammation or sepsis or in the presence of advanced HIV infection with low CD4 count and high viral load, as these are known to reduce the success rate. Inadequate tract preparation with persistent tract epithelialization and granulation tissue lining the tract, leading to its chronicity, are all attributed to failure of fistula closure associated with fibrin instillation. Fibrin clot extrusion during coughing or straining or due to liquid consistency of the glue are other possible reasons for failure. The disadvantage attributed to fibrin glue instillation is the theoretical risk associated with transmission of infectious agents to humans, including hepatitis B or HIV from human pooled blood or exposure to spongiform encephalopathy from bovine aprotinin (43).

## FISTULA PLUG

Experience with the fibrin glue instillation leads to the development of a material that could be secured to the fistula tract and improve the fistula closure rate. Fistula plus is used to obliterate the track and secure it with sutures to the internal opening. Surgisis Anal Plug (Cook Surgical, Belington, Indiana) is the first-generation bioabsorbable, xenograft made from porcine small intestinal submucosa. Fistula plug, like fibrin glue instillation, is performed when local sepsis is controlled and the tract is relatively dry. A draining seton is typically needed for approximately 8 weeks prior to fistula plug application. During the procedure, the seton is removed, and the tract is cleaned with hydrogen peroxide and debrided with fistula brush. The plug is then pulled through the internal opening until mild resistance is met and then secured in four quadrants at the internal opening with an absorbable suture. The excess plug is trimmed at the external opening. The external opening is also widened to ensure adequate drainage. Strenuous activity could still extrude the plug, and patients are advised to avoid such activities for 2 weeks postoperatively.

Newer prefabricated cone-shaped devices such as Surgisis Anal Fistula Plug (AFP) (Cook Surgical, Bloomington, Indiana) have been introduced since, which can be easily secured into the fistula track and are available now. Like fistula glue instillation, the results vary widely and are reported to be between 14% and 87% (24,51–54). Review of 20 studies (2 abstracts and 18 original articles) with 530 patients showed a fistula closure rate at 54% and plug extrusion rate at 8.7%. This review also showed no differences in the fistula closure rate between Crohn and non-Crohn patients. An absence of the preoperative seton, aggressive curettage of the track during the procedure leading to widening of the lumen, and inadequate fixation are all factors leading to extrusion of the plug. Inappropriate selection of patients also leads to higher failure rates, such as patients with multiple tracks.

Delayed absorbable synthetic plug (GORE BIO-A) was purported as an improvement with an expanded disc at one end and several tails. The disc is anchored to the internal sphincter and buried under a mucosal flap. The length of the fistula plug is adjusted to fit the length of the fistula track with studies reporting use with fistula track ranging from 1.5 to 8 cm (55,56). These delayed absorbable flaps undergo hydrolytic and enzymatic degradation, and studies have reported that polymer scaffolding is replaced by a layer of newer tissue within 7 months without generating a chronic inflammatory response (57,58). The rate of fistula healing ranges between 15.8% and 72.7%. There has been some disagreement over the use of a draining seton before insertion of the GORE BIO-A plug, with Stamos et al. reporting higher plug implantation and healing rate without the use of a prior seton (59,60).

## LIGATION OF INTERNAL FISTULA TRACT

The ligation of internal fistula tract (LIFT) procedure includes identifying the fistula tract in the intersphincteric plane, ensuring secure ligation of the tract, curetting the external portion of the tract, and performing partial fistulotomy or drainage along with laying open the distal part of the tract (Figure 20.6). Any defect in the external sphincter muscle is repaired with sutures. This procedure was first described by Rojanasakul in 2007 with healing rates of up to 94% (61,62). Although similar results are not reproduced by many, the LIFT technique continues to remain popular. A meta-analysis of 18 studies with 592 patients reported a mean healing rate of 74.6% during a mean follow-up period of 42.3 weeks with a mean healing time of 5.5 weeks. No incontinence was reported from the procedure (63). Similar results were reported from a recent meta-analysis of 24 original articles including 1,100 patients, which showed a similar result with a success rate of the repair at 76.4%, with no reported incontinence. Failure of the LIFT procedure presents as discharge from the intersphincteric incision and has the anatomy of simple fistulas and could be managed with fistulotomy or local wound care (64,65).

Modifications to improve and reinforce LIFT repair further, by insertion of a bioprosthetic graft in the intersphincteric plane to act as a physical barrier, is called the BIOLIFT procedure. The bioprosthetic graft ideally must overlap the closure of the fistula tract by 1–2 cm in all directions,

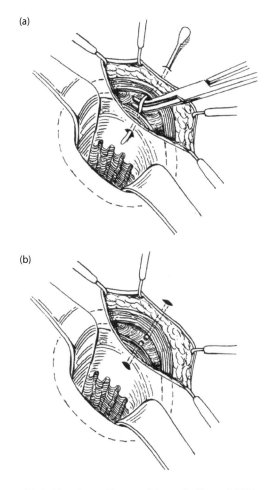

(a)

(b)

Figure 20.6 Ligation of intersphincteric Tract (LIFT). **(a)** Incision in the intersphincteric groove to expose fistula tract containing a flexible probe. **(b)** Tract is ligated. (With kind permission from Springer Science+Business Media: *Fundamentals of Anorectal Surgery*, Anorectal Abscess and Fistula-in-ano, 2018, Vogel JD, Vasilevsky CA.)

requiring more extensive dissection in the intersphincteric plane. The principle behind BIOLIFT appears to have been extrapolated from studies using biological graft in rectovaginal fistula repairs (66). Studies show the BIOLIFT procedure to have a fistula closure rate of 63%–94%, with poorer outcomes with anterior fistulas. A human acellular dermal matrix has been used as an adjunct with LIFT, called BIOLIFT plug, and has been shown to be successful in 90% of cases in a study involving 21 patients (67,68). The meta-analysis by Vergara et al. did not show enough evidence that variants in the surgical technique of the LIFT procedure showed better outcomes (63). But, the meta-analysis by Hong et al. showed the LIFT success rate to increase from 74.6% to 83.5% when all the combined LIFT procedures (LIFT, BIOLIFT, LIFT plus coring, and LIFT plus fistula plug) are included in the analysis (69).

Currently, a randomized, multicenter prospective trial (NCT01478139) is in progress comparing Bio-LIFT with LIFT alone (70).

## STEM CELLS

Autologous expanded adipose tissue derived stem cells (eADSC) has been used in the management of fistula. These cells are obtained easily with liposuction and have been proposed in suppressing inflammation and promote healing (71). After identifying the internal opening and curettage of the tract, the internal opening of the tract is closed, and eADSC suspension is injected at the level of the intersphincteric tract and into the walls of the tract. Early results from the use of eADSC have been modest at best, with 71.5% initial healing and 33% at 3 years (72–74). An autologous bone marrow–derived mesenchymal stromal cells (MSC) solution has also been evaluated in a smaller trial with intractable Crohn perianal fistulas by injecting into the lumen and the walls of the fistula tract. It has shown promising results with 70% fistula healing at 1 year (75).

## ADVANCEMENT FLAP PROCEDURES

Advancement flap procedures are indicated in more complex fistulas that are not suitable for fistulotomy without compromising continence. They are also indicated in cases with rectourethral or rectovaginal fistulas. The mechanics of the anal fistula with higher pressure on the luminal side of the anus help with the technique of flap closure as it brings a layer of healthy tissue over the internal opening (76).

The flaps are based from the rectum or perianal skin. The endorectal advancement flap is based from the rectum and the anocutaneous and transanal sleeve advancement flap and based from the perianal skin.

## ENDORECTAL ADVANCEMENT FLAP

Endorectal advancement flap (ERAF) is considered as the gold standard sphincter preserving operation and usually performed as a second-stage procedure after a seton fistulotomy for high transsphincteric or suprasphincteric fistulas. The essential principles behind ERAF includes debridement or excision of the fistula tract, and mobilization of a vascularized, tension-free mucosal flap to cover the area over the internal opening. After curetting the tract, the defect in the internal anal sphincter is closed with absorbable sutures. The broad-based flap with adequate blood supply is developed along the level of the submucosal plane and includes a few superficial fibers of the internal anal sphincter. The base of the flap should be approximately twice the width of its length to ensure absence of tension at the suture line. Adequate hemostasis and a tension-free suture line are essential to ensure success of the flap repair. Although a majority of them use a U-shaped flap, a semicircular flap avoids ischemia at the corners. It is recommended to excise a small rim of the anoderm below the internal opening to create a neodentate line (Figure 20.7).

The advantages of ERAF include avoiding division of the sphincter with less risk for incontinence, maintaining the anal contour, avoiding keyhole deformity, and promoting quicker healing. Additional procedures can be incorporated into the operation, like sphincteroplasty without the need for fecal diversion. Failure of the repair does not usually lead to worsening of symptoms, as disruption of the internal sphincter at the level of the anorectal junction is offset by more rigidity at the same level due to the scar tissue. Advancement flap techniques are not recommended when associated with anorectal sepsis, active proctitis, malignant or radiation-related fistulas, stricture of the anorectum, severe sphincter defect, or severe perianal scarring from previous fistula surgery (76,77). Smokers are associated with lower healing rates (60%) compared to nonsmokers (79%) (78).

The healing rates after ERAF were reported to be between 60% and 93% with a recurrence rate of 19.7% over a median follow-up period of 42 months (range 24–65 months) (76,79,80). The median time to relapse was 5 months (range 1–11.7 months), with no recurrences seen after 1 year of the repair. For lesions below the dentate line—fistulotomy or dermal advancement flap was preferred to avoid the creation of mucosal ectropion (81). Mitalas et al. reported the healing rate after first ERAF to be 67%, and patients with a failed previous repair had a 69% healing rate after the second repair, thus resulting in an overall success rate of 90% (82). ERAF when combined with fibrin glue injection had worse outcomes, while a combination of ERAF with platelet-rich plasma was shown to have better outcomes (83,84). Full-thickness rectal flaps were shown to have better recurrence rates compared to partial-thickness flaps without higher incontinence rates in a retrospective review involving 54 patients (85). Smoking and obesity negatively impacted the outcomes after ERAF (86).

## ANO-CUTANEOUS ADVANCEMENT FLAP

An ano-cutaneous advancement flap is an alternative to a rectal advancement flap. It includes a V-shaped incision made in the perianal skin with the base of the incision including the internal opening and the lateral edge including the external opening. The flap is raised by mobilizing along the underlying fat to allow advancement without tension (Figure 20.8). The track is cored out, including both internal and external openings. The flap is sutured to the anal mucosa above the internal opening with one side of the flap left open to ensure adequate drainage (76).

The transanal sleeve advancement flap procedure takes the concept of flap advancement further by mobilizing the circumference of the anal canal and is useful in patients with severe complex fistulas associated with Crohn disease (87). It includes a near circumferential incision at or below the dentate line to create a sleeve of full thickness of the bowel wall, which was mobilized to allow the flap to be advanced into the supralevator space without tension. The distal suture line is kept below the level of the

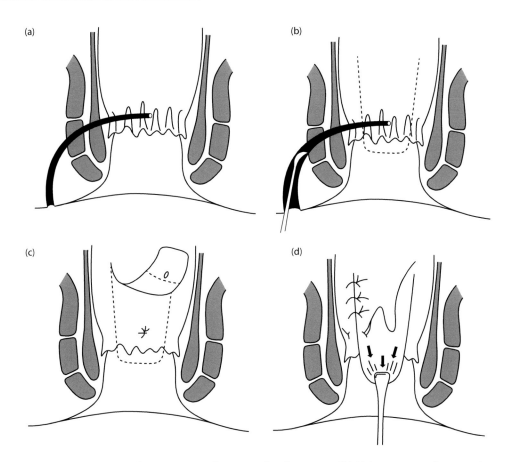

Figure 20.7 Endorectal advancement flap. **(a)** Transphincteric fistula-in-ano. **(b)** Enlargement of external opening. **(c)** Flap of muscle and muscle is mobilized. **(d)** Flap is advanced, the distal tip is removed, and the flap is sutured in place. (From Vasilevsky CA. Fistula-in-ano and abscess. In Beck DE, Wexner SD. (eds). *Fundamentals of Anorectal Surgery*, 2nd edition, 1998, Figure 10–15, p.176, with permission.)

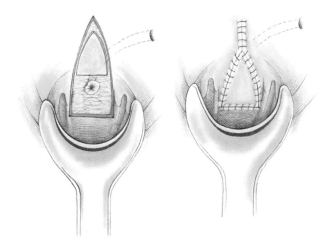

Figure 20.8 Anocutaneous flap.

internal opening with absorbable sutures. The advancement flap procedures are safe and effective in around 70% patients with minimal or no disturbance of continence. Studies show the healing rates of the fistula range from 64% to 95% with a recurrence rate ranging from 0% to 36% during a follow-up period ranging from 1 to 31 months (88–91).

## FISTULOTOMY WITH SPHINCTER RECONSTRUCTION

This is an effective management strategy when complex anal fistulas are associated with incontinence or have higher risk for incontinence, as those with a history of multiple or complicated childbirths, those who present with preexisting sphincter defect, or those women who have anterior fistulas. The first German guideline for the treatment of anal fistulas considered "fistula excision with reconstruction" as a therapeutic option (92). These radical procedures are associated with higher healing rates ranging from 83.3% to 97.4% but are associated with higher incontinence rates ranging between 3.7% and 21.4% (80,93–99). Although the results from U.S. centers are reassuring, most available data are from European centers (80).

## VIDEO-ASSISTED ANAL FISTULA MANAGEMENT

Video-assisted anal fistula treatment (VAAFT) uses a fistuloscope manufactured by Karl Storz GmbH (Tuttlingen,

Germany), obturator, unipolar electrode, endobrush, and cyanoacrylate glue. The procedure involves diagnostic fistuloscopy under irrigation, fulguration of the fistula tract, closing of the internal opening with a mucocutaneous flap, or using a stapler followed by reinforcement of the repair with cyanoacrylate glue. Cyanoacrylate glue reinforcement has not been uniformly accepted as part of VAAFT as it could contribute to impaired drainage of the tract and delay healing. Appropriate widening of the external opening is necessary with daily irrigation to ensure adequate drainage of the debrided tract. VAAFT is also helpful to identify the secondary tracts, which are one of the main reasons for failure of anal fistula surgery. The early results of VAAFT repair are promising with primary healing in 73.5% with maintenance of healing in up to 87.1% of patients who showed healing over a short period (100–102).

## FILAC

Fistula layer closure is a novel sphincter saving procedure where the primary closure of the track is achieved using laser energy from a diode laser. After identifying the track and curettage, a 14 Fr catheter was inserted into the fistula track using a guidewire. A 400 μm radial-emitting disposable laser fiber was inserted through the 14 Fr catheter and delivers laser energy (1470 nm wavelength) homogeneously at 360° while the fiber is withdrawn from the internal opening of the fistula track outward by 1 mm/s. The radial penetration depth of the energy has been shown to be 2–3 mm beyond the fistula track. Studies show a successful closure rate of 71.4% over a 20-month follow-up period, but reported a 22.9% incidence of significant postoperative pain and anismus. Öztürk and colleagues reported an 82% healing rate at 12 months of follow-up after the procedure. The FiLaC procedure remains investigational; additional data must be made available before further recommendations can be made (80,103,104).

## REFERENCES

1. Abcarian H. Clin Colon Rectal Surg 2011;24(1):14–21.
2. Eglitis J. Ohio J Sci 1961;61(2):65–79.
3. Seow-Choen F, Ho JM. Dis Colon Rectum 1994;37(12): 1215–8.
4. Shafik A. Invest Urol 1976;13:424.
5. Milligan ETC et al. Lancet 1937;2:1119.
6. Courtney H. Am J Surg 1950;79:155.
7. Milligan ETC. Proc R Soc Med 1943;36:365.
8. Haagensen CD et al. The Lymphatics in Cancer. Philadelphia, PA: Saunders, 1972.
9. Parks AG. Br Med J 1961;1:463.
10. Seow-Choen F, Ho JM. Dis Colon Rectum 1994;37: 1215–8.
11. Gosselink MP et al. Colorectal Dis 2015;17(12):1041–3.
12. Mitalas LE et al. Tech Coloproctol 2012;16:113–7.
13. Sözener U et al. Dis Colon Rectum 2011;54(8):923–9.
14. Liu CK et al. J Microbiol Immunol Infect 2011;44(3): 204–8.
15. Zinicola R, Cracco N. Colorectal Dis 2014;16(7):562.
16. Browder LK et al. Tech Coloproctol 2009;13(4):301–6.
17. Malik AI et al. Cochrane Database Syst Rev 2010;7: CD006827.
18. Ramanujam PS et al. Surg Gynecol Obstet 1983;157(5): 419–22.
19. Cariati A. Updates Surg 2013;65(3):201–5.
20. Quah HM et al. Int J Colorectal Dis 2006;21(6):602–9.
21. Cox SW et al. Am Surg 1997;63:686–9.
22. Chrabot CM et al. Dis Colon Rectum 1983;26:105–8.
23. Lunniss PJ, Phillips RK. Br J Surg 1994;81:368–9.
24. Davis BR, Kasten KR. Anorectal Abscess and Fistula. ASCRS Textbook of Colon and Rectal Surgery, 3rd Edition. New York, NY: Springer, 2016.
25. Garcia-Aguilar J et al. Dis Colon Rectum 1996;39(7): 723–9.
26. Pescatori M et al. Colorectal Dis 2006;8(1):11–4.
27. Ho YH et al. Br J Surg 1998;85(1):105–7.
28. Jain BK et al. J Korean Soc Coloproctol 2012;28(2): 78–82.
29. Williams JG et al. Br J Surg 1991;78:1159–61.
30. Awad ML et al. Colorectal Dis 2009;11:524–6.
31. Takesue Y et al. J Gastroenterol 2002;37(11):912–5.
32. Seow-Choen F. Colorectal Dis 2003;5:373.
33. Gurer A et al. American J Surg 2007;193:794–6.
34. Subhas G et al. Dig Surg 2012;29(4):292–300.
35. García Olmo D et al. Br J Surg 1994;81:136–7.
36. Durgun V et al. Dig Surg 2002;19:56–8.
37. Lentner A, Wienert V. Dis Colon Rectum 1996;39: 1097–101.
38. Sözener U et al. Dis Colon Rectum 2011;54(8):923–9.
39. de Parades V et al. Colorectal Dis 2010;12(5):459–63.
40. Hjortrup A et al. Dis Colon Rectum 1991;34:752–4.
41. Patrlj L et al. Dig Surg 2000;17:77–80.
42. Cintron JR et al. Dis Colon Rectum 2000;43:944–9. discussion 949–50.
43. Lindsey I et al. Dis Colon Rectum 2002;45:1608–15.
44. Zmora O et al. Dis Colon Rectum 2003;46:584–9.
45. Buchanan GN et al. Dis Colon Rectum 2003;46: 1167–74.
46. Maralcan G et al. Surg Today 2006;36:166–70.
47. Johnson EK et al. Dis Colon Rectum 2006;49:371–6.
48. Grimaud JC et al. Gut 2006;55(Suppl. V):A40.
49. Tyler KM et al. Dis Colon Rectum 2007;50:1535–9.
50. Singer M et al. Dis Colon Rectum 2005;48:799–808.
51. Ommer A et al. Ger Med Sci 2012;10:Doc13.
52. Heydari A et al. Dis Colon Rectum 2013;56(6):774–9.
53. Buchberg B et al. Am Surg 2010;76(10):1150–3.
54. de la Portilla F et al. Dis Colon Rectum 2011;54(11): 1419–22.
55. Ratto C et al. Colorectal Dis 2012;14(5):e264–9.
56. Narang SK et al. Colorectal Dis 2016;18(1):37–44.
57. Limura E et al. World J Gastroenterol 2015;21:12–20.
58. Katz AR et al. Surg Gynecol Obstet 1985;161:213–22.

59. Stamos MJ et al. *Dis Colon Rectum* 2015;58:344–51.
60. de la Portilla F. *Colorectal Dis* 2013;15:628–9.
61. Rojanasakul A et al. *J Med Assoc Thai* 2007;90(3):581–6.
62. Rojanasakul A. *Tech Coloproctol* 2009;13(3):237–40.
63. Vergara-Fernandez O, Espino-Urbina LA. *World J Gastroenterol* 2013;19(40):6805–13.
64. Tan KK et al. *Dis Colon Rectum* 2011;54(11):1368–72.
65. van Onkelen RS et al. *Colorectal Dis* 2013;15(5):587–91.
66. Ellis CN. *Dis Colon Rectum* 2010;53:1361–4.
67. Chew M-H et al. *Int J Colorectal Dis* 2013;28:1489–96.
68. Tan K-K, Lee PJ. *ANZ J Surg* 2014;84:280–3.
69. Hong KD et al. *Tech Coloproctol* 2014;18(8):685–91.
70. https://clinicaltrials.gov/ct2/show/NCT01478139.
71. Scoglio D et al. *Clin Colon Rectal Surg* 2014;27(4):172–81.
72. Mizuno H et al. *Plast Reconstr Surg* 2002;109(1):199–209. discussion 210–1.
73. Garcia-Olmo D et al. *Dis Colon Rectum* 2009;52(1):79–86.
74. Guadalajara H et al. *Int J Colorectal Dis* 2012;27(5):595–600.
75. Ciccocioppo R et al. *Gut* 2011;60(6):788–98.
76. Williams JG et al. *Colorectal Dis* 2007;9(Suppl 4):18–50.
77. Ozuner G et al. *Dis Colon Rectum* 1996;39:10–4.
78. Zimmerman DD et al. *Br J Surg* 2003;90:351–4.
79. Abbas MA et al. *Am Surgeon* 2008;74:921–4.
80. Santoro GA, Abbas MA. *Complex Anorectal Fistulas. ASCRS Textbook of Colon and Rectal Surgery*, 3rd Edition. Cham, Heidelerg, New York, Dordrecht, London: Springer, 2016.
81. Christante DH, Thorsen AJ. *The Management of Anorectal Abscess and Fistula. Current Surgical Therapy*, 12th Edition. Philadelphia, PA: Elsevier Health Sciences, 2016.
82. Mitalas LE et al. *Dis Colon Rectum* 2007;50(10):1508–11.
83. Jacob TJ et al. *Cochrane Database of Syst Rev* 2010;5:CD006319.
84. Gottgens KW et al. *Dis Colon Rectum* 2014;57(2):223–7.
85. Dubsky PC et al. *Dis Colon Rectum* 2008;51(6):852–7.
86. Schwandner O. *BMC Gastroenterol* 2011;11:61.
87. Marchesa P et al. *Br J Surg* 1998;85:1695–8.
88. Jun SH, Choi GS. *Br J Surg* 1999;86:490–2.
89. Amin SN et al. *Dis Colon Rectum* 2003;46:540–3.
90. Del Pino A et al. *Dis Colon Rectum* 1996;39:224–6.
91. Nelson RL et al. *Dis Colon Rectum* 2000;43:681–4.
92. Ommer A et al. *Dtsch Arztebl Int.* 2011;108:707–13.
93. Parkash S et al. *Aust N Z J Surg* 1985;55:23–7.
94. Christiansen J, Rønholt C. *Int J Colorectal Dis* 1995;10:207–9.
95. Roig JV et al. *Colorectal Dis* 2010;12:145–52.
96. Kraemer M, Picke D. *Coloproctology* 2011;33:104–8.
97. Arroyo A et al. *Ann Surg* 2012;255:935–9.
98. Perez F et al. *Am J Surg* 2006;192:34–40.
99. Ratto C et al. *Dis Colon Rectum* 2013;56:226–33.
100. Meinero P, Mori L. *Tech Coloproctol* 2011;15:417–22.
101. Wałęga P et al. *Pol Przegl Chir* 2014;86:7–10.
102. Seow-En I et al. *Tech Coloproctol* 2016;20(6):389–93.
103. Giamundo P et al. *Colorectal Dis* 2014;16:110–5.
104. Oztürk E, Gülcü B. *Dis Colon Rectum* 2014;57:360–4.
105. Vogel JD, Vasilevsky CA. Anorectal Abscess and Fistula-in-ano. Beck DE, Wexner SD, Steele SR. (eds). *Fundamentals of Anorectal Surgery*, 3rd edition. NY: Springer, 2018.
106. Vasilevsky CA. Fistula-in-ano and abscess. In Beck DE, Wexner SD. (eds). *Fundamentals of Anorectal Surgery*, 2nd edition. 1998. Figure 10–15, p.176.

# 21

# Surgery and nonoperative therapy of anal fissure

MARY T. O'DONNELL AND CARY B. AARONS

## CHALLENGING CASE

A 28-year-old female presents to your clinic with rectal bleeding and extreme anal pain with bowel movements that lasts for hours afterward. These symptoms have been present for 6 months since the birth of her first child. She reports intermittent constipation, and the pain is partially relieved with hydrocortisone creams and sitz baths. During physical exam, gentle exposure of the anal verge reveals an anteriorly located fissure. Given the chronicity of her symptoms, she desires surgery. What is your next step?

## CASE MANAGEMENT

Despite the duration of symptoms and the patient's request, treatment in this young postpartum female should begin with fiber supplementation, increased fluid intake, and lifestyle modifications. In a young female who may experience sphincter, perineal, or pudendal nerve trauma from childbirth in the future, it is especially important to pursue conservative measures as a first-line treatment due to their proven efficacy without impairment in fecal continence. Specifically, postpartum fissures are unique in that they are associated with decreased pressures in the sphincter complex, rather than hypertonia associated with the typical anal fissure. Treatment should not be focused on medication or surgery to relax the sphincter, but rather aid in healing the wound. Greater than 90% of these will heal with topical anesthetic and improved bowel habits, with the remaining patients needing procedures such as anorectal advancement flaps (1). If surgical intervention is planned, preoperative anal manometry or ultrasound should be considered.

## INTRODUCTION

Anal fissure is a common condition in which the epithelium is torn at the anal verge or distal anal canal. While true population incidence is unknown, estimates suggest 10% of referrals or up to 250 visits per year of a colorectal surgery clinic visits are for anal fissures (2). Patients present with symptoms of mild bleeding and sharp, tearing pain with defecation that can last for hours afterward. Precipitating events include constipation and passage of hard stool that causes trauma to the anal canal, though diarrhea has also been reported prior to symptoms. A history consistent with an anal fissure and visualization on external exam are usually sufficient for diagnosis. Spreading the buttocks with opposing traction of the thumbs at the anal verge usually reveals the fissure defect. Digital rectal exam and anoscopy are often not well tolerated given patient discomfort; however, they should be performed if there is concern for the accuracy of the diagnosis. In these cases, an exam under anesthesia with possible biopsy may aid in diagnosis of abnormally located fissures or other anorectal etiologies for pain.

## CLASSIFICATION

Anal fissures are classified by chronicity and etiology. A fissure that has been present for more than 4 weeks can begin to demonstrate secondary findings of chronic inflammation, including a sentinel pile (external skin tag) and/or a hypertrophied anal papilla proximal to the fissure (Figure 21.1). In some cases, the fibers of the internal sphincter are visible through the fissure opening. Once a fissure has been present for over 6 weeks, usually having been refractory to conservative lifestyle modifications, it is considered chronic. The etiologies of anal fissures are vast. While the

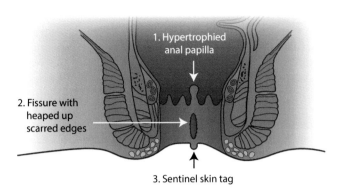

Figure 21.1 Chronic anal fissure. (Reprinted from the American Society of Colon and Rectal Surgeons website. Image provided by Robin Noel, Graphic Artist: University of Pennsylvania.)

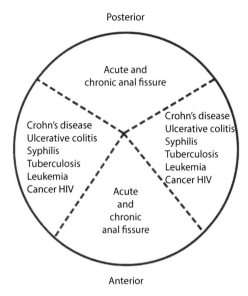

Figure 21.2 Location and etiologies of anal fissure at the anal canal.

typical acute anal fissure in a healthy person can be caused by the local trauma of a hard stool, fissures can be associated with underlying inflammatory bowel disease, cancer, sexually transmitted infections, and even childbirth.

The location or multiplicity of an anal fissure can help determine both the etiology and chronicity of a fissure. Most commonly, the acute tear leads to anal pain that precipitates patient aversion to defecation and increased sphincter tone. The problem is exacerbated by the hypertonic sphincter at rest, which in turn causes decreased perfusion of the anoderm. The posterior midline, which has the lowest perfusion of all quadrants of the anoderm, is predisposed to mild ischemia with resultant poor healing, especially in the setting of increased anal pressure (3). For this reason, up to 90% of fissures can be found at the posterior midline. Fissures have been reported anteriorly in up to 25% of women and 8% of men, with 3% being found simultaneously in anterior and posterior positions. Atypical presentations, such as lateral, painless, or multiple fissures, should raise clinical suspicion for Crohn disease, ulcerative colitis, leukemia, trauma, tuberculosis, sexually transmitted diseases, HIV/AIDS, or anal carcinoma (Figure 21.2). Women with reduced anal canal pressures more often demonstrate anteriorly located fissures, which should prompt consideration for anal manometry or endorectal ultrasound prior to surgical interventions.

## NONOPERATIVE MANAGEMENT

### DIET AND LIFESTYLE MODIFICATION

Once the diagnosis of an anal fissure is confirmed, the initial and most conservative steps in management are to improve bowel consistency and control symptoms. Fiber supplementation with adequate water intake improves consistency and bulk of stool leading to less straining and trauma to the area. In a double-blind placebo-controlled trial, fissure recurrence was 16%, 60%, and 68% in patients receiving 15 g unprocessed bran, 7.5 g unprocessed bran, and placebo (4). Studies have shown that half of acute fissures resolve with sitz baths, psyllium, topical anesthetics, or anti-inflammatory ointments, making this the current recommendation in the American Society of Colon and Rectal Surgeons (ASCRS) Clinical Practice Guideline for initial management of acute fissure (5). Unfortunately, up to 50% of these fissures will recur within 5 years, and a 2012 Cochrane Review suggests no difference between lidocaine, bran, and hydrocortisone and placebo (6). There are few, if any, side effects to these interventions, and therefore, little risk exists in recommending these simple therapies to patients as initial treatment for acute anal fissure. If diet and lifestyle modifications have failed for a period of 6–8 weeks, the fissure is classified as chronic and may only improve with topical medications or surgery.

## NITRATES

The smooth muscle tone of the internal anal sphincter is partially affected by the nonadrenergic, noncholinergic neurotransmitter nitric oxide, which is released with the application of nitroglycerin cream. A compounded diluted mixture of 0.2%–0.4% glyceryl trinitrate (GTN) or nitroglycerin cream is applied to the anus two to three times daily for 4–8 weeks to relax the internal sphincter and allow the fissure to heal. Glyceryl trinitrate has been associated with an overall healing rate of 48.9% and an overall improvement in healing rate of 13.5% when compared to placebo or lidocaine alone in patients with chronic anal fissures (6). GTN applications in different dosages (from 0.05% to 0.4%) as well as methods of administration (intraanal injection or distant dermal patch application) have been investigated with similar results.

When compared with lateral internal sphincterotomy (LIS), nitrates generally demonstrate significantly lower healing rates after 6–8 weeks of therapy. Since the previous version of this volume, which referenced six studies demonstrating large differences in healing rates between LIS and nitrate therapy, only one additional study directly comparing the two therapies has been reported. These are summarized in Table 21.1. There are a number of other studies that compare these treatments, but their data groups involve crossover treatments and are not discussed in this chapter. While side effects of nitrates are minimal, headaches are reported in up to 30% of patients using nitrates, which often results in discontinuation of therapy and poor compliance. Therefore, the available data support that topical nitrates can be used to treat anal fissures with low risk, but with the expectation of lowered success rates in more chronic fissures and an associated risk of headaches.

## CALCIUM-CHANNEL BLOCKERS

Calcium-channel blockers, which include diltiazem and nifedipine, work similarly to relax the smooth muscle of the hypertonic internal sphincter and allow a fissure to heal. These medications can be used orally or topically with similar success. Topical diltiazem 2% must be prescribed from a compounding pharmacy and applied three times daily over 8 weeks. Numerous studies have demonstrated the success of calcium channel blockers, though the heterogeneity of dosing, small study number, and short follow-up time have limited the applicability of their conclusions. Healing of fissures with diltiazem appears to be similar to that of GTN (over 85%) when treated over 8 weeks with good follow-up (15). Unfortunately, recurrence of these fissures within 6 months is common. Calcium-channel blockers have demonstrated equivalent healing rates to topical nitrates, but with fewer side effects, such as headaches. Therefore, these medications are recommended more commonly as first-line medical therapy than nitrates. However, like other medical therapies with low-risk profiles, their long-term success rates are lower than sphincterotomy. One study demonstrated a 20% difference in anal fissure healing rates between 0.3% nifedipine plus lidocaine ointment with gentle dilation and LIS (16).

## BOTULINUM TOXIN

The exotoxin of the bacterium *Clostridium botulinum* can be injected locally to cause sympathetic blockade of the internal anal sphincter. Temporary paralysis of the internal anal sphincter can allow an acute anal fissure to heal. Botulinum injection of 20 units bilaterally has demonstrated superior effectiveness to nitroglycerin ointment. Healing rates of anal fissures with botulinum injection are between 37% and 43%, though the published data demonstrate a variety of botulinum doses in use. A Cochrane Review (6) suggested that botulinum toxin was slightly superior to placebo. In a randomized controlled trial of lateral internal sphincterotomy versus botulinum injection, LIS demonstrated superior outcomes (17). This study also demonstrated the concerning finding of recurrence of 50% of fissures that had previously healed 1 year after botulinum treatment. The paralytic effect of the toxin subsides after 3–5 months, which may contribute to fissure recurrence rates. The temporary effect may be used to the clinician's advantage since any side effects will also be temporary. Because healing rates of up to 43% have been demonstrated (18) and some equivalence in topical medications has been suggested, it can be recommended for use in the treatment of chronic anal fissure. Due to the temporary and few side effects, clinicians may prefer botulinum toxin to sphincterotomy in patients over 50 years old due to the risk of incontinence.

## SURGICAL MANAGEMENT

## ANAL DILATION

Dilation of the anal sphincters was thought to decrease the maximum resting anal pressure and therefore aid in healing of fissure due to hypertonic anal sphincters. Historically, manual digital dilation or graduated serial dilations with anal dilators were often used, but complications of incontinence from diffuse sphincter damage have largely led to the abandonment of this method as it has been shown to have worse healing rates with higher rates of incontinence (5). However, balloon dilation was evaluated in comparison to LIS in a prospective randomized trial and found to demonstrate similar fissure healing rates (19). After 2 years, there was less incontinence in the balloon dilation group than in the LIS group (0% versus 16%). Therefore, balloon dilation by a physician, not manual dilation, can be considered in the treatment of fissure; however, more research must be done before it could become a recommended treatment option for chronic anal fissures.

## LATERAL INTERNAL SPHINCTEROTOMY

The surgical procedure that has shown the most efficacy in the resolution of a chronic anal fissure is the LIS. This involves the partial division of the internal sphincter to counteract the hypertonicity that is the source of the typical anal fissure. Not surprisingly, incontinence of gas or liquid stool is an associated side effect in up to 10% of patients (20). The sphincterotomy is best made laterally on the internal sphincter so as to avoid risk of incontinence in women with thinned anterior sphincter or the dreaded "keyhole" deformity posteriorly caused by division of the internal sphincter through the posterior fissure. It has been shown in a number of studies that the extent of the sphincterotomy need not be the entire length of the muscle to the dentate line. No significant difference in healing rates was

Table 21.1  Randomized controlled trials of nitrates versus surgical sphincterotomy for the treatment of chronic anal fissure

| Author/year | Number of patients | Treatment groups (% ointment) | Treatment length (weeks) | Fissure healing (%) | Overall side effects (%) | HA (%) | IC flatus (%) | Follow-up (months) | Recurrence (%) |
|---|---|---|---|---|---|---|---|---|---|
| Oettle (7) | 24 | NTG/LIS TID | 4 | 83 versus 100 ($p$ = NS) | NR | NR | NR | 1 | NR |
| Richard (8) | 82 | 0.25/0.5 GTN/LIS TID | 6 | 30 versus 90 ($p$ = 0.0) | 84 versus 29 ($p < 0.001$) | 21 | None | 6 | 38 versus 3 |
| Evans (9) | 60 | 0.2 GTN/LIS TID | 8 | 61 versus 97 ($p < 0.001$) | NR | 33 | 7.4 | 5 | 45 versus 4 |
| Libertiny (10) | 70 | 0.2 GTN/LIS TID | 8 | 54 versus 100 ($p < 0.02$) | NR | 20 | 2.9 | 24 | 16 versus 2.9 |
| Parellada (11) | 54 | 0.2 IDN/LIS TID | 6 | 67 versus 96 ($p < 0.001$) | 30 versus 44 ($p$ = NR) | NR | 44@5 wk  15@24 wk | 24 | 13 versus 0 |
| Mishra (12) | 40 | 0.2 GTN/LIS BID | 6 | 90 versus 85 ($p$ = 0.347) | 40 versus 70 ($p$ = NR) | 15 | 15 | 4 | NR |
| Brown (13) | 51 | 0.25/0.5 NTG/LIS TID | 6 | 59 versus 100 ($p < 0.01$) | NR | NR | 67 | 79.4 | 37 versus 25% |

Source: Adapted from Whitlow CB et al. Improved Outcomes in Colon and Rectal Surgery. Boca Raton, FL: CRC Press, 2009, p. 203 (14).
Note: BID, twice daily; GTN, glyceryl trinitrate; HA, headache; IC, incontinence; IDN, isosorbide dinitrate; LIS, lateral internal sphincterotomy; NR, not reported; NS, not significant; NTG, nitroglycerin; TID, three times a day.

found between patients who underwent sphincterotomy the length of dentate line versus sphincterotomy to the apex of the fissure (21). Current recommendations have moderate-quality evidence to demonstrate that this tailored LIS yields equivalent healing rates with traditional LIS to the dentate line, and further investigation is needed. In conclusion, traditional LIS remains the standard of care until more data are obtained.

The sphincterotomy procedure can be performed as a "closed" or "open" technique, and numerous studies have shown equivalency of these methods. In the operating room, an exam under anesthesia is performed and the sphincter complex digitally palpated for the intersphincteric groove. In the "open" lateral internal sphincterotomy, an anal retractor of choice (Pratt bivalve or Hill-Ferguson of appropriate size) is used to place the sphincter complex on stretch, and a radial incision is made over the intersphincteric groove. The internal sphincter is then elevated under direct visualization and divided. The anoderm is then closed with an absorbable suture or left open.

The "closed" LIS is performed by similarly palpating the sphincter anatomy, inserting an 11-blade knife through the anoderm laterally in the intersphincteric groove. The blade is then rotated 90°, and the internal sphincter is then cut medially toward a finger in the anus.

Success rates of LIS have been consistently described near 90% in multiple studies and Cochrane reviews and is the treatment of choice for chronic or medically refractory anal fissures (22–26). The decision to proceed with LIS should be made judiciously in patients at high risk for incontinence, such as women, people older than 50 years, those with a history of previous anal surgery, or patients with sphincter injury after childbirth.

Last, recurrent anal fissure after LIS can be safely treated with repeat LIS on the contralateral side. This has been evaluated in a study of 55 people with 98% healing rate demonstrated at over a year after surgery (27).

## ADVANCEMENT FLAPS

In traditional fissures associated with hypertonicity, no significant difference has been found between healing rates in patients who underwent advancement flaps versus sphincterotomy. These flaps can be combined with LIS or botulinum toxin injection for decreased postoperative pain and good primary fissure healing. Combining anocutaneous flap with injection of botulinum toxin has shown healing rates from 86.7% to 92% at 2 years with minimal fecal incontinence (28,29). Similarly, when combined with LIS, advancement flaps can lead to less postoperative pain, faster healing, and fewer soiling episodes (30).

Anocutaneous flaps are considered a safe alternative to LIS due to good fissure healing rates (81%–100%) and lower rates of minor fecal incontinence (0%–6%) (31–33). If the underlying fissure pathology is hypotonicity rather than hypertonicity, an advancement flap may be ideal. Tissue healing can be aided by advancement flap without the need for a procedure to decrease anal tone.

Different techniques have been described for anorectal advancement flaps, all of which are created with the principle of transferring healthy tissue coverage for the chronic fissure wound. The simplest of these is the Y-V anoplasty. A Y-shaped incision is made to debride the fissure bed, and then the V flap is advanced into the anal canal and sutured in place. The wide base of the V allowed for a well-vascularized flap (Figure 21.3). Alternatively, the V-Y anoplasty involves a triangular incision with the apex on the perianal skin and the base made just past the fissure. After fissurectomy, the V is mobilized from the subcutaneous tissue and advanced into the anal canal with closure of the skin behind the V aiding in advancement of the flap (Figure 21.4). Less common techniques include the "house" advancement pedicle flap (Figure 21.5) and the diamond flap (Figure 21.6), which can be used if more circumferential coverage is needed along the anal canal. The editors prefer the House flap.

(a)          (b)          (c)

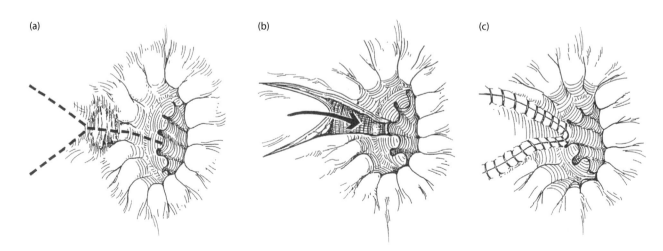

Figure 21.3 Y-V Anoplasty. (Reprinted with permission from Whitlow CB et al. *Improved Outcomes in Colon and Rectal Surgery*. Boca Raton, FL: CRC Press, 2009, pp. 199–214.)

(a)   (b)

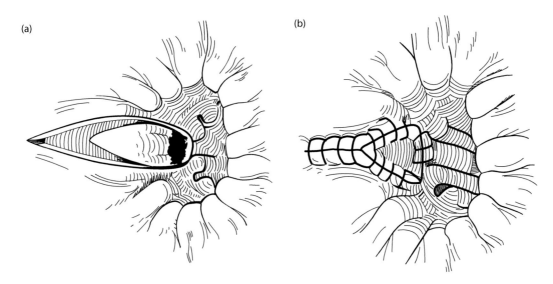

Figure 21.4  V-Y Anoplasty. (Reprinted with permission from Whitlow CB et al. *Improved Outcomes in Colon and Rectal Surgery.* Boca Raton, FL: CRC Press, 2009, pp. 199–214.)

(a)   (b)   (c)

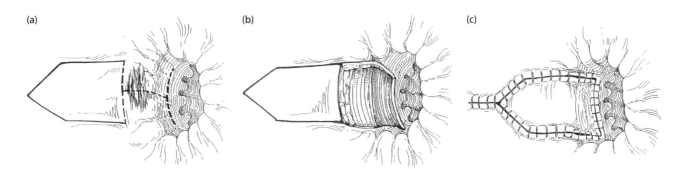

Figure 21.5  House advancement flap. (Reprinted with permission from Whitlow CB et al. *Improved Outcomes in Colon and Rectal Surgery.* Boca Raton, FL: CRC Press, 2009, pp. 199–214.)

(a)   (b)   (c)

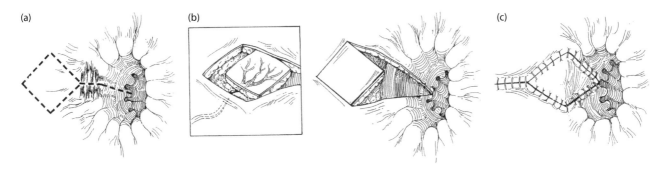

Figure 21.6  Diamond flap. (Reprinted with permission from Whitlow CB et al. *Improved Outcomes in Colon and Rectal Surgery.* Boca Raton, FL: CRC Press, 2009, pp. 199–214.)

## SPECIAL SITUATIONS

## CROHN DISEASE

Anorectal surgery for anal fissures should be avoided in patients with active Crohn disease in favor of medical management of the underlying disease. Fissures in these patients are usually a manifestation of active inflammation and should be suspected if fissures are atypical in location or appearance, or are multiple in number. Fissures in Crohn disease tend to be deeper in nature and can be associated with fistulas, which if left unmanaged can lead to significant sphincter deformity. Therefore, efforts should be directed toward continence preservation with medical management of the underlying Crohn disease.

## SEXUALLY TRANSMITTED DISEASES

Sexually transmitted diseases such as syphilis and HIV have a known association with anal fissures. HIV-related anorectal disease can manifest as ulcers or fissures in atypical locations. These fissures are unique in that instead of the typical sharp pain on defecation, patients often have painless or persistent "gnawing" pain (34). These are more often associated with poor sphincter tone. Examination under anesthesia with viral culture or biopsy should be performed to confirm acute infections and to rule out similarly presenting pathology such as HIV-related anal ulcer. Appropriate antibiotics should be used to treat syphilis or other sexually transmitted diseases. HIV-related fissure treatment should be aimed at optimizing treatment with antiretroviral therapy.

## FISSURES WITHOUT HYPERTONICITY

Acute low-pressure anal fissures are most commonly seen in postpartum patients, and these should be managed conservatively with medications and lifestyle modification. Because fissures in the presence of sphincter hypotonicity are not improved by sphincter relaxants or sphincterotomy, treatment measures should be directed toward healing of the fissure wound.

Chronic fissures in postpartum patients can be managed with fissurectomy and advancement flap with near perfect results (35). Similarly, other fissures in the setting of hypotonicity should be considered for anorectal advancement flap as therapy in the chronic setting.

## CONCLUSION

Acute anal fissure in the otherwise healthy individual with resultant hypertonic sphincter can be treated with lifestyle modifications, topical relaxants, and close clinical follow-up to determine resolution of symptoms. Chronic anal fissures in the setting of a hypertonic sphincter, including anal fissure refractory to medical management, should be considered for further therapies, including botulinum injection, lateral internal sphincterotomy, or combination of botulinum injection/LIS with anorectal advancement flap. Fissures due to inflammatory bowel disease, sexually transmitted diseases, or HIV should be managed by confirming diagnosis with examination under anesthesia and biopsy or culture, and medical management of the underlying disease process. In patients with anal fissure with suspected hypotonic sphincter mechanism or who are at high risk for incontinence (multiparous female or previous anorectal surgery), anal manometry or endorectal ultrasound should be considered. Patients with chronic anal fissure with reduced resting anal pressures should be conservatively managed, then considered for fissurectomy and anorectal advancement flap. Lateral internal sphincterotomy has consistently demonstrated high rates of healing and is considered the treatment of choice in patients with chronic anal fissure. Last, repeat contralateral LIS can be performed in patients with recurrent anal fissure who continue to demonstrate hypertonic sphincter.

## REFERENCES

1. Corby H et al. *Br J Surg.* 1997;84:86–8.
2. Beck DE et al. *The ASCRS Textbook of Colon and Rectal Surgery.* New York: Springer, 2011.
3. Schouten WR et al. *Dis Colon Rectum.* 1994;37:664–9.
4. Jensen SL. *Br Med J (Clin Res Ed).* 1986;292:1167–9.
5. Stewart DB et al. *Dis Colon Rectum.* 2017;60:7–14.
6. Nelson RL et al. *Cochrane Database Syst Rev.* 2012; Issue 2: Art. no. CD003431. DOI: 10.1002/14651858.CD003431.pub3.
7. Oettlé GJ. *Dis Colon Rectum.* 1997;40:1318–20.
8. Richard CS et al. *Dis Colon Rectum.* 2000;43:1048–57; discussion 1057.
9. Evans J et al. *Dis Colon Rectum.* 2001;44:93–7.
10. Libertiny G et al. *Eur J Surg.* 2002;168:418–21.
11. Parellada C. *Dis Colon Rectum.* 2004;47:437–43.
12. Mishra R et al. *ANZ J Surg.* 2005;75:1032–5.
13. Brown CJ et al. *Dis Colon Rectum.* 2007;50:442–8.
14. Whitlow CB et al. *Improved Outcomes in Colon and Rectal Surgery.* Boca Raton, FL: CRC Press, 2009.
15. Bielecki K, Kolodziejczak M. *Colorectal Dis.* 2003; 5:256–7.
16. de Rosa M et al. *Updates Surg.* 2013;65:197–200.
17. Arroyo A et al. *Am J Surg.* 2005;189:429–34.
18. Samim M et al. *Ann Surg.* 2012;255:18–22.
19. Renzi A et al. *Dis Colon Rectum.* 2008;51:121–7.
20. Nelson R. *Cochrane Database Syst Rev.* 2005; Issue 2: Art. no. CD002199. DOI: 10.1002/14651858.CD002199.pub2.
21. Elsebae MM. *World J Surg.* 2007;31:2052–7.
22. Saad AM, Omer A. *East Afr Med J.* 1992;69:613–5.
23. Olsen J et al. *Int J Colorectal Dis.* 1987;2:155–7.
24. Weaver RM et al. *Dis Colon Rectum.* 1987;30:420–3.
25. Ram E et al. *Tech Coloproctol.* 2007. https://doi.org/10.1007/s10151-007-0373-7
26. Nelson RL et al. *Cochrane Database Syst Rev.* 2011; Issue 11: Art. No.: CD002199. DOI: 10.1002/14651858.CD002199.pub4.
27. Leong AF, Seow-Choen F. *Dis Colon Rectum.* 1995; 38:69–71.
28. Halahakoon VC, Pitt JP. *Int J Colorectal Dis* 2014; 29(9):1175–7.
29. Patti R et al. *Updates Surg.* 2012;64:101–6.
30. Theodoropoulos GE et al. *Am Surg.* 2015;81:133–42.
31. Gupta P. *ANZ J Surg.* 2006;76:718–21.
32. Kennedy ML et al. *Dis Colon Rectum.* 1999;42:1000–6.
33. Giordano P et al. *World J Surg.* 2009;33:1058–63.
34. Viamonte M et al. *Dis Colon Rectum.* 1993;36:801–5.
35. Patti R et al. *Colorectal Dis.* 2010;12:1127–30.

# 22

# Surgery for pilonidal disease and hidradenitis suppurativa

JOHN D. HUNTER AND LEANDER M. GRIMM JR.

## PILONIDAL DISEASE

### INTRODUCTION

Pilonidal disease is a chronic inflammatory condition of the skin and associated hair follicles typically found in the sacrococcygeal region. Clinically, pilonidal disease can present on a wide spectrum, including asymptomatic incidentally found pits, acute or recurrent abscess, chronically draining sinus, or a large nonhealing wound from a previous attempted repair. The environment of the natal cleft can be moist, hirsute, unhygienic, and subject to a wide range of forces throughout the day. These characteristics can lead to a unique challenge for the surgeon treating pilonidal disease.

The true incidence of pilonidal disease is unclear. It has been reported anywhere from 26 per 100,000 to 4.6% (1,2). Typical age at presentation is in the late teens to early 30s. It is rarely found in patients older than 45 years. Classically it is found in young adult Caucasian males. However, recent military data reported a similar incidence rate among males and females (1.9 and 1.7 per 1,000 p-years) (3).

### BACKGROUND

The first description of pilonidal disease is credited to Herbert Mayo in 1833. In his chapter on fistula disease, he describes a young woman with a sinus opening an inch behind the anus and "upon examining it with a probe, I found that instead of running towards the rectum, it extended upwards for a length of five inches between the skin and os sacrum" (4). In 1844, Anderson gave a description of hair extracted from an ulcer (5). Hodges later coined the term "pilonidal" in 1880, derived from the Latin words for "hair" and "nest" (6). Pilonidal disease became much more prevalent in World War II, during which 80,000 soldiers were hospitalized with the disease for an average of 55 days each (7). Buie coined the term "jeep disease," attributing pilonidal disease to trauma to the gluteal cleft from riding long distances over rough terrain in jeeps under hot and sweaty conditions (8).

### ETIOLOGY

Pilonidal disease was initially thought to be congenital in origin. Failed involution of neural tube structures left remnants that eventually became pilonidal cysts and sinuses (9). In 1946 Patey challenged this theory, suggesting that pilonidal disease was acquired from hair piercing the skin of the gluteal cleft, leading to local inflammation and eventual cysts and sinuses. Karydakis studied over 6,000 cases and surmised three main factors leading to pilonidal disease: (1) an "invader," that is, loose hair applying a (2) force causing hair insertion, composed of factors including depth, narrowness, and friction of the gluteal cleft, and (3) vulnerability of the skin and soft tissues. Loose hairs from the head, back, and natal cleft accumulate in the natal cleft. Friction from walking drives the hairs into the skin creating a foreign-body reaction. This eventually creates a "pit" opening through which more hairs are pulled and eventually form a chronic cavity (10). Bascom also suggests that native hair follicles of the natal cleft become infected with keratin, which leads to infection and abscess formation. Friction forces then "suck" hair into the cavity, further seeding the inflammatory cycle (11). (Figure 22.1) The acquired theory is further supported by reports of pilonidal disease in the interdigital regions of the hands of barbers, pet groomers, sheep shearers, and cow milkers (12–15).

Risk factors for the development of pilonidal disease include hirsutism, deep natal cleft, obesity, poor hygiene, prolonged sitting, excessive sweating, and family history. A prospective case control study by Harlak in 2010 studied 587 patients with pilonidal disease and compared them to 2,780 healthy controls. The four most predictive factors were (from strongest to weakest) body hair stiffness, number of baths per week, hours spent seated per day, and body mass index. They showed that hirsute individuals who sit

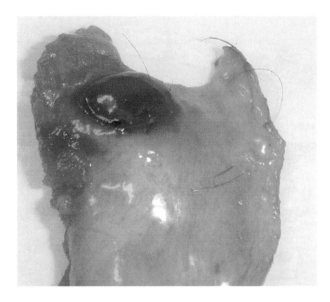

Figure 22.1 **(See color insert.)** Pilonidal cyst opened after excision showing hair inside cavity.

for >6 hours per day and bathe two or less times per week have a 219-fold increased risk of pilonidal disease. This fits with the higher incidence of the disease seen in military populations (16).

## PRESENTATION AND DIAGNOSIS

With the wide spectrum of pilonidal disease, the surgeon can see a variety of clinical presentations. Some patients are referred for an incidental finding of midline pits and are completely asymptomatic. Others may have had an acute abscess already drained and are referred for further management. Then there are patients with persistent disease that can range from minimally symptomatic to debilitating wounds that have failed multiple operations.

The diagnosis of pilonidal disease is made by history and physical. Patients often complain of a vague pain over the sacrum that is often associated with intermittent clear or bloody drainage. The drainage is sometimes confused with rectal bleeding. An acute abscess may have accompanying fevers or purulent drainage. (Figure 22.2) Classic physical examination findings are one or more midline "pits" 3–5 cm posterior to the anus (Figure 22.3). These are often associated with an acute abscess or chronic draining sinus off midline. Probing the sinus with a fine clamp will reveal numerous tufts of hair. Differential diagnosis includes hidradenitis, anorectal abscess, and anorectal fistula, and digital rectal examination and anoscopy (or proctoscopy) should be performed to exclude these diagnoses.

## MANAGEMENT OF ACUTE DISEASE

An acute abscess secondary to pilonidal disease is managed like any other abscess. Incision and drainage can be carried out at the bedside under local anesthetic or in the operating room under general or regional anesthesia. Lateral

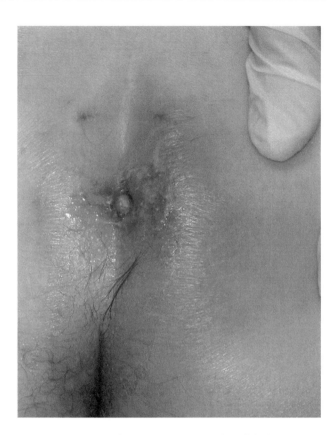

Figure 22.2 **(See color insert.)** Acute pilonidal abscess. Note midline opening with abscess slightly to the right of midline.

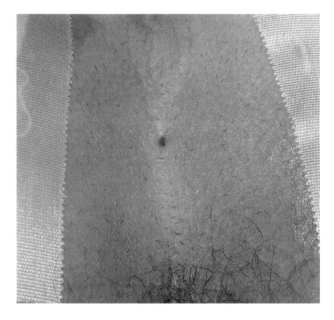

Figure 22.3 **(See color insert.)** Chronic pilonidal disease showing midline pit.

decubitus or prone positioning allows proper exposure. The area of fluctuance is typically 1–2 cm off midline; an elliptical incision is made over this area, and the cavity is debrided of all purulence and hair. Thorough irrigation, hemostasis, and packing complete the procedure. Postoperative antibiotic use is typically not needed unless significant cellulitis is encountered.

The importance of the off-midline incision was reported in a 2011 study, where 96 patients with acute presentation of pilonidal abscess were treated with midline versus off-midline incisions. This retrospective review found the patients receiving an off-midline incision healed about 3 weeks faster (17).

Incision and drainage can at times be definitive. In a series of 73 patients who underwent incision and drainage for acute abscess in the setting of first-time pilonidal presentation, 58% had healed wounds at 10 weeks. Of those patients, 21% had recurrence during the mean follow-up of 60 months. Those patients with fewer pits and tracts had a better chance of complete cure (18).

## MANAGEMENT OF CHRONIC DISEASE

In the setting of chronic disease, it is crucial for the surgeon to tailor treatment to the individual patient. Patient expectations should be managed early and often, stressing the possibility of extended periods of wound care that may be borne out of failed smaller procedures or more aggressive procedures.

## NONOPERATIVE AND MINIMALLY INVASIVE MANAGEMENT

Patients who present with asymptomatic or minimally symptomatic disease can be safely observed. Nonoperative management should focus on good hygiene with attention directed toward keeping the natal cleft clean and dry. Patients whose job requires them to sit for prolonged periods should be encouraged to briefly stand and walk around multiple times a day.

### Depilation

Given that hair is the inciting factor in pilonidal disease, removing hair from the natal cleft would intuitively lessen the progression and potentially provide an environment to heal some pilonidal disease. Weekly shaving can improve the environment of the natal cleft and aid in healing.

A pilot study in the mid-1970s compared conservative management of pilonidal disease in 101 soldiers at a single Army training hospital to the previous 2 years of excisional therapy. They applied conservative measures such as hygiene education, meticulous hair shaving, simple lateral incision and drainage for acute abscess, and avoidance of certain exercises that put stress on the sacrococcygeal region (sit-ups and leg lifts). Hair shaving consisted of a 5 cm strip shaved from the anus to the presacrum every week until healing occurred. Over the 1-year period, the conservative group required no operations, compared to the 240 operations during the 2 years prior. Number of occupied bed days decreased to 83 from 4,760 during the 2 years prior. A follow-up study applied the conservative

pilonidal protocol over a period of 17 years to the population of Tripler Army Medical Center in Hawaii. During the 17-year study period of 150 pilonidal admissions, there were only 23 excisional procedures performed. Admissions were reduced by 78% between the first 4 years and last 4 years of the study (19).

Laser depilation has been used with some success in the treatment of recurrent pilonidal disease. It offers the advantage of longer-term hair control. However, the hair loss is not permanent, and treatments can be painful and often require local anesthetic. Odili et al. reported 14 patients with recurrent pilonidal wounds after multiple surgical procedures (average three) who underwent laser depilation. Eight patients were healed by 1 year and 10 by the second year. The remaining four healed after a second treatment. They postulated that without hair present, secondary healing proceeded rapidly (20).

Razor and laser depilation have also been shown to have adverse effects on the recurrence rate of pilonidal disease. Peterson and colleagues reviewed 504 patients who were treated surgically, 113 of whom shaved the area postoperatively. They observed a 30.1% recurrence rate in those who shaved versus 19.7% in those who did not (21). Another study looked at laser depilation prior to undergoing flap reconstruction for pilonidal disease. They found a 20% recurrence rate in laser depilation group versus 4% in the control group (22).

### Fibrin

Fibrin glue injections have been used to treat chronically draining pilonidal sinuses. The idea is that forming a fibrin clot within the sinus would obliterate dead space and promote healing through clotting cascade signaling. A similar technique has been applied to anal fistulas with variable success. Lund and Leveson treated six patients with chronic draining pilonidal sinuses with fibrin glue. Half were recurrent patients, while the others were primary presentations. Under general anesthesia, they curetted the pits and then injected 2 mL of fibrin. They reported minimal postoperative discomfort, 2–3 day return to work, and one recurrence 4 months after treatment. There were no other recurrences at 18 months (23). In a similar study in 2014, Isik et al. reported on 40 patients treated with fibrin glue injection. With a patient selection that excluded more than one sinus tract, no previous sinus infection, no previous treatment, and no history of recurrence, they achieved a 10% recurrence rate at 1 year (24).

A variation on direct injection, simple excision followed by fibrin injection was performed on 25 patients by Saleem et al. in 2004. Again, these were first-time presenters with noninfected tracts numbering from 1 to 3. Simple excision of the entire pit/tract complex was performed down to the postsacral fascia with minimal skin excision, followed by injection of the cavity with fibrin glue. With a mean follow-up on 10.8 months, they achieved a 96% healing rate (25).

## Phenol

Sclerotherapy with phenol has been used to treat nonrecurrent pilonidal disease. The technique consists of first removing the hairs from the deep cavity through the pits. Phenol is then placed through the pits into the cavity, either by injection or in crystal form, and left in for 2 minutes. After, the phenol is removed through expression. Necrotic debris is then removed 24 hours later. At follow-up, if there is continued leakage, the process is repeated.

A group of 76 patients were treated with phenol sclerotherapy in a 2012 study. The overall success rate was 67%. Return to work was immediate for all patients. Patients with a previous abscess drainage or more than three sinus openings, or those who required more than one treatment were at higher risk of failure (26). A more recent prospective randomized control trial (RCT) compared phenol injection to excision and healing by secondary intent in 140 primary and recurrent pilonidal patients (27). Wound healing time, operative time, time to normal activity, and pain scale all heavily favored the phenol group. At 3 weeks, 89% of the patients in the phenol group were healed; at 6 weeks all were healed. At 40 months of follow-up, there was no significant difference in recurrence rates (18.6% versus 12.9%).

## SURGICAL TREATMENT

Recurrent, chronic, and nonhealing pilonidal disease requires a more aggressive surgical approach for cure. Complete excision of the disease leaves a large open wound that is difficult to manage given the location. Thus, many different approaches have been developed in an attempt to find the optimal operation for pilonidal disease. Of course, none of them are appropriate in every patient, and ultimately selection is based on patient parameters and surgeon comfort. The most common techniques are presented here.

In general, these procedures are performed in the prone jackknife position with the buttocks taped apart. Standard preoperative antibiotics are given. The simpler procedures can be done as an outpatient, whereas the more complex flap procedures will usually require a short hospital stay for bedrest, pain control, and wound monitoring.

## MINIMAL/MODERATE DISEASE

### Unroofing and wide local excision

Unroofing consists of laying open all sinus tracts and cysts that make up the pilonidal complex in a manner similar to fistulotomy for simple anal fistulas. This technique, along with wide local excision, is among the earlier and most common treatments for pilonidal disease.

Once the patient is positioned and prepped, the pits are probed to identify sinus tracts. The sinus tracts are then opened along the length of the probe. All extensions and tracts of the sinus are opened and then debris, hair, and granulation tissue are removed with curette. Care should

be taken to keep as much of the wound off midline as possible. Wound edges are then excised to prevent early closure. Once hemostasis is obtained, the wound is packed and covered. Patients are discharged home the same day with adequate oral analgesia. Wound care consists of daily packing and showering, with the help of a family member or home health provider. Close follow-up in the immediate postoperative phase allows for adequate monitoring and as-needed debridement and separation of wound edges.

Kepenecki and colleagues reported on their experience with this technique in 2009. In this report, 297 patients presenting with acute, chronic, or recurrent disease were subjected to the unroofing technique; 84.5% were done under local anesthesia. Return to work was 3.2 days, and average healing time was 5.4 weeks. During their average follow-up time of 54 months, they reported only a 2% recurrence rate (28).

Marsupialization involves suturing the skin edges to the base of the unroofed wound with absorbable suture. The goal is to create a smaller shallow wound that heals faster and is easier for the patient to manage (Figure 22.4). A 2007 study examined 26 patients who underwent wide local excision and 42 who underwent unroofing and marsupialization. Mean time to healing (21 versus 6 weeks), postoperative complications, and reoperative rate (35% versus 2%) all favored the unroofing and marsupialization group (29). A more recent study examined 39 patients who underwent either wide local excision or unroofing and marsupialization. Their evidence also favored unroofing and marsupialization, demonstrating a faster healing time (5.9 versus 23 weeks), reduced recurrence (4% versus 31%), and no need for reoperation (0% versus 25%) (30).

Wide local excision involves removing the entire pilonidal cyst/sinus complex. An elliptical incision is made to include all the sinus tracts and is carried down to the sacrococcygeal fascia to ensure the entire cyst cavity is removed. The resulting wound can be either closed or left open to heal by secondary intention. Closing the wound makes postoperative care simpler, but this can lead to wound breakdown or infection. Leaving the wound open lessens the chance of infection but leaves the patient with difficult and cumbersome wound care that can often take months to heal. The use of negative pressure wound therapy to augment healing of large pilonidal wounds has been investigated. A recent study treated 24 patients with wound vac therapy after wide local excision for 2 weeks postoperatively and then switched to regular dressing changes. When compared with the control group, the wound vac group had significantly smaller wounds at 2 weeks. Complete healing was achieved at 84 days versus 93 days in the control group (31).

Several RCTs have examined primary closure versus leaving the wound open to heal secondarily. A recently updated Cochrane Review of these trials showed there was no difference in wound infection between the two, and healing rates were faster in the closure group. The recurrence rate was 35% less in the open group, but when the midline closures were removed from analysis, the recurrence rates

Figure 22.4 **(See color insert.)** Marsupialization the diseased tissue is excised with electocautery **(a)**, and the cavity is debrided **(b)**. The edges of the wound are then sutured down to the base of the wound using absorbable suture **(c)**, resulting in a small open wound **(d)**.

were no different. Thus, primary off mid-line closure is recommended in wide local excision. The risk of infection and recurrence is similar to open healing, and the patient gains the benefit of faster healing with less wound care and scarring (32).

## Limited excision

Limited sinus excision was developed to minimize morbidity in the treatment of limited pilonidal disease, defined as four or less pits and no active infection. Oncel and colleagues reported a technique that excises the individual pits in an upside-down funnel-shaped manner. Methylene blue is injected into the pits to aid in identification of the tract and sinus. They stressed that only the minimum amount of tissue is removed, and there is no need to dissect all the way to the postsacral fascia. If two sinuses are connected, the fistula tract and overlying skin are also excised. The wounds are left open to heal by secondary intention (33). They later reported on 62 consecutive patients with limited pilonidal disease treated with the technique. Mean return to work was 2 days; mean healing was 43 days. At 1-year follow-up, they had only one recurrence.

Soll and colleagues described a similar technique for limited excision. Along with patients having more than four pits, they also excluded those with a distance of more than 8 cm between pits. Their initial report of 93 consecutive

patients demonstrated a median healing time of 5 weeks and a 5% recurrence rate at 2 years (34). They later reported long-term data on 257 patients. At 3.6 years, the overall recurrence was 7%, and median time to work was 7 days. They also emphasized the majority of the procedures (93%) were able to be performed under local anesthesia (35).

Mohamed and colleagues prospectively compared this limited excision technique to wide local excision left open and wide local excision with primary closure. They found the limited excision group to have shorter operative time, shorter hospital stay, and less postoperative pain. Healing time was significantly shorter for the closed incision and limited incision groups. With a minimum follow-up of 15 months, there was no difference in recurrence rates (36).

## Bascom procedure

In 1980, Bascom described a minimally invasive technique for pilonidal disease that focused on removing the midline pits rather than large amounts of tissue. He based this off the idea that the hair follicle itself was the source of the inflammation that leads to the development of the sinus and cyst. The abscess cavity is incised off midline and debrided. The cavity walls are not excised. The associated fistula tracts are dissected out and excised. The midline pits are then individually excised (sometimes referred to as "pit picking") and closed with absorbable suture. Punch biopsy devices can be

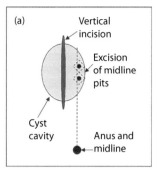
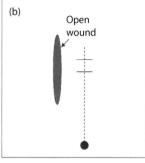

Figure 22.5 Bascom operation. **(a)** A vertical incision is made overlying the cyst, 1cm away from the gluteal cleft. The cyst cavity any communicating fistula tracts are debrided. The midline pits are excised, with the wounds communicating to the cavity. **(b)** The midline wounds are closed primarily with absorbable suture and the vertical wound is packed lightly and left to heal by secondary intention.

employed for this portion. The lateral wound is left open or closed partially to heal by secondary intention (37) (Figure 22.5). His initial experience with 149 patients showed an average healing time of 3 weeks, time to work of 1 day, and a 16% minor complication/recurrence rate at 3.5 years (38). In 2000, Senapati and colleagues performed the Bascom technique on 218 patients: 68% of the patients had more than two midline pits and/or a lateral discharging sinus. They achieved an initial success rate of 90% (39). Others have shown that for simple pilonidal disease, the Bascom procedure can be performed with minimal pain, early return to work, and an acceptable success rate (40).

## ADVANCED DISEASE

A small but significant portion of pilonidal patients will go on to develop chronic nonhealing wounds. These may be the result of wide local excision left to heal secondarily, breakdown of a closure, recurrence of disease, or unacceptable

scarring. These patients will require excision of diseased tissue and subsequent closure of the defect with various tissue transfer techniques. Here, we discuss the more common advanced techniques that can be employed by the colorectal or general surgeon. More advanced tissue transfers should involve consultation with a plastic surgeon.

## Karydakis flap

In 1973 Karydakis described his operation as one "which places resistant skin at the depth of the intergluteal fold" (41). With the patient prone and the buttocks taped apart, an off-midline elliptical incision is made in a vertical orientation centered about the bulk of the disease. This is carried down to the sacrococcygeal fascia, and all the disease tissue is removed en bloc. A skin flap is then raised across midline, such that when the tape is released the wound edges come together allowing for a closure under minimal tension. The result is an off-midline incision and a flatter gluteal cleft less prone to recurrent pilonidal disease (Figure 22.6). Given the large potential space created, drainage can be employed to help prevent fluid collections. A 2005 study showed that routine drainage decreased the risk of significant seroma formation in Karydakis flaps by 24%, avoiding painful postoperative office drainage procedures (42).

Karydakis published his initial experience with 6,545 cases and reported a <1% recurrence rate (10). Kitchen later published on a series of 141 patients with an 18-month follow-up and demonstrated a 96% success rate. Findings were that 23% of the patients presented with recurrence from previously treated disease and were all completely cured with the Karydakis flap (43). Other studies have continued to show the Karydakis flap to be a durable procedure for the treatment of pilonidal disease. A prospective randomized trial in 2015 compared 161 Karydakis flap patients to 160 undergoing excision alone with secondary healing. The recurrence rate in the flap group was 1.2% versus 7.5% in the excision alone, suggesting an important role in the flattening of the gluteal cleft to prevent

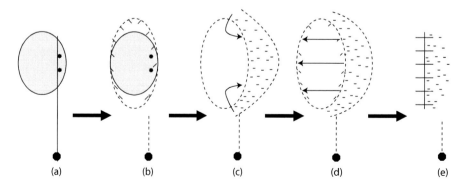

(a)  (b)  (c)  (d)  (e)

Figure 22.6 Karydakis flap. **(a)** Schematic of the operative field depicting a pilonidal cyst slightly to the left of midline with 2 midline pits. **(b)** An elliptical incision is made encompassing the cyst and pits. The excision is carried down to the sacrococcygeal fascia. **(c)** The medial edge of the wound is raised as a flap crossing the midline. **(d)** The tape retracting the buttocks is released so that the wound edges are able to be approximated without tension. **(e)** Final result showing a vertical incision closed primarily away from the midline, resulting in a flattened gluteal cleft.

recurrence (44). A 2011 prospective randomized study of 269 patients compared the Karydakis flap to the Limberg flap (discussed in the following). The Karydakis group had a lower complication rate, lower postoperative pain score, and better perceived cosmetic result. The recurrence rate was lower (3% versus 9%), but this was not statistically significant (45).

## Bascom cleft lift

In 2002 Bascom offered a modification to the Karydakis flap to use for patients with severe recurrent disease that has become known as the "cleft lift" or "Bascom II." The procedure begins with preoperative marking—the buttocks are pressed together while standing and the line of contact is marked. In the operating room, the ellipse of skin to be removed is marked to include the midline pits and previous scar but does not extend past the preoperatively marked line. The ellipse is excised into the cyst cavity, unroofing it. The cyst wall is scrubbed with gauze to promote granulation and incised in various locations to release tension, while secondary openings are enlarged to promote drainage. A flap is then raised across midline to the preoperatively marked line. When the tape is released, the edges come together and an off-midline wound is closed with minimal tension (Figure 22.7). A drain is left in place. In his initial series of 31 patients with severe recurrent pilonidal disease, all of them healed completely, and none had recurred at 20 months (11). Bascom later reported on 69 patients, all of whom had undergone at least two prior surgeries, who were treated with the cleft lift procedure. All but three were healed with a single operation. The others required one to two repeat procedures (46). Others have reproduced similar results, with or without a drain, reporting very little if any recurrence (47).

## Advanced flaps

More advanced flaps include rotational and myocutaneous flaps. The rhomboid flap, and its variants the Limberg and Dufourmental flaps, are commonly used rotational flaps. The cyst and midline pits are excised down to the sacrococcygeal fascia via a rhomboid-shaped skin incision with its long axis oriented vertically. A triangular incision with the same acute angle and side-length as the rhomboid is made based on the lateral extent of the initial incision and rotated in to fill the defect (Figure 22.8). A randomized trial comparing the Limberg flap to primary closure showed the Limberg flap patients to have shorter hospital stays, less time off work, fewer postoperative complications, and a lower recurrence rate. Equivalent outcomes have been reported between the Limberg and Karydakis flaps (48). One advantage the Limberg flap has over the Karydakis flap is the ability to excise very lateral disease without the risk of tension in the closure (49).

Other flaps used to treat extensive pilonidal disease include the V-Y flap and Z-plasty, along with other rotational flaps. Myocutaneous flaps based off the gluteus maximus can be used to fill large chronic nonhealing defects. The choice of which approach to use will depend on patient factors and surgeon comfort. When planning complex pilonidal repair with large flap coverage, consultation with a plastic surgeon is recommended. Poor flap selection in an initial operation can limit options for the patient should the patient require additional procedures.

## CONCLUSION

Pilonidal disease can present in a variety of ways. The patient who presents with a straightforward case of pilonidal disease can evolve into a complex problem with significant morbidity. It is imperative for the surgeon to understand

(a)

(b)

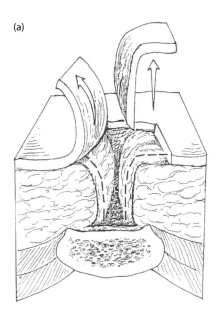
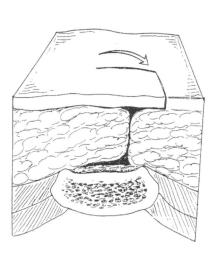

Figure 22.7 U-flap technique as described by Bascom for non-healing wounds. **(a)** One side of would is excised and the other side is elevated as a flap. **(b)** Deep wound is closed and remaining flap is advanced to allow closure of incision off midline.

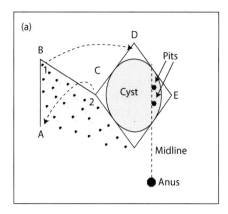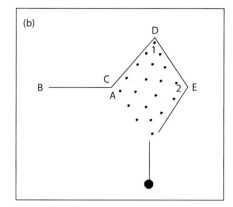

Figure 22.8 Rhomboid flap. **(a)** A rhomboid incision encompassing the pilonidal cyst and midline pits is marked on the skin, along with a lateral extension. The rhomboid is composed of 2 120° angles and 2 60° angles. Line BC is drawn at a 90° angle to Line CD. Line AB is drawn vertically down. All lines should be of equal length. The cavity is excised down to fascia and debrided. The flap is raised and mobilized to cover the defect. **(b)** The flap is rotated into the defect so that Point 2 meets Point E, Point 1 meets Point D, and Point A meets Point C. This results in a primarily closed wound and flattened gluteal cleft.

the disease process, variety of treatments, as well as unique individual patient factors when evaluating pilonidal disease. Appropriate selection of treatment early on will ultimately lead to better outcomes for the patient (Figure 22.9).

## PERIANAL HIDRADENITIS SUPPURATIVA

## BACKGROUND AND PATHOPHYSIOLOGY

Historically, hidradenitis suppurativa (HS) has long been defined as a chronic, waxing and waning disease process involving inflammation and infection of the apocrine sweat glands, which predominate in the axillary, inguinal, and perianal regions. This disease process was first described in the literature by the French physician Velpeau in 1832 (50). It was not until 1864 that another French physician, Vernuil, associated the disease process with sweat glands in the skin, thus coining the term *hidradenitis suppurativa*; however, Vernuil made this association not through histopathological

studies, but rather by noting that the most common areas of disease distribution in HS correlated with areas where these sweat glands are primarily found (51,52).

More modern histopathologic studies have argued quite vociferously and convincingly that HS is actually a disease process that begins with occlusion of hair follicles, similar to the pathogenesis of the common acne vulgaris, and that apocrine sweat glands are only involved secondarily, if at all, in cases of widespread follicular obstruction and infection. Whereas acne vulgaris is more frequently seen in areas with a predominance of sebaceous sweat glands such as the face and upper back/chest, HS tends to most commonly appear in the opposite or *inverse* anatomical areas, primarily the axilla, groin, and perianal regions, but also any other intertriginous region, such as the inframammary folds, scrotum, labia, and perineum (52). Thus, HS is now more accurately referred to as *acne inversa*, a term first used in this manner by Plewig and Stegar in 1989 (53). Despite this more accurate name, the term *hidradenitis suppurativa* has been maintained and is still used most frequently for this disease, especially in the surgical literature.

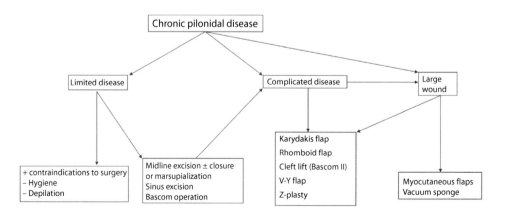

Figure 22.9 Algorithm for management of pilonidal disease.

A recent study by Danby et al. further characterized the process of follicular obstruction by identifying a defect in the basement membrane at the sebofollicular junction of the folliculopilosebaceous unit as the initiating event, which leads to bacterial colonization and subsequent inflammation and infection (54,55). When there are multiple adjacent areas of follicular obstruction, these areas may rupture and even connect via sinuses and fistulas as they become infected. This can lead to wide areas of purulent drainage and discomfort. Some mild cases may respond at least initially to a course of antibiotics or simple drainage or unroofing of the tracts, but in severe cases, the recurrent nature of the disease can often lead to areas of active infection coalescing with widespread areas of fibrosis and scar, rendering a regional catacomb of disease in a patient who is not only in a constant state of discomfort but also often severely socially isolated due to the malodor and dyshygienic appearance of those suffering from chronic severe disease (56).

## CLASSIFICATION

Most commonly, HS is classified by degree of severity according to the Hurley staging system (57). Hurley stage I disease is characterized by simple abscess formation, either single or multiple, but without sinus tracts or scarring. Stage II disease is characterized by recurrent abscesses with the formation of sinus tracts and scarring, but these occur as either single lesions or multiple lesions that are widely separated. Hurley stage III (Figure 22.10) represents the most severe stage of HS, defined by diffuse or nearly diffuse involvement of the entire affected region with numerous interconnected, honeycombing sinus tracts and abscesses throughout (55–58). Hurley III patients are those most likely to ultimately require radical surgical excision.

Recently, a group from France further stratified Hurley II/III patients into three latent classes (LC1-3) based on

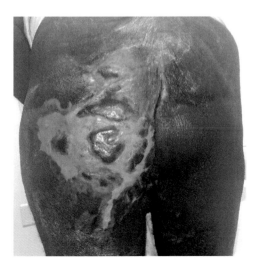

Figure 22.10 **(See color insert.)** Chronically recurrent Hurley stage III HS in the setting of multiple incision and drainage and local excision procedures.

differences in typical phenotypic expression between the groups. LC1 patients (48%) primarily express lesions in the axilla and breast, while LC2 patients (26%) display a follicular pattern more widely distributed on the body, as well as a concurrent history of pilonidal disease and a family history of HS. Most relevant to this chapter, LC3 patients (26%) are most likely to have gluteal disease, have less severe disease overall, and are less often obese (59).

## DIAGNOSIS AND NATURAL HISTORY

The prevalence of HS has frequently been reported to be around 1% (60,61); however, more recent and robust epidemiologic studies in the United States show that it is significantly rarer than previously thought, as low as 0.053% (62,63). A genetic component is frequently seen, as 34%–40% of patients with HS have a family history of the disease, and many potential gene groups have been identified (59,64–66). HS is rare in prepubertal children, with a peak onset in one's early 20s and a decline in disease after 50 (58,59). It affects women more than men at a ratio of 3:1, but a higher proportion of males have perianal disease (58,59).

The diagnosis of HS is generally a clinical one, where patients present with the classic findings as described by the Hurley classification system. In cases of perianal HS, it is important to examine the other common areas affected by HS, such as the axilla and inguinal regions, to aid in obtaining the correct diagnosis. Mild perianal HS can sometimes be confused with an anal fistula of cryptoglandular origin; however, as opposed to a classic anal fistula, HS will at most only involve the very distal anal verge and not the dentate line. Smoking (82%) and obesity are the two most common conditions associated with both the diagnosis and increasing severity of HS (55,56,58–63,67), although perianal disease is often seen in the nonobese and even underweight (59). Depilation, sweating, tight-fitting clothes, deodorant use, friction, androgen excess, and even pilonidal disease have been associated with HS (55,56). Patients with metabolic syndrome have also been shown to have an increased prevalence of HS (68,69), but this did not correlate with increased HS disease severity (69).

HS has also long seen an increased prevalence in patients with inflammatory bowel disease (IBD). A 2009 Dutch survey of patients with IBD reported that 17% of patients with Crohn disease and 14% with ulcerative colitis had coexisting HS (70). Similarly, a 2016 retrospective review from the Mayo Clinic concluded that patients with IBD were nine times more likely to suffer from HS than the general population (71). Although quite rare, transition into invasive squamous cell carcinoma (SCCA) within areas of long-standing and chronically inflamed HS has also been described (72). Due to the extremely scarred, inflamed setting in these instances, SCCA is often either a delayed diagnosis or incidental finding after radical excision, and several cases of death from metastatic disease have been reported; therefore, a high index of suspicion is necessary in individuals with a long-standing history of severe disease (73).

## NONEXCISIONAL THERAPY

In cases of milder disease, lifestyle modifications have a role in helping prevent disease progression or flares. In fact, educating patients to keep the affected areas as clean and dry as possible, promoting perianal hygiene, avoiding excessive sweating or friction, and not wearing tight-fitting clothes should be an important conversation with every patient encountered with HS. Antibiotics, both topical and systemic, have long been used in the treatment of acute flares, especially in conjunction with simple unroofing or incision and drainage of abscesses (73,74). A frequently cited 1983 RCT showed that topical clindamycin for 3 months was superior to placebo in cases of mild disease, with better resolution of flares and fewer recurrences (75). In 1998, another RCT showed no advantage of systemic tetracycline over topical clindamycin (76).

As antibiotics cannot be used indefinitely for long-term control, a myriad of more aggressive attempts at control via systemic therapy have been described (55,56,58,77). Antiandrogen therapy in females (78), immunosuppressants such as cyclosporine (79), and retinoids (80,81) have all been used with varying degrees of success at inducing remission, decreasing flares, and improving quality of life, especially in mild to moderate HS.

With the fairly common coexistence of IBD and HS, it is not surprising that biologic agents, primarily tumor necrosis factor-$\alpha$ (TNF-$\alpha$) inhibitors, have been studied extensively in the treatment of HS. A recent Dutch systematic review evaluated all papers available in the Medline and Embase databases regarding the systemic treatment of HS with immunosuppressants and retinoids (81). Included in the review were 87 papers representing 518 patients. Patients treated with infliximab (89%) and adalimumab (79%) had by far the highest response rate, while etanercept showed less of a response (56%). All three biologics included one manuscript of level A evidence and more than five of level B in their analyses. However, most patients had recurrence of active disease within a couple of months of discontinuing therapy, and to date only adalimumab has been approved for use in patients with moderate to severe HS.

There are also numerous described techniques of local invasive therapy for HS short of radical excision. In addition to unroofing and local excision techniques, both YAG and $CO_2$ laser therapies have been employed, and even radiation therapy in some instances. However, all of these options have fairly high recurrence rates, especially if used in severe disease, and can still result in the significant scarring that contributes to much of the decreased quality of life seen in recurrent disease (55,58).

## EXCISIONAL THERAPY

Despite these recent attempts at improved medical control with aggressive systemic therapy, radical wide surgical excision remains the best chance for cure or at least significant disease burden control in severe perianal HS. The excision in itself is quite straightforward, in that it requires complete excision of all the gross disease with a margin of normal-appearing tissue. The excision is carried at least into healthy subcutaneous fat, but in cases of severe disease, excision all the way down to the fascia of the gluteus muscle and exposure of the external anal sphincter may be necessary. Failure to completely excise the affected areas will ensure recurrence, though the risk of recurrence is still quite high with any modality. A retrospective review from 1998 reported a recurrence rate of 100% for incision and drainage procedures, 43% for limited excision, and only 27% for radical excision ($p < 0.05$) (82).

The more difficult decision is wound management after excision, as simple primary closure is rarely technically possible in Hurley II/III patients. When primary closure is attempted, recurrence rates are high, as the surgical margin is often compromised to allow primary closure. Many, perhaps most, surgeons still opt to allow the wounds to heal by secondary intention, with quite acceptable long-term outcomes that rarely lead to any functional disability in the perianal region. The biggest drawback is wound healing time, which usually takes 12–14 weeks (83,84).

Immediate or even delayed split-thickness skin grafting alone or in combination with myocutaneous advancement flaps if enough healthy adjacent tissue remains has been associated with decreased wound healing time and less scar contracture; however, at least partial graft loss from contamination and shearing forces is common (Figure 22.11). Others have at times employed rectal tubes and vacuum-assisted closure devices to help speed healing and decrease contamination, with mixed results. It is likely that all options are important to have in one's armamentarium to treat each patient on a case-by-case basis. An able and willing plastic surgery colleague is also helpful to tailor and employ the optimum approach for each individual patient. Only rarely is fecal diversion necessary (82–85).

A recent case series from Japan describes a two-stage approach to wound closure using artificial dermis. At the initial wide excision, attempts to preserve the deep subcutaneous fat are made to allow for a more suitable graft bed, and then the wound is immediately grafted with artificial dermis. Two weeks later, the artificial dermis is covered with split-thickness skin graft after re-excising any areas of persistent HS and lightly curetting the surface. Their results show a very high graft take rate with very low recurrence. Although they do not report wound healing time, they cite the minimal to no hypertrophic scarring or wound contracture seen with this technique as the primary advantage, leaving the grafted areas flexible and supple long term (86). This approach is similar to approaches commonly employed at our institution and many others in the management of severe burn injuries.

A newer even less invasive excisional technique described by the Dutch group of Blok et al. in 2014 is the skin-tissue-sparing excision with electrosurgical peeling (STEEP) procedure. This procedure focuses on excising all the affected areas via tangential unroofing incisions that then focus

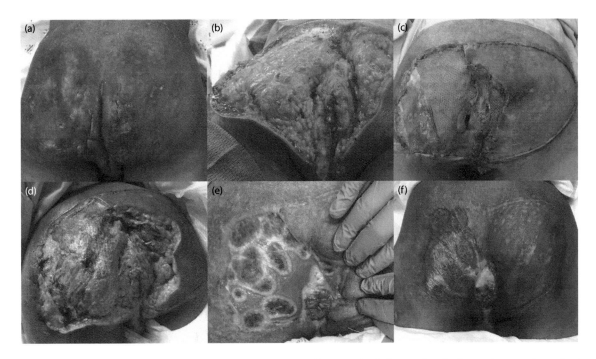

Figure 22.11 **(See color insert.)** **(a)** Severe Hurley III perianal HS affecting the left > right. **(b)** Status/post wide radical excision with exposed external sphincter. **(c)** Immediate reconstruction via a right-sided V-Y advancement flap and split-thickness skin grafting. **(d)** Early loss of large portions of the skin graft due to fecal contamination and poor patient mobility. **(e)** Excellent reepithelialization from areas of viable graft at 6 weeks. **(f)** Complete healing without disease recurrence at 16 weeks.

on minimal excision of only the inflamed sinus tracts, attempting to leave the epithelialized sinus floor and non-affected subcutaneous fat in situ to minimize wound size and shorten healing time (87). Their preliminary retrospective data of 363 operations in 133 patients with Hurley II/III HS shows a 29% recurrence rate but high satisfaction scores (8/10). The most frequent complication was hypergranulation tissue in 7% (88). Certainly more prospective studies are needed before this becomes more widely adopted.

Despite the postexcision wound management technique employed, the large majority of patients report a significantly improved quality of life after excision as well as long-term satisfaction with their decision to have undergone excision. A large quality of life survey from the Mayo Clinic was recently published in which all their patients with HS of any region who underwent operative treatment from 1976 to 2014 were surveyed. Of the 113 respondents, 83% were satisfied with their surgical result, and 96% were glad that they underwent surgery. Only a small minority of patients underwent flap of skin graft wound closure. The means quality of life for all respondents increased significantly from 5/10 to 8.4/10 after surgery. Additionally, those with isolated gluteal and perianal disease reported the greatest increase in quality of life after surgery (89).

## CONCLUSION

In summary, hidradenitis suppurativa, or acne inversa, appears to be a disease instigated by follicular occlusion rather than one of apocrine sweat gland origin. Regardless of the inciting event, HS is a chronic disease that can lead to severe disability and social withdrawal. While topical and systemic options may be successful at controlling milder disease, and while simple incision and drainage or unroofing procedures may temporize severe areas of suppuration, wide radical excision currently remains the mainstay of treatment, especially in severe disease. Radical excision allows the best chance of significant long-term disease control and quality of life improvement, regardless of the postexcision wound management decision, a decision that is best made on an individualized basis in multimodal fashion. Fecal diversion is rarely required.

## REFERENCES

1. Søndenaa K et al. *Int J Colorectal Dis.* 1995;10(1):39–42.
2. Aysan E et al. *Surg Today.* 2013 Nov;43(11):1286–9.
3. Armed Forces Health Surveillance Center (AFHSC). *MSMR.* 2013;20(12):8–11.
4. Mayo OH, *Observations on Injuries and Diseases of the Rectum.* London, UK: Burgess and Hill, 1833, pp. 115–6.
5. Anderson AW. *Boston Med Surg J.* 1847;36:74.
6. Hodges RM. *Boston Med Surg J.* 1880;103:485–6.
7. Abramson DJ. *Mil Med.* 1978;143:753–7.
8. Buie LA. *South Med J.* 1944;37:103–9.
9. da Silva JH. *Dis Colon Rectum.* 2000;43(8):1146–56.
10. Karydakis GE. *Aust N Z J Surg.* 1992;62(5):385–9.
11. Bascom J, Bascom T. *Arch Surg.* 2002;137(10):1146–50.
12. Ballas K et al. *J Hand Surg Br.* 2006;31(3):290–1.

13. Patel MR et al. *J Hand Surg Am.* 1990 Jul;15(4):652–5.
14. Phillips PJ. *Med J Aust.* 1966;2(24):1152–3.
15. Mohanna PN et al. *Br J Plast Surg.* 2001;54(2):176–8.
16. Harlak A et al. *Clinics (Sao Paulo).* 2010;65(2):125–31.
17. Webb PM, Wysocki AP. *Tech Coloproctol.* 2011;15(2): 179–83.
18. Jensen SL, Harling H. *Br J Surg.* 1988;75(1):60–1.
19. Armstrong JH, Barcia PJ. *Arch Surg.* 1994 Sep;129(9): 914–7; discussion 917–9.
20. Odili J, Gault D. *Ann R Coll Surg Engl.* 2002;84(1): 29–32.
21. Petersen S et al. *Dis Colon Rectum.* 2009;52(1):131–4.
22. Demircan F et al. *Int J Clin Exp Med.* 2015;8(2): 2929–33.
23. Lund JN, Leveson SH. *Dis Colon Rectum.* 2005;48(5): 1094–6.
24. Isik A et al. *Int J Clin Exp Med.* 2014;7(4):1047–51.
25. Seleem MI, Al-Hashemy AM. *Colorectal Dis.* 2005; 7(4):319–22.
26. Dag A et al. *Surgery.* 2012;151(1):113–7.
27. Calikoglu I et al. *Dis Colon Rectum.* 2017;60(2):161–9.
28. Kepenekci I et al. *World J Surg.* 2010;34(1):153–7.
29. Tejirian T et al. *Am Surg.* 2007;73(10):1075–8.
30. Rouch JD et al. *JAMA Surg.* 2016;151(9):877–9.
31. Biter LU et al. *Dis Colon Rectum.* 2014;57(12):1406–11.
32. Al-Khamis A et al. *Cochrane Database Syst Rev.* 2010 Jan 20; Issue 1: Art. no. CD006213.
33. Oncel M et al. *Tech Coloproctol.* 2002;6(3):165–9.
34. Soll C et al. *Int J Colorectal Dis.* 2008;23(2):177–80.
35. Soll C et al. *Surgery.* 2011;150(5):996–1001.
36. Mohamed HA et al. *Surgeon.* 2005;3(2):73–7.
37. Bascom J. *Surgery.* 1980;87(5):567–72.
38. Bascom J. *Dis Colon Rectum.* 1983;26(12):800–7.
39. Senapati A et al. *Br J Surg.* 2000;87(8):1067–70.
40. Colov EP, Bertelsen CA. *Dan Med Bull.* 2011;58(12):348.
41. Karydakis GE. *Lancet.* 1973;2(7843):1414–5.
42. Gurer A et al. *Dis Colon Rectum.* 2005;48(9):1797–9.
43. Kitchen PR. *Br J Surg.* 1996;83(10):1452–5.
44. Keshvari A et al. *J Surg Res.* 2015;198(1):260–6.
45. Ates M et al. *Am J Surg.* 2011;202(5):568–73.
46. Bascom J, Bascom T. *Am J Surg.* 2007;193(5):606–9.
47. Theodoropoulos GE et al. *Dis Colon Rectum.* 2003; 46(9):1286–91.
48. Khan PS et al. *Indian J Surg.* 2013;75(3):192–4.
49. Can MF et al. *Am J Surg.* 2010;200(3):318–27.
50. Velpeau A. *Dictionnaire de Medicine, un Repertoire General des Sciences Medicales sous la Rapport. Therique et Pratique.* Paris: Bechet Jeune, 1839.
51. Vernuil A. *Arch Gen Med Paris.* 1864;114:537–57.
52. Sellheyer K, Krahl D. *Int J Dermatol.* 2005;44:535–40.
53. Plewig G, Steger M. Acne inversa (alias acne triad, acne tetrad or hidradenitis suppurativa). In Marks R, Plewig G (eds). *Acne and Related Disorders.* London, UK: Martin Dunitz, 1989, pp. 345–57.
54. Danby FW et al. *Br J Dermatol.* 2013;168:1034–9.
55. Gill L et al. *F1000 Prime Reports* 2014;6:112.
56. Alikhan A et al. *J Am Acad Dermatol.* 2009;60(4): 539–61.
57. Hurley HJ. Axillary hyperhidrosis, apocrine bromhidrosis, hidradenitis suppurativa, and familial benign pemphigus: surgical approach. In: Roenigk RK, Roenigk HH Jr (eds). *Dermatologic Surgery: Principles and Practice.* 2nd edition. New York, NY: Marcel Dekker, 1996, pp. 623–45.
58. Jemec G. *N Engl J Med.* 2012;366(2):158–64.
59. Canoui-Poitrine F et al. *J Invest Dermatol.* 2013;133: 1506–11.
60. Revuz JE et al. *J Am Acad Dermatol.* 2008;59: 596–601.
61. Jemec G et al. *J Am Acad Dermatol.* 1996;35:191–4.
62. Cosmatos I et al. *J Am Acad Dermatol.* 2013;68(3): 412–9.
63. McMillan K. *Am J Epidemiol.* 2014;179(12):1477–83.
64. Fitzsimmons JS et al. *J Med Genet.* 1984;21:281–5.
65. Fitzsimmons JS, Guilbert PR. *J Med Genet.* 1985; 22:367–73.
66. Melnik BC, Plewig G. *Exp Dermatol.* 2013;22(3): 172–7.
67. Sartorious K et al. *Br J Dermatol* 2009;161:831–9.
68. Sabat R et al. *PLOS ONE.* 2012;7:e31810.
69. Gold DA et al. *J Am Acad Dermatol.* 2014;70: 699–703.
70. van der Zee HH et al. *Br J Dermatol.* 2010;162:195–7.
71. Yadav S et al. *Clin Gastroenterol Hepatol.* 2016;14(1): 65–70.
72. Losanoff JE. *Am Surg.* 2011;77(11):1449–53.
73. Shah N. *Am Fam Physician.* 2005;72(8):1547–52.
74. van der Zee HH et al. *J Am Acad Dermatol.* 2010;63(3): 475–80.
75. Clemmensen OJ. *Int J Dermatol.* 1983;22:325–8.
76. Jemec GB, Wendelboe P. *J Am Acad Dermatol.* 1998; 39(6):971–4.
77. Nazary M et al. *Eur J Pharmacol.* 2011;672:1–8.
78. Kraft JN. Searles, GE. *J Cutan Med Surg.* 2007;11: 125–31.
79. Buckley DA, Rogers S. *J R Soc Med.* 1995;88:289–90.
80. Boer J, Nazary M. *Br J Dermatol.* 2011;164(1):170–5.
81. Blok JL et al. *Br J Dermatol.* 2013;168:243–52.
82. Ritz J et al. *Int J Colorect Dis.* 1998;13:164–8.
83. Balik E et al. *World J Surg.* 2009;33(3):481–7.
84. Wollina U et al. *Int J Dermatol.* 2017;56:109–15.
85. Menderes A et al. *Int J Med Sci.* 2010;7(4):240–7.
86. Yamashita Y et al. *Dermatol Surg.* 2014;40(2):110–5.
87. Blok JL et al. *J Eur Acad Dermatol Venereol.* 2015; 29(2):379–82.
88. Blok JL et al. *J Eur Acad Dermatol Venereol.* 2015; 29(8):1590–7.
89. Kohorst JJ et al. *Dermatol Surg.* 2017;43(1):125–33.

# 23

# Surgical treatment of fecal incontinence

NICOLE M. SAUR AND JOSHUA I.S. BLEIER

---

## CHALLENGING CASE 1

A 30-year-old F presents to your office with complaints of incontinence to solid and liquid stool and gas. She is G2P2 (gravida 2, para 2) and had vaginal deliveries with need for perineal laceration repair after both deliveries. Her last child was delivered 1 year ago. She reports worsening passage of both solid and liquid stool, often without her knowledge. The incontinence is affecting her lifestyle, and she is wearing a pad.

## CASE MANAGEMENT 1

The remainder of her history is negative. Physical examination reveals a thin perineal body, decreased resting and squeeze pressures, and an anterior sphincter defect. Flexible sigmoidoscopy did not reveal any masses or mucosal abnormalities. Anorectal manometry shows decreased average resting and squeeze pressures (worst anteriorly), and an endoanal ultrasound revealed an anterior sphincter defect and a perineal body measurement of 6 mm. After discussion with the patient, the decision is made to proceed with overlapping sphincterotomy.

## CHALLENGING CASE 2

A 65-year-old male presents with incontinence to liquid and solid stool. He reports that he has had incontinence for "years" but describes that it has progressed from incontinence to only liquid stool and gas to incontinence to solid stool. He has a history of an excisional hemorrhoidectomy 20 years ago. He also has a diagnosis of irritable bowel syndrome. He states that the incontinence is affecting his quality of life, and he is having one to three accidents a week.

## CASE MANAGEMENT 2

A complete history is otherwise negative. Physical examination reveals weak resting and squeeze pressures. A full colonoscopy was negative for masses or mucosal abnormalities. Anorectal manometry revealed decreased resting and squeeze pressures circumferentially. Endoanal ultrasound did not reveal a sphincter defect. Pudendal nerve terminal motor latencies are prolonged bilaterally. He is counseled and started on a trial of fiber supplementation and biofeedback. He has a modest improvement in his symptoms. After further discussion, he is offered sacral nerve stimulation.

Fecal incontinence (FI) and its implications can have a major impact on a patient's quality of life. Whether it is soiling, inadvertent passage of flatus, or the leakage of stool, the symptoms can be debilitating. Therefore, the surgeons treating this condition should be well versed in the medical and surgical treatment options to offer a patient-centered approach.

## EPIDEMIOLOGY

The true incidence of FI has largely been unknown; however, a recent systematic review by Sharma et al. included 30 studies and showed a rate of FI ranging from 1.4% to 19.5%. They found that if incontinence to flatus was included in the definition, the prevalence rates were highest (15%–17%). In addition, the prevalence of FI to liquid or solid stool at least once a month was found to be 8.3%–8.4% for face-to-face interviews or phone interviews and as high as 12.4% for surveys conducted by mail (1). Groups of individuals at high risk for incontinence include the elderly, the mentally ill, institutionalized patients, those with neurologic disorders, and parous women. Macmillan et al. (2) had reported similar results in an older systematic review. The estimated prevalence of FI (including flatus incontinence) varied from 2% to 24%, and the estimated prevalence of FI (excluding flatus incontinence) varied from 0.4% to 18% in that study.

Data have been published recently on the socioeconomic impact of FI. The average yearly cost for FI was $4,110 per patient. Direct medical costs accounted for $2,353 yearly. Multivariate regression showed that more severe FI was associated with higher costs (3). In addition, we are likely not fully treating the entire appropriate patient population, as two-thirds of patients with FI symptoms do not seek care, and of those who do, more than half are seen only with their primary care physicians-clinicians who may not have a complete understanding of the workup and treatment algorithms (4–7).

## ETIOLOGY AND SCORING

Fecal continence requires coordination of learned and reflex responses to colonic and rectal stimuli. Normal individual variation in bowel habits makes the definition of abnormal defecation and incontinence difficult. Normal physiologic continence depends on a number of general (mental function), colonic (colonic stool transit, stool volume, and stool consistency), and anorectal (rectal distensibility, anal sphincter function, anorectal sensation, and anorectal reflexes) variables (8). Definitions, although imprecise, have been utilized including complete or full incontinence relating to complete loss of control of solid feces and partial incontinence involving inadvertent soiling or leakage of liquid stool or inadvertent passage of flatus. Patients may have difficulty qualitatively or quantitatively describing partial incontinence.

In an effort to more accurately classify the severity of symptoms, Browning and Parks proposed the following criteria: category A, those patients with normal continence who are continent of solid stool, liquid stool, and flatus; B, those continent of solid and usually liquid stool but not flatus; C, acceptable continence of solid stool but no control over liquid stool or flatus; and D, continued fecal leakage of solid or liquid stool (9). In addition, numerous severity scores exist and are simple to use to reflect sphincter

function: the worse the function, the higher is the score. Summary scores are considered more accurate in quantifying the patient's symptoms, comparing patients, and gauging treatment response. These scales also include items such as urgency, cleaning difficulties, the use of pads, and lifestyle alterations. Numerous summary scales have been designed, such as those according to Rockwood, Wexner, Pescatori, and Vaizey. The assignment of values to types and frequencies of incontinence varies between scales. The frequently cited and validated Wexner/Cleveland Clinic Florida Incontinence Score is outlined in Table 23.1 (10). More in-depth scoring systems have been adopted to incorporate quality of life measures (FI severity index [FISI], FI Quality of Life Scale [FIQLS]) (11,12).

Most discussions of etiology of anal incontinence have been based on the assumption that women, particularly women younger than 65 years of age, are more at risk for FI than men. Obstetric injury to the pudendal nerve or sphincter muscles is described as the primary risk factor, irritable bowel syndrome as a secondary factor (a disease thought to be more prevalent in women; secondary to urgency and frequency of bowel movements), and other etiologies such as diabetes were listed as a less common third cause. Yet, population-based surveys of anal incontinence prevalence, including that by Nelson et al., demonstrate FI in men at higher than expected rates (63% women, 37% men). Therefore, etiologies other than childbirth must be evaluated (13).

The true percentage of incontinence attributable to each of the possible causes is unknown. However, surgical and obstetric injuries are the most common. In addition, nerve damage secondary to diabetes has been reported, and spinal cord injuries also account for cases of FI (14–16). For purposes of discussion and classification, we break down the causes of FI into those involving (1) the anal sphincter, (2) the rectum, (3) the colon/stool consistency, and (4) the central nervous system.

## THE ANAL SPHINCTER

### Obstetric injury

Obstetric injury is the most common risk factor for FI in women following childbirth. In 1993 Sultan et al. published

Table 23.1 Wexner/Cleveland clinic florida fecal incontinence scale

|  | Never | Rarely | Sometimes | Usually | Always |
|---|---|---|---|---|---|
| Incontinence to solid stool | 0 | 1 | 2 | 3 | 4 |
| Incontinence to liquid stool | 0 | 1 | 2 | 3 | 4 |
| Incontinence to gas | 0 | 1 | 2 | 3 | 4 |
| Alteration of lifestyle | 0 | 1 | 2 | 3 | 4 |
| Wears a pad | 0 | 1 | 2 | 3 | 4 |

Source: Adapted from Jorge JM, Wexner SD. Dis Colon Rectum. 1993;36(1):77–97.
Note: Rarely: <1/month; sometimes: <1/week, ≥1/month; usually: <1/day, ≥1/week, always: ≥1/day. Score of 0 corresponds to perfect continence, score of 20 to complete incontinence.

their well-known article evaluating anal sphincter injuries during vaginal delivery and described the results of an endosonographic study of 79 primiparous women. Endoanal ultrasound was performed 6 weeks before and 6 months after routine vaginal delivery. After vaginal delivery, sphincter defects were detected in 35% of the patients. A similar evaluation was performed in 23 primiparous women who had undergone a cesarean section, and none of these women demonstrated a sphincter defect after delivery (17). Eason et al. (18) studied 949 women 3 months after delivery, and 3.1% reported incontinence to solid or liquid stool, while 25.5% reported gas incontinence. FI was more frequent in women who delivered vaginally with third- or fourth-degree perineal lacerations than in those without (7.8% versus 2.9%). Forceps delivery (relative risk 1.45) and sphincter tears (relative risk 2.09) were independent risk factors for all types of incontinence. Anal sphincter injury was most strongly associated with first vaginal births (relative risk 39.2) but was also independently associated with median episiotomy (relative risk 9.6), forceps delivery (relative risk 12.3), and vacuum-assisted delivery (relative risk 7.4). Birth weight (relative risk for birth weight 4000 g or more: 1.4) or length of the second stage of labor (relative risk for second stage 1.5 hours or longer compared with less than 0.5 hours: 1.2) were not strongly associated with sphincter injuries.

Seventy percent of women with postpartum sphincter defects do not demonstrate FI in the postpartum period (19). The question is whether women with an occult sphincter defect are at increased risk for FI over time. According to Rieger and Wattchow, many women remain asymptomatic because the number of occult sphincter defects is far greater than the documented prevalence of FI in the community (20). However, we must keep in mind that FI is largely underreported in community observational studies. Oberwalder et al. examined elderly females with late-onset FI, all of whom had a history of vaginal delivery. They observed sphincter defects in more than 70% of the patients (21). Despite these findings, it is still not possible to determine the exact risk for asymptomatic women with a sphincter defect to develop FI later in life. More studies including those longitudinally following these patients are necessary to determine the true incidence.

It has been theorized that elective cesarean section at term before the onset of labor protects the anal sphincters and prevents FI (22,23). However, although cesarean section performed during labor protects the anal sphincters, it does not necessarily prevent FI. This finding suggests a significant component of pudendal nerve injury during labor. A Cochrane Review evaluated almost 32,000 women, more than 6,000 of whom underwent delivery by C-section, and of the 21 studies reviewed, only 1 revealed a difference in preservation of anal continence between vaginal and cesarean deliveries. The authors concluded that preservation of anal continence should not be used as a reason for selecting C-section for delivery (24).

## Surgical injury

Surgical injuries are possible following surgery of the anal canal including lateral internal sphincterotomy (LIS), fistula surgery, anal dilatation, and hemorrhoidectomy. Injury is most common to the internal sphincter, but external sphincter injury can occur as well. Khubchandani and Reed evaluated the effect on continence with lateral internal sphincterotomy, a procedure in which the internal sphincter is purposely divided. They found that lack of control of flatus was the most common complaint (35%), followed by fecal soiling (22%) and accidental bowel movements (5%) (25). A significantly higher proportion of patients who reported accidental bowel movements were older than 40 years. Most recently, Liang and Church reported on a prospective series of 57 patients undergoing LIS for chronic fissure. Only two (4%) reported any changes in continence, and overall satisfaction in this cohort was $9.7 \pm 0.9$ out of 10 patients ($p < 0.001$) (26). The differences in reported incontinence rates between studies is likely secondary to differences in the length of internal sphincter divided. In the later study, the internal sphincter was only divided for the length of the fissure and not the entire length of the sphincter, which likely resulted in less incontinence to liquid stool and gas.

Fistula surgery is the anorectal procedure most commonly followed by postoperative incontinence. Gross incontinence of feces generally may be avoided if the anorectal ring is preserved. However, minor abnormalities in continence may result if even a small amount of sphincter muscle is divided. This complication can be reduced by avoiding division of the sphincter muscles. This goal is accomplished by placing a seton followed by utilization of the ligation of the intersphincteric fistula tract (LIFT), or the fistula plug, or endorectal advancement flap for transsphincteric fistulae. However, although the endorectal advancement flap repair is thought to heal the fistula without dividing sphincters or compromising continence, impairment of continence has been reported with an incidence between 8% and 35% (27–30). This could be secondary to inclusion of the internal sphincter in the flap mobilization. In addition, it has been suggested that anal stretch caused by the Parks' retractor is a contributing factor to sphincter injury and incontinence (31).

Currently, after surgery for hemorrhoids, incontinence is a rare complication. However, inadvertent injury of the sphincter mass (e.g., in a blind-clamping technique causing the internal sphincter to be grasped by a clamp) may lead to incontinence. In addition, minor alterations in continence can be attributed to removal of the hemorrhoidal cushions that are known to contribute to continence via anal canal occlusion at rest (32).

## Miscellaneous

Congenital malformations such as imperforate anus can disrupt normal anal sphincter structure and function.

Rectal prolapse, too, is frequently associated with FI because the rectum is intermittently or chronically distal to the sphincter mechanism. Persistence of FI after repair of rectal prolapse occurs in up to 50% of patients (33), which has been attributed, at least in part, to nerve injury (34). FI can also occur with trauma to the anus associated with pelvic trauma. Inflammatory conditions (inflammatory bowel disease [IBD], infectious proctitis, sexually transmitted diseases, etc.) can result in FI as can carcinoma of the anal canal.

## RECTUM

The rectum serves as a reservoir for the stool bolus. If the reservoir function is impaired, most commonly in the form of decreased wall compliance, this can result in FI. Mechanisms for rectal reservoir function impairment include rectal masses, radiation proctitis, infectious or inflammatory proctitis, history of proctectomy, pelvic nerve damage, and rectal prolapse, as mentioned.

## COLON/STOOL CONSISTENCY

IBD and irritable bowel syndrome (IBS) can be associated with changes in stool transit and consistency, which lead to FI. Liquid stool is more likely to be associated with FI as is stool with increased transit. In addition, constipation can be associated with overflow FI.

## CENTRAL NERVOUS SYSTEM

Patients with history of stroke or dementia are more likely to have FI and lack of awareness of need for bowel movements. In cases of myelomeningocele, the nerve supply, both sensory and motor, is disturbed in a variety of ways, leading to various forms of incontinence. Any form of trauma, neoplasm, vascular accident, infection, or demyelinating disease to the central nervous system or spinal cord can interfere with normal sensation or motor function, leading to incontinence. In addition, diabetic patients with autonomic neuropathy may have impaired reflex relaxation of the internal sphincter (35).

## DIAGNOSIS

## HISTORY AND PHYSICAL

### History

A proper history can delineate the severity of the patient's symptoms and the likely etiology. In addition, treatment recommendations are based on the cause and characteristics of the incontinence with assessment of the sphincter status. True incontinence should be distinguished from seepage and soiling, which may be associated with a variety of anorectal disorders such as hemorrhoids and prolapse. Incontinence also must be distinguished from diarrhea with urgency, in which the patient's diet or underlying bowel condition lead to frequent passage of liquid stool accompanied by a sense of urgency. In such cases, simple dietary change or the addition of medications (antispasmotics, fiber, antidiarrheals, etc.) may be all that is necessary. When these underlying diseases are treated, persistent urge incontinence has been reported to be a marker of external anal sphincter dysfunction (36).

Female patients should be asked about number of childbirths and type of delivery as well as a history of instrument-assisted vaginal deliveries. A history of anal sphincter trauma such as episiotomies, perineal tears, and prior anorectal procedures should be obtained as well as a history of the patient's continence in the postpartum period. Also notable are a history of associated conditions such as urinary incontinence, prolapsing tissue, history of associated fistulae, diabetes mellitus, medications, radiation treatment, and previous colon, anorectal, or rectal operations. A history of conditions that can lead to diarrhea such as IBD, IBS, and infectious colitis as well as food and beverage history are important to ascertain especially because, for example, some beverages such as coffee or beer can lead to frequent loose bowel movements. Inquiring about associated motor or sensory symptoms may point to a neurologic lesion (37). A clue to the severity of the problem is to determine the frequency of the incontinence and the necessity to wear a protective pad.

Grading and scoring the severity of the FI can be undertaken at the time of the history taking. It is especially useful to identify the severity of FI as well as the impact of the problem and past treatments on the patient's quality of life. Specific scoring scales and quality of life scales are discussed in more detail in the section "Etiology and Scoring."

### Physical examination

When beginning the physical examination, undergarments or pads should be inspected for staining by stool, mucus, or pus. In addition, the perineum must be inspected and the perineal body measured. A decreased length of the perineum is frequently associated with a defect of the external anal sphincter after sphincter injury. By simple retraction of the gluteal muscles, the large patulous anus, for example, that occurs with rectal prolapse can be recognized easily and large prolapsing hemorrhoids or evidence of pruritus may suggest seepage and soiling. Scars from previous anorectal operations or episiotomies may also be identified. With straining, perineal descent or mucosal or full-thickness rectal prolapse may become obvious. Examination in the sitting position or aided by Valsalva may be necessary to demonstrate prolapse.

Digital rectal examination can reveal the strength of the sphincters (resting tone and augmentation on squeeze) or large sphincter defects. However, the assessment of anal tone is, at best, a very indistinct barometer of sphincter function. The assessment of the strength of voluntary sphincter contraction is subjective. Contraction of the puborectalis at the tip of the finger versus contraction of the external sphincter over the midportion of the finger may be distinguished and the anorectal angle can be assessed. Anoscopic and proctosigmoidoscopic examinations may demonstrate inflammatory or neoplastic processes contributing to the patient's FI.

## TESTING

Multiple tests are available for the evaluation of FI, but the usefulness of each test depends on the cause of incontinence and the likely proposed treatment. Practically speaking, many investigations do not influence the choice of initial treatment. If conservative measures fail, further investigation, particularly with endorectal ultrasound or manometry may be useful.

## Ultrasonography

Endoanal ultrasound is easily available and accurate. It has been shown to be superior to electromyographic mapping, anorectal manometry, and physical examination (sensitivity for sphincter defect detection 100% versus 89% versus 67% versus 56%) (38). Based on these and other studies, endoanal ultrasound is considered to be the gold standard diagnostic tool for the assessment of sphincter injury. However, interpretation of ultrasound images of the external anal sphincter and associated defects can be subjective, operator dependent, and difficult to differentiate from normal anatomical variations. Differentiation of normal variants from sphincter defects can be difficult, especially in the upper part of the anal canal in female patients, which is due to asymmetry of the external anal sphincter at that level (39). In 75% of asymptomatic nulliparous women, Bollard et al. found a natural gap in the anterior external anal sphincter, just below the level of the puborectalis. According to these authors, the gap explains the difficulties of interpretation of postpartum ultrasounds (40). Sentovich et al. evaluated the accuracy and reliability of endoanal ultrasound for anterior sphincter defects (41). In incontinent, parous women, the sphincter defects detected by ultrasound were confirmed at the time of operation in 100% of the cases. However, in continent, nulliparous women, the two ultrasonographers identified sphincter defects in 55% and 75%, respectively, which may be partially explained by the difficulty in delineating the anterior sphincter anatomy. To reduce the rate of false positives, some advocate measuring perineal body thickness. Zetterstrom et al. reported that the perineal body thickness was $6 \pm 2$ mm in patients with an anterior sphincter defect and $12 \pm 3$ mm without (42).

Endoanal ultrasound is associated with substantial interobserver variability in assessment of the thickness of the sphincters; however, the qualitative assessment of sphincter defects is similar among observers (43). Despite several disadvantages, endoanal ultrasound is, to date, the best tool for the assessment of sphincter defects associated with FI. In the last decade, the use of three-dimensional (3D) techniques has increased, and studies have validated that compared to two-dimensional (2D) ultrasound, 3D ultrasound has an improved concordance with sphincter findings at the time of operation (44).

## Anorectal manometry

Resting and squeeze pressures, measures of rectal compliance, and the rectoanal inhibitory reflex (RAIR) are obtained during a manometry study. The absence of the RAIR raises the suspicion for Hirschsprung disease. However, in addition, the RAIR may be absent after low anterior resection. Basal pressure is thought to represent the activity of the internal sphincter, although the spontaneous activity of the external sphincter also affects maximal basal pressure. Squeeze pressure is secondary to the voluntary function of the external sphincter and the pelvic floor muscles. If both basal and squeeze pressures are low, patients are likely to be totally incontinent. If only the voluntary function (squeeze pressure) is low, the patients are likely partially incontinent (45). External sphincter function is critical for achieving continence of solid stool (46).

Penninckx et al. (47) studied the relationship between incontinence symptoms and the results of manometric data. Values >40 mmHg for maximum basal pressure and >92 mmHg for squeeze pressure could identify continent patients with 96% accuracy and incontinent patients with 88% accuracy. Unfortunately, there is a 10% overlap between the manometric values obtained from incontinent and continent patients (46). Following childbirth, pudendal nerve damage increases the risk of FI in women with anal sphincter injury, but manometric findings are not able to differentiate these patients from patients without pudendal nerve injuries and, therefore, the manometric readings do not correlate to the likelihood of incontinence (48). In addition, manometric values do not correlate with the severity of incontinence, and they do not predict the success of operative intervention (49). Finally, normal manometric readings do not fully exclude incontinence (45).

## Defecography

The anorectal angle is more obtuse (increased) in patients with incontinence (49). Voiding defecography or balloon proctography can demonstrate this increased angle. This examination will not likely add information about the etiology or treatment of fecal incontinence but has been shown to identify an occult internal intussusception.

## Pudendal nerve terminal motor latency

Although the severity of nerve injury does not appear to influence the severity of incontinence, it may affect the outcome of sphincter repair (50,51). Assessment of the pudendal nerve terminal motor latency (PNTML) provides a useful tool in defining pathology of the pudendal nerves. Roig et al. (52) found pudendal neuropathy in 70% of their patients with FI (59% in patients with a sphincter defect, 94% in patients without a sphincter defect). Therefore, pudendal neuropathy is a likely etiologic or, at least, contributing factor in FI. Laurberg et al. demonstrated that pudendal neuropathy affects surgical treatment, and in their series, sphincter repair was successful in 80% of patients without neuropathy and in only 10% of patients with neuropathy (51). However, the relationship between pudendal nerve injury and surgical outcome is not universally accepted. Rasmussen et al., Chen et al., and Young et al. were unable to identify a relationship between pudendal neuropathy and a poor outcome after sphincteroplasty (53–55).

## Magnetic resonance imaging

Magnetic resonance imaging is comparable to endoanal ultrasound in reliability of identification of sphincter defects, and its use is based on surgeon and institution preference. Magnetic resonance imaging has been shown to be more accurate in identifying sphincter atrophy than ultrasound, a finding that may correlate with the outcome of sphincter repair (56).

## TREATMENT

Underlying disorders (IBD, rectal prolapse, carcinoma, etc.) should be optimally managed prior to treatment of FI. In addition, patients should be given a trial of conservative symptomatic management prior to proceeding with surgical intervention. An algorithm is proposed in Figure 23.1.

## MEDICAL THERAPY

Initial treatment of FI should be conservative. Dietary changes, including fiber supplementation, and perineal exercises are often recommended for patients with FI, but generally are useful in patients with incontinence to liquid and not solid stool. Rosen et al. (57) reviewed the various antidiarrheal agents that can be used in patients with incontinence to liquid stool. Substances such as kaolin, activated charcoal, pectin, and bulk-forming agents such as fiber act on the intestinal contents to solidify them. Agents such as bismuth salts and astringents such as aluminum hydroxide may produce a barrier between intestinal contents and the intestinal wall, which can be particularly useful in the presence of inflammation. Anticholinergic agents such as atropine act to inhibit intestinal secretion and gut motility, but at therapeutic doses these drugs may produce troubling side effects. The opium derivatives such as tincture of opium, paregoric, and codeine act directly on the smooth muscle of the intestinal wall, but the risk of addiction limits long-term use. One of the most frequently used antidiarrheals is loperamide (Imodium), which inhibits intestinal motility by directly affecting the circular and longitudinal muscles of the intestinal wall. It both solidifies the stool and increases rectal compliance, both of which decrease urgency. In addition, it has also been shown to increase resting anal pressures (58) and, therefore, improve continence

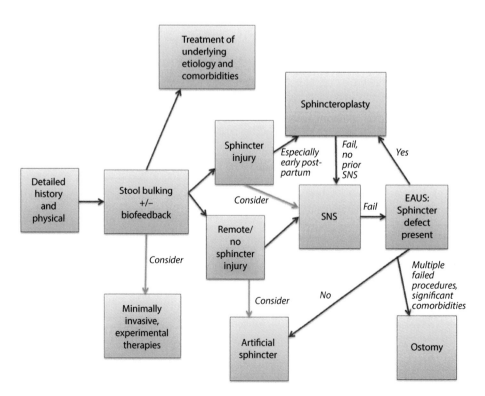

Figure 23.1 Proposed algorithm for the treatment of FI. (SNS: sacral nerve stimulation, EAUS: Endoanal ultrasound.)

after restorative proctocolectomy (59). For patients with certain neurologic conditions, the regular administration of enemas may achieve a level of social continence by emptying the rectum and left colon of stool.

Amitriptyline, a tricyclic antidepressant agent with anticholinergic and serotoninergic properties, has been used empirically in the treatment of idiopathic FI. Santoro et al. (60) conducted an open study to test the response to amitriptyline 20 mg daily for 4 weeks in 18 patients with idiopathic FI. Amitriptyline improved incontinence scores (scale 1–18; median pretreatment score 6 versus median posttreatment score 3, $p < 0.001$). Treatment also reduced the number of bowel movements per day and improved symptoms in 89% of patients with FI. The major effects of amitriptyline are a decrease in the amplitude and frequency of rectal motor complexes and an increase in colonic transit time, which lead to the formation of a more firm stool that is passed less frequently. In combination, these results may be the source of the improvement in continence in patients treated with amitriptyline.

Stool bulking with fiber plus or minus a low-dose antidiarrheal is used routinely as first-line treatment for incontinence to predominately liquid stool in our practice. This combination has a low risk of severe side effects and can be efficacious. In addition, if a patient has a history of cholecystectomy and has FI to liquid stool, a bile acid sequestrant is utilized.

## BIOFEEDBACK

Engel et al. (61) first described biofeedback training for FI, which involves screening patients for incontinence, particularly to liquid stool, and selecting motivated, cooperative patients for a three-phase instruction of voluntary control mechanisms. There are at least three components to biofeedback treatment: (1) exercise of the external sphincter muscle, (2) training in the discrimination of rectal sensations, and (3) training synchrony of the internal and external sphincter responses during rectal distention (62). All or some of these components may be effective for some patients.

Biofeedback involves placement of a balloon in the rectum and connection of pressure transducers to a graph to give the patient a visual feedback corresponding to his or her sphincter responses to command. Initially, large amounts of air are injected into the rectal balloon; gradually the volume of distention is reduced until the patient can sense small distention and contract the external anal sphincter. Subsequently, visual feedback is eliminated, and the patient is tested to respond to rectal sensations alone. Training occurs weekly generally for 4–8 weeks and is supplemented by at-home sphincter exercises. The goals of this training are to increase the strength of external sphincter contraction and detect and respond to small volumes of rectal distention.

One major disadvantage is the time required for therapy as each session takes at least 2 hours and involves a significant amount of equipment. Wald (63) reported that

diabetic patients exhibit multiple abnormalities of anorectal sensory and motor functions. Pharmacologic treatment and dietary interventions to decrease diarrhea, as well as biofeedback to improve rectal sensory thresholds and striated muscle responsiveness, may be successful especially in this patient population.

Several literature reviews have been performed to determine the efficacy of biofeedback in the management of FI. Norton et al. conducted a Cochrane Review of controlled studies of biofeedback and sphincter exercises for FI. Twenty-one studies met the inclusion criteria of being a randomized or quasi-randomized trial, which included 1,525 participants. The authors concluded that they were not able to definitively evaluate biofeedback with the number and quality of studies available. They did find that biofeedback is enhanced with electrical stimulation in addition to the exercises (64). Heymen et al. searched the Medline database for papers published between 1973 and 1999 including the terms "biofeedback" and "FI," which included 35 studies. Only six studies used a parallel treatment design, and just three of those randomized subjects to treatment groups. A meta-analysis comparing the treatment outcome of studies using coordination training (i.e., coordinating pelvic floor muscle contraction with the sensation of rectal filling) to studies using strength training (i.e., pelvic floor muscle contraction alone) failed to show any advantage for one treatment strategy over another. The mean success rate was 67% and 70%, respectively. Despite these positive results, the authors state that the conclusions of the reviewed studies are limited by the quality of the studies available (65). The largest randomized controlled trial has been conducted by Norton et al. They randomly assigned 171 patients with FI into four treatment arms: (1) standard care; (2) standard care plus instruction in sphincter exercises; (3) same as (2) plus computer-assisted biofeedback involving coordination techniques; (4) same as (3) plus daily use of an electromyography (EMG) home trainer device. About half of the participants in all four groups who completed their treatment protocol showed improvement, which was maintained at 1-year follow-up. These data indicate that improvement can be realized without sphincter exercises and without biofeedback. Patient and therapist interaction and the development of better coping strategies seem to be important factors associated with success (66). Another randomized controlled study, conducted by Solomon et al., revealed that instrument-guided biofeedback offers no advantage over simple pelvic floor retraining with digital guidance alone (67).

The mechanisms for the effect of biofeedback are not clear. It has been suggested that biofeedback is beneficial by improving the contraction of the external anal sphincter and the pelvic floor muscles due to strength training. Initial attempts to demonstrate objective manometric changes secondary to biofeedback have proved difficult. Fynes et al. conducted a randomized controlled trial to compare the effects of biofeedback alone with those of biofeedback combined with electrical stimulation. The manometric parameters did not change after the biofeedback alone, whereas anal resting and squeeze pressures increased after combined biofeedback and electrical stimulation (68). Beddy et al. observed a significant improvement in anal resting pressure, duration of the squeeze, and amplitude of the squeeze after EMG-guided biofeedback, but no improvement in the squeeze pressure (69). Biofeedback might also work by enhancing the ability to perceive and respond to rectal distensions, known as sensory training. Chiarioni et al. reported that sensory retraining is the key to biofeedback treatment of FI. Although they observed an increase of maximum squeeze pressure and squeeze duration after biofeedback, the sphincter strength alone did not separate responders from nonresponders. However, responders had lower thresholds for first sensation (70). Critics of this treatment modality argue that the improvement is a result of the supportive interaction between the physiotherapist and the patient, resulting in decreased anxiety and increased confidence. Despite many unanswered questions, it seems obvious that biofeedback is beneficial for more than half of the patients with FI, at least in the short term.

Another question that remains is whether the outcome of biofeedback can be predicted. Manometric parameters, except for increased cross-sectional asymmetry, do not predict response to biofeedback therapy (71). Another study revealed that incomplete anal relaxation during straining adversely affects the outcome of biofeedback (72). The long-term results after biofeedback have also been questioned. Most studies offer a follow-up of less than 2 years. Enck et al. posted a questionnaire to patients who were treated by biofeedback 5–6 years earlier. The same questionnaire was also sent to patients who had not entered the treatment program. In both groups 78% of the patients experienced episodes of incontinence. However, the severity of incontinence was significantly less in the treatment group. Five to 6 years after the treatment, the severity of incontinence was similar to that reported immediately after therapy (73). However, two other studies revealed deterioration over time (74,75). Ryn et al. reported an overall success rate of 60% immediately after the treatment. This dropped to 41% after a median follow-up of 44 months (76). Based on this deterioration over time, it has been suggested that it could be useful to reinitiate biofeedback training. Pager et al. were not able to demonstrate this worsening with time. At a median of 42 months after completion of the training program, 75% of their patients still perceived a symptomatic improvement, and 83% reported improved quality of life. They also observed that patients continued to improve during the years following the training, possibly due to the strong emphasis placed on them to continue the exercises on their own (77). Because biofeedback treatment is multimodal, more studies are needed to establish selection criteria, to compare different biofeedback techniques, and to establish valid endpoints and follow-up. Although biofeedback is time consuming and labor intensive, it is noninvasive and safe. Based on the reported outcomes, it can be considered as initial treatment in patients with FI, especially predominantly to liquid stool and with intermittent incontinence.

It has been suggested that biofeedback is also beneficial as an adjuvant therapy following anal sphincter repair. Davis et al. performed a randomized controlled trial where 38 patients were randomly assigned to sphincter repair or sphincter repair plus biofeedback. Shortly after surgery, there was no difference in functional outcome between the two groups. More studies are warranted to elucidate the role of adjuvant biofeedback (78).

## OPERATIVE TECHNIQUES

Once conservative management has failed, operative intervention is indicated. All operative techniques except sacral nerve stimulation involve preparing the patient by evacuation of the large bowel with laxatives and enemas or oral lavage solutions. At the time of operation, an indwelling urethral catheter is placed and maintained until decreased pain permits voluntary voiding. In all cases, perioperative broad-spectrum antibiotics are administered as per the institution's Surgical Care Improvement Project guidelines.

## OVERLAPPING SPHINCTEROPLASTY

External anal sphincter defects, most frequently in the anterior sphincter, are the principal cause of FI secondary to obstetric trauma. These anatomic defects can be treated by an anterior anal sphincter repair, which is the classic surgical procedure for an early (4 months to several years) postpartum sphincter injury. Most surgeons use an overlapping technique to repair the divided external anal sphincter; however, a primary or end-to-end repair may be employed very early (less than 3 months) after sphincter injury, as there is no significant scar, and muscle tissue is healthy.

The technique of sphincteroplasty, as applied by Fang et al. (79) and Parks and McPartlin (80), provides good to excellent results in most patients who have adequate residual muscle mass. The operation is performed with the patient in the prone jackknife position, with the buttocks elevated over a Kraske roll. Anesthesia may be either regional or general, but local anesthesia is also utilized.

The first step is the mobilization of the anoderm from the underlying sphincter mechanism and scar tissue via a curvilinear incision that parallels the outer edge of the external sphincter. The incision should extend no more than 180°, depending on the amount of scar tissue present (Figure 23.2a). Further incision risks injury to the pudendal nerves laterally. Cephalad mobilization should extend approximately to the distal edge of the anorectal ring. The entire sphincter mechanism is then dissected widely from its bed, and care is taken to preserve the branches of the pudendal nerves as they enter into the muscle posterolaterally. Wide dissection permits approximation without tension. In one approach, the entire sphincter mechanism is sectioned transversely through the middle of the scar tissue, with preservation of the scar for suture placement. The muscle ends

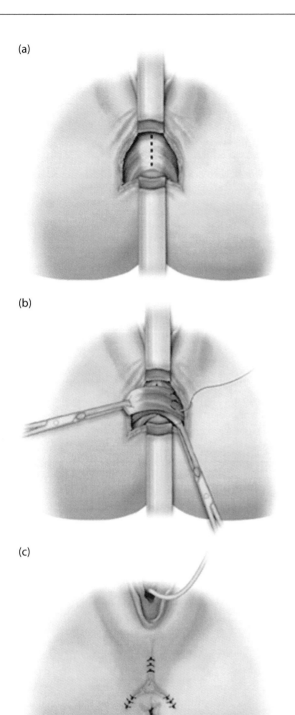

(a)

(b)

(c)

Figure 23.2 Overlapping sphincteroplasty. **(a)** The sphincter muscle is dissected free on both sides with care to preserve the scar tissue attached to the muscle to improve the strength of the repair. **(b)** The muscle is overlapped and sutured in place with mattress sutures. **(c)** The wound is closed with a drain or packing in the center to facilitate drainage. (With permission from Gurland B, Hull T. Wexner SD, Fleshman JD (eds). *Master Techniques in Surgery. Colon and Rectal Surgery: Anorectal Operations.* Philadelphia, PA: Wolters Kluwer, 2012.)

are overlapped to decrease the size of the anal aperture until it fits snugly over the index finger. Multiple mattress sutures are carefully placed to maintain the desired aperture. The suture used is generally a 2–0 synthetic slowly absorbable suture. The sphincter should lay easily overlapped, because the separation of the ends of the sphincter is a sign of inadequate mobilization of the muscle from its bed and will predispose to separation at the suture line. When all sutures have been placed, they are pulled tight, and the orifice is checked again to ensure proper placement of the sutures and properly sized aperture and the sutures are then tied. A second approach involves preservation of midline scar, and imbrication of the tissue, and then the performance of overlapping repair.

If the perineal body is thin, attempts should be made to bulk it, which is performed by an anterior levatorplasty. Tissues from each side of the perineum (transverse perinei muscles and/or scar tissue) are approximated in the midline. This reconstruction supports the anovaginal septum and effectively separates the anal orifice from the introitus. The anoderm is sutured carefully over the sphincter with interrupted or running absorbable sutures. The horseshoe-shaped defect outside the muscle is partially closed, and the remainder is packed open with gauze or over a drain (Figure 23.2c).

Postoperative management varies based on surgeon preference. The recent trend has been toward early feeding. Although there is concern for subsequent need for laxatives, we administer opiates to decrease the pain and frequency of bowel movements. Mahony et al. (81) conducted a randomized trial designed to compare a laxative regimen with a constipating regimen in early postoperative management after primary obstetric and anal sphincter repair. A total of 105 females were randomized after primary repair of a third-degree tear to receive lactulose (laxative group, 56) or codeine phosphate (constipated group, 49) for 3 days postoperatively. The first postoperative bowel movement occurred at a median of 4 days in the constipated group and 2 days in the laxative group. Patients in the constipated group had a significantly more painful first evacuation compared with the laxative group. Continence scores, anal manometry, and endoanal ultrasound findings were similar in the two groups at 3 months postoperatively. Sitz baths are given two to three times a day for comfort and to wash away secretions. Some surgeons are concerned about skin maceration and prefer to irrigate the wound with warm saline solution or even diluted hydrogen peroxide (dilute 1:4) to provide both comfort and cleanliness. With the introduction of food, fiber supplementation is started to eliminate any straining at defecation and disruption of the suture repair. Performing a diverting stoma is not required. An alternative strategy is to teach the patient to irrigate his or her rectum by sliding a catheter posteriorly along the natal cleft and into the anal canal, away from the surgical site. This may avoid issues of delayed constipation or impaction upon discharge.

Numerous reports have been published on the short-term outcomes of sphincter repair, and overall, initial success is positive, with approximately 60% of patients achieving significant benefit. However long-term success has not been as durable. In one of the larger studies published, Karoui evaluated 86 patients undergoing sphincteroplasty. At 3 months postoperatively, 30% of patients were totally continent, and an additional 33% were incontinent only to gas. However, at 40 months follow-up, <30% of patients remained fully continent and >70% were incontinent to either gas or feces (82). Malouf et al. evaluated 55 consecutive patients undergoing overlapping sphincteroplasty as a result of obstetric injury. At 15 months postoperatively, 42/55 patients were continent to both solid and liquid stool. At 5 years follow-up, no patient was fully continent to both solid and liquid stool, which shows the deterioration of continence over time (83). Similarly, Halverson reported on a series of 71 consecutive patients undergoing sphincteroplasty assessed at a median of 69 months after surgery. Forty-nine (69%) were available for follow-up, and of these patients, four patients had undergone fecal diversion and 54% were incontinent to liquid or solid stool, while only six patients (14%) remained fully continent (84).

Attempts at determining predictive factors for success have evaluated age, pudendal nerve injury, and type of repair. Despite the wealth of literature, there are no clear answers. Age of the patient at the time of sphincter repair has been assessed by several investigators. Simmang et al. evaluated 14 patients with ages ranging from 55 to 81 years, where almost all of the patients reported improvement in symptoms and half reported complete continence. In this admittedly small series, advanced age did not seem to predict failure (85). Rasmussen assessed postoperative continence in 24 women under the age of 40 years and in 14 women older than 40 years and found a significant difference in postoperative continence in the older cohort. This was hypothesized to be, at least partially, related to weakening of the pelvic floor (86). However, patient perception may also play a role. Young evaluated 57 women undergoing overlapping sphincter repair and found that 78% of patients younger than 40 deemed the repair a success compared to 93% of patients in the older group, while formal incontinence scores improved equally in both groups (54).

Pudendal nerve injury as evidenced by prolonged PNTML has often been cited as one of the etiologies of postobstetric injury incontinence. Numerous publications have attempted to assess this, and data are still divided. This is supported by studies by Barisic, Londono-Schimmer, and Giliand (87–89) comparing groups with and without pudendal neuropathy showing a significant difference in incontinence scoring after sphincteroplasty between the groups; however, this is refuted by multiple studies, including those by Bravo-Gutierrez, Halverson, Malouf, and Koroui (82–84,90). Tjandra attempted to evaluate whether repair technique, overlapping versus end-to-end repair, was associated with different functional outcomes. In this study, 23 patients with anterior defects underwent sphincter repair, 12 randomized to end-to-end repair and 11 to overlapping repair. At a median follow-up of 18 months, Wexner scores

were identical in both groups. Resting pressures and maximal squeeze pressures were no different, and subjective success scores were also no different (91).

Briel et al. conducted a prospective study looking at whether bulk overlapping repair was superior to separate internal and external sphincter repair. In this study, 31 patients underwent separate internal and external sphincter repair, and 24 patients underwent standard overlapping repair. There was no statistically significant difference in these two groups (92).

Hasegawa et al. (93) conducted a randomized trial to assess whether fecal diversion would improve primary wound healing and functional outcome after sphincter repair. Patients were randomly assigned to a defunctioning stoma ($n = 13$) or no stoma ($n = 14$). The incontinence score improved significantly in both groups (stoma 13.5–7.8; no stoma 14–9.6). There was no significant difference in the functional outcome or the number of complications of sphincter repair between the groups. However, stoma-related complications occurred in 7 of 13 patients (parastomal hernia, 2; prolapsed stoma, 1; incisional hernia at the stoma site requiring repair, 5; and wound infection at the closure site, 1). They concluded fecal diversion in sphincter repair is unnecessary because it gives no benefit for wound or functional outcomes and itself is a source of morbidity.

Despite mixed data, sphincteroplasty should remain a viable approach to address continence in patients with sphincter injuries, especially in the first years following injury (Figure 23.1). In our practice, this procedure is reserved for young women with sphincter defects with the knowledge that they may need another operation in the future when the repair loses its durability.

## OTHER SPHINCTEROPLASTIES

### Postanal repair

Prior to the introduction of endoanal ultrasound, most cases of FI were classified as "idiopathic" or neurogenic. For the treatment of patients presenting with this type of incontinence, Parks devised the postanal repair, and he believed that this procedure worked by restoring the anorectal angle and increasing the length of the anal canal. Several studies, however, have revealed that a postanal repair does not result in a significant change of the anorectal angle (94–98). However, several studies have demonstrated an increase in the length of the anal canal after successful postanal repair (9,94,99). Conflicting data have been reported regarding the impact of postanal repair on anal pressure. Some have found that resting and squeeze anal pressure increase after successful postanal repair (95–97,100,101). However, others have shown that postanal repair does not affect anal pressure (102,103). Due to the lack of consistent changes in anatomy and physiology, it is unclear why postanal repair is effective in some patients, but it might be due to lengthening and narrowing of the anal canal. Van Tets and Kuijpers suggested that this procedure might improve continence by a placebo effect and not by enhanced muscle function (104). For the reasons above and the lack of durability of the repair when it does improve symptoms, the procedure has fallen out of favor.

## GRACILIS MUSCLE TRANSPOSITION (GRACILOPLASTY)

Several advanced techniques have been described using pedicled muscle flaps to replace a damaged or nonfunctional sphincter. In general, due to technical difficulty, high rates of morbidity, and the success of newer, less invasive techniques, graciloplasty is rarely performed and may only be accessible in select situations and at specialized centers where expertise and experience may maximize results.

This technique was first described more than a century ago by Chetwood and renewed as a technique for use in pediatric FI by Pickrell (105). More recently, it was championed by Wexner as a salvage treatment after catastrophic sphincter damage in otherwise healthy patients. In this technique, the gracilis muscle is harvested as a pedicled flap. The muscle is tunneled around the sphincter complex and sutured in place. Initially described as only a muscle transposition, the wrapped muscle functions as a biologic cerclage, akin to the Thiersch procedure. In addition, patients learn techniques to voluntarily contract this muscle to augment control, at the expense of altered gait (106).

To additionally augment the procedure, electrostimulation is employed in order to convert the more easily fatigued fast-twitch skeletal muscle fibers to slow twitch fibers via neuromodulation resulting in relatively tonic contraction. This was dubbed a "dynamic graciloplasty." Isolated series produced favorable results; however, due to surgical difficulty and high complication rates, it was rarely performed. Wexner, reporting on one of the largest series, showed that at 2 years >60% of patients had a significant improvement in quality of life and incontinence scores (107). Long-term success was less favorable as Thornton and others showed a significant decrease in success at 5 years, with only 16% maintaining continence, and overall complication rates >70%. Therefore, this procedure has also largely been abandoned.

## SACRAL NEUROMODULATION

Sacral nerve stimulation (SNS) (Interstim, Medtronic, Minneapolis, Minnesota) has emerged as the most promising modality in the treatment of medically refractory FI. The treatment was originally studied and developed for the treatment of urinary incontinence, but its efficacy for the treatment of FI quickly became apparent due to the incidence of mixed urinary incontinence and FI. Clinically, it seems to be more efficacious for the treatment of FI (108). Following the 2010 American Society of Colon and Rectal Surgeons presentation and subsequent publications (109,110) based on multi-institutional trial data, SNS was approved by the U.S. Food and Drug Administration (FDA)

in 2011 for the indication of FI in patients who have failed best conservative therapy.

To provide nerve stimulation, a quadripolar lead electrode is placed transcutaneously and passed via the sacral foramen to follow the path of the S3 nerve root (Figure 23.3). An initial test phase with a temporary external pacer is

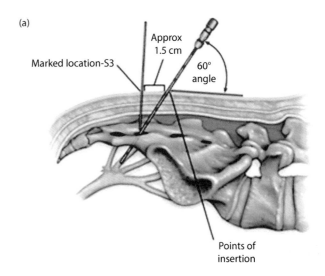

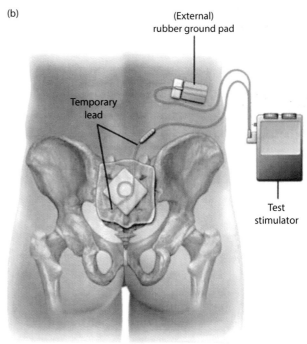

Figure 23.3 SNS. **(a)** The needle is passed at the level of the S3 nerve root at a 30° angle, and the electrode is passed through the needle. The electrode is stimulated to confirm position along the S3 nerve root. **(b)** A temporary simulator is attached to the electrode for the trial period. If the patient responds to treatment, a permanent simulator is placed in a subcutaneous pocket. (With permission from Matzel KE. In: Wexner SD, Fleshman JD (eds). *Master Techniques in Surgery. Colon and Rectal Surgery: Anorectal Operations.* Philadelphia, PA: Wolters Kluwer, 2012.)

utilized to test efficacy before the implantable stimulator is placed. The minimum definition of success of the trial period (1–3 weeks) is a 50% reduction in the number of episodes of fecal incontinence. If needed, two separate test phases can be used. If preferred, an office-based temporary unipolar nontined lead can be placed using either anatomic landmarks or with fluoroscopic guidance rather than utilizing placement in the operating room. However, as this is a nontined lead, this test phase lasts for a maximum of 3–7 days because of the high likelihood of lead dislodgment. This test is best suited for patients with frequent FI episodes, often one or more per day.

Stimulator programming is based on best motor responses obtained (therefore, if the procedure is performed in the operating room, only light sedation is performed). A successful lead placement causes bellowing of the levators and toe turning of the great toe, which indicate specific S3 stimulation. If the test period reveals a >50% reduction in the number of FI episodes, the stimulator is placed in a subcutaneous pocket just inferior to the posterior superior iliac spine. At typical settings, the current stimulator model has a battery life of approximately 5 years (111).

The seminal prospective trial validating SNS was conducted by Tjandra et al., published in 2008, and compared SNS to best medical therapy. The study included patients with FI varying etiologies and with sphincter defects of up to 120°. There were 120 patients in the initial cohort, 60 in the control group and 60 in the SNS group. Remarkably, 90% of patients reported success with initial testing and moved on to implantation. Of this group, almost 50% achieved perfect continence, compared to no improvement in the control group (112). The FDA qualifying trial echoed Tjandra's results, with an 87% success rate and an >40% rate of patients achieving perfect continence. Interim follow-up at 3 years was conducted by Mellgren and found that success was sustained: 83% of patients still reported overall success with a mean decrease in the number of FI episodes from a baseline of 9.4–1.7 (109,113). Forty percent of this cohort still reported perfect continence. Complications in this trial were minimal, the most frequent complication being implant site pain in 28%, with a 10% infection rate noted. Hull reported on 5-year follow-up in this cohort in 2013. Impressively, 89% of patients still reported success with therapy, and 36% still reported maintenance of perfect continence. Rates of complications remained similar to the earlier studies. They demonstrated that over 5 years, 24.4% of patients underwent at least one revision or replacement of the stimulator (114). It should be noted that in this trial, patients with sphincter defects of up to 60° were included, and this had no effect on overall success. Longer-term data for this therapy have been published by numerous groups, primarily from Europe. In the Italian SNS registry, Altomare published 5-year follow-up on 52 patients. Mean Wexner incontinence scores decreased from a baseline of 15 to 5. Seventy-four percent of patients had at least a 50% improvement in the number of FI episodes with full continence maintained in 20% of patients (115). Lim published

5-year follow-up for the Australian experience in 53 patients and reported that mean Wexner scores improved from a baseline of 11.5 to 8 (116). Michelsen published the Danish experience with a 6-year follow-up of 126 patients and demonstrated mean Wexner score improvement from a baseline of 20 to 7 (117). The European SNS outcomes study group reported on 7-year outcomes in a multinational study incorporating 10 European centers and 407 patients with a mean follow-up of 84 months (118). Side-by-side comparison of multiple incontinence scoring parameters including number of incontinent episodes, Wexner score, and St. Mark's score all showed dramatic and significant improvements persisting to 7 years of follow-up. George (119) published a 10-year follow-up study of 25 patients. Ninety-two percent of patients still had a >50% improvement, and full continence was maintained in almost 50%. In an attempt to define predictive variables for success, Brouwer and Duthie evaluated a cohort of patients with 4 years of follow-up looking at variables including sphincter defect, neuropathy, and prior sphincter repair. The therapy was overwhelmingly positive in all groups, regardless of these variables present (120). As a result of the overwhelming success of SNS, the effective indications of pelvic floor testing for these patients have decreased. Since no predictors of success are based on manometric values, and since the technique works irrespective of a sphincter injury, preoperative pelvic floor testing is of negligible use and should not be considered routine, or even necessary at all in patients deemed appropriate for SNS.

## POSTERIOR TIBIAL NERVE STIMULATION

Posterior tibial nerve stimulation (PTNS) was first used for the treatment of urinary incontinence in 1983 by Nakamura (121). As with SNS, it was serendipitously found to have efficacy for the use of FI as well. Either transcutaneous or percutaneous electrodes are applied over the posterior tibial nerve and stimulation is typically performed twice daily, for 20-minute sessions over a 3-month period. An early series was published by Shafik in which 32 patients with medically refractory FI were treated with percutaneous stimulation, and significant improvement in FI was achieved in >78% of the patients (122). Leroi, using a modified transcutaneous technique, performed a randomized prospective trial on 144 patients. Almost all patients in the treatment group showed improvement in FI scores compared to only 27% in the sham group, though this did not reach statistical significance (123). A more recent systematic review identified nearly 300 patients treated with tibial nerve stimulation. Success, defined by at least a 50% improvement in incontinence scores, was achieved by between 63% and 82% of patients (124). Thin et al. performed a randomized clinical trial comparing tibial nerve stimulation to SNS. Although SNS showed greater success than tibial nerve stimulation, both treatments showed clinical efficacy (125). Knowles reported on the largest randomized sham-controlled trial including 227 patients.

Compared to 31% in the sham group, 38% of patients in the treatment group achieved a >50% reduction in the number of weekly incontinent episodes (126). Edenfield recently published a systematic review inclusive of 15 studies. The group was composed of 745 patients, and although the majority of the studies were of poor quality, both percutaneous and transcutaneous approaches showed significant improvement over controls (127).

PTNS remains an interesting potential option for motivated patients who may be otherwise ineligible for standard sacral neuromodulation; however, it is not currently FDA approved for this indication.

## INJECTABLES

A recent modality used to treat FI is injection of bulking agents, which are synthetic or biomaterials injected into the tissue around the anal canal in order to bulk the area and cause a relative physical obstruction. Numerous materials have been tested including autologous fat, collagen, as well as slowly absorbable biomaterials including hydrogel cross-linked with polyacrylamide synthetic calcium hydroxyapatite ceramic microspheres, silicone biospheres (PTQ, Cogentix Medical Incorporated, Minnetonka, Minnesota), carbon-coated beads (Durasphere EXP, Coloplast Corporation, Minneapolis, Minnesota), and nonanimal stabilized dextranomer in hyaluronic acid (NASHA Dx – Solesta, Salix Pharmaceuticals, Raleigh, North Carolina) (111).

The majority of published data surrounds the use of NASHA Dx, under the trade name Solesta. The seminal study, a randomized double-blind trial, compared a treatment arm with a sham saline injection arm. In this study, 52% of patients in the treatment group experienced a 50% or more reduction in the number of incontinent episodes; however, in the sham group, 31% also achieved this endpoint (128). Some significant adverse events were reported including rectal and prostatic abscesses. Maeda performed a recent systematic review looking at all trials of injectable bulking agents. Not surprisingly, as the majority of these were industry funded, many were found to be at high risk for bias. Only the Solesta trial showed a statistically significant improvement in continence. However, one of the trials comparing silicone biospheres (PTQ) to carbon-coated beads (Durasphere) showed some short-term advantages (129). Some of the key questions that have yet to be well answered include optimum dose and delivery method. In Maeda's review, ultrasound-guided delivery was found to be superior to manually guided injection. A study of Solesta conducted by La Torre (130), looking at longer-term results, found some durable efficacy at 24 and 36 months with just over half of patients still maintaining a >50% reduction in fecal incontinent episodes.

In order to identify predictors for failure, Hussain conducted a systematic review of all injectable materials and found that the only significant predictors for failure were the use of local anesthetic for injection as well as the failure to use laxatives in the postoperative period (131). There is little positive data reflecting any durable success with this modality. Guerra followed a cohort of 19 patients with a mean follow-up of 7 years who underwent treatment with Durasphere, PTQ, or Solesta. Patients underwent clinical assessment, anal manometry, and ultrasound evaluation. In this group, the vast majority of implants were no longer detectable or clinically effective (132).

Bulking agents have largely been abandoned by colorectal surgeons for the treatment of FI. A niche may still exist in patients with seepage and soilage, especially after anorectal surgery.

## ARTIFICIAL BOWEL SPHINCTER

The artificial bowel sphincter (ABS), developed by American Medical Systems (Minnetonka, Minnesota), utilizes an inflatable cuff that is tunneled around the native sphincter complex. The cuff is controlled by a fluid-filled pressure-regulated balloon that is implanted anterior to the bladder and controlled manually by an actuator implanted in the scrotum or labia majora. First reported on by Christiansen and Sparso (133), 12 patients with anal incontinence due to neurologic disease or failure of previous incontinence surgery underwent implantation of an artificial bowel sphincter. The system used was a modification of the AMS 800 artificial urinary sphincter. In two patients, infection necessitated removal of the system, and in four patients eight revisional procedures had to be performed because of mechanical failure. Erosion through the anal canal did not occur. Among 10 patients with the system in place for more than 6 months, the result was considered excellent in five, with only occasional leakage of flatus; good in three, with occasional leaked liquid feces and flatus; and acceptable in two, in whom the cuff obstructed defecation. The authors concluded that implantation of an artificial bowel sphincter is a valid alternative to permanent colostomy in patients with anal incontinence due to neurologic disorders and in patients in whom other types of incontinence surgery have failed. Since the initial report, more data cast a question of device safety. Mundy published a systematic review in 2004 (134) showing encouraging initial functional success in two-thirds of patients. However, complication rates were unacceptably high, including infection rates >20% as well as mechanical failures resulting in explantation in more than half of patients. Darnis published an even more ominous series showing a >75% complication rate (135). Wong published a more balanced series of 52 patients with a greater than 5-year follow-up with a revision rate of 50%, but explantation in only 27%, In this series, more than two-thirds of patients who retained their implants at 5 years had a significant improvement in FI scores and quality of life scores (136). In order to better determine predictors of success, Wexner followed a cohort of 51 patients over a 9-year period. In this study, there was a 41% rate of infection, 18/23 of which were early postop. Multivariate analysis showed that prior perianal infection and time between implant and first bowel movement were predictive of infection (137).

Overall, despite success in a highly select population, the overwhelming technical and infectious complications have resulted in the device no longer being implanted except at select centers.

## MAGNETIC ANAL SPHINCTER (FENIX)

With SNS successfully treating the majority of patients, the group of patients who still fail has become smaller and more difficult to treat. Not surprisingly, new techniques have taken inspiration from past failure. The magnetic anal sphincter is a modern update of the cerclage technique popularized by Thiersch called the FENIX (Torax Medical Inc., Shoreview, Minnesota). This technique involves the implantation of a string of titanium beads with magnetic cores linked together by wire. As in the Thiersch procedure, this wire is tunneled around the native sphincter complex and secured in place. At rest, the magnetic cores are drawn together, providing an occlusive force. The technology was first used (and abandoned) for esophageal closure to prevent reflux. Force generated in the rectum during Valsalva is enough to overcome the magnetic forces, and allow passage of stool (111).

Lehur first published a feasibility study in 2010, reporting on 14 patients. Complications were reported in 7/14 patients including one erosion into the anal canal. Of those who maintained their implants, 5 patients at 6-month follow-up had a >90% reduction in the number of FI episodes, and a significant improvement in the Wexner score (17.8 to 7.8) (138). Barussaud published a prospective study on 23 patients implanted with the magnetic anal sphincter with an 18-month follow-up. They reported that median incontinence scores decreased from 15.2 to 6.9 at 6 months. With follow-up as long as 36 months, they reported that FI scores remained low, with a Wexner score of 5.3. Only two patients required explantation due to infection (139). This device has been FDA approved under the Humanitarian Device Exception. There is an ongoing SaFaRI trial comparing the FENIX to SNS for FI (140).

## RADIOFREQUENCY THERAPY

Radiofrequency (RF) therapy is a technique that was originally described for use to treat gastroesophageal reflux disease and was termed the Stretta technique. The adaptation for use in the anal sphincter is termed the Secca procedure (Curon Medical Incorporated, Fremont, California). This technique uses submucosally applied RF energy to induce tissue remodeling. The Secca procedure can be performed on an ambulatory basis using conscious sedation and local anesthesia. The patient is positioned in the prone jack-knife position. A special RF energy device that utilizes an anoscopic barrel with four nickel-titanium curved needle electrodes is used. Within the tip and at the base of each electrode, thermocouples are present to monitor tissue and mucosal temperature during RF delivery. The instrument is introduced into the anal canal under direct visualization, so

that the needle electrodes start to penetrate the tissue 1 cm distal to the dentate line. Additional lesions are created up to 1.5 cm above the dentate line in all four quadrants. Mucosal temperature is cooled by surface irrigation. In this way, thermal lesions are created in the muscle below the mucosa, while preserving the mucosal integrity. In contrast to the belief that RF therapy would cause scarring and tightening of the anal canal, essentially causing mild obstruction akin to cerclage, new or histologic assessment of RF-treated tissue reveals that nonablative RF energy causes morphologic changes in damaged sphincter muscle to become more histologically normal (141). Efron published some of the earliest data in a multicenter trial involving 50 patients. In this cohort, mean Wexner scores improved from a baseline of 14.5 to 11.1 at 6 months. All quality of life parameters were also improved, and only minor complications were noted (142). Five-year data were reported by Takahashi showing that mean Wexner scores remain significantly improved from baseline of 14 to 8 with nearly 85% of patients showing a >50% improvement (143). Ruiz reported on more modest results at 2-year follow-up showing mild improvement in incontinence scores from 15.6 to 12.9 (144). Currently, few centers are employing this modality, in favor of the more reliable results achieved with sacral neuromodulation.

## ANTEGRADE CONTINENCE ENEMA (ACE PROCEDURE)

The ACE procedure was first described by Malone in 1990 (145). This treatment was developed for patients with disabling colonic motility disorders and difficulty with evacuation of solid stool. In this description, the appendix is reversed and tunneled into the wall of the cecum, creating a one-way valve. The proximal end is brought through the abdominal wall as a small stoma in the right lower quadrant, flush with the skin. In order to eliminate, the appendicostomy is intubated, and the colon is flushed in an antegrade manner with fluid in order to clear the colon of stool. This has been employed primarily in the pediatric population, afflicted with congenital motility disorders, but is also rarely used in adults. Several modifications of this procedure have been described in order to simplify the technical rigors. Several reports have shown good results (146,147). Worsoe reported long-term results on a series of 80 patients with a mean follow-up of 75 months. In this cohort, there was an overall success rate of 74%, with very positive subjective results (148). ACE can be considered in select patients as an option prior to colostomy.

## COLOSTOMY

For patients with anal incontinence so severe that they are disabled by their symptoms and unable to maintain continence by either conservative or surgical modalities, construction of a colostomy or ileostomy may become necessary. Despite the assumed negative associations with a stoma, the patient's quality of life may be significantly enhanced, and self-imposed isolation corrected. A colostomy is especially appropriate in patients with profound incontinence related to anorectal disease or tumor, and in whom other surgical approaches are contraindicated, or in situations where reconstruction is impossible. Norton et al. (149) reviewed the formation of a permanent stoma as a last resort when all other interventions for FI have failed. Questionnaires were sent asking about the stoma, previous incontinence, anxiety, depression, and quality of life. Sixty-nine replies were received from 11 males and 58 females with a median age of 64 years and a median of 59 months since the operation. Rating their ability to live with their stoma on a scale of 0–10, the median response was 8. The majority (83%) felt that the stoma restricted their life "a little" or "not at all," a significant improvement from perceived restriction from former incontinence. Satisfaction with the stoma was a median score of 9. Eighty-four percent would "probably" or "definitely" choose to have the stoma again. They concluded the majority of previously incontinent people felt positively about the stoma and the difference it had made to their life. However, a few had not adapted and disliked the stoma intensely.

## ONGOING INVESTIGATIONS

Other modalities are currently being tested in order to increase our armamentarium for the treatment of this debilitating issue. Current clinical trials include the TOPAS device (American Medical Systems), which is a polypropylene mesh sling implanted to reinforce the puborectal angle, as well as the LIBERATE trial (Pelvilon, Inc.), which employs an inflatable vaginal insert used to occlude the anal canal. In addition, the use of an occlusive anal plug has been employed as a minimally invasive option. Examples include the Peristeen anal plug (Coloplast UK), and the Procon-2 device.

## CONCLUSIONS

Modern surgery is experiencing an increase in the number of modalities available to treat fecal incontinence. Especially regarding the success of SNS, there has been a profound paradigm shift in the more conservative, yet equally effective management of all but the most extreme cases of FI. Despite the wide range of surgical options, most patients with FI can be treated very successfully with appropriate conservative management and the use of stool bulking agents and antidiarrheal medications. For those who failed conservative treatment, there are a wide variety of surgical options. The classical historical gold standard of sphincter repair has been largely supplanted with much less invasive and much more effective techniques, with SNS leading the way. Nevertheless, a thorough understanding of all of the medical and surgical options for management of FI is required of all surgeons who may evaluate and treat these patients.

## REFERENCES

1. Sharma A et al. *Br J Surg* 2016;103:1589–97.
2. Macmillan AK et al. *Dis Colon Rectum* 2004;47(8): 1341–9.
3. Xu X et al. *Dis Colon Rectum* 2012;55(5):586–98.
4. Brown HW et al. *Female Pelvic Med Reconstr Surg* 2013;19(2):66–71.
5. Damon H et al. *Dis Colon Rectum* 2002;45(11):1445–50; discussion 1450–1.
6. Perry S et al. *Gut* 2002;50(4):480–4.
7. Brown HW et al. *Int J Clin Pract* 2012;66(11):1109–16.
8. Madoff RD et al. *N Engl J Med* 1992;326(15):1002–7.
9. Browning GG, Parks AG. *Br J Surg* 1983;70(2):101–4.
10. Jorge JM, Wexner SD. *Dis Colon Rectum* 1993;36(1): 77–97.
11. Rockwood TH et al. *Dis Colon Rectum* 1999;42(12): 1525–32.
12. Rockwood TH. *Gastroenterology* 2004;126(1 Suppl 1): S106–13.
13. Nelson R et al. *JAMA* 1995;274(7):559–61.
14. Cerulli MA et al. *Gastroenterology* 1979;76(4):742–6.
15. Ctercteko GC et al. *Aust N Z J Surg* 1988;58(9): 703–10.
16. Keighley MR, Fielding JW. *Br J Surg* 1983;70(8): 463–8.
17. Sultan AH et al. *N Engl J Med* 1993;329(26):1905–11.
18. Eason E et al. *CMAJ* 2002;166(3):326–30.
19. Oberwalder M et al. *Br J Surg* 2003;90(11):1333–7.
20. Rieger N, Wattchow D. *Aust N Z J Surg* 1999;69(3): 172–7.
21. Oberwalder M et al. *Arch Surg* 2004;139(4):429–32.
22. Faridi A et al. *J Perinat Med* 2002;30(5):379–87.
23. Fynes M et al. *Obstet Gynecol* 1998;92(4 Pt 1):496–500.
24. Nelson RL et al. *Cochrane Database Syst Rev* 2010; (2):CD006756.
25. Khubchandani IT, Reed JF. *Br J Surg* 1989;76(5): 431–4.
26. Liang J, Church JM. *Am J Surg* 2015;210(4):715–9.
27. Aguilar PS et al. *Dis Colon Rectum* 1985;28(7):496–8.
28. Golub RW et al. *J Gastrointest Surg* 1997;1(5):487–91.
29. Ortiz H, Marzo J. *Br J Surg* 2000;87(12):1680–3.
30. Schouten WR et al. *Dis Colon Rectum* 1999;42(11): 1419–22; discussion 1422–3.
31. van Tets WF et al. *Dis Colon Rectum* 1997;40(9): 1042–5.
32. Stelzner F. *Prog Pediatr Surg* 1976;9:1–6.
33. Parks AG. *Proc R Soc Med* 1975;68(11):681–90.
34. Suilleabhain CB et al. *Dis Colon Rectum* 2001;44(5): 666–71.
35. Schiller LR et al. *N Engl J Med* 1982;307(27):1666–71.
36. Gee AS, Durdey P. *Br J Surg* 1995;82(9):1179–82.
37. Henry MM. *Gastroenterol Clin North Am* 1987;16(1): 35–45.
38. Sultan AH et al. *Br J Surg* 1993;80(4):508–11.
39. Bharucha AE. *Gastroenterology* 2004;126(1 Suppl 1): S90–8.

40. Bollard RC et al. *Dis Colon Rectum* 2002;45(2):171–5.
41. Sentovich SM et al. *Dis Colon Rectum* 1998;41(8):1000–4.
42. Zetterstrom JP et al. *Dis Colon Rectum* 1998;41(6):705–13.
43. Gold DM et al. *Br J Surg* 1999;86(3):371–5.
44. Xue Y et al. *Zhonghua Wei Chang Wai Ke Za Zhi* 2014;17(12):1187–9.
45. Hiltunen KM. *Dis Colon Rectum* 1985;28(12):925–8.
46. Read NW et al. *Br J Surg* 1984;71(1):39–42.
47. Penninckx F et al. *Acta Gastroenterol Belg* 1995;58(1):51–9.
48. Tetzschner T et al. *Acta Obstet Gynecol Scand* 1995;74(6):434–40.
49. Bartolo DC et al. *Br J Surg* 1983;70(11):664–7.
50. Baig MK, Wexner SD. *Br J Surg* 2000;87(10):1316–30.
51. Laurberg S et al. *Br J Surg* 1988;75(8):786–8.
52. Roig JV et al. *Dis Colon Rectum* 1995;38(9):952–8.
53. Rasmussen OO et al. *Int J Colorectal Dis* 1990;5(3):135–41.
54. Young CJ et al. *Dis Colon Rectum* 1998;41(3):344–9.
55. Chen AS et al. *Dis Colon Rectum* 1998;41(8):1005–9.
56. Briel JW et al. *Int J Colorectal Dis* 2000;15(2):87–90.
57. Rosen L et al. *Am Fam Physician* 1986;33(3):129–37.
58. Bannister JJ et al. *Br J Surg* 1989;76(6):617–21.
59. Hallgren T et al. *Dig Dis Sci* 1994;39(12):2612–8.
60. Santoro GA et al. *Dis Colon Rectum* 2000;43(12):1676–81; discussion 1681–2.
61. Engel BT et al. *N Engl J Med* 1974;290(12):646–9.
62. Loening-Baucke V. *Dig Dis* 1990;8(2):112–24.
63. Wald A. *Eur J Gastroenterol Hepatol* 1995;7(8):737–9.
64. Norton C, Cody JD. *Cochrane Database Syst Rev* 2012;(7):CD002111.
65. Heymen S et al. *Dis Colon Rectum* 2001;44(5):728–36.
66. Norton C et al. *Gastroenterology* 2003;125(5):1320–9.
67. Solomon MJ et al. *Dis Colon Rectum* 2003;46(6):703–10.
68. Fynes MM et al. *Dis Colon Rectum* 1999;42(6):753–8; discussion 758–61.
69. Beddy P et al. *J Gastrointest Surg* 2004;8(1):64–72; discussion 71–2.
70. Chiarioni G et al. *Am J Gastroenterol* 2002;97(1):109–17.
71. Sangwan YP et al. *Dis Colon Rectum* 1995;38(10):1021–5.
72. Fernandez-Fraga X et al. *Dis Colon Rectum* 2003;46(9):1218–25.
73. Enck P et al. *Dis Colon Rectum* 1994;37(10):997–1001.
74. Guillemot F et al. *Dis Colon Rectum* 1995;38(4):393–7.
75. Glia A et al. *Dis Colon Rectum* 1998;41(3):359–64.
76. Ryn AK et al. *Dis Colon Rectum* 2000;43(9):1262–6.
77. Pager CK et al. *Dis Colon Rectum* 2002;45(8):997–1003.
78. Davis KJ et al. *Aliment Pharmacol Ther* 2004;20(5):539–49.
79. Fang DT et al. *Dis Colon Rectum* 1984;27(11):720–2.
80. Parks AG, McPartlin JF. *Proc R Soc Med* 1971;64(12):1187–9.
81. Mahony R et al. *Dis Colon Rectum* 2004;47(1):12–7.
82. Karoui S et al. *Dis Colon Rectum* 2000;43(6):813–20.
83. Malouf AJ et al. *Lancet* 2000;355(9200):260–5.
84. Halverson AL, Hull TL. *Dis Colon Rectum* 2002;45(3):345–8.
85. Simmang C et al. *Dis Colon Rectum* 1994;37(11):1065–9.
86. Rasmussen OO et al. *Dis Colon Rectum* 1999;42(2):193–5.
87. Gilliland R et al. *Dis Colon Rectum* 1998;41(12):1516–22.
88. Londono-Schimmer EE et al. *Int J Colorectal Dis* 1994;9(2):110–3.
89. Barisic GI et al. *Int J Colorectal Dis* 2006;21(1):52–6.
90. Bravo Gutierrez A et al. *Dis Colon Rectum* 2004;47(5):727–31; discussion 731–2.
91. Tjandra JJ et al. *Dis Colon Rectum* 2003;46(7):937–42; discussion 942–3.
92. Briel JW et al. *Dis Colon Rectum* 1998;41(2):209–14.
93. Hasegawa H et al. *Dis Colon Rectum* 2000;43(7):961–4; discussion 964–5.
94. Womack NR et al. *Br J Surg* 1988;75(1):48–52.
95. Miller R et al. *Br J Surg* 1988;75(2):101–5.
96. Orrom WJ et al. *Dis Colon Rectum* 1991;34(4):305–10.
97. Athanasiadis S et al. *Langenbecks Arch Chir* 1995;380(1):22–30.
98. Healy JC et al. *Dis Colon Rectum* 2002;45(12):1629–34.
99. Setti Carraro P et al. *Br J Surg* 1994;81(1):140–4.
100. Browning GG, Motson RW. *Ann Surg* 1984;199(3):351–7.
101. Jameson JS et al. *Dis Colon Rectum* 1994;37(4):369–72.
102. Keighley MR. *Int J Colorectal Dis* 1987;2(4):236–9.
103. Laurberg S et al. *Br J Surg* 1990;77(5):519–22.
104. van Tets WF, Kuijpers JH. *Dis Colon Rectum* 1998;41(3):365–9.
105. Pickrell K et al. *Am J Surg* 1955;90(5):721–6.
106. Wexner SD et al. *Dis Colon Rectum* 1996;39(9):957–64.
107. Matzel KE et al. *Dis Colon Rectum* 2001;44(10):1427–35.
108. Chodez M et al. *Tech Coloproctol* 2014;18(12):1147–51.
109. Wexner SD et al. *Ann Surg* 2010;251(3):441–9.
110. Wexner SD et al. *J Gastrointest Surg* 2010;14(7):1081–9.
111. Wexner SD, Bleier J. *Expert Rev Gastroenterol Hepatol.* 2015;9:1577–89.
112. Tjandra JJ et al. *Dis Colon Rectum* 2008;51(5):494–502.
113. Mellgren A et al. *Dis Colon Rectum* 2011;54(9):1065–75.
114. Hull T et al. *Dis Colon Rectum* 2013;56(2):234–45.
115. Altomare DF et al. *Dis Colon Rectum* 2009;52(1):11–7.
116. Lim JT et al. *Dis Colon Rectum* 2011;54(8):969–74.

117. Michelsen HB et al. *Dis Colon Rectum* 2010;53(4): 414–21.
118. Altomare DF et al. *Br J Surg* 2015;102(4):407–15.
119. George AT et al. *Dis Colon Rectum* 2012;55(3): 302–6.
120. Brouwer R, Duthie G. *Dis Colon Rectum* 2010;53(3): 273–8.
121. Nakamura M et al. *Hinyokika Kiyo* 1983;29(9):1053–9.
122. Shafik A et al. *Eur Surg Res* 2003;35(2):103–7.
123. Leroi AM et al. *Am J Gastroenterol* 2012;107(12): 1888–96.
124. Thomas GP et al. *Colorectal Dis* 2013;15(5):519–26.
125. Thin NN et al. *Br J Surg* 2015;102(4):349–58.
126. Knowles CH et al. *Lancet* 2015 Oct 24;386(10004): 1640–8.
127. Edenfield AL et al. *Obstet Gynecol Surv* 2015;70(5): 329–41.
128. Graf W et al. *Lancet* 2011;377(9770):997–1003.
129. Maeda Y et al. *Cochrane Database Syst Rev* 2013;2: CD007959.
130. LaTorre F, de la Portilla F. *Colorectal Dis* 2013;15(5): 569–74.
131. Hussain ZI et al. *Br J Surg* 2011;98(11):1526–36.
132. Guerra F et al. *Tech Coloproctol* 2015;19(1):23–7.
133. Christiansen J, Sparso B. *Ann Surg* 1992;215(4):383–6.
134. Mundy L et al. *Br J Surg* 2004;91(6):665–72.
135. Darnis B et al. *Dis Colon Rectum* 2013;56(4):505–10.
136. Wong MT et al. *Ann Surg* 2011;254(6):951–6.
137. Wexner SD et al. *Dis Colon Rectum* 2009;52(9): 1550–7.
138. Lehur PA et al. *Dis Colon Rectum* 2010;53(12): 1604–10.
139. Barussaud ML et al. *Colorectal Dis* 2013;15(12): 1499–1503.
140. Williams A et al. *Int J Colorectal Dis* 2016;31(2): 465–72.
141. Herman RM et al. *Colorectal Dis* 2015;17(5):433–40.
142. Efron JE. *Surg Technol Int* 2004;13:107–10.
143. Takahashi-Monroy T et al. *Dis Colon Rectum* 2008; 51(3):355–9.
144. Ruiz D et al. *Dis Colon Rectum* 2010;53(7):1041–6.
145. Malone PS et al. *Lancet* 1990;336(8725):1217–8.
146. Lawal TA et al. *J Laparoendosc Adv Surg Tech A* 2011;21(5):455–9.
147. Ellison JS et al. *J Urol* 2013;190(4 Suppl):1529–33.
148. Worsoe J et al. *Dis Colon Rectum* 2008;51(10): 1523–8.
149. Norton C et al. *Dis Colon Rectum* 2005;48(5):1062–9.

# 24

# Surgery for rectal prolapse

STEVEN R. HUNT

**CHALLENGING CASE**

A 75-year-old woman with a history of chronic obstructive pulmonary disease (COPD) and congestive heart failure (CHF) presents with full-thickness rectal prolapse. Her colonoscopy was normal.

**CASE MANAGEMENT**

The patient is offered a perineal proctosigmoidectomy (Altmeier procedure).

## INTRODUCTION

Rectal prolapse (rectal procidentia) is defined as the full-thickness intussusception of the rectum through the anal canal. The annual incidence of rectal prolapse is estimated to be 2.5 per 100,000 population (1). The disorder tends to affect elderly women, psychiatric patients, and patients with neurologic disorders. Presenting symptoms are usually referable to the prolapse itself. Additional presenting complaints include constipation, straining, incontinence, and mucous soilage of the undergarments.

Surgery remains the only definitive therapy for rectal prolapse. Over 100 operations have been described for the treatment of procidentia. Generally, these procedures can be divided into peritoneal and abdominal approaches. The optimal procedure for each patient should be determined by presenting symptoms and patient comorbid disease.

## CLASSIFICATION

In the strictest sense, rectal prolapse refers only to full-thickness, circumferential protrusion of the rectum beyond the anal canal. While it is often clinically obvious, several other anorectal disorders can imitate the condition. Circumferential prolapsed internal hemorrhoids, when large, are frequently diagnosed as prolapse, and prolapse is often diagnosed as hemorrhoids. Rectal polyps or cancer can protrude through the anus and mimic prolapse. It is important to differentiate between true procidentia and mucosal prolapse, as the entities may have similar presenting symptoms. Patients with mucosal prolapse frequently have a history of prior anorectal procedures or trauma, and the prolapse is often asymmetric. Solitary rectal ulcers and colitis cystica profunda can present with symptoms similar to rectal prolapse. These disorders are associated with internal intussusception of the rectum but may coexist in patients with rectal prolapse. Both solitary rectal ulcer and colitis cystica profunda are hypothesized to result from repeated mucosal trauma and ischemia at the lead point of the prolapse. Significant rectal bleeding is relatively rare in patients with procidentia, although it is a common presentation in solitary rectal ulcer syndrome and colitis cystica profunda.

Internal rectal intussusception without prolapse may be a predecessor to rectal prolapse, although this association has not been proven (2). Rectal intussusception is frequently identified during defecography performed to evaluate obstructed defecation or constipation. It is also a common finding in asymptomatic patients (3). While it is clear that surgery is the mainstay of treatment for complete rectal prolapse, the indications for surgical intervention in cases of internal intussusception are less clear. Some authors advocate surgical intervention in cases of symptomatic intussusception, while others are more cautious in their approach (4,5). In the author's section, the initial approach to patients with rectal intussusception is dietary modification and pelvic floor retraining through biofeedback. Surgery is generally reserved for patients with complications of internal prolapse (solitary rectal ulcers and colitis cystica profunda) who have failed conservative therapy.

## PATIENT EVALUATION AND INVESTIGATIONS

As rectal prolapse is a benign disease, surgery need only be considered if the symptoms are debilitating. Frequency of the prolapse and initiating factors (defecation, straining, or standing) should be documented. The presence of severe constipation or symptoms of obstructed defecation should be noted, as these patients may require further evaluation. Fecal incontinence occurs in 60%–80% of patients, and a frank discussion should ensue regarding expected surgical outcomes with regard to continence. Most large series show improvement in fecal incontinence in greater than 40% of procidentia patients after surgery, regardless of the approach (6). Continence may continue to improve over the first 6–12 months postoperatively.

A detailed surgical history should be obtained, with special attention to anorectal and pelvic operations, as this may influence the ultimate surgical approach. In patients with recurrent rectal prolapse, operative notes from the prior procedures should be obtained and scrutinized. Female patients may have a history of bladder or uterine prolapse, requiring consultation with a urogynecologist and a combined approach. All patients with prolapse should have a recent colonoscopy to rule out any mucosal lesions.

## PHYSICAL EXAM

The diagnosis of procidentia is made by demonstration of the prolapse in the surgeon's office. Patients with advanced prolapse may be able to produce the prolapse on the examination table with minimal straining. If the patient cannot prolapse on the examination table, he or she should be examined after straining on the toilet. Once the prolapse has been achieved, the examiner should first differentiate between full-thickness prolapse and hemorrhoidal or mucosal prolapse. Full-thickness prolapse is characterized by concentric mucosal rings, as opposed to the radially oriented sulci seen with mucosal and hemorrhoidal prolapse.

The digital rectal exam should exclude other anorectal pathology, and the sphincter tone and the squeeze pressure should be evaluated. Female patients should be evaluated for the presence of an enterocele or rectocele. Rigid proctoscopy should be performed in the office to rule out any rectal tumors, and to evaluate for solitary ulcer and colitis cystica profunda.

Generally, a physical exam and demonstration of the complete prolapse in the office are sufficient evaluation prior to surgery. Additional studies are sometimes required in certain cases.

## ANAL PHYSIOLOGY

Patients with chronic severe straining at stool should be evaluated with anal physiology testing. Electromyography that demonstrates a nonrelaxing puborectalis should prompt initiation of biofeedback therapy as an adjunct to surgery.

Postoperative continence can also be predicted on the basis of a prolonged pudendal nerve terminal motor latency (PNTML) and poor resting sphincter tone (7,8). We do not routinely obtain physiologic studies in the evaluation of procidentia, as they are expensive and a prolonged PNTML is not a contraindication for surgery.

## ADDITIONAL STUDIES

When the patient is unable to reproduce the rectal prolapse in the office, defecography may be used to evaluate for internal prolapse or other defecatory pathology. In patients with severe constipation and prolapse, a colonic transit study may be obtained. Concentration of the markers in the left and sigmoid colon on day 5, in the setting of severe constipation, is an indication for a resection rectopexy.

## OPERATIVE REPAIRS

Although the modern operative procedures for rectal prolapse are not particularly morbid, the patients are frequently elderly, and morbidity is not trivial. Some series report mortalities as high as 7%. These patients often have significant comorbid conditions, and the operative approach (perineal, open, or laparoscopic) should take these factors into account. The choice of procedure is frequently dictated by surgeon preference and experience; however, a one-size-fits-all approach may not be suitable for all patients.

In addition to the morbidity of the procedure, evaluation of the various surgical approaches to rectal prolapse must take efficacy and functional outcomes into account. Some techniques have excellent results in terms of recurrence but can predispose the patients to constipation or evacuatory difficulties, trading one problem for another.

## PERINEAL REPAIRS

The preponderance of the historical literature suggests that the abdominal approach to rectal prolapse is superior to the perineal approach in terms of recurrence rates. While most single institution studies report better outcomes for abdominal procedures, this difference is not demonstrated in meta-analysis (9,10).

The major advantage of the perineal approach is the ability to conduct the operation under spinal or even local, anesthetic. The avoidance of general anesthesia and an abdominal dissection makes this the preferred approach for patients with significant comorbidities.

### Perineal proctosigmoidectomy (Altmeier procedure)

The technique of perineal proctosigmoidectomy involves mobilization and resection of the prolapsed rectosigmoid colon via a perineal approach. Patients should have a complete mechanical bowel preparation. The prone-jackknife or left lateral position is preferred over lithotomy, as it allows easy access to the operative field for the surgeon and assistant. While general anesthetic provides more comfort for the patient, it is often necessary to use local or spinal anesthesia in frail patients. The buttocks should be taped apart, and a Lonestar retractor is used to efface the anus and provide optimal exposure.

The procedure is begun by recreating the prolapse. Once the bowel has been completely prolapsed, a circumferential incision is made in the rectum approximately 1.5–2 cm proximal to the dentate line. Using the electrocautery, this incision should be continued until the full thickness of the rectal wall has been incised circumferentially. The incised rectum is then everted and pulled downward. The vaginal wall is frequently adherent to the prolapsed segment and should be dissected away from the rectum to avoid the devastating complication of a postoperative colovaginal fistula. The peritoneal cavity is then entered by incising the peritoneum of the pouch of Douglas anteriorly. Entrance into the peritoneal cavity facilitates delivery of the prolapsed rectum and division of the mesorectum. The mesorectum is then divided and ligated with ligatures, or alternatively, a vessel-sealing device may be used. Division of the mesorectum should be continued, advancing proximally on the bowel until tension is encountered (Figure 24.1).

Once the redundant rectosigmoid has been mobilized, the anterior peritoneum should be repaired, including seromuscular bites of the anterior bowel wall, with a running absorbable suture to obliterate the pouch. A levatorplasty should be considered if a defect is present in the pelvic floor. If the levator muscles can be identified without extensive dissection, plication should be performed anteriorly and posteriorly. The redundant bowel is then divided and a hand-sewn anastomosis is fashioned using interrupted absorbable sutures. Alternatively, the anastomosis may be created using an EEA stapler with acceptable results (11,12).

Generally, patients have minimal narcotic requirements postoperatively and ileus is exceedingly rare. Patients should be ambulated and their diet is advanced on postoperative day 1. Constipating regimens have no proven beneficial

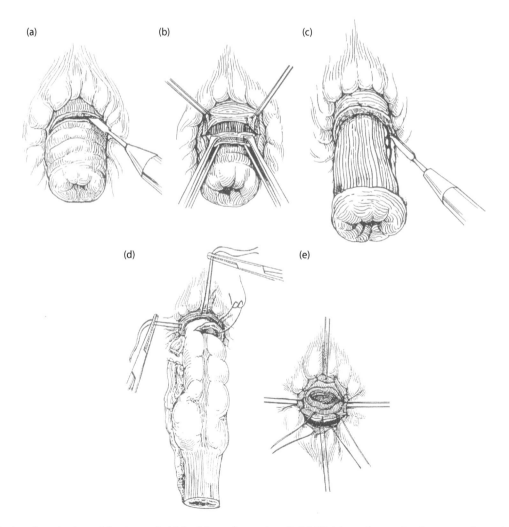

(a) (b) (c)

(d) (e)

Figure 24.1 Perineal rectosigmoidectomy. **(a,b)** Incision of rectal wall. **(c)** Division of vessel adjacent to bowel wall. **(d)** Mesenteric vessels ligated. Stay sutures previously placed in distal edge of outer cylinder are placed in cut edge of inner cylinder. **(e)** Anastomosis of distal aspect of remaining colon to the short rectal stump.

results. It is the author's practice to discharge patients after the first bowel movement, but in some centers, the Altmeier procedure is performed on an outpatient basis (11).

In experienced hands, the Altmeier procedure has excellent results, rivaling the abdominal procedures for recurrence rates. Several recent large series report recurrence rates ranging from 6% to 16% (7,9,11). Both incontinence and constipation are also significantly improved after perineal proctectomy (7,9,13). Some authors describe significant improvement in recurrence rates if a levatorplasty is performed (14).

Fortunately, major morbidity and mortality for this procedure are rare. The anastomotic leak rates are reportedly 1%–2%, with significant bleeding occurring in a similar percentage of patients (7,9,14).

## Delorme procedure

Delorme procedure offers another alternative to the Altmeier repair. The technique involves a submucosal resection of the prolapsed rectum, with plication of the muscularis propria. The submucosal nature of the dissection in this procedure does not allow for a concomitant levatorplasty.

As with the Altmeier procedure, mechanical bowel preparation should be performed and the procedure conducted in the prone-jackknife or left lateral position with effacement of the anus. Again, local or spinal anesthesia may be used for infirm patients. The rectal prolapse is delivered, and the submucosal plane is infiltrated with local anesthetic containing epinephrine. A circumferential mucosal incision is made 1 cm proximal to the dentate line. The submucosal plane is identified, and downward traction is applied to the mucosal tube. Dissection is carried out within this plane to the apex of the prolapsed segment of rectum. At this point, the exposed muscularis propria is plicated with multiple bites in four quadrants using an absorbable monofilament or braided suture. The redundant mucosa is then excised and the plication sutures are tied. The mucosal edges are then reapproximated using interrupted absorbable sutures (Figure 24.2).

The recurrence rate in most recent large series ranges from 13% to 27% (15–17). The morbidity and mortality rates are similar to those of the Altmeier repair. Improvement is reported in both continence and constipation in most series where these functional outcomes were evaluated (16–18).

Given the uniformly inferior results of Delorme procedure relative to the Altmeier repair, it is the author's feeling that this approach should not be used as a first-line perineal procedure. Many advocate this procedure for the treatment of mucosal prolapse; however, other, less involved

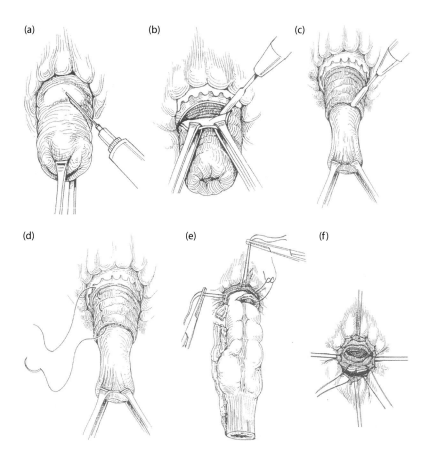

Figure 24.2 Delorme procedure. **(a)** Subcutaneous infiltration of dilute epinephrine solution. **(b)** Circumferential mucosal incision. **(c)** Dissection of mucosa off muscular layer. **(d)** Plicating stitch approximating cut edge of mucosa, muscular wall, and mucosa just proximal to dentate line. **(e)** Plicating stitch tied. **(f)** Completed anastomosis.

techniques exist for this disorder. Elastic rubber band ligation is frequently adequate for modest mucosal prolapse. The circular stapler technique used in the treatment of hemorrhoids is a second appealing option for more advanced mucosal prolapse.

## Anal encirclement (Thiersch repair)

Anal encirclement has almost reached the status of historical interest, as it has been replaced by other procedures with more favorable results. The procedure can be performed in a short period of time with only local anesthetic. The original repair described by Thiersch used a silver wire to encircle the anal sphincter complex. The wire encirclement has fallen out of favor as the wire can break or erode through the sphincters and anoderm. Marlex or Mersilene mesh are the preferred alternatives to wire, as they are softer and less prone to breakage or erosion.

The operation can be performed in the prone-jackknife or lithotomy position. After meticulous antiseptic preparation, small posterior and anterior incisions are made 1 cm outside the anal verge. A curved clamp is then tunneled through the ischiorectal fossa from the anterior incision to the posterior incision, and one end of the mesh is then pulled through the tunnel. This is duplicated on the opposite side, and the other end of the mesh is delivered. The redundant mesh is pulled through and the prosthetic is tightened around an 18F Hegar dilator. The mesh is then overlapped anteriorly and sewn to itself with a nonabsorbable suture. The small incisions are then closed with absorbable subcuticular sutures, and the wounds are sealed with Dermabond, to prevent subsequent soilage of the wounds (Figure 24.3).

Anal encirclement procedures do not repair the prolapse but merely prevent external prolapse. Infectious complications are common with the synthetic mesh, occurring in up to 33% of patients (19). Postoperatively, these patients frequently experience tenesmus and difficulty with evacuation (20). This procedure should be reserved for patients who have significant contraindications to more formal repairs. One relative indication for this repair is the patient with significant hepatic ascites (not amenable to transjugular intrahepatic portosystemic shunt) and debilitating rectal prolapse.

## OPEN ABDOMINAL REPAIRS

A prerequisite to the open approach is the patient's ability to tolerate a general anesthetic and laparotomy. A variety of abdominal repairs are described in the literature, but only a few have withstood the test of time. The common theme among these time-tested procedures is complete rectal mobilization and fixation of the rectum to the sacrum. It is suggested that the fibrosis resulting from the rectal mobilization is responsible for the long-term fixation of the rectum and avoidance of recurrence (21).

All of the large series involving abdominal procedures show improvement in fecal continence. The same cannot

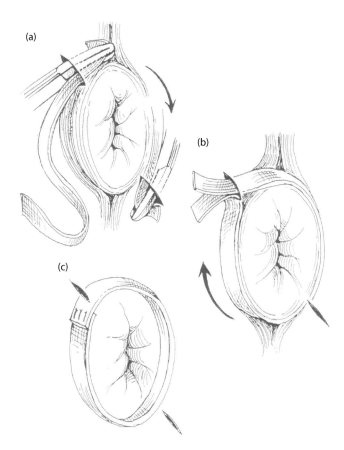

**Figure 24.3** Anal encirclement (Thiersch). **(a)** Lateral incisions with prosthetic mesh tunneled around the anus. **(b)** Mesh completely encircling the anal opening. **(c)** Completed anal encirclement procedure.

be said for constipation, as rectopexy alone tends to worsen constipation. In cases of severe constipation preoperatively, a sigmoidectomy may be combined with rectal fixation.

The repairs discussed in the following all involve complete rectal mobilization. In all cases, the rectal mobilization should be carried out in the avascular plane outside the mesorectal fascia. The peritoneum at the sacral promontory is incised, and the plane posterior to the superior rectal artery is identified. Great care should be taken to prevent injury to the hypogastric plexus, and the ureters should be identified and avoided. When rectal fixation sutures are placed, the position of the ureters should be reconfirmed to prevent inclusion in the suture. These approaches are not immune to the usual pitfalls of open laparotomy, with complications including small bowel obstruction, prolonged ileus, and wound complications.

There is some controversy regarding the extent of rectal mobilization. While some authors advocate division of the lateral rectal ligaments to improve recurrence rates, there are some reports of worsening constipation if the lateral ligaments are divided (22). In a small randomized prospective study comparing rectal mobilization with and without division of the lateral ligaments, Mollen et al. reported no difference between the two groups with regard to constipation scores or to total colonic transit time. Anterior rectal mobilization is recommended with all of these procedures, but this is generally a minimal dissection as these patients tend to have a deep pouch of Douglas.

## Mesh sling repair (Ripstein procedure)

The Ripstein procedure involves the posterior mobilization of the rectum down to the pelvic floor followed by fixation of the rectum to the sacrum using a mesh sling. Before the advent of the laparoscopic approach, this procedure was one of the most commonly employed abdominal techniques for rectal prolapse.

Patients should undergo a complete mechanical bowel preparation, and the operation is performed in the lithotomy position. A complete rectal mobilization is carried down to the pelvic floor. A 3–4 cm wide piece of polytetrafluoroethylene (PTFE) or polypropylene mesh is then fixed to the sacrum approximately 1 cm to the right of the midline using several nonabsorbable sutures. Traction is then applied to the rectum in a cephalad direction, and the mesh is fixed at multiple points to the anterior rectum by seromuscular bites of nonabsorbable suture. The mesh is then secured to the left side of the sacrum approximately 1 cm off the midline, taking care to ensure that the mesh does not constrict the rectum (Figure 24.4).

The results of the Ripstein repair are excellent in terms of recurrence, with recurrence rates of 0%–7% reported in large series (6,23,24). In spite of these enviable results,

enthusiasm for this procedure has waned because of reports of mesh erosion into the rectum, late colovaginal fistulas, stenosis, and significant constipation following the procedure (23). In light of these complications and the success of other alternative therapies, the Ripstein procedure's role in the modern treatment of rectal prolapse should be limited.

## Ventral mesh rectopexy

A variation of an anterior mesh rectopexy is to use an anteriorly placed vertical strip attached posteriorly, secured to one side of the sacral promontory. This approach is known as a ventral mesh rectopexy (25). This differs substantially from a traditional Ripstein in that the posterior dissection is typically limited to exposure of the sacral promontory. With this technique, the right aspect of the distal sigmoid mesentery and upper rectum are mobilized by incising the right side of the peritoneal reflection at the level of the sacral promontory and then sweeping the mesentery off of the retroperitoneum in order to expose a site of fixation of the mesh to the sacral promontory. The left side of the peritoneum is left intact, while the right peritoneum is incised in a curvilinear fashion, over the lateral ligaments and into the anterior peritoneal reflection. The anterior dissection is undertaken to the level of the mid-vagina or seminal vesicles. The mesh is fashioned to the appropriate width and length and is then secured to the anterior rectum with interrupted suture. The mesh then courses along the right

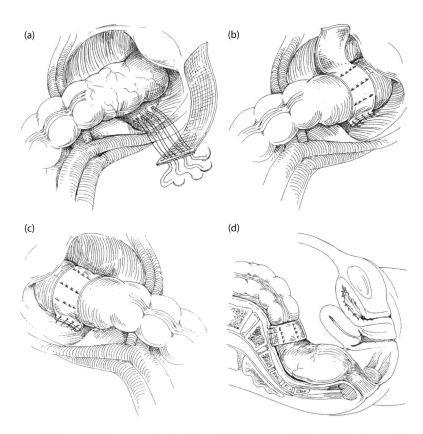

Figure 24.4 Mesh rectopexy (Ripstein): **(a)** posterior fixation of sling on one side, **(b)** sling brought anteriorly around mobilized rectum, **(c)** sling fixed posteriorly on the opposite side, and **(d)** sagittal view of the completed rectopexy.

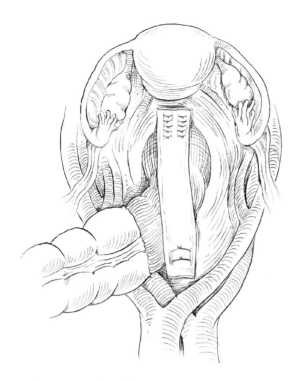

Figure 24.5 Ventral mesh rectopexy.

anterior rectum and is ultimately fixed to the sacral promontory (Figure 24.5). Drains are not routinely placed.

In most mesh procedures, the mesh is extraperitonealized, typically by closing the peritoneum with a running, absorbable suture. This step theoretically minimizes the potential for small bowel obstruction secondary to adhesions to the mesh as well as minimizes the potential for mesh erosion and fistula formation. Every patient with rectal prolapse has, by definition, an element of pelvic floor dysfunction. The various components of pelvic floor dysfunction (e.g., rectocele, enterocele, cystocele, uterine or vaginal prolapse) often coexist. Another advantage of a ventral rectopexy is that if the dissection is carried low enough, it can concomitantly address a symptomatic rectocele as well with low recurrence rates (26,27).

### LAPAROSCOPIC MESH RECTOPEXY

The principles, anatomy, and landmarks for laparoscopic mesh rectopexy are identical to those for open mesh rectopexy, as previously detailed. One impact the use of mesh will have on a laparoscopic case may be port selection, as a 12 mm port is typically required for introduction of the mesh. While most synthetic mesh products can be laparoscopically handled with similar ease as in open procedures, many biologic grafts are thick, and the handling and suturing of such materials laparoscopically can pose a challenge. For that reason, when selecting a biologic mesh for laparoscopic rectopexy, a thinner and partially transparent mesh may reduce some of the difficulty and clumsiness when handling and securing the mesh.

Robotic-assisted surgery in rectal prolapse repair uses the same dissection and points of fixation as a laparoscopic repair. Some surgeons prefer the robotic approach for ease of deep pelvic dissection and knot tying.

### Results of mesh rectopexy

In its various iterations, mesh rectopexy has performed well in terms of low recurrence rates, but occasionally high morbidity rates have led to evolution of the procedure over time (6,28–32). With the original Ripstein repair, recurrence rates ranged from 4% to 10%, but the morbidity was high, with complications including mesh erosion, large bowel obstruction, fecal impaction, and rectovaginal fistula in up to 50% of patients (30,33,34). Secondary to this relatively high complication rate, Ripstein modified the procedure to involve posterior fixation of the mesh with anterolateral fixation to the rectum/mesorectum with improved results (35). Ventral mesh rectopexy has demonstrated excellent results in terms of low rates of major morbidity and mortality with recurrence rates of 0%–6% and no higher than 8.2% in long-term follow-up (36–43). A multi-institutional review of 2,203 patients undergoing laparoscopic ventral rectopexy with either synthetic mesh (80.1%) or biologic grafts (19.9%) examined the incidence of mesh-related complications in either group (40). The authors report erosion of mesh in 2.4% of cases using synthetic mesh and 0.7% of those using biologic mesh. The median time to mesh erosion was 23 months. Recurrences of rectal prolapse were not included in the outcomes and were not reported in either group.

The use of an Ivalon sponge was later abandoned following a randomized control trial demonstrating significant complication rates, including increased constipation and pelvic abscess formation (29). The principles of this technique have persisted, however, with use of various synthetic and absorbable mesh products, used in both open and laparoscopic approaches (44–47). Due to increased rates of complications, we believe that mesh should likely only be utilized in a laparoscopic ventral rectopexy procedure, or in a repair of a recurrent prolapse.

### Posterior mesh fixation (Wells operation)

The technique of posterior fixation of the rectum to the sacrum with insertion of an Ivalon sponge was first described by Wells with excellent results and a low complication rate (48). The technique of the Wells operation is similar to that of the Ripstein procedure, except the mesh fixation to the sacral promontory is posterior. Theoretically, this posterior mesh orientation may reduce the problems typically associated with the anterior sling. The procedure was originally described using an Ivalon (polyvinyl alcohol) sponge. In the United States, experience with the Ivalon sponge is limited, as it has not been approved for implantation. Instead, many centers perform the procedure using polypropylene mesh.

Full mechanical bowel preparation is performed, and the patient is positioned in lithotomy position. The rectum is mobilized down to the pelvic floor. Retracting the rectum anteriorly, a 5 × 8 cm piece of mesh is then anchored to the sacrum in the midline using nonabsorbable suture.

The rectum is then retracted cephalad, and the redundancy is eliminated. With the rectum under traction, the mesh is sutured bilaterally to the lateral rectal mesentery. The mesh wrap forms a trough around the dorsal half of the rectum and does not cover the anterior rectal wall. The peritoneum is then closed over the mesh to exclude it from the abdominal cavity (Figure 24.6).

With regard to recurrence, the Wells operation has exceptional results with recurrence rates generally between 0% and 5% for most large open series (49–51). While there are fewer reported mesh complications, these series uniformly show a worsening of constipation after the procedure (44,49–51).

## Suture rectopexy

Prior to the laparoscopic era, suture rectopexy alone was not a common procedure. This technique involves rectal mobilization followed by suture fixation to the sacral promontory. Its appeal lies in the fact that no foreign bodies are used, thus negating the complications of mesh infection and erosion. A prospective randomized trial comparing open suture rectopexy to the Wells operation found no difference in the two procedures in terms of recurrence (49). This

procedure will be described in more detail under laparoscopy, as it has evolved primarily as a laparoscopic technique.

## Resection rectopexy (Frykman-Goldberg procedure)

Constipation clearly worsens after rectopexy alone. Many authors advocate sigmoid colectomy with rectopexy to alleviate postoperative constipation. This technique, termed the Frykman-Goldberg procedure, involves full rectal mobilization, sigmoid colectomy with colorectal anastomosis, and suture fixation of the rectum to the sacrum.

Patients require a complete mechanical bowel preparation and are positioned in lithotomy. The rectum is completely mobilized to the pelvic floor posteriorly. The lateral stalks are left intact. The rectum is then retracted into the abdomen, and the posterolateral mesorectum is fixed to the presacral fascia using nonabsorbable sutures. The sigmoid colon and upper rectum are then resected. Mobilization of the splenic flexure is usually not required, as the redundant sigmoid colon allows for resection and subsequent anastomosis without tension. The anastomosis is created with an EEA stapler. The original description of this procedure involved fixation of the anterior rectum to the endopelvic fascia to eliminate

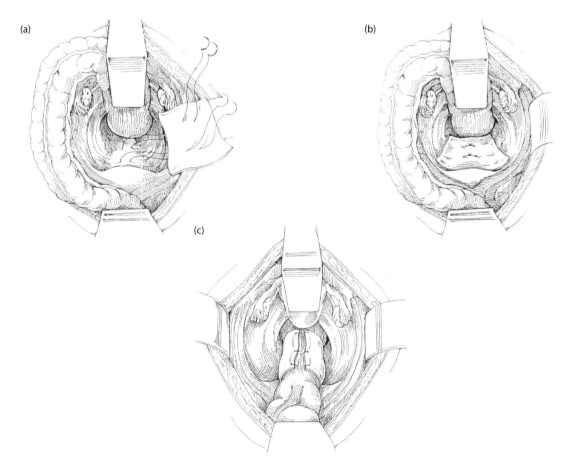

Figure 24.6 Ivalalon (polyvinyl alcohol) sponge rectopexy (Wells): **(a)** polyvinyl sponge being fixed to the sacrum, **(b)** sponge in place before fixation to the rectum, and **(c)** incomplete encirclement of the rectum anteriorly with the sponge sutured in place.

the cul-de-sac. Most modern proponents of this operation have abandoned these anterior sutures as they have no proven benefit and can be difficult to place safely.

The resection rectopexy has superior results with respect to both recurrence and constipation. Most large series report recurrence rates in the low single digits (9,52–54). Morbidity rates range from 0% to 35% and mortality from this procedure is low (9,52). This remains the only commonly employed abdominal procedure with significant improvement in postoperative constipation. One relative contraindication to resection rectopexy is severe incontinence with compromise of the anal sphincter, as sigmoidectomy can worsen incontinence in this patient population.

The addition of a sigmoid resection confers a significantly increased risk of anastomotic complications when compared to rectopexy alone. Careful adherence to the usual tenets of a safe colorectal anastomosis (a good proximal and distal blood supply, a tension-free anastomosis, and air testing of the anastomosis) should allow safe practice of this procedure.

## LAPAROSCOPY

Over the last decade, the laparoscopic approach to colorectal diseases has become pervasive. The literature has been flooded with series reporting the successful treatment of rectal prolapse through minimally invasive techniques. Rectal prolapse lends itself extraordinarily well to the laparoscopic approach, as the procedure is isolated to one sector of the abdomen, and there is frequently no specimen removal or anastomosis required, avoiding a conventional incision altogether. Recent reports comparing open to laparoscopic treatment of rectal prolapse find that there are significant patient benefits to laparoscopy, including decreased pain, quicker resumption of diet, earlier return of bowel function, shorter length of stay, reduced hernia rates, and a lower incidence of small bowel obstruction (45,55,56). Mortality rates for the laparoscopic approach are low. All of the open procedures discussed previously can be performed laparoscopically; however, the Ripstein procedure has proven tedious to complete laparoscopically and is seldom performed.

In general, these laparoscopic procedures require a steep Trendelenburg position to keep the small bowel and sigmoid colon out of the pelvis. The mesorectum is frequently elongated and thin in these patients. The mesorectal peritoneum is scored at the sacral promontory, and the plane behind the superior rectal artery is identified with the aid of pneumoperitoneum. The hypogastric nerves should be spared and the ureters identified. The initial mesorectal mobilization should be posterior in the avascular plane. As with the open approach, division of the lateral ligaments is controversial. The author performs a circumferential mobilization to the pelvic floor, including division of the lateral ligaments. The editors prefer to leave the lateral ligaments intact.

The Wells repair has proven more amenable to the laparoscopic approach than the Ripstein procedure. The laparoscopic technique is similar to the open technique. Three or four laparoscopic ports are required, and the procedure is most easily accomplished with a 30° camera to allow for visualization deep in the pelvis. This approach requires skill in laparoscopic sewing and knot tying. As with the open Wells procedure, the recurrence rate is excellent, with recurrence rates ranging from 0% to 4% in recent series (46,47,57). Functional outcomes were also analogous to the open procedure in these series, with improvement in continence but worsening of constipation. Morbidity and mortality are low.

Laparoscopists, forever testing the premise that less is more, have trended toward more suture repairs without mesh. The laparoscopic suture rectopexy is more manageable, as it does not require challenging manipulations of mesh and involves less suturing. Again, three to four ports are required, and a 30° camera is recommended. After the rectum is mobilized, it should be pulled in a cephalad direction, and the lateral stalks are sutured to the sacral promontory using nonabsorbable sutures. One suture on each side of the rectum is generally sufficient. The patient's diet may be advanced rapidly, and the patient should be ambulated early after surgery. It has been our practice to discharge patients after their first bowel movement; however, many centers perform this procedure with only a short postoperative stay.

The laparoscopic suture rectopexy has been proven effective in several recently published series, with recurrence rates from 0% to 6% (58–60). Continence is improved postoperatively, but the benefit of this simple technique may be found in improvement in postoperative constipation (59–61). These series provide hope that the suture rectopexy alone, without mesh, may rival the mesh repair in efficacy, without the long-term complication of constipation. This may obviate the need for a concomitant resection and thus decrease the difficulty and morbidity of the repair.

Some centers still favor laparoscopic resection rectopexy as the primary procedure for rectal prolapse. As with the open technique, splenic flexure mobilization is usually not required. The addition of sigmoidectomy increases the operative time relative to suture rectopexy alone by nearly 100 minutes (61,62). Results, as with the open technique, are excellent, with recurrence rates from 0% to 2.5% (4,63). Both constipation and incontinence are improved postoperatively.

No comparative studies between open and laparoscopic techniques have proven a significant reduction in morbidity or mortality for the laparoscopic approach, but trends seem to favor the laparoscopic approach (64,65). What is clear from the literature is that the minimally invasive approach to rectal prolapse is not inferior. The clear benefits of the laparoscopic approach in terms of cost, length of stay, and decreased pain mandate consideration of this approach when it is feasible.

## RECURRENT PROLAPSE

Recurrent rectal prolapse occurs with every procedure, and the surgical approach to repair of the recurrence requires consideration of the initial procedure. The mean time to recurrence is between 18 and 24 months. Patients who have recurred require physiologic testing and defecography to evaluate for anismus. If anismus is identified, these patients should be referred for biofeedback prior to any surgical therapy.

There is no clear algorithm for management of recurrent prolapse. Some authors advocate for a change in approach, performing perineal procedures if the initial approach was abdominal, and vice versa. Others promote the use of the same approach for repair of the recurrence. No definitive published data exist on the proper selection of the second procedure. The only absolute principle in the treatment of recurrent prolapse is that if a resection is planned, any prior anastomoses must be resected in order to avoid an intervening ischemic segment. Again, comorbid disease should play a role in the selection of the procedure. Patients unfit for general anesthetic should be offered a perineal approach if at all possible.

The few published series on the treatment of recurrent prolapse offer little to no insight on the best approach. A series from the University of Minnesota suggests that the abdominal approach is superior to the perineal approach in terms of re-recurrence (65). The Cleveland Clinic Florida has published one of the larger series on treatment of recurrent prolapse. Various surgical approaches were used, and it is not clear how the procedures are selected. Compared to primary operations for rectal prolapse, there was no difference in terms of recurrence, morbidity, and bowel function (66).

A difficult situation arises in the patient who has had a prior abdominal resection rectopexy but is now unfit for general anesthetic. Before undertaking a perineal proctectomy in such a patient, the surgeon must be sure the prior anastomosis can be mobilized and resected. If not, the surgeon is left with three less than desirable options. The patient may be counseled that an operation is not in his or her best interest. A Delorme procedure may be performed, or the patient may be offered anal encirclement.

## CONCLUSION

While many procedures exist for rectal prolapse, only a few offer acceptable results in terms of recurrence, postoperative bowel function, and morbidity. Of the perineal techniques, the Altmeier procedure appears to offer superior outcomes in terms of these principles. All of the described open abdominal approaches have satisfactory recurrence rates, but only the resection rectopexy shows improvement in postoperative bowel function. Laparoscopy, with all of its inherent advantages, may be the preferred approach. Of these procedures, the laparoscopic suture rectopexy appears to offer the best hope of achieving favored status, given the relative simplicity of the procedure and its exceptional outcomes with minimal morbidity.

The surgeon who treats this disease should possess the flexibility and breadth of skills to tailor the procedure to the individual patient. Surgeon preference and experience should play a role in the choice of procedure but should not justify a single procedure for a complex disease. An algorithm used in our section is to offer laparoscopic suture rectopexy as the default technique. If a patient has severe constipation, a laparoscopic resection rectopexy is performed. The patient with a hostile abdomen or the patient who is too infirm to undergo an abdominal procedure is offered a perineal proctosigmoidectomy.

## REFERENCES

1. Kairaluoma MV, Kellokumpu IH. *Scand J Surg.* 2005; 94(3):207–10.
2. Mellgren A et al. *Dis Colon Rectum.* 1997;40(7): 817–20.
3. Dvorkin LS et al. *Br J Surg.* 2005;92(7):866–72.
4. Ashari LH et al. *Dis Colon Rectum.* 2005;48(5):982–7.
5. Kruyt RH et al. *Br J Surg.* 1990;77(10):1183–4.
6. Tjandra JJ et al. *Dis Colon Rectum.* 1993;36(5): 501–7.
7. Glasgow SC et al. *Dis Colon Rectum.* 2006;49(7): 1052–8.
8. Birnbaum EH et al. *Dis Colon Rectum.* 1996;39(11): 1215–21.
9. Kim DS et al. *Dis Colon Rectum.* 1999;42(4):460–6; discussion 6–9.
10. Bachoo P et al. *Cochrane Database Syst Rev.* 2000; (2):CD001758.
11. Kimmins MH et al. *Dis Colon Rectum.* 2001;44(4): 565–70.
12. Boccasanta P et al. *Dis Colon Rectum.* 2006;49(5): 652–60.
13. Whitlow CB et al. *J La State Med Soc.* 1997;149(1): 22–6.
14. Chun SW et al. *Tech Coloproctol.* 2004;8(1):3–8; discussion 9.
15. Marchal F et al. *Dis Colon Rectum.* 2005;48(9): 1785–90.
16. Watts AM, Thompson MR. *Br J Surg.* 2000;87(2): 218–22.
17. Tsunoda A et al. *Dis Colon Rectum.* 2003;46(9): 1260–5.
18. Lechaux JP et al. *Am J Surg.* 2001;182(5):465–9.
19. Lomas MI, Cooperman H. *Dis Colon Rectum.* 1972; 15(6):416–9.
20. Corman M. *Rectal Prolapse, Solitary Rectal Ulcer, Syndrome of the Descending Perineum, and Rectocele,* 5th Edition. Philadelphia, PA: Lippincott, Williams, and Wilkins, 2005.
21. Nelson R et al. *Tech Coloproctol.* 2001;5(1):33–5.
22. McKee RF et al. *Surg Gynecol Obstet.* 1992;174(2): 145–8.
23. Schultz I et al. *Dis Colon Rectum.* 2000;43(1):35–43.
24. Winde G et al. *Eur J Surg.* 1993;159(5):301–5.

25. Snyder JR, Paquette IM. Rectal prolapse and intussusception. In Beck DE, Wexner SD. (eds). *Fundamentals of Anorectal Surgery*, 3rd Edition. New York: Springer, In press.
26. Wong M et al. *Colorectal Dis.* 2011;13:1019–23.
27. Maggiori L et al. *Tech Coloproctol.* 2013;17:431–6.
28. Sahoo MR et al. *J Minim Access Surg.* 2014;10:18–22.
29. Ripstein CB. *Dis Colon Rectum.* 1972;15:334–6.
30. Gordon PH, Hoexter B. *Dis Colon Rectum.* 1978;21: 277–80.
31. Dyrberg DL et al. *Scand J Surg.* 2015;104:227–32.
32. Dulucq JL et al. *Surg Endosc.* 2007;21:2226–30.
33. Kupfer CA, Goligher JC. *Br J Surg.* 1970;57:482–7.
34. Roberts PL et al. *Arch Surg.* 1988;123:554–7.
35. McMahan JD, Ripstein CB. *Am Surg.* 1987;53:37–40.
36. D'Hoore A et al. *Br J Surg.* 2004;91:1500–5.
37. Bloemendaal AL et al. *Colorectal Dis.* 2015;17: O198–201.
38. Boons P et al. *Colorectal Dis.* 2010;12:526–32.
39. Consten EC et al. *Ann Surg.* 2015;262:742–8.
40. Evans C et al. *Dis Colon Rectum.* 2015;58:799–807.
41. Randall J et al. *Colorectal Dis.* 2014;16:914–9.
42. Sileri P et al. *J Gastrointest Surg.* 2012;16:622–8.
43. Owais AE et al. *Colorectal Dis.* 2014;16:995–1000.
44. Allen-Mersh TG et al. *Dis Colon Rectum.* 1990;33(7): 550–3.
45. Purkayastha S et al. *Dis Colon Rectum.* 2005;48(10): 1930–40.
46. Zittel TT et al. *J Gastrointest Surg.* 2000;4(6):632–41.
47. Himpens J et al. *Surg Endosc.* 1999;13(2):139–41.
48. Wells C. *Proc R Soc Med.* 1959;52:602–3.
49. Novell JR et al. *Br J Surg.* 1994;81(6):904–6.
50. Mann CV, Hoffman C. *Br J Surg.* 1988;75(1):34–7.
51. Aitola PT et al. *Dis Colon Rectum.* 1999;42(5): 655–60.
52. Watts JD et al. *Dis Colon Rectum.* 1985;28(2):96–102.
53. Huber FT et al. *World J Surg.* 1995;19(1):138–43; discussion 43.
54. Husa A et al. *Acta Chir Scand.* 1988;154(3):221–4.
55. Duepree HJ et al. *J Am Coll Surg.* 2003;197(2): 177–81.
56. Solomon MJ et al. *Br J Surg.* 2002;89(1):35–9.
57. Dulucq JL et al. *Surg Endosc.* 2007;21(12):2226–30.
58. Heah SM et al. *Dis Colon Rectum.* 2000;43(5): 638–43.
59. Kessler H et al. *Surg Endosc.* 1999;13(9):858–61.
60. Bruch HP et al. *Dis Colon Rectum.* 1999;42(9):1189–94; discussion 94–5.
61. Kellokumpu IH et al. *Surg Endosc.* 2000;14(7):634–40.
62. Baker R et al. *Dis Colon Rectum.* 1995;38(2):199–201.
63. Benoist S et al. *Am J Surg.* 2001;182(2):168–73.
64. Kairaluoma MV et al. *Dis Colon Rectum.* 2003;46(3): 353–60.
65. Steele SR et al. *Dis Colon Rectum.* 2006;49(4):440–5.
66. Pikarsky AJ et al. *Dis Colon Rectum.* 2000;43(9): 1273–6.

# 25

# Management of diverticulitis

DAVID E. BECK, H. DAVID VARGAS, AND MOLLY M. FORD

## CHALLENGING CASE

A 52-year-old male presents to the emergency department with complaints of left lower quadrant abdominal pain for the last 16 hours. The patient describes the pain as escalating in nature, unrelieved with a bowel movement. History is unremarkable except for hypertension, which is treated with a beta-blocker. The patient denies any similar symptoms previously. Past medical history includes a left inguinal hernia repair 25 years ago. Abdominal exam reveals a mildly distended abdomen, with tenderness to the left lower quadrant, but no guarding or rigidity. A basic metabolic profile is normal, and complete blood count reveals a leukocytosis at 14,000. Computed tomography (CT) scan of the abdomen and pelvis with oral and rectal contrast demonstrates thickening of the sigmoid colon with mesenteric thickening but no identifiable abscess or perforation.

## CASE MANAGEMENT

Treatment should consist of broad-spectrum antibiotics, typically, ciprofloxacin and metronidazole; IV fluids; and bowel rest. Admission to the hospital is based on physical examination, comorbidities, and CT findings. Treatment should be continued until the patient's pain has resolved or symptomatic improvement is noted, and then oral intake may resume. Antibiotics are typically continued for 7–10 days following resolution of pain.

## INTRODUCTION

Diverticulosis coli represents a physical outpouching of the colonic wall. While a true diverticulum involves all layers of the bowel wall, most common colonic diverticulum involve a false or "pseudo" diverticulum where the mucosa and submucosa protrude through the muscular and serosal layers. This condition was first described by Curveihier in the mid-1800s, while the first significant case series of diverticulitis did not appear in the literature until 1899 (1,2).

The impact of diverticular disease on health care is substantial and increasing in both incidence and cost. Peery et al. surveyed the Health Care Utilization Project and revealed that diverticular disease represented the sixth most common gastrointestinal diagnosis among patients being seen in outpatient clinics in the United States, exceeding those presenting with inflammatory bowel disease or colorectal cancer (3). A report querying a database of U.S. emergency departments revealed that from 2006 to 2013, emergency department visits for diverticulitis increased by 40% (3). This same survey indicated that admissions to the hospital remained constant, suggesting a shift toward outpatient management of diverticulitis. Health-care cost of diverticulitis over this period of time rose accordingly and can be measured in many ways, including by hospital admissions, office visits, and total health-care costs.

## EPIDEMIOLOGY

This condition afflicts people of Western industrialized countries more frequently than their counterparts in underdeveloped, more agrarian-based economies, and points to the long-standing belief that diets higher in fiber content serve as a protective effect (4). In addition to fiber, newer theories for pathogenesis include increased elastin deposition and variations in collagen cross-linking serving to reduce wall compliance (5). Last, there appears to be a genetic component that predisposes individuals to diverticulitis (6).

A genetic influence in diverticular disease is supported by the anatomic observation that in Western countries, diverticulosis is most often localized to the left colon, whereas it is predominantly localized in the right colon in Asian countries (7). In addition, studies of population migration suggest that despite populations adopting new environmental factors, there may not be subsequent changes in diverticular disease incidence. A study of Turkish migrants to the Zaanstreek region of the Netherlands found a much lower incidence of diverticulosis than the native Dutch population of 7.5% compared to 50% (8). In the Japanese population living in Hawaii and eating a more Westernized diet, diverticula remain predominantly right sided (9). Most recently, two large twin studies found that genetic factors are a strong contributor to developing diverticular disease. A study of the Swedish Twin Registry found that the odds ratio (OR) of developing diverticular disease if one's co-twin was affected was 7.15 in monozygotic twins as compared to 3.2 for dizygotic twins (10). The Danish twin study found a relative risk (RR) for diverticulosis in twin siblings was 2.92 as compared to the general population (11). Both studies estimate the contribution of heredity to be roughly 40%–50%.

The development of colonic diverticulum increases with age; at 50 years old approximately 40% of the population in the United States will harbor diverticulosis, and this rises to 70% by age 80 years (12). Complications of diverticulosis coli include bleeding or inflammation. Lifetime risks of such complications are difficult to accurately estimate but are probably less than the previously held belief of 15%–20%, and recent reports indicate that a 5% lifetime risk of both bleeding and inflammation is more likely (13).

## PATHOPHYSIOLOGY

Diverticulitis refers to inflammation and initial local sepsis of the peridiverticular colonic tissues. The pathophysiologic mechanism underlying diverticulitis is not well understood. The most commonly held theory involves increased pressure in the lumen of the diverticulum that leads to ischemia, perforation, and inflammation (14). The loss of integrity with local contamination with colonic microorganisms leads to local inflammation and infection. Predisposing local factors may facilitate this development.

The actual role of infection and sepsis has been challenged, giving rise to treatment paradigms not involving antimicrobials. In addition, randomized prospective trials performed in European centers have shown that CT scan proven, uncomplicated diverticulitis can be successfully treated with supportive measures and bowel rest without antibiotics (15). This challenges our conventional and long-held beliefs of local sepsis and perhaps would indicate that there exists a spectrum of the pathologic condition. Symptom development and the timing of clinical presentation may identify the process at a preinfectious phase. Such thinking has led to the alternative treatment paradigm involving anti-inflammatory agents such as aminosalicylates.

## CLINICAL PRESENTATION AND DIAGNOSIS

Clinically, patients report abdominal pain in the left lower quadrant or lower abdomen that progresses to increasing pain with movement or palpation. There is often an associated change in bowel habits preceding the pain, and symptoms of fever and chills. Rectal bleeding can coincide with pain but is rare and would be the exception rather than the rule.

During recent decades, a significant change in both diagnostics and treatment of acute colonic diverticulitis has evolved. The initial evaluation should include a problem-specific history and physical examination, a complete blood count, urinalysis, and abdominal radiographs in selected clinical scenarios (16). As a supplement to clinical evaluation (history and physical examination), CT scans verify and determine the stage of acute colonic diverticulitis and improve decision-making in nonoperative and operative management (17). CT scan is a cost-effective way to diagnose acute abdominal conditions; however, radiation exposure remains a concern (18). CT findings in diverticulitis are discussed in Chapter 12.

The rate of complicated acute colonic diverticulitis is highest during the primary admission. Most patients who experience a free perforation do so during their first presentation. In contrast, the majority of readmitted patients have uncomplicated disease (19,20). In these patients with clinical recurrent disease and a C-reactive protein <50 mg/mL, a repeated CT scan may be omitted (21). A clinical diagnosis of uncomplicated diverticulitis, which comprises the majority of these patients, remains a major component of outpatient management (22–24).

A prospective study on the capability of clinical findings, temperature, C-reactive protein, and white blood cell count to discern patients with acute colonic diverticulitis from all other patients admitted with acute abdominal pain found that evaluation by nonspecialist doctors had a high degree of diagnostic precision (25). The accuracy of the clinical diagnosis was slightly better in younger patients. Elderly patients tend to have more vague and nonspecific symptoms, broader alternatives of differential diagnosis, altered clinical signs that do not correlate with disease severity, higher incidence of comorbidity and multipharmacy, and communication difficulties because of hearing and cognitive impairment (26,27). This makes elderly patients more prone to misdiagnosis than younger patients (28).

High-risk patients include the morbidly obese, elderly, and immunocompromised (29–31). A review of the American College of Surgeons National Surgical Quality Improvement Program data set from 2005 to 2010 found that morbidly obese patients undergoing surgery for diverticulitis were nearly 10 years younger than normal weight patients and more likely to require emergency surgery, ostomy creation, and open surgery, and to undergo procedures without an anastomosis (29). Morbidly obese patients undergoing emergency surgery were also more likely to have preoperative systemic inflammatory response syndrome, sepsis, and septic shock.

Immunosuppression is commonly related to transplant status and chemotherapy. The surgery rate at the first episode of acute colonic diverticulitis appears high in this population and results in a high morbidity (30). However, if medical treatment is successful, this group of patients appears to have a low recurrence rate, and a follow-up elective resection is not recommended (31).

## CLASSIFICATION

Classification of the disease severity helps determine how to treat patients with diverticular disease. Older classifications systems were based on barium enema, physical examination, and pathology reports (32). While all three methods are sufficient to make a diagnose, the improved sensitivity and specificity of newer technology have changed the way we diagnosis, classify, and treat this disease. CT scanning currently provides practical and predictive information that assists in the classification of severity of the disease process. A number of useful classification systems have been developed to assist the physician in deciding on a course of treatment (33,34). These classification systems can be based on CT scan findings (Ambrosetti, Table 25.1), intraoperative findings (Hinchey, Table 25.2), or a more global view of the disease (Thorson and Goldberg, Table 25.3).

Ambrosetti did extensive work on CT findings of diverticular disease and developed a classification system based on the appearance of the inflamed colon (38). His work is simple and divides patients into two groups; uncomplicated or complicated (Table 25.1). Other studies have looked at the size of the abscess and amount of mesenteric air to

Table 25.1 Ambrosetti classification of diverticulitis based on CT findings

Uncomplicated—Colonic wall thickening, pericolic fat stranding, inflammatory changes
Complicated—Extracolonic air, abscess, perforation

Source: Aydin HN, Remzi FH. Dig Liver Dis. 2004;36:435–45.

Table 25.2 Intraoperative classification: Hinchey classifications

Type I—Diverticulitis with no or local peritonitis
Type II—Diverticulitis with a small pericolic abscess
Type III—Diverticulitis with local purulent or fecal peritonitis
Type IV—Diverticulitis with diffuse purulent or fecal peritonitis

Source: Golfieri R, Cappelli A. Tech Coloproctol. 2007;11: 197–208.

Table 25.3 Definitions of diverticular disease

Diverticulosis
• *Asymptomatic*
Diverticulitis
• *Noninflammatory*
  • Symptoms without inflammation
• *Acute*
  • Complicated
    Perforation, abscess, phlegmon, fistula bleeding
  • Uncomplicated (simple)
    Localized, thickening, fat stranding
• *Chronic*
  • Recurring or persistent disease
    Symptoms with systemic signs (may be intermittent)
  • Atypical
    Symptoms without systemic signs
• *Complex*
  • Fistula, stricture, obstruction, fibrosing

Source: Boulos PB. Best Pract Res Clin Gastroenterol. 2002;16: 649–62.

determine if those are predictors of failure of nonoperative therapy (34).

In 1978, Hinchey classified patients using the findings at surgery and recommended surgical intervention based on his classification system (39). His formula divided the intraoperative findings into four categories based on the amount and type of peritonitis (Table 25.2).

However, not all diverticular disease can be classified by CT scan or operative findings. Thorson and Goldberg described diverticular disease based on the presentation, timing and duration of disease, and complexity (40) (Table 25.3).

## TREATMENT

Diverticulitis patients present with a spectrum of disease from uncomplicated acute disease, to complicated disease, to complex or recurrent disease. Treatment should be individualized to the specific patient and his or her disease.

## ACUTE UNCOMPLICATED DISEASE

Clinically stable, reliable patients with uncomplicated colonic diverticulitis are usually treated conservatively with antibiotics. Patients who can tolerate oral antibiotics can be treated initially as outpatients (41,42). A systemic review of one randomized controlled trial, six clinical controlled trials, and three case series found no difference in failure rates of medical treatment (6.5% versus 4.6%, $p = 0.32$) or in recurrence rates (13% versus 12.1%, $p = 0.81$) between those receiving ambulatory care and inpatient care for uncomplicated diverticulitis (43). Ambulatory treatment was associated with an estimated daily cost savings of between 600 and

1,900 euros per patient treated. Treatment in an ambulatory setting was related to a higher failure rate of medical treatment at immediate follow-up in comparison to an inpatient setting (6.5% versus 4.6%). However, all patients who failed after the initial medical treatment were managed successfully without surgical interventions. Similar recurrence rates at longer periods of follow-up were noted between both those who were ambulatory and those in an inpatient setting (13% versus 12.1%). Jackson and Hammond conducted a systemic review that showed similar favorable outcomes with IV compared to oral antibiotics in an inpatient setting and concluded that these results justify ambulatory treatment of uncomplicated diverticulitis (44).

However, the role of antibiotics in diverticulitis has been disputed (45) The Swedish AVOD study prospectively compared 623 inpatients with CT-confirmed uncomplicated left-sided diverticulitis with IV fluids to IV fluids with antibiotics and found that antibiotics did not prevent complications, accelerate recovery, or prevent recurrences (46). A subsequent Cochrane Review of three randomized trials also found no significant difference between antibiotics and no antibiotics for the treatment of uncomplicated diverticulitis (15).

After resolution of an episode of diverticulitis, a variety of agents may be effective in preventing future attacks. Supplemental fiber, rifaximin, antispasmodics, mesalamine, and probiotics have been studied in randomized, controlled trials as well as in less rigorous studies. Many of these studies included heterogeneous patients and poorly characterized the history of diverticulitis in the study subjects. Although some of the literature suggests a protective benefit for these agents, their role in prevention of diverticulitis remains to be defined (47). Another study suggests that a family history of diverticulitis may predict recurrence (48).

## ACUTE COMPLICATED DISEASE

Patients with complicated disease (i.e., free perforation, larger abscesses, fistula, or stricture) who cannot tolerate oral hydration, who have relevant comorbidities, or who do not have adequate support at home require hospital admission and, typically, IV antibiotics and bowel rest. Antibiotics should cover gram-negatives and anaerobes. Multidisciplinary, nonoperative management of inpatients with acute diverticulitis is successful in as many as 91% of patients (49).

Patients with free perforations and diffuse peritonitis are resuscitated and taken for urgent/emergent surgery. A select group of patients with free and localized peritonitis may be managed with close observation and antibiotics (50).

CT-guided percutaneous transabdominal drainage of intraabdominal abscesses was introduced in the 1980s and has been widely adopted (51,52). Large localized abscesses (>4–5 cm) are primarily drained by a percutaneous approach in order to resolve the sepsis. Those with smaller abscesses are often treated with IV antibiotic therapy alone

(51). Percutaneous abscess drainage is a safe and effective alternative to surgery for draining infected fluid collections, with a higher success rate (70%–90%), lower complication rate, and shorter hospital stay compared to surgical drainage (35,36). However, 20%–25% of patients are either not suitable for radiological drainage (multiloculated, anatomically inaccessible) or do not respond to drainage and will require surgical intervention (37). Deep pelvic abscesses not accessible for transabdominal percutaneous drainage are managed by transvaginal or transrectal drainage under radiological (ultrasound/CT/fluoroscopy) or endoscopic guidance.

Gastrointestinal hemorrhage associated with diverticular disease is covered in Chapter 37.

## EVALUATION AFTER RECOVERY FROM ACUTE DIVERTICULITIS

After resolution of an episode of acute diverticulitis, the colon should typically be endoscopically evaluated to confirm the diagnosis, if this is a first episode or recent colonoscopy has not been performed (16). The purpose of the investigation is to exclude other diagnoses, because patients with simple thickening on imaging may be found to have ischemia, inflammatory bowel disease, or neoplasia (53). Although the discovery of a mass lesion associated with colon wall thickening is highly suggestive of an underlying neoplasm, the absence of a mass on CT does not preclude neoplasia (54,55). When fat stranding is more severe than expected for the degree of bowel wall thickening, an inflammatory condition such as diverticulitis is most likely (56). Patients with presumed diverticulitis who have not had a recent colon evaluation should undergo colonoscopy, typically within 6–8 weeks following resolution of the acute episode (although data supporting this time interval are lacking). The absence of neoplasia on colonoscopy may confirm the diagnosis of diverticulitis suspected on CT (57).

Long-term perforations or abscesses may develop into fistulas. The common areas affected by fistula from diverticular disease are the bladder (colovesical), the vagina (colovaginal), and the skin (colocutaneous). Symptoms will be determined by the organs involved: stool or gas per vagina for colovaginal and skin for colocutaneous, pneumaturia or fecalurrea, or urinary tract infections for colovesical fistula. Many of these can be confirmed by contrast-enhanced CT scans or contrast enemas. Bullous edema on cystoscopy can also confirm colovesical fistula. The primary treatment is resection of the involved segment of bowel.

## ACUTE/URGENT SURGERY

Peritonitis, free intraabdominal air with diffuse peritonitis, or obstruction unrelieved by other methods is an indication for operation. Patients with signs of peritonitis or hemodynamic instability are not candidates for medical management and should be resuscitated and taken to the operating room. Three different operations have been proposed for the treatment of complicated diverticulitis with peritonitis. The first operative approach described was the three-stage procedure encompassing drainage with stoma, followed by resection and anastomosis with continued diversion, and finally by restoration of continuity. The second approach involved resection and diversion or the traditional Hartmann procedure. However, this approach is being challenged by the third approach of resection with primary anastomosis. Primary resection with anastomosis (PRA) can be performed with or without a covering stoma, and/or on table lavage. The three-stage procedure will not be discussed here as it is not considered standard of care and should be used only in infrequent situations.

In 1921, Hartmann advocated his two-stage resection that was superior and quickly became the standard of care (58). However, early in the 1960s, there were eight reports with a total of 50 patients who underwent resection and primary anastomosis for generalized peritonitis with a low mortality of 10%. Not much debate is raised now with respect to patients presenting with recurrent or chronic diverticulitis. They are typically managed in an elective fashion with primary anastomosis. Patients are given a bowel preparation prior to surgery, although the role of mechanical preparation continues to be discussed.

Patients who present with acute symptoms, typically Hinchey stages III or IV, are taken to the operating room urgently. These patients constitute approximately 3.2 per 100,000 patients (59). These patients present a dilemma, because typically they are older, have a high number of comorbidities, and suffer a greater number of complications. In a review by Salem and Flum of 98 articles on the outcome of complicated diverticulitis based on the type of operation performed, the authors identified 1,051 patients who underwent a Hartmann procedure from 54 studies, and 569 patients having undergone a primary anastomosis from 50 studies (60). Of the patients undergoing a primary anastomosis, 16% had covering stomas and 10% had on-table lavage. The mortality rates of those in the Hartmann group (19.6%) were much higher than those undergoing a primary anastomosis (9.9%). The anastomotic leak rate in patients with a primary anastomosis ranged from 6.3% to 19.3%. If a diverting proximal stoma was performed at the time of a primary anastomosis, the anastomotic dehiscence rate fell to 6.3%. Wound infections were also more frequently seen in the Hartmann group (24.2%) versus the primary anastomosis group (9.6%). Again, patients with covering stomas had the lowest wound infection rate at 4%. Patients undergoing a Hartmann procedure also required a larger second operation than those who had PRA with or without a covering stoma. Complications from a Hartmann reversal were associated with a mortality of 0.8%, a wound infection rate of 4.9%, and an anastomotic leak rate of 4.3%. These patients also experienced stoma complications (10.3%) that required medical attention. The conclusion was that primary anastomosis is no worse than a Hartmann procedure and has several advantages,

including higher restoration of continuity rate, less hospitalization, and fewer infectious complications.

Multiple studies have evaluated the morbidity and mortality of the Hartmann procedure as well as the risks incumbent with takedown. Most seasoned surgeons realize that at times restoration of continuity can be more of a challenge to both patient and surgeon than the original operation. This was demonstrated in a multicenter prospective trial involving 415 patients with complicated diverticulitis (61). In this trial, 248 patients underwent resection with primary anastomosis. The other 167 had a Hartmann procedure. The mortality rate for those undergoing primary anastomosis was 4%, while those with resection and diverting colostomy was 23.4%. After case adjustment, the data suggested that the Hartmann procedure was associated with a 1.8-fold increase in likelihood of death. This was not statistically significant. However a 2.1-fold increase in morbidity was found between the two groups, and this was significant. In part this is due to the fact that surgeons typically reserved a Hartmann procedure for those older patients with more comorbidities and thus predisposed to a poorer outcome.

## RISKS ASSOCIATED WITH HARTMANN REVERSAL

Reversal of a Hartmann colostomy also carries with it a significant risk that must be entertained when considering this operation for patients who will desire continuity in the future. Failure to reverse the colostomy has been reported in 20%–50% (62) of patients, and leak rates on reversal are around 2%–30% (60,62). Mortality has been reported anywhere from 0% to 10%, and wound infection rates range from 12% to 50%.

A strong interest in primary anastomosis has been revived in the literature with papers describing the successful outcomes of patients undergoing this type of operation. However, few papers are prospective and less are randomized, and such a trial is still needed today to definitively answer the questions of safety and efficacy. Multiple trials have shown that the outcomes of primary anastomosis are indeed as safe as a Hartmann and in many cases better. In a recent review, Constantinides et al. reviewed the outcomes of patients undergoing Hartmann (63), PRA (135 patients), and primary resection with anastomosis and diversion (126 patients) (59). Patients undergoing a Hartmann procedure had a morbidity and mortality of 35% and 20%, respectively. Primary anastomosis showed a slightly higher morbidity and mortality at 55% and 30%, while those with a primary anastomosis with diverting stoma demonstrated morbidity and mortality rates of 40% and 25%, respectively. Stomas were permanent in 27% of patients undergoing a Hartmann procedure and 8% of those having a primary anastomosis with diversion. They concluded that primary anastomosis with defunctioning stoma may be an optimal strategy for selected patients. The Hartmann procedure should be reserved for patients with an extremely high risk of perioperative complications and only after consideration of long-term implications.

Patients undergoing on-table lavage have been analyzed as well, which showed similar outcomes to those who did not undergo on-table lavage. Regenet described 60 patients, all Hinchey III or greater: 27 underwent primary anastomosis with intraoperative lavage and 33 had a Hartmann procedure (63). In this prospective observational study, they found that the Hartmann procedure took much less time to perform, but that the mortality and morbidity for both groups were equal. Three patients in the intraoperative lavage group had an anastomotic leak (11%). A Hartmann reversal occurred in 69% of the patients. The reversal had its own associated morbidity of 24%, an anastomotic leak rate of 7%, and no deaths. Postoperative stay after primary anastomosis and intraoperative lavage was 18.4 days and Hartmann procedure was 38 days. They concluded that primary anastomosis with intraoperative lavage and a Hartmann procedure are both adequate approaches for generalized peritonitis complicating diverticulitis. Covering stomas have been recommended by most studies when primary anastomosis is performed because of the variable anastomotic leak rate. Both diverting colostomies and ileostomies have been described with equal success. Most of the poor outcomes noted are not necessarily due to the operation performed but to the comorbidities and peritonitis associated with the patient and disease. These risks play more into the outcome of patients than the type of operation performed.

# ELECTIVE SURGERY

In the past, there was a fear that subsequent attacks of diverticulitis carried increased risk of perforation and the potential need for stoma creation. This widely held belief motivated surgeons and patients to proceed with prophylactic elective resection to reduce the need for an urgent operation and the limited operative options therein. Subsequent studies of the natural history of recurrent diverticulitis and the likelihood of perforation found the risk to be low even in elderly populations (64). Traditionally, elective colectomy has been recommended for young patients (<50 years at initial presentation), patients who have had complicated disease (abscess, fistula, or perforation), and patients who have experienced two or more episodes of uncomplicated diverticulitis (65,66).

However, there is increasing evidence to suggest that the natural history of the disease may be more commonly benign, and the risk of experiencing complicated recurrence requiring emergency operation may be low, leading many to challenge the traditional indications for elective colectomy (67–72). These data are reflected in more contemporary practice guidelines that favor individualized treatment decisions and more selective use of elective colectomy (12,16).

A population-based analysis by Li and colleagues found a significant decline in the use of elective colectomy following diverticulitis; the proportion of patients undergoing elective colectomy within 1 year of discharge declined from 9.6% in 2002 to 3.9% by 2011 (73). The observed decrease in

elective surgery was most pronounced for younger patients and those with complicated disease.

Young age has traditionally been considered a risk factor for more virulent disease, but increasing evidence has accumulated to contradict this theory. Two meta-analyses suggest that younger patients are at increased risk of recurrence, but the relationship between age and risk of emergency operation remains unclear. Katz et al. found no association between young age and risk of emergency operation following initial nonoperative management, and two studies by Li and colleagues did not find any association between young age and risk of emergency operation at index presentation or during follow-up after nonoperative management (74–76). These studies suggest that young age does not appear to confer a more virulent disease trajectory, and the practice of elective surgical resection based on age criteria alone should be discouraged (16).

Complicated diverticulitis accounts for up to 35% of admissions for diverticulitis, yet little is known about the clinical course of such patients managed nonoperatively (75). Older practice guidelines recommend elective colectomy following nonoperative management of complicated diverticulitis, supported by evidence suggesting that such patients are at increased risk of recurrent disease and sepsis (16,34,77). However, the risk of subsequent disease-related events in this subset of patients has not been well studied, with data limited to a few single or multi-institutional cohort studies with small sample sizes and high loss to follow-up, with reported recurrence rates ranging from 24% to 53% (34,78,79). More recently, the success of managing complicated diverticulitis without elective colectomy has led some to question the necessity of routine elective surgery, particularly in patients at high operative risk (68,69,80). In a study by Li and colleagues, the 5-year cumulative incidence of readmission and emergency surgery was only 12% and 4.3% among patients with complicated diverticulitis (76). This suggests that elective colectomy may not be necessary for many patients with complicated disease. Surgical recommendations may remain for high-risk patient subgroups, such as patients with multiple recurrent episodes, persistent abdominal symptoms, high-risk medical comorbidities, and large pelvic abscesses. Certainly, the rationale for resection must be balanced by the risk of complication of surgery and the best estimate of actual reduction of risk of recurrent episodes. With regard to operative risk, Salem et al. examined a decision analysis tool that revealed a minimum of three to four attacks could justify the operative risk (81).

## Technical considerations

The extent of elective resection is determined intraoperatively based on the anatomy and the quality of the tissues. The distal margin is an important determinant in minimizing the recurrence of diverticulitis and must extend to the proximal rectum to enable a colorectal anastomosis, because a colo-colonic anastomosis significantly increases the risk of recurrence (82,83). Patients in whom the proximal rectum is secondarily inflamed may require more extensive rectal resection with a lower rectal anastomosis. The proximal extent of resection in the descending colon is chosen by the absence of thickened, hypertrophic tissue and inflammation. Although it is not necessary to remove all diverticula-bearing colon, care should be taken to avoid incorporating any false diverticula in the proximal side of the anastomosis, because this will increase the risk of leak.

Randomized controlled trials demonstrate that laparoscopic colectomy by experienced surgeons is safe and results in better short-term outcomes compared with open surgery. Specifically, laparoscopy is associated with decreased operative blood loss, less pain, shorter hospitalization, reduced duration of ileus, reduced complication rates, and improved quality of life (84,85). A meta-analysis of 25 randomized controlled trials comparing open and laparoscopic colorectal resection for any indication also documents superior short-term outcomes associated with the laparoscopic approach (86). National inpatient sample data also strongly support laparoscopy over open elective colectomy for diverticulitis (87). Although the majority of published reports included patients with uncomplicated disease, the surgical literature supports the laparoscopic approach to complicated diverticulitis as well (88–90). Hand-assisted laparoscopic colectomy may be particularly useful in this setting (91). Long-term follow-up data from a previously published open versus laparoscopic randomized controlled trial with a median follow-up of 30 months reported comparable gastrointestinal quality of life index scores and comparable diverticulitis recurrence rates after surgery (92). In addition, the hernia rate in patients who had laparoscopic resection was one-third of the hernia rate in patients who had open or converted operations. Laparoscopic sigmoid resection for diverticulitis is technically challenging and requires training and adequate experience. The open approach to diverticulitis should be performed at the discretion of the surgeon as determined by unique patient factors and the individual surgeon's judgment and experience.

## COMPLICATIONS

## ANASTOMOTIC LEAK

Elective colectomy has been well documented to carry a very low anastomotic leak rate, of about 1%–3% (60). However, in the face of active inflammation or peritonitis, attempts at performing a primary anastomosis carry a higher risk of anastomotic dehiscence. Primary anastomosis in the setting of Hinchey stage III or IV carries a leak rate from 8% to 22% (60,61,93–95).

## MORTALITY

Elective colectomy also carries with it a low mortality rate, typically less than 1%. A majority of postoperative deaths result from cardiovascular problems. However, patients involved with complicated diverticulitis face greater risks that can be evaluated with numerous scoring systems. Mortality rates range from 0% to 36% in patients presenting with peritonitis and depend greatly on their comorbidities and time to operation (96).

## FAILURE TO REVERSE

Maggard looked at colostomy reversal at the population level for the state of California (97). Of the 1,176 patients who had a Hartmann procedure for diverticular disease, only 65% had a reversal at a mean of 143 days. Younger men were more likely to have their ostomy reversed, as opposed to older patients, and women. Patients with more comorbid risk factors also had fewer reversals. When evaluating all patients, 35% never had their ostomy reversed during the 4-year study. Complication rates following Hartmann reversal were quite high and included an overall rate of 57.4%. Infection (9.1%), aspiration pneumonia (8.7%), pulmonary edema (6%), and acute renal failure (4.9%) were all problematic.

Most of the literature quotes a 20%–50% failure of reversal rate on patients for a number of factors, including comorbidities, age, and failed attempts at reversal (97–100). Boland et al. found that 38% of patients suffered a major complication after their reversal (98). Failure to restore continuity in their population was 10.3%. Due to the morbidity of the Hartmann reversal as well as the number of patients who either are not reversed or fail an operative attempt at reversal, they recommended always trying a primary anastomosis first with diversion if possible. In another similar study, Aydin et al. found that Hartmann reversal was associated with a higher prevalence of surgical or medical complications when compared with primary resection and anastomosis (99). The overall postoperative morbidity and 30-day mortality rates for Hartmann reversal were 48.5% and 1.7%, respectively. Patients undergoing a primary resection with anastomosis suffered a morbidity rate of 26% and mortality rate of 0.7%. Having controlled for the number of comorbid conditions, extent of diverticular disease, severity of peritoneal contamination, and operative urgency, patients who underwent Hartmann reversal were 2.1 times more likely to have an adverse surgical event during their postoperative period.

The difficulty with these comparative studies is that despite attempting to find similar cohorts, patients who undergo a Hartmann procedure are usually older, frailer, and sicker than those who undergo a primary anastomosis. Surgeons generally wish to correct the problem as fast as possible and get the patient off of the operating room table. This creates the possibility of bias in evaluating the literature, as patients undergoing Hartmann's versus primary anastomosis typically have a worse outcome. However, when added with the risks of a second complex and morbid operation of future stoma takedown, primary anastomosis and diversion with a loop ileostomy appears much friendlier. If the patient is able to tolerate the extra 30 minutes required to perform a primary anastomosis, one should be performed with diversion.

## RECURRENCE OF DIVERTICULITIS AFTER PREVIOUS SURGICAL RESECTION

Recurrence of diverticulitis or its symptoms following resection has been reported in 3%–13% of elective cases (83,101,102). Factors that have been found to contribute to the recurrence of diverticulitis after a resection include shorter resection length and the leaving behind of a cuff of distal sigmoid (101,102). Most recently, Thaler demonstrated that the level of the anastomosis is the only significant determinant of recurrence after laparoscopic resection (83). The practice parameters of the American Society of Colon and Rectal Surgeons set out several general recommendations regarding resection of diverticular disease. For elective resection, all thickened, diseased colon, but not necessarily the entire proximal diverticula bearing colon, should be removed. It may be acceptable to retain proximal diverticular colon as long as the remaining bowel is not hypertrophied. Distally, all of the sigmoid colon should be removed to the level of the rectum (12).

## TIMING OF CLOSURE

Timing of closure continues to be a contentious issue and has not been fully settled. Traditional teaching is to wait 3–4 months to allow the inflammatory process to subside and the patient to heal prior to performing another major operation. Mean time intervals in the literature range from 120 to 210 days. One study did compare closure at 4 and 8 months. Complication rates associated with timing of reoperation were 2.5 and 5 times higher at 4 and 8 months, respectively (99). Complications from the reversal included anastomotic leak, and rectovaginal fistulas in women. These fistulas are attributed to improper dissection of the vagina and failure to carefully mobilize the rectum.

## CONCLUSION

Diverticular disease appears to be increasing in incidence in an ever-widening spectrum of ages throughout the United States and other developed countries. However, with more experience with the disease process, coupled with better medical therapies and diagnostic measures, more patients are able to be managed conservatively than ever before. Uncomplicated diverticular disease may be treated medically without fear that recurrent episodes will lead to more complicated findings. Complicated disease is being managed medically more aggressively than ever before in an effort to prevent emergent operations. Primary anastomosis with diversion as opposed to the traditional two-staged Hartmann procedure appears to be equally effective without the downside of a second major operation. Certainly, the trends today for diverticular disease are to be less aggressive with operative management, and treat each individual case based on its own merits as opposed to the more stringent guidelines of the past.

## REFERENCES

1. Cruveillhier J. *Paris.* 1849;1:590.
2. Graser E. *München Med Wchnschr.* 1899;46:721–3.
3. Peery AF et al. *Gastroenterology.* 2012;143(5):1179–87.e3.
4. Hobson KG, Roberts PL. *Clin Colon Rectum.* 2004; 17:147–53.
5. Wess, L et al. *Gut.* 1995;37:91–4.
6. Sheth A et al. *Am J Gastroenterol.* 2008;103:1550–6.
7. Rajendra S, Ho JJ. *Eur J Gastroenterol Hepatol.* 2005; 17:871–5.
8. Loffeld RJ. *Colorectal Dis.* 2005;7:559–62.
9. Stemmermann GN. *Arch Environ Health.* 1970;20: 266–73.
10. Granlund J et al. *A P & T May.* 2012;35(9):1103–7.
11. Strate LS et al. *Gastroenterology.* 2013;144(4):e14.
12. Rafferty J et al. *DCR.* 2006;49:939–44.
13. Somasekar K et al. *J R Coll Sur Edinb.* 2002;47:481–4.
14. Gordon PH. Diverticular disease of the colon. In Gordon PH, Nivatvongs S (eds). *Principles and Practice of Surgery for the Colon, Rectum, and Anus.* New York, NY: Informa Health Care, 2007, pp. 909–70.
15. Shabanzadeh DM, Wille-Jorgensen P. *Cochrane Database Syst Rev.* 2012;11:CD009092.
16. Feingold D et al. *Dis Colon Rectum.* 2014;57:284–94.
17. Andeweg CS et al. *Dig Surg.* 2013;30(4–6):278–92.
18. Brenner DJ. *Rev Environ Health.* 2010;25(1):63–8.
19. Talabani AJ et al. *Int J Colorectal Dis.* 2014;29: 937–45.
20. Ritz JP et al. *Surgery.* 2011;149(5):606–13.
21. Nizri E et al. *Tech Coloproctol.* 2014;18(2):145–9.
22. Laméris W et al. *Dis Colon Rectum.* 2010;53(6): 896–904.
23. Isacson D et al. *Scand J Gastroenterol.* 2014;49(12): 1441–6.
24. Isacson D et al. *Int J Color Dis.* 2015;30(9):1229–34.
25. Talabani AJ et al. *Int J Colorectal Dis.* 2017;32:41–7.
26. Lyon C, Clark DC. *Am Fam Physician.* 2006;74(9): 1537–44.
27. Chang C-C, Wang S-S. *Int J Gerontolog.* 2007;1(2): 77–82.
28. Laurell H et al. *Gerontology.* 2006;52(6):339–44.
29. Bailey MB et al. *J Am Coll Surg.* 2013;217(5):874–80.
30. Biondo S et al. *Am J Surg.* 2016;212(3):384–90.
31. Biondo S et al. *Am J Surg.* 2012;204:172–9.
32. Nelson RS, Thorson AG. Operative and nonoperative therapy for diverticuar disease. In Whitlow CB, Beck DE, Margolin DA, Hicks TC, Timmcke AE. (eds). *Improved Outcomes in Colon and Rectal Surgery.* London: Informa Healthcare, 2010, pp. 249–62.

33. Rafferty J et al. *DCR.* 2006;49:939–44.
34. Kaiser AM et al. *Am J Gast.* 2005;100:910–7.
35. Aydin HN, Remzi FH. *Dig Liver Dis.* 2004;36:435–45.
36. Golfieri R, Cappelli A. *Tech Coloproctol.* 2007;11: 197–208.
37. Boulos PB. *Best Pract Res Clin Gastroenterol.* 2002; 16:649–62.
38. Ambrosetti P et al. *Dis Colon Rectum.* 2000;43: 1363–7.
39. Hinchey EJ et al. *Adv Surg.* 1978;12:85–109.
40. Thorson, AG, Goldberg SM. Benign colon: Diverticular disease. In Wolff BG, Fleshman JW, Beck DE, Pemberton JH, Wexner SD (eds). *The ASCRS Textbook of Colon and Rectal Surgery.* New York: Springer-Verlag, 2007, p. 271.
41. Alonso S et al. *Colorectal Dis.* 2010;12:278–82.
42. Etzioni DA et al. *Dis Colon Rectum.* 2010;53:861–5.
43. Balasubramanian I et al. *Dig Surg.* 2017;34:151–60.
44. Jackson JD, Hammond T. *Int J Colorectal Dis.* 2014; 29:775–81.
45. Isacson D et al. *Scand J Gastroenterol.* 2014;49(12): 1441–6.
46. Chabok A et al. *Br J Surg.* 2012;99:532–9.
47. Maconi G et al. *Dis Colon Rectum.* 2011;54:1326–38.
48. Hall JF et al. *Dis Colon Rectum.* 2011;54:283–8.
49. Dharmarajan S et al. *Dis Colon Rectum.* 2011;54: 663–71.
50. Sallinen VJ et al. *Dis Colon Rectum.* 2014;5(7):875–81.
51. Siewert B et al. *Am J Roentol.* 2006;186:680–6.
52. Singh B et al. *Ann R Coll Surg Engl.* 2008;90(4): 297–301.
53. Wolff JH et al. *J Clin Gastroenterol.* 2008;42:472–5.
54. Eskaros S et al. *Emerg Radiol.* 2009;16:473–6.
55. Moraitis D et al. *Am Surg.* 2006;72:269–71.
56. Pereira JM et al. *Radiographics.* 2004;24:703–15.
57. Lau KC et al. *Dis Colon Rectum.* 2011;54:1265–70.
58. Wong WD et al. *Dis Colon Rectum.* 2000;43:290–7.
59. Constantinides VA et al. *Ann Surg.* 2007;245:94–103.
60. Salem L, Flum DR. *DCR.* 2004;47:1953–64.
61. Constantinides VA et al. *BJS.* 2006;93:1503–13.
62. Wigmore SJ et al. *Br J Surg.* 1995;82:27–30.
63. Regenet N et al. *Int J Colorectal Dis.* 2003;18:503–7.
64. Buchs NC et al. *World J Gastrointest Surg.* 2015;7(11): 313–8.
65. Wong WD et al. *Dis Colon Rectum.* 2000;43:290–7.
66. Köhler L et al. *Surg Endosc.* 1999;13:430–6.
67. Biondo S et al. *Br J Surg.* 2002;89:1137–41.
68. Chapman J et al. *Ann Surg.* 2005;242:576–81.
69. Gaertner WB et al. *Dis Colon Rectum.* 2013;56: 622–6.
70. Janes S et al. *Br J Surg.* 2005;92:133–42.
71. Chapman JR et al. *Ann Surg.* 2006;243:876–80.
72. Pittet O et al. *World J Surg.* 2009;33:547–52.
73. Li D et al. *Dis Colon Rectum.* 2016;59:332–39.
74. Katz LH et al. *J Gastroenterol Hepatol.* 2013;28: 1274–81.
75. Li D et al. *Dis Colon Rectum.* 2014;57:1397–405.
76. Li D et al. *Ann Surg.* 2014;260:423–30.
77. Mueller MH et al. *Eur J Gastroenterol Hepatol.* 2005; 17:649–54.
78. Elagili F et al. *Dis Colon Rectum.* 2014;57:331–6.
79. Eglinton T et al. *Br J Surg.* 2010;97:952–7.
80. Nelson RS et al. *Am J Surg.* 2008;196:969–73.
81. Salem L et al. *JACS.* 2004;199:904–12.
82. Dozois EJ. *J Gastrointest Surg.* 2008;12:1321–3.
83. Thaler K et al. *Dis Colon Rectum.* 2003;46:385–8.
84. Klarenbeek BR et al. *Ann Surg.* 2009;249:39–44.
85. Gervaz P et al. *Ann Surg.* 2010;252:3–8.
86. Schwenk W et al. *Cochrane Database Syst Rev.* 2005: CD003145.
87. Masoomi H et al. *World J Surg.* 2011;35:2143–8.
88. Scheidbach H et al. *Dis Colon Rectum.* 2004;47: 1883–8.
89. Bartus CM et al. *Dis Colon Rectum.* 2005;48:233–6.
90. Jones OM et al. *Ann Surg.* 2008;248:1092–7.
91. Lee SW et al. *Dis Colon Rectum.* 2006;49:464–9.
92. Gervaz P et al. *Surg Endosc.* 2011;25:3373–8.
93. Stumpf MJ et al. *Am Surg.* 2007;73:787–91.
94. Gooszen AW et al. *Eur J Surg.* 2001;167:35–9.
95. Richter S et al. *World J Surg.* 2006;30:1027–32.
96. Landen S, Nafteux P. *Acta Chir Belg.* 2002;102: 24–9.
97. Maggard MA et al. *Am Surg.* 2004;70:928–31.
98. Boland E et al. *Am Surg July.* 2007;73:664–8.
99. Aydin HN et al. *DCR.* 2005;48:2117–26.
100. Oomen JT et al. *Dig Surg.* 2005;22:419–25.
101. Benn PL et al. *Am J Surg.* 1986;151:269–71.
102. Leigh JE et al. *Am J Surg.* 1962;103:51–4.

# 26

# Abdominal surgery for colorectal cancer

JASON F. HALL AND ROCCO RICCIARDI

## CHALLENGING CASE

A 65-year-old woman with no significant past medical history underwent a laparoscopic sigmoid colectomy for colon cancer. The patient had delayed return of bowel function and on postoperative day 7, developed a fever as well as increasing abdominal pain. A contrast enema revealed an anastomotic leak.

## CASE MANAGEMENT

The patient was returned to the operating room for a laparotomy, abdominal washout, and end colostomy. The anastomosis had a pinpoint defect posteriorly without evidence of tension or ischemia. She responded well to antibiotics and was discharged 16 days following her initial procedure.

## INTRODUCTION

The need for improved quality in health care has reached the consciousness of policymakers, providers, payers, and patients. Following the publication of two Institute of Medicine reports: *To Err Is Human: Building a Safer Health System* and *Crossing the Quality Chasm: A New Health System for the Twenty-First Century*, the quality of our nation's health care has been critically examined while outcomes have been questioned. Increased attention to health care has led to demands for better access and distribution of care. Rigorous monitoring and quality assessment, as well as pay for reporting and potentially pay for performance are likely inevitable. In order to accelerate the diffusion and pace of quality improvement efforts, the Institute of Medicine launched the Redesigning Health Insurance

Performance Measures, Payment, and Performance Improvement Project. With an aim toward equitable and reliable high-quality care, our nation has started down the road of more measurement in order to gain better outcomes.

Quality has always been a major focus of attention for surgeons, but with the advent of pay for reporting, attempts to measure quality of care have accelerated. Presently, the focus of quality assessment is on process measures such as antibiotic prophylaxis and venous thrombosis prophylaxis. In time, however, it is likely that morbidity, mortality, quality of life, and patient satisfaction will become increasingly important components of our assessment. Many of the aforementioned metrics are currently in use in the field of colon and rectal surgery. Oncologic measures are under active development and will likely standardize the way we manage colon and rectal cancer. It is for this reason that our chapter on improving outcomes for abdominal surgery in colorectal cancer is particularly important to readers of this book and, in particular, surgeons who perform these procedures. Procedures of the colon and rectum are characterized by high rates of morbidity and mortality; thus, techniques to reduce the burden of disease from colon and rectal surgery are important.

Surgical resection remains the standard of care for curative treatment of colorectal cancer. In order to improve outcomes, numerous surgical techniques have been proposed to reduce complications. However, as with all surgical procedures, complications related to preoperative, intraoperative, and postoperative factors occur more frequently than most practitioners recognize. As the collective interest in surgical outcomes has increased, surgeons have been charged not only with improving their outcomes but also with documenting that improvements in surgical care are real and generalizable to the population served. This chapter provides a systematic overview of the major recent developments in outcomes and quality in colorectal cancer. It also provides an evidence-based platform for the minimization and management of common surgical complications in order to improve outcomes.

## ONCOLOGIC OUTCOMES IN COLORECTAL CANCER

A number of factors affect prognosis after colorectal resection for cancer. Generally, oncologic outcomes for colorectal cancer resection are inversely proportional to the patients' stage of disease. Following attempted curative resection, survival parallels the TNM stage (I, well above 90%; II, 65%–90%; and III, 45%–75%) (1,2). More specifically, local extent of disease, the presence of metastatic disease, nodal involvement, adequacy of regional node harvest, incomplete resection, preoperative carcinoembryonic antigen level, tumor grade, and tumor biology have all been correlated with oncologic outcomes (3–7). Conversely, tumor size and gross tumor configuration have not been correlated with prognosis following surgery. Despite these patient and tumor factors, the surgeon can greatly influence oncologic outcomes by performing a proper preoperative oncologic evaluation, adequate tumor resection, and satisfactory nodal harvest.

## PREOPERATIVE EVALUATION

Following the diagnosis of colorectal cancer, the surgeon should assess the patients' surgical risk while determining local and distant extent of disease. Despite the lack of consensus for preoperative testing of colorectal cancer, we adhere to a thorough evaluation of the abdomen and chest to rule out distant disease while determining the local extent of disease, especially when planning a laparoscopic resection. Most importantly, however, prior to completing a colorectal resection, colorectal cancer patients should have a complete assessment of the colon. Approximately 5% of patients will have a synchronous colorectal cancer, and 25%–76% patients will have a synchronous adenomatous polyp (8). Colonoscopy is advantageous for identifying the position of the lesion while permitting tattooing for intraoperative localization during laparoscopic resections. Also, some lesions are prohibitively large, and thus the planned operation may require alteration to ensure a complete resection. Virtual computed tomography (CT) and barium enema are other methods that may be applied if a colonoscopy cannot be performed for technical reasons. In addition, we have had excellent results with intraoperative $CO_2$ colonoscopy. Thus, an adequate assessment of the patients' colonic disease reduces the likelihood that the patient may require another procedure for missed lesion.

## SURGICAL TECHNIQUE

In addition to an adequate preoperative assessment, adequate tumor resection is critical to ensuring a good prognosis. Appropriate surgical margins critically influence outcome after colorectal cancer resection. In addition to the proximal and distal bowel margins, the radial or circumferential margin is particularly important in the treatment of both colon and rectal cancers (9). A 5 cm proximal and distal bowel margin is generally adhered to for colon cancers, despite data suggesting that mural tumor migration rarely occurs beyond a 2 cm margin in either the proximal or distal direction to cancer (10). In the setting of rectal cancer, a distal margin of as little as 1–2 cm has become the rule in lower tumors, while it is important to note that survival is adversely affected by a distal margin of less than 0.8 cm (11).

Controversy regarding the point of ligation of the vascular pedicle has been a point of contention for years. Many surgeons argue that a high ligation of the vascular pedicle is critical to ensuring good oncologic outcomes. However, a comparison of high versus more distal ligation for left-sided cancers by the French Association for Surgical Research demonstrated no difference in survival (12). Despite the fact that advocates of proximal vascular ligation have little evidence to support improved outcomes, the net effect of high ligation may be to improve lymph node sampling. An adequate mesenteric resection to include an appropriate nodal sample importantly predicts survival (5). Given the overwhelming data in this area, the College of American Pathologists has recommended additional techniques to enhance nodal recovery if less than 12 nodes are identified on initial examination (6). Similarly, several national organizations have proposed setting benchmarks of 12 lymph nodes as a proxy of an adequate oncologic resection for colorectal cancer (13–17). This proposed benchmark may someday serve as an important quality measure to compare surgeons and providers treating colorectal cancer. At this time, however, advocates of lymph node benchmarks have no evidence that such thresholds will result in real measurable improvement in patient outcome.

Surgical advances in laparoscopic technique have resulted in rising enthusiasm for applications of this technique to cancer resections. These advances have resulted in some improvement in short-term outcomes, such as postoperative pain, length of ileus, and hospital stay. Most importantly, multicenter trials of laparoscopic resection versus open resections for colon cancer reveal no compromise in oncologic outcomes (18). Despite early reports of port site recurrences from laparoscopic oncologic resections, well-designed trials support the oncologic equivalency of laparoscopic colectomy in the hands of experienced surgeons (18,19). Thus, oncologic outcomes are comparable for the experienced laparoscopic surgeon as compared to open surgery for colon cancer, with the proviso that population-based data are unavailable at this time. At this time, oncologic results for laparoscopic proctectomy for rectal cancer have been concerning (20). Further data are needed to demonstrate oncologic equivalency for laparoscopic approaches to proctectomy.

## SURGICAL OUTCOMES IN COLORECTAL CANCER

There are a number of complications that occur following colorectal resections for cancer. Although some are difficult to avoid, we stress methods to reduce the frequency of these complications and improve outcomes.

## ANASTOMOTIC COMPLICATIONS

Anastomotic complications are some of the most feared complications in colorectal surgery patients. Although rare, the development of anastomotic complications results in a prolonged postoperative stay with a high cost to the patient, the health care system, and society. Perioperative anastomotic complications can also lead to long-term consequences including stricture, abdominal wall hernia, permanent diversion, poor functional outcome, and need for reoperative therapy. A number of variables have been linked to the development of anastomotic complications, particularly the technique employed, the conditions under which the anastomosis is constructed, and other patient characteristics.

### Anastomotic leak

One of the most devastating outcomes of a new anastomosis for colorectal cancer is anastomotic leak, occurring in 3%–6% of all colorectal cases. These leaks occur more commonly with more distal resections and are reported to be as high as 15.3% for low rectal reconstructions (21). Although the development of leak is frequently attributed to surgeon error, patient characteristics also importantly influence the development of leaks. For example, renal failure, chronic obstructive pulmonary disease, steroid use, elevated white blood count, and malnutrition have all been attributed to anastomotic leak (22,23). In addition, operative factors such as low rectal anastomoses, intraoperative septic conditions, difficulties encountered during the anastomosis, and use of blood transfusion have been implicated (22). Although surgical construction of the anastomosis is an important variable, there is no difference in the development of anastomotic leak whether the reconstruction is stapled, hand-sewn in one layer, or even two layers (24,25).

With respect to anastomotic technique, emphasis should be placed on providing an adequate blood supply and ensuring a tension-free anastomosis. Adequate blood supply can be confirmed with multiple methods: by dividing the marginal artery of Drummond or other arcades and encountering pulsatile bleeding or by confirming bleeding at the cut edge of the colon. A tension-free anastomosis is also critical and can be facilitated by high ligation of the feeding vessel, although this maneuver is not always critical. Other techniques to reduce tension and increase mobility include separation of the greater omentum from the transverse colon and adequate mobilization of the approximating ends. In the setting of low pelvic anastomoses, especially those anastomoses constructed following the use of neoadjuvant therapy, a protective proximal intestinal stoma should be considered in order to reduce the life-threatening consequences of anastomotic leak (26).

In addition to lack of tension and adequate blood flow, the local conditions under which an anastomosis is created can affect outcome. Attention should be focused on the patient's preoperative nutritional status. Golub et al. have demonstrated that an albumin concentration less than 3 g/L is associated with anastomotic leakage (22). In a multivariate analysis, these authors also demonstrated a relationship between preoperative corticosteroid use, peritonitis, bowel obstruction, and chronic obstructive pulmonary disease, as well as perioperative transfusion and the incidence of anastomotic leakage (22). Other authors have identified perioperative conditions that increase the risk of anastomotic leakage, and they include obesity, malnutrition, weight loss greater than 5 kg, and use of alcohol (27). If the patient's nutritional status is in question or the local conditions are not favorable, it advisable not to construct an anastomosis. Once the unfavorable circumstances have been corrected, the patient can undergo restoration of intestinal continuity under more favorable circumstances.

Bowel preparations have traditionally been employed to clear the bowel of feces before colorectal operations. This practice was thought to decrease the likelihood of anastomotic leak by limiting the passage of stool through the newly constructed anastomosis. More recent data reveal an increase in anastomotic complications with the routine use of bowel preparations (28). Others have similarly demonstrated more wound infections in addition to increased rates of anastomotic leak in patients receiving mechanical bowel preparations (29). Because of the temporary starvation and electrolyte imbalance sometimes associated with mechanical bowel preparations, it is not clear that this practice represents anything more than surgical dogma. Despite the growing body of evidence against the routine use of bowel preparation, surgeons in North America seem slow to move away from this long-held practice, with many suggesting that colonic manipulation of an unprepped bowel during laparoscopic surgery is difficult.

Once an anastomotic leak develops, it usually becomes evident within 5–8 days following the procedure. However, in a recent series of 1,223 patients with intestinal anastomoses, 36% were identified more than 30 days postoperatively (30). The diagnosis is usually suspected by clinical factors and often confirmed by radiologic examination. Patients with early clinical evidence of anastomotic leak can present with fever, tachycardia, abdominal distention and tenderness, ileus, early diarrhea, or possibly septic shock. Depending on the patient's clinical condition, the presence of any one of these factors is indication for examination with a radiologic study. If there are obvious signs of peritonitis or hemodynamic collapse, then urgent exploratory laparotomy is often preferable. Radiological investigation can be performed with either abdominopelvic CT or with a soluble contrast enema (Figure 26.1). There have been conflicting reports as to the superiority of each technique (31,32); however, CT scans have the additional benefit of demonstrating other intraabdominal pathology such as hematoma or abscess.

If an anastomotic leak is demonstrated by clinical or radiologic means, antibiotics should be administered and

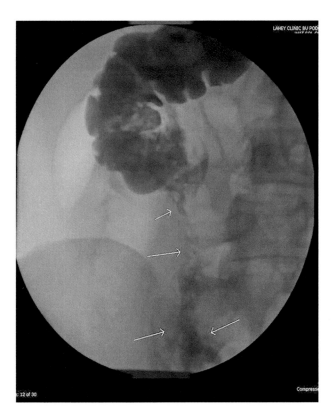

Figure 26.1 Contrast radiograph demonstrating anastomotic leak.

the patient resuscitated. Surgical exploration is then indicated to wash out the abdominal cavity and examine the anastomosis. If conditions are favorable, an intraperitoneal anastomosis can be reconstructed, although most anastomotic leaks generally require the construction of a stoma. Alternatively, the management of left-sided and low pelvic anastomoses is more complex. If the leak is secondary to bowel necrosis or ischemia and there is not sufficient bowel for reanastomosis, a colostomy should be created with a Hartmann pouch. This procedure should be performed with consideration of the fact that the majority of these patients will be left with permanent stoma (33). If there is sufficient bowel for reanastomosis and local conditions are favorable, revision of the anastomosis can be considered with the protection of a proximal loop ileostomy. If there is dense inflammation surrounding the anastomosis, a loop ileostomy should be constructed and a large drain placed in the perianastomotic area. A number of anastomotic leaks associated with localized peritonitis and abscess formation can often be managed nonoperatively (32). If there is a contained collection, the patient should be treated with IV antibiotics, and drainage of the abscess should be considered by radiologic means (34).

## Anastomotic stricture

Anastomotic stricture is a common occurrence following colorectal anastomosis and has been reported in up to 30% of cases in some series (35). Strictures are often asymptomatic but may also present with partial or complete large bowel obstruction. The mechanism of stricture formation is not completely understood but may be related to anastomotic leakage, pelvic sepsis, radiation injury, or local ischemia (36,37). Numerous nonrandomized trials and meta-analyses have demonstrated a higher rate of stenosis with end-to-end stapled anastomosis. The presence of a proximal diverting colostomy also seems to increase the risk of stricture, possibly due to the lack of dilation by the fecal stream (38–40). However, patients who undergo proximal diverting ileostomy have generally more difficult anastomoses, and often the ileostomy is formed because of the potentially higher risk for leakage. Thus, the higher risk of leakage in these patients may be confounded by local factors or patient variables that have been difficult to describe to date.

Strictures typically present within the first postoperative year (41) and can be managed with a number of different modalities depending on the anastomotic site. Many are asymptomatic and will resolve on their own as the bulk of the fecal stream slowly dilates the stenosis over the course of a few months. Before any therapeutic procedure is undertaken, the operator should be confident that a new stricture does not represent a cancer recurrence. If there is uncertainty by visual inspection, the diagnosis can easily be ascertained through a formal biopsy of the anastomosis. Most colonic strictures following surgery can be managed with sequential digital manipulation, bougeinage, or hydrostatic balloon dilation. Patients often require several treatments before complete resolution as repeat dilations are more common following resections for cancer than for benign causes (42). Newer techniques involve the use of endoscopic stents as well as endoscopic transanal resection of strictures. Small published series using these techniques report safe and satisfactory long-term outcomes (43). Surgical revision of the anastomosis is occasionally necessary when the stricture is not accessible by endoscopic means or recurs after numerous less invasive procedures.

## Anastomotic bleeding

Postoperative bleeding related to intestinal anastomosis is a relatively rare but potentially serious event. The incidence in stapled colorectal anastomoses is 1.8%–5% (44,45). The method of construction, whether stapled or hand-sewn, appears to be unrelated to the development of this complication (46). The diagnosis of anastomotic bleeding is typically inductive as patients will pass variable amounts of maroon-colored blood with their first bowel movement. More active bleeding commonly presents with large amounts of blood per rectum. To prevent this complication, we perform a simple examination of the staple line through the enterotomy. All visible bleeding is controlled with sutures rather than electrocautery as applying thermal energy to the staple line may increase the likelihood of a full-thickness burn injury.

The initial management of postoperative hemorrhage is typically nonoperative. Greater than 80% of patients will stop bleeding without intervention, but nearly 50% of patients will require a transfusion (47). Often, simple techniques such as correcting the coagulopathy and halting unfractionated or low molecular weight heparin are sufficient. Alternatively, treatment for hemodynamically stable patients includes endoscopic electrocoagulation of the anastomotic line (48) or injection of the staple line with epinephrine or clips (49). Although others have proposed that proximal colonic anastomoses should not be treated endoscopically (48), the data against this belief are minimal. If endoscopic methods fail, some patients are candidates for angiographic embolization or vasopressin treatment. Obviously, angiographic options should be exercised with care as embolization may interrupt the blood supply to the anastomosis and thus result in bowel infarction as well as anastomotic leak (50). In addition, the use of vasopressin is also associated with myocardial and intestinal ischemia and should be employed with caution in patients with risk factors for heart disease (51,52). Failure of the aforementioned hemostasis methods will often require exploratory laparotomy and revision of the anastomosis.

## PELVIC HEMORRHAGE

Massive pelvic bleeding is a difficult complication that can occur rarely during proctectomy or retroperitoneal dissection. This bleeding usually results from inadvertent violation of the avascular presacral plane and resultant damage to the presacral veins. Presacral venous hemorrhage is difficult to control and can be a significant source of postoperative morbidity and mortality (53). Conventional methods of hemostasis rarely are effective and usually result in increased bleeding. If encountered, bleeding should be controlled with direct pressure while the anesthesiology team appropriately resuscitates the patient. Laparotomy sponges are used to tamponade bleeding, while microfibrillar collagen and absorbable gelatin can be used. If simple tamponade does not control the bleeding, then sterile titanium thumbtacks can be inserted into the bleeding point on the sacrum (54). In addition, endoscopic multifeed staplers used in laparoscopic mesh hernia repairs can be used (55). Others have described fixing a 4 cm² piece of rectus muscle to the bleeding vessel while applying a high-frequency electrical current to the muscle until it adheres to the presacral fascia (56). Alternatively, bonewax can be used with some efficacy on the sacrum. In the most difficult circumstances, the pelvis is packed with sponges, and the patient returned to the operating room in 1–2 days for laparotomy pad removal (57).

## SPLENIC INJURY

Iatrogenic injury to the spleen is a potentially serious complication of colectomy with significant long-term adverse consequences. It is defined as any injury to the spleen caused by the operating team during a surgical procedure. Splenic injury occurs during 1.2%–8% of colorectal resections

(21,57,58), although these figures likely underestimate the incidence of the problem as conservatively managed splenic injuries are rarely reported. Splenic injury is associated with the proximity of the lesion to the splenic flexure as traction on the peritoneal band attaching the greater omentum and spleen appears to be the most common mechanism by which the spleen is injured (59–61). Other mechanisms of injury include retractor and direct instrumental damage (62). Langevin reported no injuries to the spleen in 733 procedures in which the splenic flexure was not mobilized, but 3.1% of patients requiring splenic flexure takedown sustained splenic injuries (21). Mortality rates are higher in patients who sustain splenic injury after gastrointestinal surgery, particularly colorectal surgery (63,64). Splenic injury is associated with a higher incidence of early infections, potentially from hematoma formation and subsequent superinfection (58) or loss of splenic function. In a recent review of California Cancer Registry and California Patient Discharge Data, patients undergoing colorectal cancer resection with inadvertent splenectomy had an increased length of stay and a 40% increase in the probability of death (65).

There are few evidence-based recommendations for avoiding intraoperative splenic injury, but basic surgical principles are obviously essential. To maximize exposure, the surgical incision should be appropriately elongated in order to obtain adequate, tension-free visualization of the appropriate structures in open surgery. All hand-held and self-retaining retractors should be placed with care and under direct visualization. Some authors have recommended a modified lithotomy position with the surgeon standing between the patient's legs during flexure mobilization. This positioning permits clearer visualization of the structures in the left upper quadrant (21). Unnecessary traction on the transverse and left colon should be avoided. Consideration should be given to dividing the lienocolic ligaments before commencing any left colonic resection (62). If there is suspicion of tumor invasion into the spleen, an en bloc resection should be performed. There are some data to suggest the benefits of laparoscopy in mobilization of the spleen. Malek reported a review of iatrogenic splenectomies following open and laparoscopic colon resections. The authors found 13 iatrogenic splenectomies in 5,477 open resections, but none following 1,911 laparoscopic resections (66). Although the authors were unable to adjust for operative difficulty, it would seem that laparoscopic mobilization may clarify splenic flexure visualization (Figure 26.2).

Prompt recognition at the time of surgery is the first step to the successful management of iatrogenic splenic injuries. Once an injury to the spleen is recognized, there are two options, either splenectomy or splenic preservation. Timely management allows the surgeon to manage bleeding at the first operation, while delayed recognition results in reduced chances of splenic salvage (67). Optimally, the surgeon should attempt to salvage the spleen unless blood loss prohibits the more time-intensive salvage methods. Techniques for splenic salvage are generally extrapolated from the trauma literature. Minor bleeding from capsular

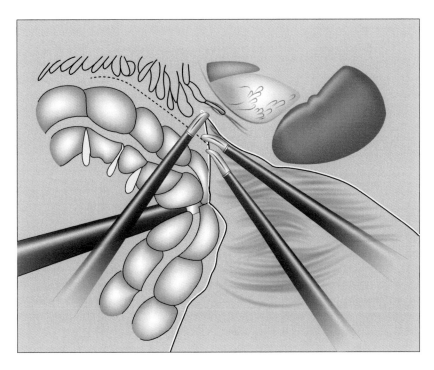

Figure 26.2 Laparoscopic mobilization of splenic flexure.

tears generally improves with gentle tamponade, whereas more active bleeders may require more intervention to achieve hemostasis. There is a long experience with various hemostatic agents such as thrombin, absorbable regenerated cellulose, and microfibrillar collagen. These are often placed on top of the bleeder and underneath a surgical pack for tamponade (68). If these simple measures fail, bleeding can be controlled by segmental ligation of the feeding hilar vessels or splenorrhaphy. With severe splenic injury, complicated by continued hemorrhage and hemodynamic instability, the surgeon should obviously consider splenectomy. If splenectomy is performed, the patient should be administered pneumococcal, meningococcal, and *Haemophilus influenzae* vaccine in order to prevent overwhelming postsplenectomy sepsis (69).

## URETERAL INJURIES

Due to the proximity of the ureters to the colon, injury is a common concern during colorectal operations. Although injuries to the ureters are uncommon during simple resections, when they occur, they can lead to significant difficulty. The ureters are most commonly injured in colorectal procedures during one of several maneuvers: while ligating the inferior mesenteric artery or dissecting at the sacral promontory or laterally in the pelvis during division of the lateral stalks of the rectum. Unfortunately only 20%–30% of intraoperative ureteral injuries are recognized at the time of the transgression (70). Despite the fact that few injuries are recognized intraoperatively, ureteral injuries are best treated during the initial operation as the local conditions are likely to be the most favorable for a successful repair. Prompt diagnosis and institution of appropriate corrective

surgical procedures often result in a very satisfactory outcome in the about 94% of cases (71).

In order to prevent ureteral injuries, patients with difficult anatomy, such as extensive pelvic adhesions after proctectomy, a large pelvic mass, or a phlegmon that makes identification of normal anatomy difficult, should be considered for preoperative stent placement. Ureteral stents permit quicker intraoperative ureter identification but do not completely eliminate the risk of injury; rather, ureteral stents permit quicker recognition of ureteral injuries and immediate repair. Since these repairs can be technically challenging, they should be performed by a surgeon who is well versed with ureteral repair techniques. General guidelines include debridement of necrotic tissues, ensuring excellent blood supply, and performing a tension-free anastomosis. More distal injuries of the pelvic portion of the ureter may be handled by reimplantation (72). Additional discussion on urologic injuries is presented in Chapter 41.

## AUTONOMIC NERVE INJURY

Genitourinary function can be greatly altered by injury to the pelvic parasympathetic and sympathetic nerves during colorectal resections. Proper oncologic resection for rectal cancer has been associated with a significant incidence (10%–69%) of urinary and sexual dysfunction (73). Although urinary dysfunction is often limited to the first few postoperative days, sexual dysfunction may persist for months or indefinitely. Both forms of postoperative dysfunction are related to the patients' preoperative function. Total mesorectal excision with autonomic nerve preservation has been advocated as an effective approach to the minimization of pelvic nerve injury. This technique mobilizes the

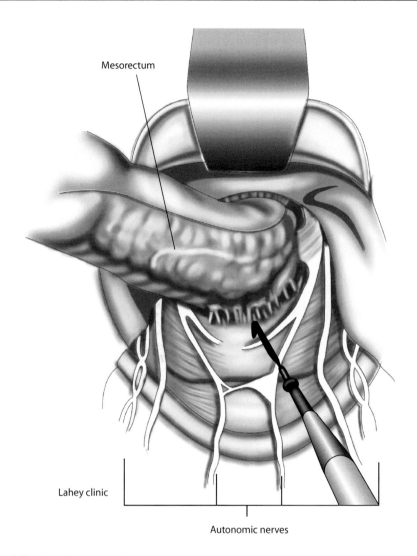

Figure 26.3 Rectal mobilization demonstrating autonomic nerves.

mesorectum circumferentially with sharp dissection along the correct pelvic parietal planes while avoiding the pelvic nerves (Figure 26.3) (73). In addition, damage to the sympathetic plexus is often encountered during high ligation of the inferior mesenteric artery. The hypogastric nerves should be identified as they course over the sacral promontory and preserved. Anterior dissection should be avoided when unnecessary as dissecting in Denonvilliers fascia places the nervi erigentes at risk. We preserve Denonvilliers fascia unless the tumor is anterior or circumferential. When total mesorectal excision and autonomic nerve preservation are combined, several authors have demonstrated a low frequency of bladder and sexual dysfunction (74,75). Both of these techniques should be considered standard when undertaking resection of the rectum.

## FUNCTIONAL OUTCOMES

Gastrointestinal function following rectal cancer resection is quite variable depending on the patients' preoperative status, use of chemoradiation, anastomotic technique and local factors, and the development of anastomotic complications. Today, sphincter preservation procedures are being performed with increasing frequency for the management of midrectal and low rectal cancers. However, preservation of intestinal continuity frequently leads to continence disturbances, which range from inadvertent passage of flatus to frank leakage of stool necessitating pad use (76–82). Patients with a straight low anastomosis may also suffer from urgency, frequency, and clustering of bowel movements. Poor function after sphincter salvage largely results from a combination of four factors: damage to the sphincter complex, loss of normal anorectal sensation, a reduced rectal capacity and compliance, and a reduction in large intestine length resulting in more liquid effluent reaching the anal canal (83). Increased effort has thus been exerted to minimize dysfunction following proctectomy with a focus toward good technique and reconstruction using a neorectum.

In recent years, improved functional outcomes have been reported following anastomotic reconstruction with a colonic J-pouch or coloplasty. The most studied and accepted reconstruction option at this time is the colonic

J-pouch, which is associated with improved physiological and functional outcomes as compared to the straight anastomosis (83). Until recently, the advantages of a J-pouch were thought to be short-lived, but a recent multicentered study revealed sustained functional advantages after 2 years postoperatively compared to both the straight colo-anal anastomosis and the coloplasty (84). Another common technique is the use of a side-to-end Baker anastomosis, which in the short term has equivalent functional results to the colonic J-pouch or coloplasty (85). Unfortunately, recent data suggest difficulty with complete evacuation of the Baker anastomosis as compared to the colonic J-pouch (85). It is for these reasons that we recommend colonic J-pouch reconstruction for low anastomoses at 6 cm or closer to the anal verge.

## PATIENT-CENTERED OUTCOMES

There has been a growing interest in medical and surgical outcomes that are most important to patients rather than traditional measures of morbidity and mortality. This interest has developed from the growing concern that medical care fails to properly assess all of the needs of the patient. Patient-centered outcomes, such as patient satisfaction or quality of life, are particularly meaningful for colorectal cancer patients. Despite the embryonic status of patient-centered outcomes in surgical fields, the Agency for Healthcare Research and Quality has developed the Consumer Assessment of Healthcare Providers and Systems (CAHPS) program, a joint public and private initiative to develop standardized surveys of patients' experiences with ambulatory and facility-level care (86). CAHPS surveys provide information about patients' care experiences rather than traditional clinical performance indicators, such as cured of disease or morbidity and mortality.

Surgeons' ability to measure and understand quality of life and other patient-centered outcome would be of great value to the colorectal cancer patient undergoing surgery. In practical terms, patient expectations would be clearer. Unfortunately, few validated and useful patient-centered metrics have been evaluated and even fewer are in use today (87). Despite the lack of real progress in this area, insurers, patients, and others are very interested in determining what patients think of the treatments we provide them. At this time, surgeons need to work closely with others to provide more comprehensive and nontraditional outcomes following surgical care.

## CONCLUSION

In summary, this chapter on improving outcomes for abdominal surgery in colorectal cancer provides an overview of potential complications, methods to reduce complications, methods to improve outcomes, surgical outcome metrics, and the future of patient-centered outcomes in colorectal cancer surgery. We have particularly emphasized the impact of the quality movement and the role of outcomes on quality measurement and assurance. The information presented in this chapter is critical as quality metrics and measurement are likely to become more and more important to the individual practitioner. Given emerging refinements of open as well as laparoscopic techniques, as well as postoperative care, outcomes measurement will become more and more important as we prove to our patients, payers, Congress, and ourselves that our outcomes are sufficient. Although payers and other government groups have become the drivers of quality improvement, it is our duty to measure our own outcomes, assess the quality of care that we provide, and compare our own results with those of our colleagues. Internal efforts to improve quality are the most likely to bring about real meaningful changes in outcomes for colorectal cancer.

## REFERENCES

1. Jagoditsch M et al. *World J Surg* 2000;24:1264–70.
2. Mcdermott FT et al. *Br J Surg* 1981;68:850.
3. Chapuis PH et al. *Br J Surg* 1985;72:698–702.
4. Tominaga T et al. Five-year follow-up report. *Cancer* 1996;78:403–8.
5. Swanson RS et al. *Ann Surg Oncol* 2003;10:65–71.
6. Compton CC et al. College of American Pathologists Consensus Statement 1999. *Arch Pathol Lab Med* 2000;124:979–94.
7. Wolmark N et al. *Ann Surg* 1984;199:375–82.
8. Langevin JM, Nivatvongs S. *Am J Surg* 1984;147:330–3.
9. Nagtegaal ID, Quirke P. *J Clin Oncol* 2008;26:303–12.
10. Quirke P et al. *Lancet* 1986;2:996–8.
11. Vernava AM et al. *Surg Gynecol Obstet* 1992;175:333–6.
12. Rouffet F et al. *Dis Colon Rectum* 1994;37:651–9.
13. Nelson H et al. *J Natl Cancer Inst* 2001;93:583–96.
14. Otchy D et al. *Dis Colon Rectum* 2004;47:1269–84.
15. Hermanek P. *Langenbecks Arch Chir Suppl Kongressbd* 1991;277–81.
16. ASCO/NCCN Quality Measures: http://ascopubs.org/doi/abs/10.1200/jco.2008.16.5068
17. Compton CC. *Arch Pathol Lab Med* 2000;124:1016–25.
18. Bonjer HJ et al. *Arch Surg* 2007;142:298–303.
19. The Clinical Outcomes of Surgical Therapy Study Group. *NEJM* 2004;350:2050–59.
20. Guillou PJ et al. *Lancet* 2005;365:1718–26.
21. Langevin JM et al. *Surg Gynecol Obstet* 1984;159:139–44.
22. Golub R et al. *J Am Coll Surg* 1997;184:364–72.
23. Alves A et al. *World J Surg* 2002;26:499–502.

24. Suturing or stapling in gastrointestinal surgery: A prospective randomized study. *Br J Surg* 1991;78: 337–41.
25. Docherty JG et al. West of Scotland and Highland Anastomosis Study Group. *Ann Surg* 1995;221: 176–84.
26. Walstad PM. *Am Surg* 1974;40:586–90.
27. Makela JT et al. *Dis Colon Rectum* 2003;46:653–60.
28. Bucher P et al. *Arch Surg* 2004;139:1359–64.
29. Bucher P et al. *Br J Surg* 2005;92:409–14.
30. Hyman N et al. *Ann Surg* 2007;245:254–8.
31. Nicksa GA et al. *Dis Col Rectum* 2007;50:197–203.
32. Hyman N et al. *Ann Surg* 2007;245:254–8.
33. Khan AA et al. *Colorectal Dis.* 2008;10(6):587–92.
34. Schecter S et al. *Dis Col Rectum* 1994;37:984–8.
35. Lutchfeld MA et al. *Dis Colon Rectum* 1989; 32: 733–6.
36. Tuson JR, Everett WG. *Int J Colorectal Dis* 1990;5: 44–8.
37. Chung RS et al. *Surgery* 1988;104:824–9.
38. Graffner H et al. *Dis Colon Rectum* 1983;26:87–90.
39. Virgilio C et al. *Endoscopy* 1995;27:219–22.
40. Waxman BP, Ramsay AH. *Aust N Z Surg* 1986;56: 797–801.
41. Matos DDM et al. *Cochrane Database Syst Rev* 2001;(3):CD003144.
42. Suchan KL et al. *Surg Endosc* 2003;17:1110–3.
43. Forshaw MJ et al. *Tech Coloproctol* 2006;10:21–7.
44. Cirocco WC, Golub RW. *American Surgeon* 1995;61: 460–3.
45. Malik AH et al. *Colorectal Dis* 2008;10(6):616–8.
46. Choy PYG et al. *Cochrane Database Syst Rev* 2007; 3:CD004320.
47. Murray JJ, Schoetz DJJr. Stapling techniques in rectal surgery. In: Fazio VW (ed). *Current Therapy in Colon and Rectal Surgery.* Philadelphia, PA: BC Decker, 1990, pp. 384–90.
48. Chardavoyne R et al. *Am Surgeon* 1991;57:734–6.
49. Chassin JL et al. *Surg Clin N Am* 1984;64:441–59.
50. Charlmers AG et al. *Clin Radiol* 1986;37:379–81.
51. Dubois JJ et al. *Military Med* 1989;154:505–7.
52. Atabek U et al. Report of two cases. *Dis Colon Rectum* 1992;35:1180–2.
53. Wang QY et al. *Arch Surg* 1985;120:1013–20.
54. Khan FA et al. *Surg Obst Gyn* 1987;165:275–6.
55. Hill AD et al. *JACS* 1994;178:183–4.
56. Xu J, Lin J. *JACS* 1994;179:351–2.
57. Civelek A et al. *Surg Today* 2002;32:944–5.
58. Konstadoulakis MM et al. *Eur J Surg* 1999;165:583–7.
59. Lord MD, Gourevitch A. *Br J Surg* 1965;52:202–4.
60. Cioffiro W et al. *Arch Surg* 1976;111:167–71.
61. Olsen W, Beaudoin D. *Surg, Gynecol, Obstet* 1970; 131:57–62.
62. Cassar K, Munro A. *J R Coll Surg Edin* 2002;6: 731–41.
63. Fabri PJ et al. *Arch Surg* 1974;108:569–75.
64. Rodkey GV, Welch CE. *Ann Surg* 1984;200:466–78.
65. McGory ML et al. *Arch Surg* 2007;142:668–74.
66. Malek MM et al. *Sur Laparosc Endosc Percutan Tech* 2007;17:385–7.
67. Falsetto A et al. *Ann Ital Chir* 2005;76:175–81.
68. Scheele J et al. *Surgery* 1984;95:6–13.
69. Working Party of the British Committee for Standards Clinical Hematology Task Force. *Br Med J* 1996;312:430–3.
70. Higgins CC. *JAMA* 1967;199:82–8.
71. Al-Awadi K et al. *Int Urol Nephrol* 2005;37:235–41.
72. Hamawy K et al. *Seminar Colon Rectal Surg* 2000;11: 163–79.
73. Pocard M et al. *Surgery* 2002;131:368–72.
74. Heald RJ, Ryall RD. *Lancet* 1986;1479–82.
75. Nesbakken A et al. *Br J Surg* 2000;87:206–10.
76. McDonald PJ, Heald RJ. *Br J Surg* 1983;70:727–9.
77. McAnena OJ et al. *Surg Gynecol Obstet* 1990;170: 517–21.
78. Batignani G et al. *Dis Colon Rectum* 1991;34:329–35.
79. Lewis WG et al. *Br J Surg* 1992;79:1082–6.
80. Karanjia ND et al. *Br J Surg* 1992;79:114–6.
81. Lewis WG et al. *Dis Colon Rectum* 1995;38:259–63.
82. Miller AS et al. *Br J Surg* 1995;82:1327–30.
83. Brown SR, Seow-Choen F. *Semin Surg Oncol* 2000; 19:376–85.
84. Fazio VW et al. *Ann Surg* 2007;246:481–90.
85. Machado M et al. *Ann Surg* 2003;238:214–20.
86. Consumer Assessment of Healthcare Providers and Systems. https://www.cahps.ahrq.gov/default.asp.
87. Morris AM. *Surg Oncol Clin N Am* 2006;15: 195–211, viii.

# 27

# Abdominal restorative surgery for rectal cancer

CHARLES C. VINING AND NIJJIA N. MAHMOUD

## CHALLENGING CASE

A 54-year-old male presents with an adenocarcinoma of the middle rectum on colonoscopy for rectal bleeding. Computed tomography (CT) of the chest, abdomen, and pelvis documented the tumor without evidence of metastatic disease. Magnetic resonance imaging (MRI) documented a T3N1 tumor.

## CASE MANAGEMENT

The patient was presented to a multidisciplinary tumor board who recommended a course of preoperative chemoradiotherapy followed by a low anterior resection and diverting loop ileostomy.

## INTRODUCTION

The morbidity associated with proctectomy, including incontinence, sexual dysfunction, functional disruption, and the possibility of permanent ostomy has been the driver of development of new techniques in rectal cancer surgery and improvement of old ones. While the description of total mesorectal excision (TME) in the 1980s in conjunction with improved neoadjuvant therapy contemporized the field and is the cornerstone for modern-day rectal cancer surgery, the avoidance of permanent ostomy has motivated several generations of surgeons to explore better ways of reestablishing gastrointestinal continuity without compromising oncologic results, while minimizing impact on function.

This chapter discusses the advances in abdominal restorative surgery for rectal cancer with a focus on the contributions of the use of neoadjuvant chemoradiotherapy, technical considerations, oncologic outcomes, and functional results. Careful preoperative planning with a multidisciplinary team can improve outcomes and chances of sphincter preservation. While there is still a role for abdominoperineal resection, the use of this technique is now reserved overwhelmingly, especially among experienced rectal surgeons in specialty centers, for those who have anal sphincter involvement, preoperative incontinence, or severe comorbidities precluding sphincter conservation. The ability to reestablish gastrointestinal continuity has been rising over the last 80 years. Efforts today focus on reduction of both short- and long-term morbidity associated with rectal resection and anastomosis.

## A CENTURY OF RECTAL CANCER TECHNICAL IMPROVEMENTS

There has been continuous evolution and advancement over the course of the twentieth century in the treatment of rectal cancer, especially with regard to improvement in quality of life, sphincter conservation, and oncologic outcomes. Advances in rectal cancer are based on improved comprehension of the disease biology and technical advancements. These improvements can be directly attributed to pioneers in the field of colorectal surgery.

Until the late 1800s, rectal cancer surgery was performed solely for symptom palliation (Figure 27.1). In 1826, Lisfrank described a perineal approach to remove the distal 3–4 cm of rectum along with the sphincter complex, essentially converting the anus to a stoma (2). Rectal resection with a combined rectal and abdominal approach was described in 1884 by Czerny, and then again by Mayo in 1904. Both recurrence rates and morbidity were dismally high. From 1899 to 1906, Miles performed 57 perineal resections for rectal cancer. Of those, 54 of 57 (95%) had early recurrences. Miles did postmortem examinations of these patients and saw that the recurrences were composed of pelvic implants, mesocolon nodules, and enlarged, malignant lymph nodes along the inferior mesenteric artery (IMA). In 1908, he revised his approach based on these observations, detailing an abdominal approach to rectal surgery with low ligation

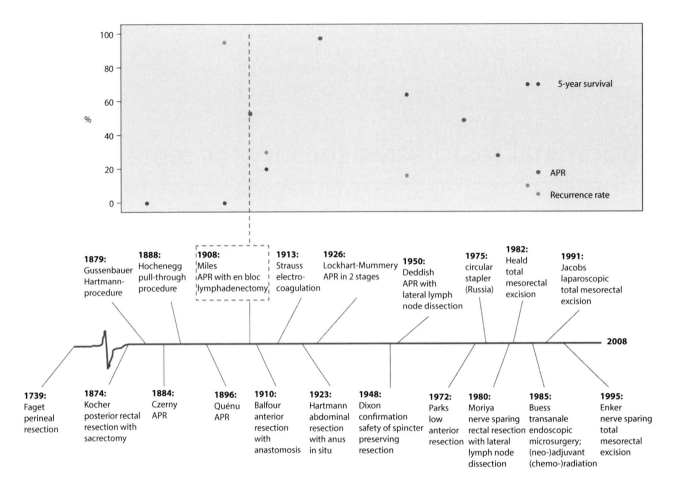

Figure 27.1 Milestones in the development of restorative proctocolectomy for rectal cancer. (From Lange M. et al. *Eur J Surg Oncol* 2009;35[5]:456–63.)

of the IMA, sigmoid diversion, and rectal dissection done transabdominally prior to completing the anal resection transperineally. This technique eventually became the gold standard operation for rectal cancer, because local recurrence rates were dramatically reduced (29.5%) as the lymph node basin was excised along with the entire rectum and sphincter complex. Despite this major breakthrough, early morbidity and mortality were high with an estimated 1-year survival of 58% (1).

It would take another decade of what amounted to direct observation and trial and error for the treatment of rectal cancer to include attempts at sphincter conservation and consideration of functional results. In the 1920s, Dr. Henri Hartmann introduced "anterior resection" of the rectum, preserving the distal third of the rectum and sphincter complex with the creation of a sigmoid colostomy for proximal rectal tumors with the goal of decreasing the complications and mortality associated with perineal wounds while improving lymphadenectomy by including a high IMA ligation. This technique mandated ostomy creation, because pull-through methods for sphincter preservation, still in their infancy, were plagued with high leak rates and perioperative mortality rates as high as 20%. Reliability of the anastomosis was still an issue, as were the technical aspects of establishing gastrointestinal continuity in the confines of the deep pelvis

where access and exposure are difficult at best (1). Claude Dixon, at the Mayo Clinic, describes eloquently his pelvic anastomotic technique—he put curved clamps side by side on both the stump of the rectum as well as the colon. Since the posterior aspect of the rectum is thin, he placed a single row of posterior interrupted sutures there. Anteriorly, an inverting row of sutures was placed as well. He commented, "Any so-called aseptic anastomosis in this region is a gymnastic feat attended by difficult clamp maneuvers deep in the pelvis, danger of tearing the rectum, the hazard of catching the opposite mucosa to create a persistent diaphragm or of perforating the rectum in forcing the anastomosis open, and finally the possibility of a poor anastomosis" (3).

Until the late 1930s, rectal resection was performed with an intraoperative change in the patients' position from supine to the prone or semiprone position. The introduction of leg rests allowed for simultaneous performance of the abdominal and perineal dissections. Introduction of simple stirrups also facilitated the advent of restorative techniques that circumvented the need for a permanent ostomy. Dixon presented results for restorative anterior resection for tumors of the proximal rectum and distal sigmoid in 1948. He demonstrated a 64% 5-year survival, prompting widespread adoption of this technique for treating cancer of the proximal rectum while preserving continuity by creating a hand-sewn distal anastomosis. Of 426 cases in his series of anterior resection of lesions between 6 and 20 cm from the dentate line, there were 25 deaths (5.9%). Eighteen occurred after the first stage of the operation and seven following closure of the stoma. Seven of the 18 deaths followed peritonitis, two after pelvic abscesses, and then the rest from perioperative issues unrelated to the technical aspects of the case. Of the seven deaths after closure of the stoma, four resulted from peritonitis. This represents a 3% operative mortality rate—remarkable for its time. For lesions proximal to 10 cm from the dentate line, the resectability rate was 10% by anterior resection. For lesions 10 cm from the dentate, it dropped to 80%, and for those at 8 cm it dropped to 44%. Dixon felt that 8 cm was the lowest level of general applicability of the operation or his ability to accurately predict his ability to reestablish continuity. Below 8 cm, there must be favorable anatomy—"a thin person with a broad, flat pelvis." Above 8–10 cm, involvement of adjacent organs did not impact resectability. Almost all of these cases were diverted—a transverse loop colostomy was the most common strategy. Analysis of other series published at the time demonstrated that with anterior resection without colostomy, 10%–20% of cases were complicated by the need for an emergent colostomy in the early postoperative period because of anastomotic leak. Stricture of the anastomosis occurred in five cases, and long-term outcomes as well as the nuances of postoperative function were not reported (3).

## PREOPERATIVE EVALUATION—IS SPHINCTER CONSERVATION POSSIBLE?

In Dixons' 1948 analysis of rectal cancer surgery, he emphasized the need for surgeons to preoperatively physically evaluate the distance of the tumor from the anal verge and dentate line by digital rectal exam and proctoscopy. Those guidelines have not changed 70 years later. Physical examination should include digital rectal examination and direct visualization via proctoscopy or flexible sigmoidoscopy to assess the size, degree of luminal obstruction, location with regard to the anal margin or anorectal ring/sphincter, distal-most aspect of the tumor, and orientation and fixation to surrounding structures such as the vagina, prostate, and sphincter complex. Digital rectal exam can also be beneficial in assessing sphincter tone and function. These factors can help determine the need for neoadjuvant treatment and address the possibility of maintaining continuity. Examination is an important aspect of clinical staging. Approximately 6% of patients with colorectal malignancies have a synchronous colorectal neoplasm. Complete colonoscopy to assess the colon preoperatively is necessary. If colonoscopy cannot be completed, a virtual colonoscopy or barium enema can substitute. A complete blood count, basic metabolic panel, liver function tests, and baseline carcinoembryonic antigen should be obtained. Clinical staging should be completed with a CT of the chest, abdomen,

and pelvis, and either MRI of the pelvis or endorectal ultrasound (ERUS). Regional imaging with MRI (most commonly performed) or ERUS assesses depth of invasion and nodal involvement and is essential in determining need for preoperative treatment either with or without radiation depending on protocol used and size, symptomatology, and characteristics of the tumor as well as clinical stage.

The ultimate goal of preoperative assessment is to most accurately determine stage, characterize the lesion, assess resectability, and determine the need for neoadjuvant treatment. Large administrative cancer databases such as Surveillance, Epidemiology, and End Results and National Cancer Database analysis demonstrate that sphincter preservation varies based on surgical volume, education, region, and sociodemographic factors. It has been demonstrated that age, insurance status, National Comprehensive Cancer Network institution, tumor fixation, level of tumor, and history of preoperative radiotherapy are all predictors of sphincter preservation. Standardization and dissemination of knowledge regarding approach to evaluation, staging, and surgery may help (4,5).

## MARGINS

The discussion of margin adequacy has been an area of evolution in the past 20 years. A satisfactory oncologic resection is predicated on an R0 resection with clear distal and circumferential margins. That said, the minimum acceptable distal margin has steadily shrunk with better data documenting acceptable clearances less than 1 cm and the importance of the circumferential radial margin (CRM) as a prognostic indicator has become manifest. Surgical techniques allowing lower connections and the advent of neoadjuvant chemotherapy facilitating shrinkage of bulky tumors made ultralow anastomoses possible and drove research to determine the absolute distal and radial spread of tumor.

### DISTAL MARGIN

In the past, a minimum of 2–5 cm distal margin on the rectum was recommended for nonirradiated patients because of the belief that intramural tumor extension was present. In 1951, Golligher, Dukes, and Bussey demonstrated local tumor spread in the vast majority of rectal cancer did not exceed 2 cm from the tumor margin by showing that tumor cells >2 cm from margin were seen in only 2% of specimens. It was therefore hypothesized that a 5 cm margin was more than sufficient from an oncologic perspective (6). Studies by Williams and colleagues in the early 1980s, however, revealed that in a cohort of more than 50 nonirradiated abdominal perineal resection (APR) specimens, 76% of patients had no intramural spread of tumor beyond the cancer itself, and in 14%, the spread was less than 1 cm distal to the tumor and most commonly in the submucosa compared with the muscularis propria. Only five patients had tumor extension beyond 1 cm, and those patients had large poorly differentiated neoplasms (7,8). Other studies and reviews done contemporaneously by Pollett and Nichols as well as the Large Bowel Cancer Group Project demonstrated similar results in patients who had not been pretreated with chemoradiotherapy. Still other data demonstrate that there is no difference in either 5-year survival rates or local recurrence (LR) in patients who had <2, 2–5, or >5 cm distal margins. Others found that while there is a difference in survival and LR in those with positive versus negative distal margins, there is no difference in LR between those with negative margins of <1 cm or >1 cm. Most recently, margins of <1 cm have demonstrated no difference in oncologic outcomes (9–11).

Data published within the past 5 years demonstrate that margins of <5 mm are acceptable in those with good risk pretreated tumors. Whole-mount pathologic examination of specimens in patients who underwent chemoradiotherapy (CRT) followed by resection found intramural extension beyond gross tumor in only 2 of 109 patients (1.8%) with a maximum distance of 0.95 mm (12). Moreover, the rate of local recurrence and 3-year recurrence-free survival are similar in patients with distal margins greater or less than 1 cm following CRT. In contrast, patients with advanced disease (T4 or N1+ tumors) are more likely to have intramural extension beyond 1 cm (9–11). All of these factors have facilitated creative and innovative approaches to sphincter conservation in the past decade by alleviating oncologic concerns and highlighting the necessity of good patient selection.

## CIRCUMFERENTIAL RADIAL MARGIN

CRM and the fascia propria emerged as very important anatomic landmarks when the importance of TME was recognized. Negative CRM is a major prognostic factor for rectal cancer as local recurrence and long-term survival are highly correlated with the presence or absence of tumor at the mesorectal margin. The CRM is defined as the shortest distance between the outer edge of the tumor and the mesorectal fascia (fascia propria). Quirke reviewed 52 specimens and found that 25% had positive margins and almost 80% of those recurred locally. A CRM of <1 mm is considered a positive margin. Studies have shown that margins <1 mm have a local recurrence rate of 25%–75%. By contrast, those with CRM >1 mm have a LR rate of less than 10%. Additionally, CRMs 1 mm or less were associated with a higher rate of distant metastasis and shorter survival. Finally, radial margin invasion risk is increased with lack of response to neoadjuvant chemoradiotherapy, palpable fixation on DRE posttreatment, and proximity to the dentate line (11,13,14).

Recognition of the role of total mesorectal excision was facilitated and complemented by pathologic data documenting the role of CRM in the rate of local recurrence. Careful dissection in the plane between the fascia propria of the rectum and the presacral fascia investing the sacrum dramatically decreased the rate of positive CRM, and subsequently improved local recurrence rates. The Dutch TME study (where TME was carefully controlled for) reported a recurrence rate of 16% versus 6% if the margins were less than or greater than 2 mm, respectively. Additionally, the widespread adoption of TME correlated with a dramatic drop in the rate of APR (15). Recognition that the proper TME plane extends to the intersphincteric groove coupled with the rise of specific technology to allow gastrointestinal continuity set the stage for transanal-transabdominal as well as transanal-TME (Ta-TME) techniques for resection of low rectal cancers.

## TECHNICAL ADVANCES ALLOW LOWER ANASTOMOSES

The development of stapling devices in the late 1960s changed nearly every surgical field, including colon and rectal surgery. Specifically, this technology improved techniques for tissue division, construction of anastomosis, and improved time efficiency. Ravitch, in 1972, published *Technics of Staple Suturing in the Gastrointestinal Tract* and triggered the near universal adoption of stapling devices. Although the development of stapling devices had been underway for several years by this time, it was this seminal publication that helped disseminate the technology (16).

In 1975, Fain demonstrated that use of the circular stapler for low colorectal anastomoses had a similar leak rate compared with hand-sewn anastomoses. These staplers lay down two staggered rows of staples to create a circular anastomosis and cut simultaneously (17). Colorectal surgery typically requires anything from a 25 mm to a 33 mm end-to-end anastomosis stapler. Circular staplers come in a variety of sizes and must be fit to both the size of the descending colon and according to what the anal canal/rectal stump can accommodate. The double stapling technique for low colorectal anastomosis was introduced in 1980, which accelerated the procedure, minimized intraoperative contamination, and avoided the disadvantage of joining bowel segments with significant size disparities. The following decade saw the introduction of techniques aimed at creating ever lower connections with the advent of the colo-anal anastomosis, the intersphincteric transanal/transabdominal rectal dissection with hand-sewn anastomosis, and introduction of the colonic pouch in an attempt to improve functional results that were (and are) frequently compromised. These techniques and instruments allow modern surgeons to perform anastomoses far below the 8 cm cutoff described by Dixon with a high degree of reliability, low complication rate, and maximized oncologic outcomes.

## NEOADJUVANT CHEMORADIOTHERAPY AND SPHINCTER CONSERVATION

While oncologic outcomes remain the main goal of rectal cancer treatment, avoiding permanent stoma and maximizing functional outcomes is a recent additional quality of life–related outcome most patients demand. There is no question that advancements in technology and data-driven reassessment of distal margin requirements have made sphincter conservation possible. Neoadjuvant therapy in rectal cancer treatment has improved clinical outcomes, facilitated resection to help with safe sphincter conservation, and become the standard of care in advanced disease. It has the potential to downstage tumors, shrink locally advanced neoplasms, and improve R0 resection rates. Its role in sphincter conservation for low-lying tumors is controversial and complex, dependent on the position and location of the tumor, the body habitus of the patient, the skill and training of the surgeon, and the patient's preoperative anorectal function.

Over the last several decades, randomized trials have investigated the role of neoadjuvant radiotherapy (RT) in the treatment of rectal cancer. Neoadjuvant RT has the potential for less acute and late toxicity with more patients receiving full-dose radiation therapy compared with the adjuvant (postoperative) setting. Preoperative radiation can be administered via two techniques: the intensive short-course radiation with large fractions ($5 \times 5$ Gy) for 1 week followed by resection within 1 week—or 5–6 weeks of conventional fractions (1.8–2 Gy), with concurrent chemotherapy followed by resection in approximately 6–10 weeks. The Swedish Rectal Cancer Trial conducted between 1987 and 1990 randomized 1,168 patients to preoperative radiotherapy (25 Gy in five fractions, short course) followed by surgery in 1 week versus surgery alone. The group that was randomized to RT demonstrated decreased local recurrence at 5 years (11% versus 27%; $p < 0.001$), and increased overall survival (58% versus 48%; $p = 0.004$). This benefit was seen in all ages and supported the idea that oncological survival is predicated on improved local control. Additionally, the Uppsala trial between 1980 and 1985 randomized patients to preoperative short-course ($5 \times 5.1$ Gy) versus postoperative conventional (total 60 Gy) radiotherapy. Preoperative radiotherapy was associated with significantly decreased local failure (13% versus 22%; $p = 0.02$) without a significant improvement in 5-year survival. Duplicating the finding that radiotherapy confers a survival benefit in other trials has been elusive (18).

Criticisms of short-course radiation include an insignificant time for downstaging, particularly in bulky tumors with threatened margins, increased acute and late toxicity, and inability to add concurrent chemotherapy. A French trial randomized patients with low-lying rectal tumors to either short (within 2 weeks) or long (6 weeks) intervals between radiation and surgery. The long interval group demonstrated a significantly better clinical tumor response (71.7% versus 51.3%; $p = 0.007$), improved pathological downstaging (26% versus 10.3%; $p = 0.005$) and a trend toward increased sphincter preservation (76% versus 68%; $p = 0.27$) (19).

Neoadjuvant chemoradiotherapy with the goal of downsizing clinically unresectable rectal cancers was investigated as well. A comparison of patients receiving combined preoperative radiotherapy (50.4 Gy) with or without concurrent chemotherapy (5-FU) demonstrated that 90% of patients who were initially unresectable converted to resectability versus only 64% of those in the radiation-only group. Additionally, combined chemoradiotherapy demonstrated complete pathological response in 20% of patients versus 6% of those receiving radiation alone. This in addition to other trials confirm the enhancement of downstaging when chemotherapy is administered concurrently with radiation for locally advanced rectal cancer (20–22).

The German Rectal Cancer Group compared preoperative and postoperative long-course CRT combined with TME for patients with stages II and III disease who were candidates for low anterior resection and found that preoperative CRT demonstrated improved 5-year local recurrence rate (6% versus 13%) and remained significant after 10 years without an effect on overall survival. They also noted less acute and chronic toxicities associated with preoperative versus postoperative CRT. Therefore, neoadjuvant CRT followed by TME is the treatment of choice for patients with locally advanced rectal cancer. Local recurrences with preoperative CRT and TME are now <10%, and in patients with complete pathological response, 10-year disease-free survival is >80%. Moreover, patients with complete or nearly complete tumor regression with neoadjuvant CRT demonstrate better long-term survival (23).

Gerard and colleagues recently did a meta-analysis of 17 randomized clinical trials of rectal cancer treatment involving chemoradiotherapy in an attempt to analyze sphincter conservation (24). Only three of the studies included sphincter conservation as an endpoint. Although there was significant heterogeneity among the studies, some generalized conclusions could be drawn regarding the role of chemoradiotherapy. Rates of sphincter conservation in general have gone up considerably from the late 1970s when it was less than 30% to the present where it exceeds 75% (Figure 27.2). Predictably, short-course radiation and chemotherapy has no impact on sphincter conservation, since no time interval is allowed for tumor downsizing prior to surgery. In the five large trials of long-course chemoradiotherapy with more than 5 weeks between the end of therapy and surgery, no increase in sphincter conservation was seen despite an increased rate of pathologic complete response up to 16%–19%. Alternatively, it is evident from these trials that the 5-year local recurrence rate has decreased from about 25% to close to 5%. While the role of preoperative chemoradiation in local control is well supported by all trials thus far, even controlling for good surgery, the role of downstaging in the facilitation of restorative surgery is unproven (25,26) (see Chapter 34).

The increase in sphincter preservation appears to be most dependent on advances in surgical techniques. The expertise of the operating surgeon is important—advanced training in rectal cancer surgery is directly correlated with improvement in sphincter conservation and the ability to perform restorative surgery. Evolving emphasis on multidisciplinary

**Differences in sphinter saving surgery rate (odds ratio) and 95% confidence intervals**

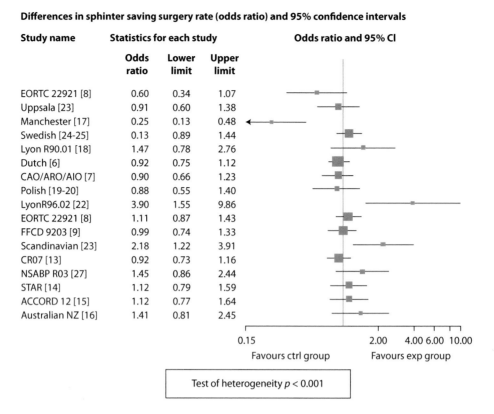

| Study name | Statistics for each study | | | Odds ratio and 95% CI |
|---|---|---|---|---|
| | Odds ratio | Lower limit | Upper limit | |
| EORTC 22921 [8] | 0.60 | 0.34 | 1.07 | |
| Uppsala [23] | 0.91 | 0.60 | 1.38 | |
| Manchester [17] | 0.25 | 0.13 | 0.48 | |
| Swedish [24-25] | 0.13 | 0.89 | 1.44 | |
| Lyon R90.01 [18] | 1.47 | 0.78 | 2.76 | |
| Dutch [6] | 0.92 | 0.75 | 1.12 | |
| CAO/ARO/AIO [7] | 0.90 | 0.66 | 1.23 | |
| Polish [19-20] | 0.88 | 0.55 | 1.40 | |
| LyonR96.02 [22] | 3.90 | 1.55 | 9.86 | |
| EORTC 22921 [8] | 1.11 | 0.87 | 1.43 | |
| FFCD 9203 [9] | 0.99 | 0.74 | 1.33 | |
| Scandinavian [23] | 2.18 | 1.22 | 3.91 | |
| CR07 [13] | 0.92 | 0.73 | 1.16 | |
| NSABP R03 [27] | 1.45 | 0.86 | 2.44 | |
| STAR [14] | 1.12 | 0.79 | 1.59 | |
| ACCORD 12 [15] | 1.12 | 0.77 | 1.64 | |
| Australian NZ [16] | 1.41 | 0.81 | 2.45 | |

0.15    2.00  4.00 6.00  10.00

Favours ctrl group          Favours exp group

Test of heterogeneity $p < 0.001$

Figure 27.2 Sphincter preservation and neoadjuvant treatment. (From Gerard JP et al. *Crit Rev Oncol Hematol* 2012[1]:21–8.)

assessment of patients preoperatively by all practitioners involved in the care of rectal cancer patients impacts patient selection for restorative surgery and local control.

There remains controversy regarding early low-risk stage II patients (small tumors with good histopathologic characteristics) regarding whether neoadjuvant CRT is beneficial. Unfortunately, limitations in clinical staging make it difficult to determine those with low-risk T3 disease. It should be noted that approximately 22% of patients who undergo preoperative imaging with MRI or ERUS diagnosed with T3N0 disease are found to have positive lymph nodes on final pathology. Moreover, approximately 18% of patients diagnosed with T3N0 disease on preoperative imaging are overstaged and found to be T2N0 on final review. At some institutions (e.g., Europe), patients with tumors with clear circumferential margins on MRI will be offered surgery without neoadjuvant CRT. However in the United States, neoadjuvant CRT is still favored for T3N0 disease due to concern for understaging, inferior local control, increased toxicity, and worse functional outcomes with postoperative CRT (27).

## SURGICAL TECHNIQUES FOR SPHINCTER CONSERVATION

The surgical management of rectal cancer should be individually tailored to the patient and disease. Early rectal cancers (stage 1) can be definitively treated by surgery alone. More advanced neoplasms should be managed by a multidisciplinary team for best outcomes. When deciding on treatment modality, staging and patient factors as well as baseline anorectal function must be considered.

## GENERAL CONCEPTS AND PREPARATION

Rectal neoplasms exist in the narrow confines of the deep pelvis. Obese body habitus, abundant visceral fat, and narrow android pelvis all challenge sphincter conservation. Besides the preoperative treatment and evaluation already discussed, a patient undergoing rectal cancer surgery should be preoperatively marked and counseled by a stoma therapist, and the concept of postoperative functional changes should be thoroughly discussed. A bowel continence history and assessment of mobility, ability to manage and handle a temporary ileostomy, renal function, and general performance status is essential.

In the operating room, lithotomy positioning for most approaches is necessary. Special attention to padding the extremities to prevent nerve injury is crucial. If approaching the dissection in an open or laparoscopically assisted fashion, lighted retractors such as the St. Mark's retractor, or a headlight, long instruments, and access to help with exposure via good retraction are essential. If approaching the tumor purely laparoscopically or robotically, many of these same concepts apply. A specially trained team that understands how to set up and troubleshoot the robot is a necessity.

Radical resection involves removal of the tumor and rectum en bloc with the lymphatics and vascular supply located in the mesorectum and is known as a TME. In radical rectal surgery with intent to cure, the goals include preservation of the autonomic nerves, negative circumferential and distal margins, preservation of sphincter function, and restoration of continuity when possible. Radical resections include sphincter-preserving surgery such as low anterior resection (LAR) and transanal transabdominal ultra-low hand-sewn approaches also described as intersphincteric proctectomy (ISP) and the sphincter-sacrificing surgery APR. As long as technically and oncologically appropriate, LAR or one of its modifications is the preferred approach to radical resection. Technical limitations include visceral obesity, a narrow and long pelvis, and low tumor location <1 cm from the sphincter complex. Anterior location can also challenge sphincter conservation. If the tumor invades either the sphincter complex or levators, sphincter preservation is contraindicated. Moreover, patients with baseline poor or marginal anorectal control are inappropriate for LAR due to worsened postoperative anorectal function.

## TOTAL MESORECTAL EXCISION

The pillar of modern rectal cancer surgery is based on the work of Heald who popularized TME as a key concept in 1982 (28). Previous to TME, many surgeons performed low anterior resections with a blunt dissection technique of the mid- and distal rectum as described by Dixon. This technique was burdened with poor 5-year disease-free survival for all stages treated with curative intent (<50%) and local recurrence up to 20%. The poor outcomes were due to breaches in the mesorectal fascia (fascia propria) during the blunt dissection with positive circumferential margins seen in up to 85% of local recurrences. Heald described "one distinct lymphovascular entity" in which the rectum and mesorectum, derived from the same embryologic origin, are removed en bloc from the surrounding parietal fascia covering the sacrum and pelvic sidewall via the avascular loose areolar *holy plane* via sharp dissection under direct vision (Figure 27.3). Heald realized that by staying away from the lateral sidewalls, bleeding, nerve injury, and positive margins were minimized, thereby dropping rates of local recurrence, improving bladder and sexual functional outcomes, and dramatically increasing rates of sphincter preservation. Although there has never been a prospective randomized trial investigating the TME technique, it is consistently associated with lower local recurrence and improved 5-year survival. Heald reported outcomes for 519 patients in 1998 demonstrating an astounding 3% local recurrence rate in patients treated with curative intent. In this study, only 49 patients had undergone chemoradiotherapy. Also, only 37 patients needed an APR. Strict attention to nerve preservation and failure to disrupt the periprostatic plexus and nervi erigentes results in vast

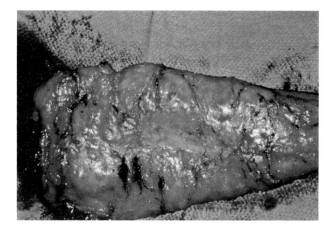

Figure 27.3 **(See color insert.)** Total mesorectal excision specimen with a smooth, intact fascia propria. (Courtesy of the author.)

improvement in sexual and urinary function. In the past, blunt dissection was associated with sexual dysfunction in up to 75% of men and nearly half of women. Urinary retention or incontinence was seen in 80% of patients (29). Currently, rates of sexual dysfunction are less than 10%–20%, and long-term bladder dysfunction is 5% or less (30). Heald deserves credit for popularizing the components of TME; however, several contemporary surgeons at institutions such as the Cleveland Clinic were performing rectal resections using the techniques of TME.

TME begins with mobilization of the sigmoid colon, careful identification of ureters and hypogastric nerves, and high ligation of the inferior mesenteric pedicle. Medial mobilization starting with ligation of the pedicle is perfectly acceptable. For the vast majority of patients requiring restorative surgery, mobilization of the splenic flexure is a must—while this can be done after the TME and vascular ligation, it typically precedes the pelvic operation when approached in a minimally invasive fashion. After vascular ligation and division of the bowel at the distal descending colon/sigmoid border, the TME proceeds by sharp dissection under direct visualization, either open, with the use of retractors, or in a minimally invasive fashion. Either way, staying in the avascular plane defined by the fascia propria of the rectum and the presacral fascia is essential. As the operation extends downward, the fascia propria investing the mesorectum becomes somewhat thinner, particularly anteriorly and laterally. At the levators, the mesorectum ends and the rectum itself extends through the levator hiatus as a bare muscular tube. The muscularis propria of the rectum is a direct extension of the internal sphincter. It is at the point just above the levator plate and directly adjacent to and distal to the mesorectum that the bowel is divided for a complete TME (Figure 27.4). Typically, this division takes place with a 30 mm TA or PI stapling device and leaves a small amount of distal rectum right at the levators about 1.5–3 cm above the dentate line depending on the body habitus of the patient and the length of the anal canal.

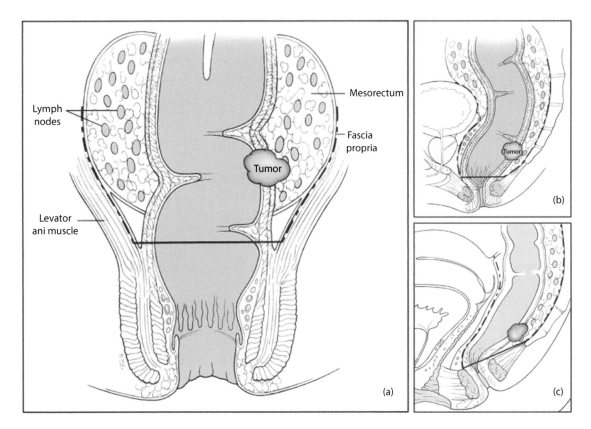

**Figure 27.4** Appropriate dissection planes for a low anterior resection. **(a)** Coronal view with distal margin delineated. **(b)** Sagittal view of dissection plane in male. **(c)** Sagittal view of dissection plane in female. (From Bordeianou L. et al. *J Gastrointest Surg* 2014;18[7]:1358–72.)

## Anterior resection in upper rectal cancers

In low and middle rectal cancers, a complete TME is performed, whereas in tumors of the upper rectum, a more localized TME can be performed with a distal division approximately 5 cm from the tumor margin. Upper rectal cancers are generally those defined as the upper one-third of the rectum, above the peritoneal reflection or above a certain distance such as 12–13 cm, which is somewhat arbitrary. Generally, those tumors in the upper rectum that are smaller (<3 cm) can undergo partial TME, dividing both the rectum and the mesorectum at minimum 5 cm distal to the bottom edge of the tumor. This leaves about 5–7 cm of rectum to perform the colorectal anastomosis. It is critical that the mesorectum is completely and cleanly resected at the same level as the rectum to ensure a good resection of the mesorectal lymph node basin and reduce the incidence of local nodal recurrence.

## Transanal transabdominal or intersphincteric proctectomy

Transanal transabdominal (TATA) or ISP is simply a way of reestablishing gastrointestinal continuity in patients whose tumors are so low that standard staplers cannot be placed below them with any confidence that negative margins would be obtained. In general, these tumors exist at the top of the anal canal at the very edge of the sphincter complex

(Figure 27.5). Surgery commences in the prone position, although it can also be done in lithotomy—transanal TME (TaTME) cases start in lithotomy as a rule. The advantage of this approach is that a negative margin can be established immediately under direct visualization. An incision is made in the intersphincteric plane or just proximal to it with electrocautery. It is relatively straightforward to get into the mesorectal plane from this approach, because the intersphincteric plane is contiguous with the plane between the mesorectum and the presacral fascia, and the internal sphincter is in continuity with the rectal wall. The surgeon can dissect all the way up into the pelvis, beyond the levator plate with this dissection. A Lone Star self-retaining retractor can be quite helpful as can anorectal retractors such as Hill-Ferguson or Pratt anal bivalve instruments (Figure 27.6). After dissecting beyond the levators circumferentially, the rectum is closed with a running suture to prevent contamination, and a moist gauze is inserted into the anal canal. The patient is placed into the lithotomy position, and a standard laparoscopic or open LAR with TME is performed. The entire specimen is brought out the abdominal incision after the abdominal TME plane meets the perineal TME plane. The colon is then mobilized such that the end of the colon is able to be pulled all the way out of the anus from the perineal side without tension. The retractor is placed back in, and orientation and pull-through of the colon take place. After a centimeter or two of colon is gently pulled out of the anus, the staple line is removed, and

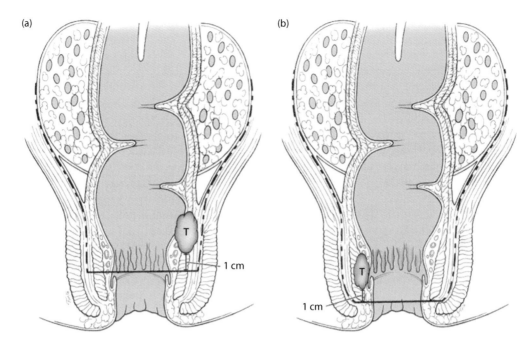

Figure 27.5 Appropriate planes for intersphincteric resection—TME plane created from above intersects intersphincteric plane. **(a)** Partial ISP. **(b)** Complete ISP. (From Bordeianou L. et al. *J Gastrointest Surg* 2014;18[7]:1358–72.)

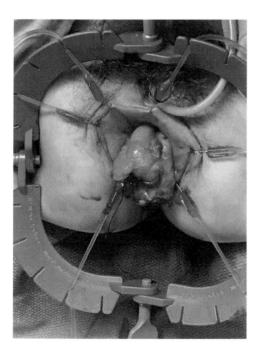

Figure 27.6 **(See color insert.)** Intraoperative positioning and retraction for establishing a hand-sewn anastomosis following an intersphincteric proctectomy. (Courtesy of the author.)

the colon is gently pushed back into the anal canal until the cut edge of the well-vascularized, viable distal rectum is at the level of the distal margin. An interrupted hand-sewn anastomosis is then performed with 3 or 2 Vicryl suture. This technique is challenging in individuals with narrow pelvises and a large amount of visceral fat that make it difficult to mobilize the colon and pull it through the anal canal.

Local recurrence after ISP is not statistically different from that of LAR or APR. Additionally, ISP and LAR have shown equivalent 5-year local recurrence-free survival suggesting that ISP is a suitable technique from an oncologic perspective. Those patients with bulky tumors and those with microscopic positive resection margins are more likely to have local recurrence after ISP (31–33).

Postoperative defecation functional outcomes such as frequency, urgency, ability to distinguish between flatus and stool, and perianal skin irritation have been demonstrated to be similar between ISP and LAR. A study by Yamada showed that patient age was the only factor associated with risk of fecal incontinence following ISP. Ito reported neo-adjuvant CRT as a risk factor in ISP for poor postoperative anal function. Koyama reported no difference in average defecation frequency between LAR and ISP, no difference in urgency or differentiation between gas and stool, and no difference in the use of antidiarrheal agents or perianal erosion. Overall, bowel functional results between ISP and LAR were not statistically different (31–33).

## Transanal total mesorectal excision (TaTME)

Challenging circumstances associated with restorative rectal cancer surgery were the main drivers of development of the TaTME approach, which is quite similar to the TATA (ISP) procedure conceptually. Male gender, high body mass index, visceral obesity, bulky distal tumors, and narrow pelvic anatomy all contribute to the difficulty of minimally invasive approaches to rectal cancer when approached transabdominally. The TaTME technique was identified as a way to overcome some of these anatomic and tumor-related challenges by starting transanally and completing the pelvic aspect of the dissection from this approach, thereby eliminating the need for deep pelvic retraction for visualization necessary for laparoscopic, robotic, and open approaches. In 2014 at a consensus conference of experts in the technique, it was agreed that the TaTME approach works well for male gender, narrow or deep pelvic anatomy, low and mid-rectal cancers 12 cm or less from the anal verge that are bulky, those with prostatic hypertrophy, high BME, and visceral obesity, and those whose tumors are 1.5 cm from the dentate line or top of the anorectal ring who may require ISP/TATA. Contraindications to TaTME are obstructing rectal cancers, emergency surgery, and most T4 tumors (34).

TaTME is dependent on a combination of laparoscopic and transanal techniques to get into the appropriate mesorectal plane from a transanal approach. The patient is typically put into lithotomy position and a purse-string suture using a 1.0 or 0.0 monofilament is placed >1 cm from the gross distal margin of the tumor. Carbon dioxide ($CO_2$) is used to insufflate via a platform similar to transanal endoscopic microsurgery instrumentation. Dissection with standard laparoscopic instruments takes place first posteriorly, where dissection starts below the level of the mesorectum and follows the mesorectal plane posteriorly until visualization of the fibers of Waldeyer fascia is observed. Anterior mobilization follows taking great care to stay in the plane between the rectal wall and the prostate or vagina. Injury to anterior structures is a hazard, and careful attention to the plane of dissection, especially with anterior tumors, is paramount. Most advocate for lateral dissection last as it can be most difficult to identify the lateral planes in very distal dissections. Dissection too laterally, a common problem with perineal approaches, can result in injury to the nervi erigentes and result in urinary and sexual dysfunction. Hand-sewn or stapled anastomoses are possible depending on the level of initial dissection. The insufflation of $CO_2$ in the developing TME plane makes visualization clear and actually aids in dissection. The entire pelvic portion of the TME takes place in this manner, obviating the need for a transabdominal pelvic approach.

The main disadvantage of TaTME currently is that there is little data on the oncologic safety of the approach, although in many ways, it mimics conceptually the ISP/TATA technique that has been in use since 1994. There have been many small institutional reviews of data (more than 36 to date) which, cumulatively have resulted in over 500 evaluable patients. These data have demonstrated rates of morbidity and mortality comparable to laparoscopic TME. The positive CRM rate was 5%, and the distal margin rate was 0.3% with intact mesorectal fascia seen on 94% of specimens. The technique shows promise and has good utility in selected patients (35).

## SPLENIC FLEXURE AND LEFT COLON MOBILIZATION

Splenic flexure mobilization (SFM) in rectal cancer is used to obtain additional length, ensure a tension-free anastomosis, and preserve blood supply. The routine use of SFM for anterior or low anterior resection after obtaining an adequate surgical margin and high ligation of the IMA in both laparoscopic and open cases has been debated, with some advocating for a selective approach (36,37). Because the sigmoid colon is frequently partially in the field of neoadjuvant radiation and can be thickened, affected by diverticulitis or diverticulosis, and marginally perfused after high IMA ligation, most surgeons favor routine resection of the sigmoid colon for proctectomy involving an anastomosis. Resection of the sigmoid requires SFM in order to create a tension-free, well-vascularized anastomosis. SFM requires additional time (15–45 minutes) and may require an additional laparoscopic port in minimally invasive cases or a longer incision in open cases. Those who argue for selective mobilization point to data showing no increased anastomotic leak rate and comparable oncologic outcomes. Data on selective use of SFM are mostly case series (36,37). The technique does not lend itself to randomized testing. Although debate remains, a selective approach to SFM requires experienced intraoperative judgement, adequate assessment of the vascularity, and a tension-free anastomosis. Over 75% of low anterior resections require SFM to achieve these goals.

Mobilizing the colon to reach the pelvis requires both SFM in most cases as well as medial mobilization with ligation of the left colic artery as it comes off the IMA and ligation of the IMV at the lower border of the pancreas. The blood supply to the left colon is therefore based off the middle colic vessels, and medial mobilization that extends to the base of these vessels is often necessary to achieve this. This extensive mobilization results in "straightening" of the left colon while preserving the marginal artery and blood supply. Occasionally, in cases of reoperative surgery, or when the left colon is exceptionally short, the middle colic vessels can be ligated so that the entire blood supply to the colon is based off the ileocolic pedicle. Placing a clamp on the middle colic pedicle prior to ligation with monitoring of the marginal arterial blood flow for a few minutes is helpful to establish that flow is sufficient. Creating a window in the mesentery of the terminal ileum (ileal window) can help with extending the reach of the colon *through* rather than *over* the small bowel mesentery, thereby saving several centimeters of valuable length. As stated before, ensuring good blood supply and pulsatile flow in the marginal artery is essential. Direct observation and palpation are key, and Doppler confirmation of flow is necessary selectively in bulky mesenteries where visualization and palpation may be difficult.

## MINIMALLY INVASIVE TECHNIQUES FOR RESTORATIVE RECTAL CANCER SURGERY

Laparoscopic and robotic radical rectal resections have had a large impact on patient quality of life outcomes in the last 15 years. Decreased pain scores and length of ileus have translated into decreased length of hospital stay, improved mobility, and faster return to normal activities of daily living. Challenges to transabdominal minimally invasive techniques revolve around the difficulty presented by operating in the deep pelvis. Many studies have reported on differences between traditional open LAR versus laparoscopic or robotic techniques.

In spite of their obvious advantages, minimally invasive techniques are still on trial with regard to their oncologic outcomes. The recent randomized clinical trials ACOSOG Z6041 and ALaCarT failed to demonstrate noninferiority of laparoscopic TME over the standard open approach (38,39). The rate of CRM positivity was 7 compared to 12.1% (lap) and 3 compared to 7.7% (lap) for each trial, respectively. The results were quite consistent. Predecessor trials have also found that CRM positivity can be challenged by minimally invasive approaches with rates in some studies as high as 16%, but this has not been consistently worse than open approaches and translation into longer-term cancer-specific outcomes such as disease-specific survival and local recurrence is either not available or not significantly different.

The prospective randomized COLOR II trial reported on the differences between open versus laparoscopic LAR in patients with rectal cancer within 15 cm of the anal verge from 30 international centers (40). Local recurrence, disease-free survival, and overall survival were nearly identical between groups at 3 years. Additionally, the COREAN trial compared open versus laparoscopic LAR following neoadjuvant CRT and found that 3-year disease-free survival and overall survival were similar (41). The CLASICC trial from the UK Medical Research Council compared open versus laparoscopic resection for rectal cancer. There was no difference between groups with regard to local control, 3-year disease-free survival, or overall survival, although a subgroup analysis of the laparoscopic LAR group noted a trend toward worsened sexual function in men following laparoscopic LAR. Additionally, there was a trend toward higher positive CRMs in the minimally invasive compared to the open group (42).

Rates of conversion from a minimally invasive to open technique by experienced surgeons are in the range of 15% and seem to be lower in those employing robotic instrumentation. Better retraction and resulting improved visualization seem to favor a robotic approach for minimally invasive pelvic surgery, and ongoing laparoscopic versus robotic rectal cancer surgery trials will help define the respective roles of these technologies (43). The development of TaTME was a direct response to the challenges of transabdominal minimally invasive approaches and an attempt to improve visualization and decrease conversion rates. It is quite clear that the considerable advantages of minimally invasive surgery make it compelling, useful, and necessary. Directions for the future clearly point to development of technical advances to facilitate easier, more reliable deep pelvic dissection.

## RESERVOIR AND POUCH RECONSTRUCTION

The reservoir techniques were developed in an attempt to improve functional outcomes associated with

proctocolectomy after LAR. Reconstruction techniques following LAR are most commonly done as a straight colo-anal anastomosis (SCA) either end to end or end to side. Frequently, however, if anatomy is favorable, creation of a colonic reservoir with a colonic J-pouch (CJP) or transverse coloplasty pouch (TCP) is possible. A concern with colonic reservoir techniques is they can be technically challenging and may be associated with a higher leak rate. A meta-analysis of reconstruction techniques following LAR reported a decreased frequency in antidiarrheal medications and improved function in the first postoperative year with CJP, whereas TCP and SCA had similar functional outcomes (44). All the techniques had similar leak rates. Additionally, prospective randomized trials have demonstrated that CJP reconstruction is associated with better short-term functional outcomes (urgency and frequency), but long-term continence and overall quality of life are similar to a straight anastomosis. A CJP is typically about 5 cm in length and creates a small, bulbous reservoir just above the anastomosis. This reconstruction may not be possible in those patients with narrow pelvic anatomy or bulky, foreshortened mesenteries. Although the TCP technique helps overcome these limitations, functional outcomes have not been as promising or consistent.

## TEMPORARY DIVERSION

Temporary diversion with a proximal diverting loop ileostomy (DLI) is employed in rectal cancer surgery to decrease the rate of symptomatic anastomotic leak. Anastomotic leak following restorative LAR in a large population-based study suggested male gender, low anastomosis (<6 cm from the anal verge), preoperative radiotherapy, and adverse intraoperative events as factors that increase leak rate.

Several randomized studies have suggested that a proximal DLI may prevent anastomotic leakage and rate of reoperation. In a randomized multicenter Swedish trial, a defunctioning stoma decreased the leak rate from 28% to 10.3% in mid- and low rectal cancer patients. Moreover, this trial reported a low likelihood of stoma reversal in patients who underwent subsequent proximal diversion following anastomotic leak (45). Forty percent of these patients were reconstructed with a colonic J-pouch. This was reinforced in another study where 256 patients were randomized to diversion or none with a straight anastomotic technique and reported a significantly lower symptomatic anastomotic leak rate among patients who were defunctionalized (46). In general, diversion with a low pelvic anastomosis is recommended.

Prior to reversal of the ileostomy, a water-soluble contrast enema and visual examination of the anastomosis should be performed to rule out subclinical anastomotic leak or stricture. Assuming no leak and normal anatomy, ileostomy reversal can be scheduled for 6–12 weeks following LAR.

## FUNCTIONAL OUTCOMES

Technical and medical advances in rectal cancer treatment and surgery have improved oncological outcomes to the extent that relatively small gains in outcomes from technical advancements are expected. Therefore, posttreatment quality of life has become an increasingly important focus of emerging research in this field. Investigation of bowel and sexual functional outcomes is specific to restorative rectal cancer surgery.

## BOWEL FUNCTION

While sphincter preservation for low rectal cancers has increased dramatically, and approaches to resection and sphincter conservation are multiplying, the same basic problems plague all techniques. All result in removal of the rectal reservoir; take place in proximity to sympathetic and parasympathetic nerves affecting sexual, bowel, and urinary function; and result in a low connection that challenges continence and sensation. While patients experience a wide range of symptoms and are differentially affected, nearly all experience some disruption in normal function. Low anterior resection syndrome (LARS) describes incomplete evacuation, clustering, frequency, and stool and gas incontinence after sphincter preservation. Shorter colonic length, small or nonexistent reservoir with diminished capacity, and nerve impairment affecting sensation account for these changes. Most studies report rates of LARS in excess of 50%, but rates widely range from 10% to 74% (47). Moreover, nearly half (43%) of patients are dissatisfied with their functional outcome in the short term (48). Improvement in function does take place over time with better function evolving over the course of 24 months. Creation of a colonic J-pouch is associated with early remediation of LARS, but long-term results are similar to a straight or end-to-end anastomosis (49).

## AUTONOMIC NERVE PRESERVATION

Preservation of autonomic nerve function is important to patient overall quality of life and satisfaction. In the early 1990s, Warren Enker, a colorectal surgeon at Memorial Sloan Kettering Cancer Center, was a vocal proponent of the preservation of the autonomic nerve sympathetic fibers, which arise from T12 to L3 ventral nerve roots. He recognized the functional consequences of nerve injury and promoted active intraoperative recognition and preservation of these structures. He showed that nerve preservation and oncologic efficacy were not mutually exclusive. These sympathetic fibers join to form the superior hypogastric plexus, and distal to the aortic bifurcation give off the hypogastric nerves. Injury to these nerves can occur during ligation of the IMA or during the TME if the plane is dissected too close to the sacrum. Injury to the sympathetic fibers can result in increased bladder tone, decreased capacity, and retrograde ejaculation. Parasympathetic nerve fibers from S2 to S4 ventral roots join the hypogastric nerves on the pelvic sidewall and form the inferior hypogastric plexus. Injury to the parasympathetic plexus can result from traction in the deep pelvis or encroachment on the deep lateral pelvic sidewalls. Parasympathetic fiber injury can result in urinary retention from increased bladder neck tone. Additionally, parasympathetic fiber injury can result in erectile dysfunction in men and impaired vaginal lubrication in women.

## SEXUAL FUNCTION

Following rectal cancer surgery and chemoradiation for advanced tumors, sexual function can be significantly altered. Current literature suggests that APR, low rectal cancers, and the use of radiation are risk factors associated with sexual dysfunction (48,49). Typically, men and elderly patients are more likely to report postoperative sexual problems. There are several possible causes of sexual impairment following rectal cancer surgery, but intraoperative injury to the autonomic plexus is the most important factor, as previously described.

Laparoscopy may be associated with increased sexual dysfunction in men. Jayne reported similar bladder function following laparoscopic versus open rectal cancer operations, with overall sexual function and erectile function worse in men following laparoscopic surgery compared to an open approach (50). This is contrary to findings by others who reported a lower incidence of erectile and bladder dysfunction in patients who undergo laparoscopic TME. Theoretically, increased exposure, illumination, and magnification can help facilitate the identification and preservation of the pelvic autonomic nerves (51). Better data are needed specifically examining functional outcomes and reported rates of intraoperative autonomic nerve identification. Intraoperative nerve identification and preservation have been proposed as an intraoperative quality metric for rectal cancer surgery by the American Society of Colon and Rectal Surgeons Quality Committee (52,53). The recognition of nerve and sphincter preservation as markers of quality surgery is a step forward for patients suffering from rectal cancer and its effects.

## REFERENCES

1. Lange M et al. *Eur J Surg Oncol* 2009;35(5):456–63.
2. Corman M. *Dis Colon Rectum* 2000;43(Supp 6): S1–29.
3. Dixon CF. *Ann Surg* 1948;128(3):425–42.
4. Abdelsattar ZM et al. *Ann Surg Oncol* 2014;21(13): 4075–80.
5. Temple LK et al. *Ann Surg* 2009;250(2):260–7.
6. Goligher JC et al. *Br J Surg.* 1951;39(155):199–211.
7. Ludwig KA. Sphincter sparing resection for rectal cancer. *Clin Colon Rectal Surg* 2007;20(3):203–212.

8. Bordeianou L et al. *J Gastrointest Surg* 2014;18: 1358–72.
9. Pollett WG, Nicholls RJ. *Ann Surg* 1983;198(2): 159–63.
10. Bujko K et al. *Ann Surg Oncol* 2012;19(3):801–8.
11. Quirke P et al. *Lancet* 1986;2(8514):996–9.
12. Guillem J. et al. *Ann Surg* 2007;245(1):88–93.
13. Nagtegaal I et al. *Am J Surg Pathol* 2002;26(3):350–7.
14. Wibe A et al. *British J Surg* 2002;89(3):327–33.
15. Kapiteijn E. et al. *N Engl J Med* 2001;345(9):638–46.
16. Ravitch M, Steichen F. *Ann Surg* 1972;175(6):815–37.
17. Fain S. *Arch Surg* 1975;110(9):1079.
18. Cedermark B et al. *N Engl J Med* 1997;336(14):980–7.
19. Francois Y et al. *J Clin. Oncol* 1999;7(8):2396.
20. Minsky BD et al. *Int J Radiat Oncol Biol Phys* 1997; 37(2):289–95.
21. Frykholm G et al. *Dis Colon Rectum* 1993;36(6): 564–72.
22. Trakarnsanga A et al. *J Natl Cancer Inst* 2014;106(10): [Abstract].
23. Sauer R et al. *N Engl J Med* 2004;351(17):1731–40.
24. Gerard JP et al. *Crit Rev Oncol Hematol* 2012;81(1): 21–8.
25. Bujko K et al. *Radiother Oncol* 2006;80(1):4–12.
26. Baker B et al. *Surg Oncol* 2012;21(3):103–9.
27. Smallwood N, Fleshman J. *Clin Colon Rectal Surg* 2015;28:5–11.
28. Heald R et al. *Br J Surg* 1982;69(10):613–16.
29. Heald RJ, Ryall RD. *Lancet* 1986;1(8496):1479–82.
30. Ho VP et al. *Dis Colon Rectum* 2011;54(1):113–25.
31. Schiessel R et al. *Br J Surg* 1994;81(9):1376–8.
32. Kuo LJ et al. *J Surg Res* 2013;183(2):524–30.
33. Schiessel R et al., Feil W, Urban M. *Dis Colon Rectum* 2005;48(10):1856–65.
34. Motson RW et al. *Colorectal Dis* 2016;18:13–8.
35. Penna M et al. *Clin Colon Rectal Surg* 2017;30(5): 339–45.
36. Park J et al. *Surg Laparosc Endosc Percutan Tech* 2009;19(1):62–8.
37. Marsden M et al. *Colorect Dis* 2012;14(10):1255–61.
38. Fleshman J et al. *The ACOSOG Z6051 Randomized Clinical Trial* 2015;314(13):1346–55.
39. Stevenson AR et al. ALaCaRT investigators. *JAMA* 2015;314(13):1356–63.
40. Van der Pas MH et al. Colorectal cancer Laparoscopic or Open Resection II (COLOR II) Study Group. *Lancet Oncol* 2013;14(03):210–8.
41. Jeong SY et al. *Lancet Oncol* 2014;15(7):767–74.
42. Jayne DG et al. *J Clin Oncol* 2007;25(21):3061–8.
43. Jayne D et al. *JAMA* 2017;318(16):1569–80.
44. Brown CJ et al. *Cochrane Database Syst Rev* 2008;(2).
45. Matthiessen P et al. *Ann Surg* 2007;246(2):207–14.
46. Chude GG et al. *Hepatogastroenterology* 2008; 55(8687):1562–7.
47. Bryant CL et al. *Lancet Oncol* 2012;13(9):e403–8.
48. Lundby L et al. *Dis Colon Rectum* 2005;48(7):1343–9.
49. Fish D, Temple LK. *Surg Oncol Clin N Am* 2014;23(1): 127–49.
50. Jayne DG et al. *Br J Surg* 2005;92(9):1124–32.
51. Wallner C et al. *J Clin Oncol.* 2008;26(27):4466–72.
52. Manwaring ML et al. *Dis Colon Rectum.* 2012;55(3): 294–301.
53. Glasgow SC et al. *Dis Colon Rectum* 2016;59(7): 601–6.

# 28

# Transanal approaches to rectal cancer

CHARLES B. WHITLOW AND LARA MCKEAN BASTÉ

## CHALLENGING CASE

A 64 year-old moderately obese man is found to have a 1 cm moderately differentiated adenocarcinoma of the rectum approximately 9 cm above the anal verge. Intra-anal ultrasound and MRI stages the lesion as T1N0.

## CASE MANAGEMENT

After presentation at a multidisciplinary tumor conference, surgical options are discussed with the patient, eg. Low anterior resection or Transanal minimally invasive surgery (TAMIS). The patient selected a TAMIS.

## INTRODUCTION

Rectal cancer is diagnosed in roughly 39,000 patients every year in the United States. The management of rectal cancer is multidisciplinary, but surgical resection is still the mainstay of treatment. The incidence of early colorectal cancers has increased in the past years as a result of the expansion of advanced endoscopic techniques and the widespread use of colorectal screening. Standard of treatment of rectal cancer involves major radical abdominal surgery including total mesorectal excision (TME) to treat locally advance or node-positive rectal cancer. This technique achieves removal of the primary tumor and the mesorectum with the associated regional lymph nodes. It has demonstrated excellent long-term results that approach 4.5% local recurrence rates at 5 years and 90% 5-year disease-free survival rates (1). However, proctectomy is associated with significant morbidity, mortality, and impact on quality of life from complications such as anastomotic leak, wound infection

or dehiscence, genitourinary dysfunction, low anterior resection syndrome, and need for temporary or permanent ostomy.

The significant morbidity resulting from proctectomy makes less invasive and less morbid treatment attractive. In order to be an acceptable option as a treatment for cure, the oncologic outcomes of any treatment and salvage after failure should be similar to the outcomes of initial proctectomy. In addition to treatment for cure, these less morbid procedures have found a place in the treatment of patients who are poor candidates for proctectomy because of comorbidities or metastatic disease. Transanal fulguration, endocavitary radiation, transsacral and transsphincteric surgical approaches have been described, but local excision (LE) by one of several techniques has been the most widely accepted. Standard transanal excision (TAE), transanal endoscopic microsurgery (TEM), transanal minimally invasive surgery (TAMIS), and more recently endoscopic submucosal dissection (ESD) all have been used to treat rectal cancer with acceptable morbidity and mortality.

Several organizations have published statements on the appropriateness of LE. National Comprehensive Cancer Network (NCCN) guidelines for rectal cancer recommend observation for patients who, after appropriate pretreatment staging, undergo LE and on pathology are found to have T1NX adenocarcinoma without high-risk features (positive margins, lymphovascular invasion, poor differentiation, and sm3 invasion) (2). The Practice Parameters for the American Society of Colon and Rectal Surgeons (ASCRS) state that "local excision is an appropriate treatment modality for carefully selected T1 rectal cancers without high-risk features" (well to moderately differentiated, no lymphovascular invasion, no perineural invasions, less than 3 cm diameter, and less than one-third rectal luminal circumference) (3). The European Association for Endoscopic Surgery (EAES) published a consensus statement on this topic. This statement describes LE as a "valid treatment option for early rectal cancer" which should be offered for T1N0 cancers with favorable features. Depth of invasion beyond sm1 was considered unfavorable. LE alone for any lesions outside of the described criteria "should be considered only as a compromise procedure" (4).

Though the guidelines discussed previously describe narrow selection criteria and the literature as a whole advises caution in local excision except for superficial lesions without risk factors, the use of local excision in the United States has continued to increase. Data from the National Cancer Data Base (NCDB) from 1998 to 2010 reported 46.5% of T1 and 16.8% of T2 rectal cancers were treated by LE (5). The increase in the use of LE from 1998 to 2010 was dramatic, with an increase of 40%–62% for T1 tumors and 12%–24% for T2 tumors.

## INITIAL EVALUATION

Patients with rectal cancer come to surgical evaluation via several avenues, the most common being a mass biopsied or excised as part of a complete colonoscopy or a mass detected on rectal exam or imaging study. A histologic diagnosis of a cancer is mandatory prior to initiation of neoadjuvant treatment or radical excision. A complete colonoscopy should be performed if not previously done. The surgeon who will be making the recommendations for surgical treatment should perform a physical exam to include proctosigmoidoscopy and digital rectal exam to assess tumor location, size, mobility, relation to levators, and anal sphincter function. Absence of induration and ulceration on exam suggest there is no invasive component, and lack of fixation indicates a superficial tumor.

Local staging of the tumor can be accomplished with endorectal ultrasound (EUS) or magnetic resonance imaging (MRI). While both of these modalities assess T stage, EUS appears to be better for superficial tumors, and MRI is superior for deeper ones. A recognized limitation of EUS is for very distal tumors where the ability to get an acceptable image is compromised by anatomic features. Both MRI and EUS have a lack of specificity and sensitivity for detecting metastases to lymph nodes. Local availability and expertise dictate which imaging technique is preferred or they may be used as complementary exams. Additional or alternative assessment of tumor depth can be acquired by examining tumor morphology and using enhanced endoscopic techniques (such as magnifying chromoendoscopy) to examine mucosal pit patterns.

Computed tomography (CT) is less accurate than EUS or MRI for local staging. However, it is the most common imaging modality for staging of distant metastases. CT of the chest, abdomen, and pelvis is routinely performed as part of complete staging. The exams of the chest and abdomen give information not included in the pelvic MRI. The pelvic CT exam is complementary to other pelvic imaging. Positron emission tomography is not indicated in routine initial staging.

In addition to tumor staging, individual patient factors, such as comorbidities and sphincter function, impact the decision-making for local excision. Patients with an unacceptably high risk for morbidity and mortality from proctectomy may elect local excision for palliation or prevention of symptoms with the understanding that local recurrence may require additional treatment. Patients who are being considered for local excision with curative intent should be counseled thoroughly on the risk, benefits, and alternatives to this treatment. Because the choice between local excision and radial resection frequently represents a choice between quality of oncologic treatment versus quality of life, the value the patient places on these factors is an important part of the decision. Additionally, adjuvant treatment, surveillance strategies, and possible salvage treatment require a commitment from the patient. This is a lengthy and complicated discussion that challenges the surgeon to present the salient data in an understandable form. The ensuing paragraphs deal with many of these issues.

## LOCAL RECURRENCE AND SURVIVAL

Recurrence after local excision has been attributed to several factors: imprecise preoperative staging, incomplete excision, tumor factors, and failure to treat regional/systemic disease (especially mesosrectal lymph node metastases) at time of presentation. The presence of lymph node metastases (LNM) increases with tumor depth of invasion. T1 rectal cancers as a whole have a LMN incidence of approximately 10%–13%, and for T2 rectal cancers the incidence is 17%–23% (6). The depth of invasion in the submucosa can be further used to predict the risk of LNM. While subjective terms such as "scant" or "slight" invasion have been used, more objective descriptions of the amount of submucosal invasion are preferred. However, there has not been uniform reporting of this data that has been published by the sm1, sm2, sm3 categorization or by absolute depth of invasion. The absolute depth of invasion is typically reported in microns, but the depth that correlates to lower risk of LNM has been variously reported as <500, <1,000, <1,500, or <2,000 (7). When depth alone is considered, superficial T1 tumors are associated with a risk of LNM of 3% or lower.

Other histopathologic tumor features associated with LNM include poor differentiation, lymphovascular or perineural invasion, and tumor budding. Location in the distal third of the rectum is an independent risk factor for LNM. Because tumors may be heterogenous, biopsy alone may not demonstrate the presence of adverse features that are found on examination of a complete excised tumor. Glasgow et al. performed a meta-analysis of histopathological features of primary colorectal cancers that predict lymph node metastases. In looking at rectal cancers specifically, they reported that tumor stage, tumor differentiation, vascular invasion, lymphatic invasion, and differentiation at the invasive front were statistically significant predictors of lymph node metastases (8).

Most of the data on LE alone for treatment of rectal cancer are from standard transanal excision, and no prospective randomized data exist on this topic. The data for LE of T1 cancers from retrospective single institution studies show 5-year local recurrence (LR) rates ranging from 13% to 18% and overall survival (OS) rates at 5 years range from 72% to 89%. Both ranges are lower than comparisons to standard resection—0%–3% and 80%–96%, respectively. Similarly, several large registries have reported 5-year LR rates of 7%–12% and 5-year OS of 70%–87%. LE alone for T2 cancers has a LR rate of 20%–30% with OS of 63%–75% (9–11).

Radical surgery performed immediately after finding adverse pathologic features by LE results in outcomes similar to initial radical resection. However, the results of radical surgery as a salvage procedure have not been as good as radical surgery as initial treatment. Median time to recurrence varies from 11 to 35 months. While most recurrences are identified within the first 36 months, recurrence after that is reported and highlights the need for prolonged surveillance. Microscopically clear margins (R0) are obtained in 82%–94% of salvage resections, although Madbouly reported that only 40% of patients underwent surgery for curative intent (12). Weiser et al. reported 55% of their radical salvage procedures required extended dissections compared to standard resections, but pelvic exenteration has only been necessary in 7%–8% of cases (13). 5-year OS rates of 53%–62% are reported. Stipa et al. reported 144 patients with rectal cancer initially treated by TEM of which 86 were T1, 38 were T2, and 20 were T3 (14). Twenty-four of 26 recurrences were endoluminal.

## TECHNICAL

## PREOPERATIVE PREPARATION

The preoperative evaluation of patients undergoing LE for rectal cancer involves the standard assessment of comorbidities as any other major surgical procedure. Additionally, a precise description of the location of the tumor should be written in the preoperative note, as well as an assessment of anal sphincter function, invasion into adjacent structures, and relationship to the anterior peritoneal reflection. It is the authors' preference to have patients complete a full mechanical bowel prep and oral antibiotic prep on the day prior to surgery. Standard preoperative IV antibiotics for bowel surgery and appropriate venous thromboembolism prophylaxis are given immediately prior to beginning the procedure.

## TRANSANAL EXCISION

While this procedure is commonly performed under general endotracheal anesthesia, TAE can be accomplished under local anesthetic with monitored anesthesia care. Positioning is based on individual surgeon preference. Most lesions can be addressed from prone jackknife, lateral, or lithotomy. Some surgeons prefer to have all patients

consistently in the same position regardless of the positional orientation of the lesion, while others prefer to position the patient so that the lesion is in the dependent position. For extremely distal tumors, standard lighted half-cylinder anoscopes (e.g., Hill-Ferguson) provide adequate exposure. Removal of larger and more proximal tumors is facilitated by placement of a Lone Star retractor with the hooks placed in the anal canal at the level of the dentate line. Additional exposure is obtained with plastic cylindrical Ferguson anoscopes, which are available in a variety of lengths and diameters. The mucosa is scored with electrocautery to outline the extent of the excision with a 1 cm margin of grossly normal mucosa. In general, cancers should be removed with a full-thickness excision of the rectal wall using electrocautery, ultrasonic shears, or bipolar vessel sealers. Hemostasis is obtained and then full-thickness wounds are typically closed in a transverse manner using an absorbable suture. The authors' preference is to use a running barbed suture with a loop at the tail end and a clip at the other, obviating the need for knot tying. While closure can be performed via a plastic Ferguson anoscopy, switching to a Hill-Ferguson anoscope is sometimes helpful in the distal rectum. Stenosis of the rectal lumen should be assessed by anoscopy, proctoscopy, or digital exam. If the distal edge of the tumor is more than 1 cm from the dentate line, no local anesthetic is needed. For lower lesions, bupivacaine (liposomal or plain) is infiltrated to perform a complete anal block. No packing is needed. Patients are observed overnight for evidence of bleeding or fever. Antibiotics are not given beyond the initial perioperative dose except in the case of fever on the night of surgery. Patients are allowed liquids immediately after surgery and advanced to a regular diet as tolerated.

Complications after TAE are uncommon but include immediate and delayed bleeding, pain, abscess, disturbances of continence, and on rare occasion perineal sepsis. Abscesses are treated by opening the rectal wall suture line, and perineal sepsis is treated with antibiotics or incision, drainage, and debridement if indicated.

## TRANSANAL ENDOSCOPIC MICROSURGERY AND TRANSANAL MINIMALLY INVASIVE SURGERY

Both TEM and TAMIS use endorectal carbon dioxide ($CO_2$) insufflation and an occluding transanally placed platform to allow access to the rectum. TEM was first described by Buess in 1984 (15). A 40 mm metal operating rectoscope is secured to the table via a mechanical adjustable mount. A detachable faceplate acts as the working attachment and an insufflation port, a channel for a standard laparoscope (or stereoscopic telescope), and two 5 mm channels for instruments. Proprietary instrumentation for grasping, cautery, and suturing is available for the commercially available TEM devices.

TAMIS differs in that a single access port is used, which does not require attachment to the operative table. Some authors recommend that all such procedures be performed in the lithotomy position and in slight Trendelenburg position (16,17). The commonly available ports for TAMIS are the GelPOINT Path (Applied Medical, Rancho Santa Margarita, California) and the SILS Port (Covidien, Mansfield, Massachusetts). Standard laparoscopes and laparoscopic instrumentation including alternative energy sources are used through the working channels.

Two technical notes are of use in TEM and TAMIS with regard to optimal visualization. First, neuromuscular blockade of the patient is critical to maintaining adequate pneumorectum. Second, an insufflation system that produces constant intrarectal pressure avoids the bellows effect encountered with standard insufflators used in laparoscopy, for example, SurgiQuest AirSeal (ConMed, Utica, New York).

Regardless of the platform used, the technique of excision is the same. Typically the mucosa is scored with cautery to outline the extent of the excision. An epinephrine-containing solution can be injected into the submucosal plane if a mucosal resection is being performed but is not necessary for full-thickness excision. Traction is placed in a manner that facilitates perpendicular dissection for the initial portion of dissection as a full-thickness incision is made using electrocautery. This incision can be extended partially or completely around the circumference of the lesion, but care should be taken to avoid "coning" and thus decreasing the margin on the deeper portion of the lesion. Mesorectal fat is encountered in full-thickness excisions and is the visual cue to begin excision in a plane parallel to the rectal wall. This can be done with monopolar electrocautery A bipolar sealing device or ultrasonic shears are sometimes used, as this part of the dissection can produce substantial hemorrhage. After complete excision, the lesion should be pinned to avoid contraction during fixation. Hemostasis should be obtained. As with TAE, it is not necessary to close extraperitoneal defects; however, many surgeons choose to do so. A variety of laparoscopic closure devices have been used including Endostitch (Covidien, Norwalk, Connecticut) and RD-180/ TK Knot Device (LSI Solutions, Victor, New York). Suturing with laparoscopic needle drivers is technically more challenging with TEM as opposed to TAMIS, especially with knot tying. The use of barbed suture with a looped tail is particularly useful in this setting. Alternatively, a suture fixation device such as silver beads or Lapra-Ty (Ethicon, Cincinnati, Ohio) can be used. If standard laparoscopic suturing is done, a knot pusher may be useful. More distal defects can frequently be approached using the transanal "open" approach. Again, the lumen should be inspected after closure to check for stenosis. The senior author has experienced clinically significant stenosis with large defects that were closed or left open. The postoperative care after TEM or TAMIS is similar to TAE.

While these techniques allow for removal of proximal rectal or rectosigmoid lesions, there is at least a theoretical concern about tumor spread with a full-thickness intraperitoneal injury and ongoing exposure to $CO_2$ insufflation. Peritoneal entry mandates complete defect closure. If this cannot be accomplished transanally, laparoscopy or laparotomy should be performed and adequate bowel closure completed.

## COMPLICATIONS

Postoperative bleeding (up to 9%), urinary retention, or urinary tract infection (up to 11%) are the most common postoperative complications (18). Fecal incontinence is infrequent and typically temporary. Abscess may occur with defects that are closed. If abscess develops in this situation, the suture line should be opened to obtain adequate drainage. Perineal sepsis has been reported in up to 3% of patients and is associated with lesions within 2 cm of the dentate line. The senior author has seen two such cases. Both of these occurred in elderly infirm patients with tumors that extended distally to the proximal anal canal. Because of this location, the distal dissection was performed by TAE and the proximal resection with TAMIS. In one case the wound was left open, and in the other it was closed. Because the dissection in the distal portion of the rectum and anal canal is below the mesorectal fat, full-thickness closure is recommended in this location.

## COMPARISON OF TECHNIQUES

A meta-analysis demonstrated similar complication rates between TAE and TEM (16). Additionally, tumors removed by TEM were more likely to have negative microscopic margins and less likely to undergo fragmentation during removal. These factors may result in lower local recurrence with TEM. The largest TAMIS experience to date reported on 200 patients for benign and malignant lesions. The positive margin rate was 7%, and fragmentation occurred in 5%. Overall morbidity was 11% with urinary retention, hemorrhage, and subcutaneous/scrotal emphysema being the most common complications (19).

## ADJUVANT TREATMENT

Data on adjuvant radiation therapy +/− chemotherapy (typically radiosensitizing 5-FU) is retrospective commonly from small series. A meta-analysis that included 14 studies showed weighted local recurrence rates of 10% for T1 tumors and 15% of T2 tumors treated with chemoradiation after LE (20). The recurrence rates for tumors treated by TEM after LE were 6% for T1 cancers and 10% for T2 lesions. Pooled survival data were not reported, but the 5-year disease-free survival was 75%–100% for patients receiving adjuvant radiation (six studies). For patients treated with TEM, two studies reported 5-year and 10-year disease-free survival of 94% and 86%, respectively. Rackley et al. reported on 93 patients who received adjuvant radiation following LE. They found T1 cancers had a 5-year overall survival of 84% and 5-year local control of 92.5% (21).

## ENDOSCOPIC TREATMENT

Endoscopic treatment of rectal adenocarcinomas is being reported with greater frequency. Endoscopic mucosal resection (saline lift polypectomy) results in a higher proportion of piecemeal resections than any of the surgical excision techniques or endoscopic submucosal dissection. The technique of submucosal dissection involves using a needle knife to incise circumferentially around the lesion. Several techniques are used to achieve mucosal lift, including the use of a hybrid needle knife with cautering and cutting capability combined with an injection port (Erbejet 2, Erbe Elekromedizin GmbH, Tübingen, Germany). An increasing number of tools are available to accomplish the actual dissection in the submucosal plain. Typically, the procedure is performed using a plastic cap on the end of the scope that facilitates visualization and dissection. One meta-analysis showed a lower recurrence rate for benign rectal lesions removed by TEM versus those removed by ESD (22). This comparison showed no differences in en bloc resections, R0 resections, and complications. Several authors have commented on the technical challenges of ESD in the distal rectum and proximal anal canal. The ESD rectal cancer literature is immature, and there are many case reports describing excision, recurrences, and complications that are already well described in the surgical literature. It is inevitable that ESD for rectal cancer will be used more frequently. The advent of new instrumentation may make it technically easier than the current version. There is no reason to expect the complications related to this approach should be any more common or severe than surgical techniques. Those who use this technique should have a thorough understanding of the nuances of the management of superficial rectal cancers as has been outlined above.

## LOCAL EXCISION AFTER CHEMORADIATION

A complete discussion of this topic is beyond the scope of this chapter. However, there has been interest in full-thickness rectal wall excision following a complete clinical response to neoadjuvant chemoradiation. The rationale for this is that residual tumor in the rectum is a source of potential local recurrence. Two systematic reviews have been published. Hallam et al. identified 20 studies, which encompassed 1,068 patients (23). They reported a local recurrence rate of 4% and a median disease-free survival of 95% for patients with ypT0 tumors. ypT1 and higher tumors had a local recurrence rate of 21.9% and a 68% median disease-free survival. The pooled complication incidence was 23.2%. Smith et al. reported data from 25 studies with 1,001 patients (24). Their main conclusions were the significant variability they identified with regard to many important technical issues including pathologic assessment, appropriate staging, and pretreatment marking. They noted substantial morbidity from TAE in the radiated rectum including abscess, fistulas, and severe pain. Additionally, subsequent radical salvage surgery for local recurrence after local excision is technically challenging because the planes of dissection have been violated. Additionally, the practice of watch and wait for complete clinical responders would seem to question the value of the practice of LE after radiation. The conclusions from this report were that if this practice is going to continue, additional study is warranted along with standardization.

## REFERENCES

1. Mellgren A et al. *Dis Colon Rectum* 2000;43: 1064–71.
2. National Comprehensive Cancer Network. Rectal Cancer (Version 3.2017). https://www.nccn.org/ professional_gls/pdf/rectal.pdf. Accessed March 25, 2017.
3. Monson JRT et al. *Dis Colon Rectum* 2013;56:535–50.
4. Morino M et al. *Surg Endosc* 2015;29:755–73.
5. Stitzenberg KB et al. *J Clin Onc* 2013;31:4276–82.
6. Ricciardi R et al. *Clin Gastroenterol Hepatol* 2006;4: 1522–7.
7. Maeda K et al. *Surg Today* 2014;44:2000–14.
8. Glasgow SC et al. *J Gastrointest Surg* 2012;16: 1019–28.
9. You NY. *Semin Radiat Oncol* 2011;21:178–84.
10. Althumairi AA, Gearhart SL. *J Gastrointest Oncol* 2015;6:296–306.
11. Heafner TA, Glasgow SC. *J Gastrointest Oncol* 2014; 5:345–52.
12. Madbouly KM et al. *Dis Colon Rectum* 2005;48: 711–21.
13. Weiser MR et al. *Dis Colon Rectum* 2005;48:1169–75.
14. Stipa F, Giaccaglia V. *Dis Colon Rectum* 2012;55: 262–9.
15. Buess G et al. *Chirurg* 1984;55:677–80.
16. deBech-Adams T, Nassif G. *Clin Colon Rectal Surg* 2015;28:176–80.
17. Gill S et al. *J Gastrointest Surg* 2015;19:1528–36.
18. Lee L et al. *Ann Surg* 2017;267(5):1.
19. Clancy C et al. *Dis Colon Rectum* 2015;58:254–61.
20. Borstlap WAA et al. *Br J Surg.* 2016;103(9):1105–16.
21. Rackley TP et al. *Dis Colon Rectum* 2016;59:173–8.
22. Arezzo A et al. *Surg Endosc* 2014;28:427–38.
23. Hallam S et al. *Dis Colon Rectum* 2016;59:984–97.
24. Smith FM et al. *Dis Colon Rectum* 2017;60:228–39.

# 29

# Abdominoperineal resection

W. BRIAN PERRY AND HUISAR DAO CAMPI

## CHALLENGING CASE

A 64-year-old woman is 7 days after an abdomino-perineal resection for a T2N1 rectal adenocarcinoma. She had received preoperative care. Her perineal wound has developed increased tenderness, is swollen, and is draining pus.

## CASE MANAGEMENT

The patient's wound is opened and the patient is started on three times a day dressing changes. After 2 days the wound is clean and a VAC dressing is placed.

## INTRODUCTION

Abdominoperineal resection (APR) completely removes the distal colon, rectum, and anal sphincter complex using both anterior abdominal and perineal incisions, resulting in a permanent colostomy. Developed more than 100 years ago, it remains an important tool in the treatment of rectal cancer despite advances in sphincter-sparing procedures. Recent reports have noted an increase in the use of sphincter-sparing options for patients diagnosed with rectal cancer. Abraham and colleagues found a 10% decrease (60.1%–49.9%) in the rate of APR from 1989 to 2001 as compared with low anterior resection (LAR) using national administrative data (1). When controlled for several variables, including patient demographics and hospital volume, patients were 28% more likely to have an LAR later in the study period. Schoetz notes that LAR outnumbers APR three to one in the submitted case logs of recent colorectal fellows (2). This ratio is similar to that found in the Swedish rectal cancer registry, where approximately 25% of over 12,000 patients with rectal cancer underwent APR from 1995 to 2002 (3). In no study or registry, however, has APR been eliminated.

## HISTORY

Early in the twentieth century, most patients with rectal cancer underwent palliative perineal procedures to address advanced disease. These included the transcoccygeal Kraske approach and the transsphincteric approach developed by Bevan in America, later attributed to A. York Mason. Patients were often left with profound sphincter dysfunction or fistulae following a protracted recovery. A two-staged operation, consisting of an initial laparotomy and colostomy followed by perineal excision, was used until the 1930s with reasonable results.

In 1908 Miles first described the operation we now know as APR, but initial reports showed a high operative mortality, up to 42%. Refinements in technique were made through the first half of the twentieth century. Gabriel described a one-stage operation with the abdominal portion done supine and the perineal portion done in the left lateral position. Lloyd-Davies' synchronous approach to the abdomen and perineum with the patient in the lithotomy position eliminated the cumbersome and sometimes dangerous need to reposition the patient while under anesthesia (4). Recent advances include total mesorectal excision and methods to enhance perineal wound healing, especially in patients who have received neoadjuvant chemoradiation. Minimally invasive techniques are also being applied to APR, with good results.

## PATIENT PREPARATION AND POSITIONING

Preparation for abdominoperineal resection starts with marking the ideal placement of the colostomy by the primary surgeon or enterostomal nurse (5). Patients take a mechanical bowel preparation the day before surgery, typically polyethylene glycol. Placement of an epidural catheter may be considered to improve postoperative analgesia and to reduce postoperative ileus (6). Prior to induction of general anesthesia,

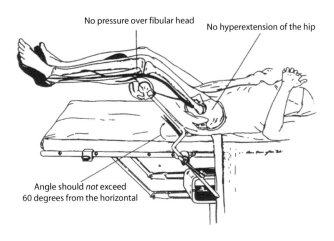

No pressure over fibular head

No hyperextension of the hip

Angle should *not* exceed
60 degrees from the horizontal

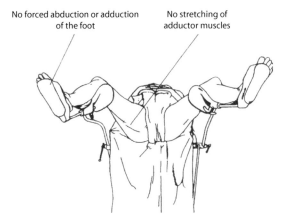

No forced abduction or adduction
of the foot

No stretching of
adductor muscles

Figure 29.1 Leg positioning for abdominoperineal resection.

intermittent pneumatic compression devices are placed on the lower extremities to reduce the risk of venous thromboembolism (7). IV antibiotics with efficacy against enteric flora administered 60 minutes before incision decrease the rate of surgical site infection (8). The abdomen and perineum are prepped, and appropriate monitoring is placed.

After induction of anesthesia, a urinary catheter is inserted; ureteral stents should be considered if the patient has had prior pelvic surgery, tumor extension into the urinary tract, or prior pelvic radiation. The patient is placed in the lithotomy position with symmetric hip extension, knee flexion, and thigh abduction using Allen stirrups with padding to prevent lower limb acute compartment syndrome (9) (Figure 29.1). A rectal exam is performed under anesthesia followed by irrigation with dilute betadine solution to remove any residual stool.

## OPEN ABDOMINAL OPERATIVE TECHNIQUE

The operative technique used today varies little from Ernest Miles' description in 1908 (10). Unlike Miles' method, we prefer the two-team approach with the patient in lithotomy position rather than lateral semiprone position. A nonabsorbable purse-string suture is placed around the anus. The abdomen and perineum are prepared with antiseptic solution and draped with openings to allow synchronous dissection. The abdomen and pelvis are accessed through a midline hypogastric incision that extends to the right of or through the umbilicus. The abdomen is explored for metastatic disease and synchronous colon lesions. After confirmation of resectability, a self-retaining retractor is placed.

The small bowel is packed into the upper abdomen with a moist towel. The sigmoid and descending colon is mobilized from the retroperitoneum in the left lateral paracolic gutter. The left ureter is identified and preserved, and the descending colon is adequately mobilized for creation of an end colostomy. The peritoneal incision is carried anteriorly followed by incision of the right lateral peritoneum. The right ureter is identified and preserved, and the peritoneal incisions are connected anteriorly at the base of the bladder. For convenience, the proximal sigmoid can be divided with a linear stapling device and the cut end used as a handle to aid with the dissection. A finger is passed below the inferior mesenteric vessels preserving the sigmoid branches, minimizing vascular compromise of the stoma. It is unnecessary to ligate the inferior mesenteric artery at its origin as this has not been shown to increase survival (11).

The superior hemorrhoidal vessels are transected. The presacral space is entered with preservation of the investing mesorectal fascia consistent with Heald's description of total mesorectal excision (12). A lighted St. Mark's retractor holding the mesorectum anteriorly helps identify the avascular plane of dissection. As the dissection continues distally, Waldeyer fascia is divided sharply to avoid injuring the presacral venous plexus minimizing bleeding.

The lateral ligaments are divided close to the pelvic side wall to maximize the radial margins. Denonvilliers fascia in males is dissected down to the pelvic floor anteriorly. Unless the tumor is anterior, it is not necessary to expose the seminal vesicles thus avoiding injury to the nervi erigentes. In females, the presence of an anteriorly based tumor may require a posterior vaginectomy. When the pelvic floor is reached circumferentially around the rectum, the abdominal portion of the dissection is completed, a colostomy is created, and the abdomen is closed.

## LAPAROSCOPIC ABDOMINAL OPERATIVE TECHNIQUE

The indications for laparoscopic APR are the same as for the open technique; it is employed in distal rectal or anal malignancies with sphincter invasion or in those patients in whom an acceptable functional result cannot be achieved by the use of sphincter-sparing surgical techniques.

The use of laparoscopy to treat patients with colon cancer has increased significantly since the publication of the COST trial (13,14). Data analyzing the outcomes of those patients undergoing laparoscopic surgery for rectal cancer are less clear with regard to long-term oncologic outcomes, and its adoption has been slower among surgeons. A recent publication by Fleshman et al. states that laparoscopic resection of patients with stages II–III rectal cancer failed to meet their set criteria for noninferiority pathologic outcomes when compared to the open technique (15). Other trials, with longer patient follow-up, state that oncologic outcomes are similar between laparoscopic and open surgical techniques (16,17).

The operation starts by entering the abdomen under direct vision in the supraumbilical area; three additional ports are placed, a 12 mm port in the right lower quadrant, a 5 mm port in the right upper quadrant, and a 5 mm port in the left lower quadrant. The dissection follows a standard medial to lateral technique. The peritoneum at the level of the sacral promontory is incised, and the dissection continues medially, identifying the ureter, gonadal, and iliac vessels. The IMA is identified, and ligation is performed distal to the takeoff of the left colic artery, this step can be achieved by the use of either an endoscopic stapler or a vessel-sealing device. High ligation of the IMV and full mobilization of the splenic flexure is seldom needed in these patients. After the medial dissection has been completed, the lateral peritoneal attachments of the colon are incised completing full colonic mobilization. The sigmoid colon is then transected with the aid of an endoscopic stapler.

Pelvic dissection is started by entering the presacral space with great care not to violate the endopelvic fascia and preserving an intact mesorectum. Dissection is carried posteriorly to the level of the levator ani complex. Once this has been achieved, the lateral ligaments are mobilized as close to the pelvic side wall as possible to maximize the radial margin. Last, anterior mobilization is performed by entering the anterior areolar plane and carrying the dissection down to the pelvic floor. Once this step is achieved, the abdominal portion of the operation is concluded, a colostomy is created, the abdomen is closed, and the perineal dissection commences.

## ROBOTIC ABDOMINAL OPERATIVE TECHNIQUE

Since the introduction of robotic-assisted surgery, this technology has been increasingly applied to the specialty of colon and rectal surgery. The advantages of using the robotic platform for rectal operations are improved ergonomics for the surgeon, excellent three-dimensional deep pelvic visualization, and articulated instruments that allow for an improved freedom of movement in a small space, as it is the deep pelvis (18). From an oncological standpoint, robotic-assisted operations appear to have similar oncologic outcomes, in terms of circumferential margins and lymph node harvest, as open or laparoscopic operations (19). The

disadvantages tied to the use of robotic platforms include loss of haptic feedback, increased costs, and increased operative time.

Robotic-assisted APR follows the same principles as laparoscopic APR except for port placement, as this will vary depending on the robotic system employed. Once the abdomen has been entered and ports placed, the patient is placed on steep Trendelenburg position with the right side down to aid in exposure of the pelvis. The abdominal cavity is inspected, and the pelvis is emptied laparoscopically, proceeding afterward to docking the robotic unit between the patient's legs. It is important to know that once the robot is docked, the table cannot be adjusted without undocking the robotic system. A standard medial-to-lateral dissection is started by incising the peritoneum at the level of the sacral promontory. Once this plane is entered, the superior rectal artery is dissected and the left ureter and gonadal vessel identified. TME is completed in the same fashion as in the open or laparoscopic technique. The initial dissection is posterior, moving toward the lateral stalks, and is completed anteriorly. Once at the level of the levators, the dissection plane proceeds in an extralevator fashion, to avoiding coning at this level to avoid a "waist" in the specimen. Once the abdominal portion of the surgery is concluded, the robot is undocked and the perineal dissection performed until the two planes of dissection meet.

## PRESERVATION OF SEXUAL AND URINARY FUNCTION

Sympathetic nerve fibers travel through the lumbar splanchnic nerves to the superior hypogastric plexus and then divide into two hypogastric nerves. Parasympathetic fibers emerge from the second, third, and fourth sacral spinal nerves as the pelvic splanchnic nerves and join the hypogastric nerves to form the inferior hypogastric (pelvic) plexus. The pelvic plexus is rectangular, and its midpoint is located at the tips of the seminal vesicles on either side of the rectum (Figure 29.2). The most caudal portion of the pelvic plexus travels at the posterolateral border of the prostate, lateral to the prostatic capsular arteries and veins, and reaches the hilum of the penis (20).

The rate of urinary dysfunction and impotence after rectal surgery ranges from 33% to 70% and 20% to 46%, respectively, while 20%–60% of potent patients are unable to ejaculate (21). A surprisingly large proportion of patients suffer various urinary tract problems and sexual problems due to extended lymphadenectomy involving the hypogastric nerve plexus. Therefore, preservation of the pelvic autonomic nerves lowers the incidence of sexual and urinary morbidity. With preservation of the superior hypogastric nerve plexus, ejaculation is maintained in 90% of the patients (22).

Utilizing precise dissection with preservation of autonomic nerves, Kim et al. noted an erection rate of 80%,

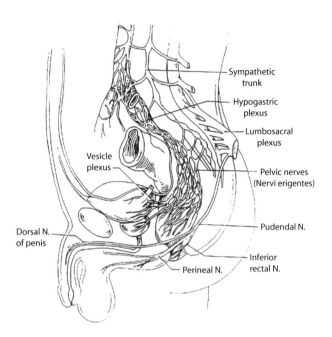

Figure 29.2 Nerve supply to the rectum.

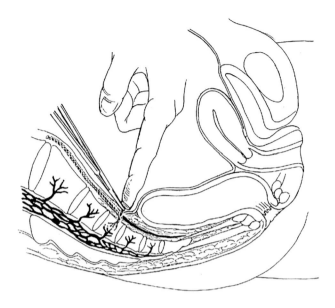

Figure 29.3 Thumbtack occlusion of bleeding basivertebral vein.

penetration ability rate of 75% with only 5.5% of patients in their study reporting complete inability for erection and intercourse (22). Study by Shirouzu et al. showed oncologic equivalence between previously described extensive resection pre-1984 and plexus preserving low rectal surgery post-1985 with local recurrence rates of 9.1% and 3.9%, respectively, and 10-year, disease-free survival rates of 77% and 81.5%, respectively. No significant difference was noted among the groups (23).

## INTRAOPERATIVE HEMORRHAGE

Hemorrhage during surgery can usually be attributed to an error in technique, but when faced with a pelvis that had previously received radiation therapy, hemorrhage may be unavoidable.

Bleeding may occur when dissection begins at the sigmoid. This is usually easily identified and controlled. In the previously irradiated pelvis, planes become distorted, making it difficult to identify vital structures. It is easy to stray laterally, which may result in iliac vessel injury. These must be repaired immediately to avoid prolonged hemorrhage. In a pelvis that has not received radiation or if there is minimal fibrosis, meticulous dissection in the proper plane down to the lateral stalks usually yields minimal bleeding.

The most troublesome bleeding in the pelvis comes from the posterior dissection along the sacrum. Very rarely there will be a prominent medial sacral artery that may be injured. More commonly, the bleeding on the sacrum will come from the venous plexus. If present, the basivertebral vein, which connects the internal vertebral venous system to the presacral system, can bleed profusely and be difficult to control.

Ideally, by taking sharp dissection down the presacral plane, there should be little to no bleeding (24,25). Unfortunately, this space may be nonexistent in certain patients or obliterated in an irradiated field. Bleeding from the sacrum can be controlled by packing, suture ligation, electrocautery, finger compression, or thumbtack compression.

Thumbtack compression is a quick, safe, and effective method of controlling sacral bleeding. There are several commercial application devices available; however, using a clamp or forceps with finger applications works equally as well (Figure 29.3). Thumbtacks also prevent damage to the surround venous plexus that may occur when using the other methods of attempting hemostasis, such as direct suture ligation or excessive cauterization (25,26).

## STANDARD PERINEAL OPERATIVE TECHNIQUE

When the abdominal operator has determined that the lesion is resectable, the perineal dissection may begin simultaneously with the abdominal portion of the case or sequentially if necessary. The perineal dissection begins with an elliptical incision from the perineal body in males or the posterior vaginal introitus in females to a point midway between the anus and coccyx. The incision should include the entirety of the external sphincter muscle but does not need to extend laterally to the ischial tuberosities. Dissection is carried down to the levator ani muscles with cautery to minimize bleeding. The inferior hemorrhoidal arteries located posterior laterally are ligated. Using a finger on the tip of the coccyx as a guide, the posterior dissection is directed anterior to the coccyx, and the anococcygeal raphe is divided. When all that remains is the anterior attachments, the specimen is drawn through the opening and used to provide traction to continue the remaining dissection. The specimen is then removed and the pelvis is irrigated. If sufficient levator muscle remains, the pelvic floor is reapproximated to reduce the risk for perineal herniation. Drains are placed and secured followed by closure of the skin with interrupted permanent or absorbable monofilament suture in a vertical mattress fashion.

## EXTRALEVATOR OPERATIVE TECHNIQUE

Since the description of total mesorectal excision by Heald in 1982, the local recurrence and survival rates from rectal cancer have improved greatly (12). However, those patients undergoing APR had worse oncologic outcomes than those patients undergoing sphincter sparing procedures, mainly due to higher rates of inadvertent tumor perforation and positive circumferential margin (27).

Extralevator APR has been credited with oncologic superiority with reduction of local recurrence and improving survival. This has been attributed to the wider resection margin that avoids "wasting" at the level of the levators and increases the circumferential margin of the specimen (28).

Patients undergoing extralevator APR can be placed in lithotomy position, or they can be flipped into prone jack-knife position once the abdominal phase of the operation is concluded. The anus is closed with a purse-string suture and the perianal skin incised. Once the skin is incised, exposure can be aided by the use of a commercial self-retraction device.

The anterior margin of the dissection will be the transverse perineal muscle, and the posterior margin the tip of the coccyx. Lateral dissection is extended into the ischiorectal fossa on both sides. Dissection is continued laterally to the pelvic side wall and includes the soft tissues around the anorectal ring. Dissection can be performed with a combination of monopolar energy and a vessel sealing device.

Extralevator abdominoperineal resection will leave a large perineal defect in patients with prior history of radiation therapy. The perineal wound can be closed primarily in multiple layers, but this is often not possible. For this reason, closure of the defect can be aided by the use of biologic mesh or by the use of muscle-cutaneous pedicle flaps, minimizing tension at the closure site, with decreased healing time and wound failure rates (29,30).

## METHODS OF CLOSURE

The perineal wound can be packed open, partially closed, or completely closed. The peritoneal defect above the pelvic space can also be sutured closed or left open. Adjunctive procedures such as drainage of the pelvic space, with or without continuous irrigation, and omental plugging may also be considered.

Rates of primary healing after perineal wounds are closed range from 4% to 92% (10,31,32). Open packing relegates all wounds to secondary healing, is inconvenient, and is often painful but may result in a lower rate of chronic perineal sinus formation (33). Closure of the pelvic peritoneum has been advocated to prevent perineal evisceration and postoperative small bowel obstruction. However, it may prevent obliteration of the pelvic cavity, leading to formation of a persistent perineal sinus (34). Loops of small bowel may also become incarcerated in small defects in the peritoneal closure, resulting in postoperative bowel obstruction.

Two studies compared various methods of peritoneal and perineal closure. Irvin and Goligher (33) prospectively randomized 106 patients undergoing proctectomy to one of three methods of perineal closure: open packing of the perineal wound; primary closure of the perineal wound without closure of the pelvic peritoneum with suction drainage of the pelvis; and primary closure of the peritoneal and perineal wounds. The overall complication rate was high; repeated surgery was necessary in 21% of patients in the open packing group, most often because of hemorrhage, and in 25% and 19% of the two closed groups, most commonly for drainage of abscesses. Primary healing occurred in 45% of the patients with primary closure of both the perineum and peritoneum and in 43% of patients with open peritoneal and closed perineal wounds.

In a prospective study part of a multicenter trial in Germany, Meyer et al. published a standardized technique of perineal closure that reduced wound complication rates from 17% to 5.4%. The perineal wound was closed tightly in multiple layers utilizing the levator muscles and subcutaneous fat, which helped to avoid the accumulation of fluid within the wound cavity. Any residual fluid was removed by closed suction drainage. Additionally, it is thought that the addition of antibiotic carriers provides local infectious prophylaxis leading to lower rates of perineal wound infection (35). This has also been demonstrated in two other prospective randomized studies and can be considered an adjunct in decreasing the overall morbidity of the perineal wound (36).

Myocutaneous flaps have been increasingly utilized in the initial closure of the perineal defect, especially in patients who have had preoperative radiation therapy. Chessin et al. at Memorial Sloan Kettering reviewed their experience with rectus abdominis myocutaneous flap closures of the perineal defect. They found the incidence of perineal wound complications was 15.8% in the rectus abdominis myocutaneous flap group compared to the 44.1% in historical controls (37). Butler et al. also looked at vertical rectus abdominis myocutaneous flaps in previously irradiated patients undergoing APR. There was a significantly lower incidence of perineal abscess (9% versus 37%), major perineal wound dehiscence (9% versus 30%), and drainage procedures required for perineal or pelvic fluid collections (3% versus 25%) (38).

In an effort to fill the pelvic space after rectal resection, Page advocates an omental plug. The omentum is mobilized on the left gastroepiploic arterial pedicle and placed in the pelvis, which increases local blood flow, increases lymphatic drainage, and helps obliterate the pelvic space. The omental plug also keeps the small bowel out of the pelvis, decreasing the chance of radiation enteritis in patients who require postoperative radiotherapy. Primary healing was noted in 26 of 34 patients (77%) (39). Nilsson reviewed all available English-language publications on the use of omentoplasty in APR wound closure with primary wound healing as the primary outcome measure. Most authors reported positive results after omentoplasty; one study showed significant improvement in perineal healing rate at 6 months. Significant reduction in sinus formation and wound dehiscence also was reported (40). Despite these promising results, there need to be randomized trials with well-described patient categories, endpoints, and follow-up to firmly assess whether omentoplasty should be a standard part of the wound closure.

## ABSCESS

Abscess formation, either intraperitoneal or perineal, is the most common major complication after APR (31). Incidence of abscess formation ranges from 11% to 16% (31,32,41). In some small series, the incidence of perineal wound infection is 100% (33). This can be attributed to the large dead space remaining after resection of the rectum and from fecal contamination.

Incision and drainage with local wound care are the treatment of choice for local perineal wound abscesses. There is a small increased risk of developing a perineal sinus after opening the skin of a subcutaneous abscess (42). Thus, if the incision is healing well, the abscess may be amenable to percutaneous drainage. In addition, percutaneous drainage is the preferred treatment of presacral and pelvic abscesses (43).

## NONHEALING WOUND AND PERINEAL SINUS

Perineal sinus is defined as a perineal wound that remains unhealed for a minimum of 6 months. Characteristics include a fixed fibrotic pelvic cavity, a long, narrow track lined with a thick unyielding peel, and a small external opening (44).

Silen and Glotzer compared the pelvic space after APR with the fixed pleural space after pneumonectomy. The pelvic space is bound posteriorly and laterally by the rigid bony pelvis, anteriorly by the relatively unyielding genitourinary structures, inferiorly by the slightly mobile perineal floor, and superiorly by the peritoneal contents. Of all these borders, certainly the peritoneal structures are the most mobile. They contend that the pelvic space after APR is filled not with granulation tissue but with a combination of upward migration of the perineal soft tissues and descent of the peritoneal contents and argue that any forces that produce a fixed fibrotic cavity are likely to result in a nonhealing perineal wound (34). Artioukh et al. reviewed their series of APR nonhealing wounds and found several possible contributing factors, including distant metastases, excessive alcohol consumption, cigarette smoking, transfusion requirement, and chemoradiation (45).

Other studies have also observed the increased risk in perineal wound infection and nonhealing in those who had radiotherapy. The Swedish Rectal Cancer trial showed an increase in wound infection from 10% to 20%, and the Dutch Colorectal Cancer Group had a 31% perineal complication rate even in those exposed to short-course radiation (46,47).

Silen and Glotzer recommended that the peritoneal contents be allowed to descend into the pelvis, the space be kept irrigated and well drained to prevent fluid accumulation, and any packing used in the perineal wound be removed early to prevent development of fibrotic wound edges. Despite the excellent description of perineal healing by Silen and Glotzer and the development of multiple techniques for perineal closure, nonhealing perineal wounds remain a common problem. Bacon and Nuguid noted a 40% incidence of persistent perineal sinus in 1,042 patients after rectal resection (48). In almost 500 patients who underwent APR at the Lahey and Mayo Clinics, 14%–24% had unhealed perineal wounds at 6 months.

Many techniques have been developed to ensure complete healing. Early efforts included operative debridement with wide drainage, including coccygectomy and even partial sacral resection (34). These measures were designed to eliminate the rigid fibrotic space that always accompanies a nonhealing perineal wound. Often these measures resulted in eventual healing but required extensive wound care for many months. Despite this treatment, some wounds failed to heal.

Oomen et al. published a set of guidelines in treating persistent perineal sinuses or complex perineal wounds with an overall 80% success rate in healing. Their algorithm consisted of VAC therapy for large defects prior to placing muscle flaps in order to decrease the size of the defect. Depending on sinus length, they either placed a transposition of rectus abdominal muscle (for sinuses >10 cm) or a gracilis muscle/gluteal thigh flap (sinus <8 cm). Initially the success rate was 57%, but after secondary surgery in some of the patients, their success rate increased to 80%. Ultimately, the best outcomes were in patients who received the gracilis or gluteal thigh flap (49).

The VAC closure system has been used to deal with complex perineal wounds following extensive operative debridement for persistent perineal sinuses. Pemberton at the Mayo Clinic (50) showed that in difficult perineal sinuses requiring debridement and removal of the coccyx and caudal part of the sacrum, the VAC system had complete resolution of the sinus in nearly all of their patients. While their evidence is anecdotal, there are documented reports with healing rates up to 95% (51,52).

Omentoplasty has been evaluated in both the primary repair of the perineal wound as well as in complex perineal sinus disease. Yamamoto et al. reported six patients with persistent perineal sinuses who underwent omentoplasty. The perineal sinus tract was completely excised and communication with the pelvis attained. The left or right gastroepiploic vessels were then ligated and the omentum brought down to the perineum where it was lightly sutured to the skin. After a 28-month follow-up period, 83% of the patients had completely healed wounds without any complications (53).

## PERINEAL HERNIA AND EVISCERATION

Perineal hernias are fortunately very rare and often troublesome to diagnose. Perineal hernia after abdominoperineal resection is defined as bulging of peritoneal contents through an intact perineal wound, and perineal evisceration describes extrusion of small or large bowel through an open perineal wound. However, other unusual contents have been described, including a leiomyoma, an aggressive angiomyoma, and a large bladder diverticulum (54). Evisceration typically occurs immediately after surgery and necessitates repeat surgery with reduction of intestines and repeat packing. Perineal hernias are a rare complication and occur in about 1% of patients after APR. This figure increases to 3% after pelvic exenteration. Initial symptoms include perineal bulging, often associated with fullness or pain on sitting (55,56). Occasionally, patients complain of voiding problems if herniated bowel compresses the bladder (57). Rarely, skin breakdown occurs, resulting in exposed bowel in the perineum. Perineal hernias, like parastomal and incisional hernias, do not always require repair. Indications for surgery are similar for all three postoperative hernias: patient discomfort refractory to conservative therapy, bowel obstruction, incarceration, and impending skin loss. Cosmesis alone should rarely merit surgical repair.

Risk factors that predispose patients to developing perineal hernias are not entirely clear. Coccygectomy, previous hysterectomy, pelvic irradiation, excessive length of the small-bowel mesentery, the larger size of the female pelvis, and possibly the failure to close the peritoneal defect have been implicated as possible causes (58,60). So et al. described 80% of their patients having perineal wounds that were laid open or had multiple large drains inserted through the wound, which they postulate may weaken the wound and allow hernia formation (61).

Diagnosis of perineal hernias can be difficult as traditional fluoroscopic imaging techniques often do not identify them. Other modalities have been used to include herniography, computed tomography, and dynamic magnetic resonance imaging (MRI). A comparative study of dynamic MRI and dynamic cystocolpoproctography showed that MRI was the only modality that identified levator ani hernias (54).

There are few large published series to describe which technique of perineal defect closure is superior. Various case reports and retrospective reviews provide much of the literature in this respect. In a review of the literature, closure techniques have ranged from the use of simple suture closure, prosthetic mesh, human dura mater allograft (62), gracilis myocutaneous flap (63), gluteus flap, and retroflexion of the uterus or bladder (64). So et al. described their experience with closures and ultimately found that recurrence rates were equal (20%) between simple and mesh closures (60). Their repair consisted of simple closure of the levator defect with nonabsorbable sutures. The approach to the repair was also felt to be a point of consideration in planning the operation. For the most part, a perineal approach was adequate with the abdominal approach reserved for recurrent hernias, or those in whom laparotomy is necessary for other reasons. The abdominal approach also provides good visualization when suturing the mesh to the bony pelvis. A combined AP approach is rarely necessary except under unusual circumstances. Skipworth et al. published their experience and technique of perineal hernia repair using Permacol mesh. Using a perineal approach, they isolated and ligated the sac in the standard fashion before proceeding to close the perineal defect. The mesh was then fashioned to the contours of the defect and sutured in place, tension free, with interrupted sutures. A small suction drain was then left superficial to the mesh and the thin, residual perineal fascia closed. They reported no recurrence in the 18 months following the repair. There are also a growing number of case reports and prospective studies in the use of laparoscopy for perineal hernia repairs. Dulucq et al. describe their experience in a prospective study done over the course of a year with three patients who had received laparoscopic mesh repairs of their perineal hernia defects. A composite mesh was fixed laterally to the border of the levator muscle, anteriorly to the posterior face of the vagina with nonabsorbable sutures and posteriorly with tacks to the sacral periosteum. One suction drain was placed. The reported benefits include adequate visualization of pelvic anatomy, the ability to look for recurrence, and fast recovery. Long-term results have yet to be published for laparoscopic perineal hernia repairs, but this may be an attractive option for patients and surgeons as it often avoids making large incisions in areas that have already been irradiated and can therefore be difficult to heal (65). Prior to embarking on a repair of any postoperative perineal hernia, it is imperative to exclude the possibility of cancer recurrence.

## REFERENCES

1. Abraham NS et al. *Aliment Pharmacol Ther.* 2001; 21(1):35–41.
2. Shoetz Jr. DJ. *J Am Coll Surg.* 2006;203(3):322–27.

3. Swedish Colorectal Cancer Registry. Available at: http://kvalitetsregister.se/englishpages/findaregistry/registerarkivenglish/swedishcolorectalcancerregistry scrcr.2156.html. Accessed June 1, 2018.

4. Ruo L, Guillem JG. *Dis Colon Rectum.* 1999;42(5): 563–78.

5. American Society of Colon and Rectal Surgeons Committee Members; Wound Ostomy Continence Nurses Society Committee Members. *J Wound Ostomy Continence Nurs.* 2007;34(6):627–8.

6. Marret E et al. Postoperative Pain Forum Group. *Br J Surg.* 2007;94(6):665–73.

7. Geerts WH et al. *Chest.* 2008;133(Suppl. 6): 381S–453S.

8. Bratzler DW, Houck PM. *Clin Infect Dis.* 2004; 38:1706–15.

9. Beraldo S, Dodds SR. *Dis Colon Rectum.* 2006; 49(11):1772–80.

10. Miles WE. *Lancet.* 1908;2:1812.

11. Corman ML. Ed. Carcinoma of the rectum. In *Colon and Rectal Surgery*, 5th Edition. Philadelphia, PA: Lippincott, Williams, and Wilkins, 2005, pp. 905–1061.

12. Heald RJ et al. *Br J Surg.* 1982;69:613–6.

13. Clinical Outcomes of Surgical Therapy Study Group. *N Eng J Med.* 2004;350(20):2050–9.

14. Moghadamyeqhanez Z et al. *Dis Colon Rectum.* 2015;58(10):950–6.

15. Fleshman J et al. *JAMA.* 2015;314(13):1346–55.

16. Ng SS et al. *Surg Endosc.* 2014;28(1):297–306.

17. Kang SB et al. *Lancet Oncol.* 2010;11(7):637–45.

18. Yamaguchi T et al. *Surg Today.* 2016;46(8):957–62.

19. Barnajian M et al. *Colorectal Dis.* 2014;16(8):603–9.

20. Kyo K et al. *World J Surg.* 2006;30(6):1014–9.

21. Moriya Y. *Int J Clin Oncol.* 2006;11(5):339–43.

22. Kim NK et al. *Dis Colon Rectum.* 2002;45: 1178–85.

23. Shirouzu K et al. *Dis Colon Rectum.* 2004;47(9): 1442–7.

24. Wang O et al. *Arch Surg.* 1985;120:1013–20.

25. Arnaud JP et al. *Dig Sur.* 2000;17(6):651–2.

26. Nivatvongs S, Fang DT. *Dis Colon Rectum.* 1986;29: 589–90.

27. Wibe A et al. *Dis Colon Rectum.* 2004;47(1):48–58.

28. Marr R et al. *Ann Surg.* 2005;242(1):74–82.

29. Howell AM et al. *Int J Surg.* 2013;11(7):514–7.

30. Devulapalli C et al. *Plast Reconstr Surg.* 2016;137(5): 1602–13.

31. Murrell ZA et al. *Am Surg.* 2005;71(10):837–40.

32. Rosen L et al. *Dis Colon Rectum.* 1982;25:202–8.

33. Irvin IT, Goligher JC. *Br J Surg.* 1975;62:287–91.

34. Silen W, Glotzer DJ. *Surgery.* 1974;75:535–42.

35. Meyer L et al. *Tech Coloproctol.* 2004;8(Suppl. 1): s230–4.

36. Gruessner U et al. *Am J Surg.* 2001;182:502–9.

37. Chessin DB et al. *Ann of Surg Onc.* 2005;12(2):104–10.

38. Butler CE et al. *J Am Coll Surg.* 2008;206(4): 694–702.

39. Page CP et al. *Dis Colon Rectum.* 1980;23:2–9.

40. Nilsson PJ. *Dis Colon Rectum.* 2006;49:1354–61.

41. Pollard CW et al. *Dis Colon Rectum.* 1994;37:866–74.

42. Baudot PE et al. *Br J Surg.* 1980;67:275–6.

43. Michalson AE et al. *Radiology.* 1994;190:574–5.

44. Anthony JP, Mathes SJ. *Arch Surg.* 1990;125:1371–7.

45. Artioukh DY et al. *Colorectal Dis.* 2007;9(4):362–7.

46. Fasth S et al. *Ann Chir Gynaecol.* 1977;66:181–3.

47. Scott H, Brown AC. *Am Surg.* 1996;62:452–7.

48. Bacon HE, Nuguid TP. *Dis Colon Rectum.* 1962;5: 370–2.

49. Oomen JW et al. *Int J Colorectal Dis.* 2007;22(2): 225–30.

50. Permberton JH. *Colorectal Dis.* 2003;5(5):486–9.

51. Argenta LC, Morykwas MJ. *Ann Plastic Surg.* 1997; 38:563–77.

52. Deva AK et al. *Med J Aust.* 2000;173:128–31.

53. Yamamoto T et al. *Am J Surg.* 2001;181(3):265–7.

54. Skipworth RJ et al. *Hernia.* 2007;11:541–5.

55. McMullin ND et al. *Aust N Z J Surg.* 1985;55:69.

56. Rutledge RN et al. *Am J Obstet Gynecol.* 1977; 129:881.

57. Brotschi E et al. *Am J Surg.* 1985;149:301–5.

58. Cattell RB, Cunningham RM. *Surg Clin North Am.* 1944;24:679–83.

59. Kelly AR. *Aust N Z J Surg.* 1960;29:243–45.

60. Frydman GM, Polglase AL. *Aust N Z Surg.* 1989;59: 895–7.

61. So JB et al. *Dis Colon Rectum.* 1997;40:954–7.

62. Delmore JE et al. *Obstet Gynecol.* 1987;70:507–8.

63. Bell JG et al. *Obstet Gynecol.* 1980;56:377–80.

64. Remzi FH et al. *Tech Colo-proctol.* 2005;9:142–4.

65. Dulucq JL et al. *Surg Endosc.* 2006;20(3):414–8.

# 30

# Management of rectal cancer after complete clinical response to neoadjuvant chemoradiotherapy

RODRIGO O. PEREZ AND LAURA MELINA FERNANDEZ

## CHALLENGING CASE

A 69 yr women with a clinical T3N1 rectal cancer undergoes neoadjuvant chemoradiation therapy after review at a multi-disciplinary tumor conference (MDT). Eight weeks after completing the therapy, a digital and endoscopic evaluation reveals no residual tumor. An MRI and PET scan fails to demonstrate any tumor.

## CASE MANAGEMENT

The patient's case is again discussed at a MDT. She appears to have a complete clinical response. She is offered an oncologic resection or enrollment into a strict surveillance program.

## INTRODUCTION

Incorporation of new treatment modalities has significantly increased complexity in the management of rectal cancer (1). Surgical treatment is still the main pillar in the management of rectal cancer. We continue to have a better understanding of the different approaches for total mesorectal excision (TME), including standard, laparoscopic, robotic, and, most recently, transanal TME. In addition to evolving surgical approaches, neoadjuvant therapy and the management of patients after assessment of tumor response to neoadjuvant therapy are also undergoing widespread changes. Neoadjuvant chemoradiation therapy (nCRT) may lead to significant tumor regression, and ultimately complete pathological response in up to 42% of patients (2). Assessment of tumor response following nCRT and prior to radical surgery may identify patients with complete clinical response who could be managed nonoperatively with strict follow-up, the "watch and wait" (WW) strategy, which in select cases may help to avoid unnecessary postoperative morbidity and maintain good long-term oncological outcomes and excellent functional results (3). In addition, close surveillance may allow for early detection of local recurrences and salvage alternatives without oncological compromise (4). The present chapter discusses the management of rectal cancer following complete clinical response after nCRT.

## RATIONALE FOR ORGAN PRESERVATION IN RECTAL CANCER

Different organ-preserving strategies in the treatment of rectal cancer have gained popularity in recent years. The main reasons for avoiding a proctectomy include the significant postoperative morbidity, including long-term urinary, sexual, and fecal continence dysfunction in addition to the requirement for temporary or definitive stomas associated with the procedure. Also, depending on associated comorbidities and patient's age, postoperative mortality may also be significant (5). Therefore, in selected patients with evidence of complete primary tumor regression, less invasive surgical and even nonsurgical approaches have been suggested (6).

The observation that rectal cancers could develop significant tumor regression with reduction in primary tumor size (downsizing), depth of tumor penetration, and even potential nodal sterilization (downstaging) set the ideal stage for organ-preserving alternatives, including local excision of small and superficial residual tumors (7). In some cases, regression of the primary tumor can result in complete disappearance of the tumor in the resected specimen (complete pathological response [pCR]). In a subset of these patients, complete disappearance of the primary tumor may be clinically detected prior to surgical resection, referred to as complete clinical response (cCR) (8). These patients with complete tumor regression of their primary rectal cancers to nCRT may be ideal patients to consider nonoperative organ-preserving strategies (9). In order to consider this approach, colorectal surgeons have to take into consideration several aspects of the disease, the patient, and treatment modalities that may be quite relevant during their clinical decision-making process.

## PREDICTION OF RESPONSE TO nCRT AND INTRATUMORAL HETEROGENEITY

Several studies have attempted to provide a clinically useful tool based on molecular biology features of rectal cancers undergoing nCRT to predict response to treatment up front (10). This would allow more precise selection of patients who would benefit the most from CRT, spare patients from potentially unnecessary treatment, and identify ideal candidates for nonoperative management. Unfortunately, however, these studies have failed to provide any clinically relevant information to be implemented into clinical practice so far. First, published gene signatures rarely present specific genes overlapping between them. Second, validation of findings between these signatures in independent cohorts often results in inaccurate identification of complete responders to nCRT (10–13).

The presence of significant intratumoral heterogeneity may have accounted at least in part for these disappointing results (14,15). The coexistence of subpopulations of cancer cells within a single rectal cancer with distinct morphological features and genetic mutations may render single biopsy samples simply not representative of the entirety of the primary tumor. Therefore, a single biopsy sample from one area of the primary tumor may contain cancer cells that are resistant to nCRT, while biopsy taken from other areas may contain cancer cells that are sensitive to nCRT (16).

## BASELINE STAGING AND INDICATIONS FOR NEOADJUVANT CHEMORADIATION

Following the results of the German trial, chemoradiation was considered the preferred initial approach for cT3–4 or cN+ rectal cancers due to the potential benefits in local disease control after radical surgery (17,18). However, data from the Mercury study suggested that after proper or optimal total mesorectal excision, local recurrence was unlikely to develop for most cT3 cancers, even in the presence of nodal disease (cN1) (19). Instead, patients at higher risk for local recurrence, and therefore, those who would most benefit from nCRT in order to improve local disease control would include radiological evidence of a positive circumferential margin (cCRM+), presence of extramural venous invasion

(cEMVI+), and ≥3 positive lymph nodes (cN2). In addition, radical surgery after nCRT was shown to result in worse functional outcomes and increased surgical morbidity when compared to surgery alone (20,21). Altogether, these data suggested that nCRT was to be restricted for high-risk patients (also referred to as the "ugly" tumors) for the development of local recurrence only. Considering that baseline staging features may influence development of complete response to nCRT, one could expect that very few patients with such advanced disease would do so.

However, the possibility of avoiding radical surgery and its related comorbidities after a cCR raised the issue of offering nCRT to more early stage rectal cancers, particularly for the most distal tumors. Ultimately, patients with cT2N0 or early cT3N0 are more likely to develop a cCR following nCRT and could benefit the most from nCRT if organ preservation is considered (22–24).

The use of nCRT should be considered only for high-risk patients (cCRM+, cEMVI, and cN2) if radical surgery is to be performed regardless of response to treatment. However, if organ-preserving strategies are an option according to tumor response, nCRT may be offered to most rectal cancers (except for cT1N0) (25). Here tumor location or height may be of significant importance. As discussed in the following sections of the chapter, clinical assessment including digital rectal examination (DRE) is crucial for the identification and surveillance of cCR, and only baseline cancers accessible to DRE (usually up to 7–8 cm from the anal verge) would be appropriate candidates for organ-preserving strategies without immediate surgery (1).

## NEOADJUVANT TREATMENT OPTIONS

Specific features of a neoadjuvant therapy regimen may ultimately affect the odds of developing a cCR and should be considered in the setting of organ-preservation strategies. Initially, it was thought that long-course CRT was the only strategy that could result in significant rates of complete response, whereas short-course CRT would only rarely have such clinical outcome. However, with the understanding of the influence of time in the development of complete response to therapy, it has been suggested that short-course RT followed by delayed assessment of response may result in similar rates of complete response to the observed after long-course CRT (2,26,27).

The dose of radiation therapy (RT) may also influence the odds of patients with rectal cancer in developing complete response to treatment. Dose-escalation studies have demonstrated progressive increase in complete response rates with higher doses of RT delivered to the primary tumor (28,29). In addition to the actual dose delivered, the method of delivery may also affect the development of a complete response. Therefore, the combination of external beam RT or intensity modulated RT with endorectal brachytherapy or even with contact RT may further increase the total dose of radiation delivered, maximizing the chances of developing cCR and still avoiding major treatment-related toxicity (30–32).

More recently a strategy has been suggested to provide neoadjuvant therapy with chemotherapy alone prior to RT in an attempt to avoid the toxic and potential morbidity resulted from RT in these patients (33). The delivery of chemotherapy alone would allow the control of possible micrometastatic foci of the disease while still providing significant response to the primary tumor in a good proportion of patients. Standard CRT could be restricted to patients showing minimal response to chemotherapy alone, therefore minimizing the amount of patients receiving RT (34).

Finally, combinations of standard CRT and more aggressive chemotherapy regimens have been suggested that include additional cycles of chemotherapy being delivered during the resting period after RT completion in standard CRT regimens (consolidation CRT regimens). One study adding additional cycles of 5FU-based chemotherapy during the resting period after 54 Gy of RT suggested an increase of CR rates to >50% in patients with T2/T3 rectal cancer (25,35). Data from a prospective study using standard CRT followed by progressively higher numbers of FOLFOX cycles during the resting periods after RT completion have demonstrated a significant increase in pCR rates after radical surgery (42).

Altogether, these data may suggest that if organ preservation is an option, optimization of RT and chemotherapy should be considered up front rather than after standard CRT.

## ASSESSMENT OF TUMOR RESPONSE

Considering that patients may develop significant tumor regression after nCRT, which may provide an appropriate setting for an organ-preserving strategy, one issue becomes crucial in this process: assessment of tumor response. However, assessment of tumor response may be quite challenging due to numerous uncertainties including optimal timing and clinical/radiological tools for such purpose.

Assessment of tumor response is also recommended even if an organ-preserving strategy is not being considered. Even if the plan after nCRT is a radical resection, one needs to consider that after nCRT the surgeon may be facing a considerably different tumor. Knowing this potentially new "anatomy" ahead of time may allow the surgeon to optimize intraoperative surgical strategy and to know in advance what challenges could be anticipated during the procedure (36). Therefore, the reassessment of tumor response should be performed in all patients.

## TIMING FOR THE ASSESSMENT OF TUMOR RESPONSE

The grade of tumor regression after nCRT appears to be a time-dependent phenomenon. The first randomized trial to consider the effect of different time intervals in the response to CRT was a French study comparing 2 versus 6 weeks from nCRT. In this study, all patients underwent radical surgery after these two time intervals, and patients with 6-week intervals presented significantly more tumor regression after nCRT (37). Due to this study, a 6-week time interval between nCRT completion and performance of radical surgery has been considered the standard of care for many years. However, retrospective studies consistently reported that patients undergoing radical surgery after longer than 6–8 weeks from nCRT were more likely to develop pCR (38–41). One of these studies suggested that the rates of pCR after nCRT may keep rising after nCRT for as long as 12 weeks from treatment completion (39). However, there was a question whether these prolonged intervals from nCRT would result in excessive tissue fibrosis in the area included in the RT field that could lead to increased technical difficulty and postoperative morbidity after radical surgery. One study included patients in nCRT regimens with progressively longer interval periods prior to surgery. Even though this was not a randomized study, patients in different groups were comparable (74). Curiously, patients undergoing surgery after 12 weeks developed similar postoperative complication rates when compared to the standard 6-week interval. The study then kept on recruiting patients for progressively longer intervals: 6, 12, 18, and 24 weeks between nCRT and surgery. Even though additional systemic chemotherapy has been offered to patients undergoing surgery after longer interval periods, delaying surgical resection to ≥20 weeks resulted in significantly higher pCR rates with no negative impact on postoperative morbidity (42). Altogether, these data seem to suggest that the longer you wait, the more tumor regression is observed, and that longer intervals than 6–8 weeks would clearly benefit patients after nCRT. However, another recently published randomized study failed to demonstrate the benefits of longer intervals after nCRT. In this study, patients undergoing 7-week intervals developed similar pCR rates to patients undergoing 11-week intervals. Moreover, patients undergoing 11-week intervals developed increased rates of postoperative complications and ended up with worse quality of the resected specimen (quality of the mesorectum), suggesting the detrimental effects of prolonged time after nCRT on fibrotic changes in the surgical and previously irradiated fields (43).

The optimal interval after nCRT remains undetermined, and additional ongoing trials will definitely provide more data to allow us to understand the benefits and risks of using prolonged intervals after treatment. In fact, it may be the case that a single and fixed interval may not be appropriate for all patients. Instead, patients/tumors may respond differently as a function of time to nCRT. Ultimately, responsive tumors may require and actually benefit from prolonged intervals from nCRT, whereas unresponsive tumors may not. It is likely that responsive tumors that are being considered for organ-preserving strategies should have their assessment of response and ultimately surgical strategy decision deferred to longer than 12 weeks. But tumors with little response that still require radical TME may benefit from 6- to 8-week intervals between nCRT completion and radical surgery (44).

## TOOLS IN ASSESSMENT OF TUMOR RESPONSE

### Clinical and endoscopic assessment

Clinical assessment is one of the most important tools to evaluate tumor response. Commonly, patients with tumor regression would have relief of their symptoms. DRE is an irreplaceable tool for the evaluation of response. The stringent criteria to consider a cCR include the absence of any irregularity, mass, ulceration, or stenosis during the DRE. The surface has to be regular and smooth (8).

Endoscopic evaluation of the area harboring the original tumor is the remaining key component of clinical assessment. It is important to look for any irregularity or superficial ulcers missed during DRE. A flat white scar and telangiectasia are common endoscopic findings among patients with a cCR (Figure 30.1). Even though flexible scopes may provide photographic documentation of endoscopic response, rigid proctoscopy may suffice for the majority of patients (8).

In the presence of a cCR by DRE and proctoscopy, endoscopic biopsies are not recommended. Even in the setting of incomplete clinical response, endoscopic biopsy results should be interpreted with caution. Among patients with significant response, negative predictive values of these endoscopic biopsies have been reported to be consistently low (45). Therefore, a negative biopsy in the setting of incomplete clinical response does not rule out microscopic residual cancer.

### Radiological assessment

Even though historically the definition of a cCR has been based on clinical and endoscopic findings by direct assessment of rectal wall, radiological studies have always attempted to provide additional information unavailable to the finger or the proctoscope, particularly regarding nodal or mesorectal status of the disease. Currently, however, significant developments in imaging definition and interpretation have resulted in significant increases in accuracy for the assessment of response not only within the mesorectum compartment, but also within the rectal wall.

High-resolution magnetic resonance (MR) is now routinely used for the assessment of response. The ability to discriminate between fibrosis and residual disease has improved with advances in technology, placing the resonance as an essential tool to confirm clinical and endoscopic findings of a cCR (46). MR may provide an accurate radiological (mrTRG) estimate of the pathological tumor regression grade (TRG). The utilization of this mrTRG score may identify good and poor responders with significant impact in disease-free and overall survival (47,48) (Figure 30.2).

Even though clinical and endoscopic assessment using stringent criteria will result in high specificity rates for the detection of a pCR, a significant amount of patients with incomplete clinical response will still harbor complete pathological response (49,50). In fact, it seems that the majority of patients with pCR after nCRT have incomplete clinical response after 8–12 weeks from nCRT (50). Therefore, there is a potential role for MR studies to identify patients with incomplete clinical response who may ultimately harbor pCR. Currently, these patients would be referred to immediate radical surgery. However, radiological tools may be able to accurately identify these patients and avoid potentially unnecessary surgery (51).

Recently, a study that compared mrTRG and residual mucosal abnormalities following nCRT suggested that mrTRG system may identify nearly 10× more complete pathological responses compared to clinical endoscopic findings.

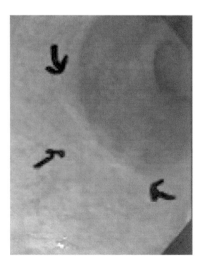

Figure 30.1 **(See color insert.)** Endoscopic view of a complete clinical response with whitening of the mucosa within the area of the scar (original area of the primary tumor).

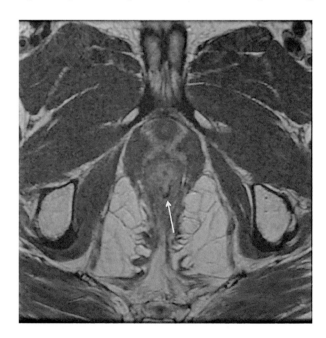

Figure 30.2 Magnetic resonance showing low-signal intensity area in the posterior rectal wall (arrow) consistent with mgTRG1 (suggestive of a complete response).

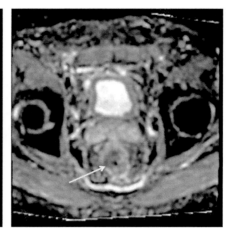

**Figure 30.3** Diffusion-weighted magnetic resonance with high-signal intensity area (left-arrow) and its corresponding low-signal intensity area in the ADC map (right-arrow).

These findings may improve the selection of patients with pCR despite initial incomplete clinical response and patients who may be appropriate candidates for deferral of surgery (51).

Diffusion-weighted MR imaging may add significant functional information to standard MR imaging. The fact that diffusion properties of water molecules may vary in areas of tissue necrosis, high cellularity (frequently observed within tumor tissues), or fibrosis, may be used to help assess tumor response to nCRT (Figure 30.3). The absence of restriction to diffusion of water molecules has been associated with the absence of residual cancer (complete response). Restriction to diffusion of water molecules (seen as high signal intensity in the area of the previous tumor) may indicate the presence of residual cancer cells (incomplete response). Initial reports with diffusion-weighted MR imaging for the assessment of response to nCRT has shown promising results with high accuracy rates and may constitute a useful tool during assessment of response (52,53).

Positron emission tomography/computed tomography (PET/CT) imaging has been studied for the prediction of response to CRT. The use of molecular imaging may provide additional information to standard structural/anatomical features to help distinguish between fibrosis or residual tumor. The use of fluorodeoxyglucose allows for the estimation of tissue metabolism (standard uptake values [SUV])

within areas of interest, and fused images of PET and CT may indicate precise anatomical areas of residual cancer cells, even among mucinous histological subtypes (22,54).

Most of the available studies have focused on SUV variation for the identification of complete responders to nCRT using variable interval periods and sequential PET/CT imaging (22,55,56). Accuracies, however, have been insufficient for its routine recommendation into clinical practice. A recently reported study has suggested the role of combination of SUV variation and volumetric reduction in tumors to predict complete response to nCRT. Using individual technical calibration for determining metabolic tumor volumes estimates, variation in total lesion glycolysis (determined by metabolic tumor volume and mean SUV values) was found to be the best predictor of response to nCRT using sequential PET/CT imaging at baseline and 12 weeks from nCRT completion (57) (Figure 30.4).

## COMPLETE RESPONSE: WATCH AND WAIT STRATEGY

### Watch and wait strategy: Follow-up

When a nonoperative strategy for cCR in rectal cancer is considered, a relatively intensive follow-up is certainly

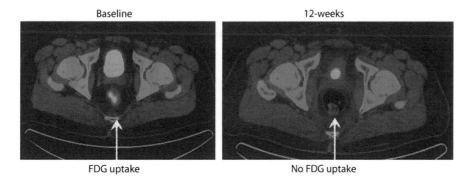

Baseline  12-weeks

FDG uptake  No FDG uptake

**Figure 30.4 (See color insert.)** PET/CT images performed at baseline (showing FDG uptake) and after 12 weeks from nCRT completion (showing no residual FDG uptake) consistent with a complete response to treatment.

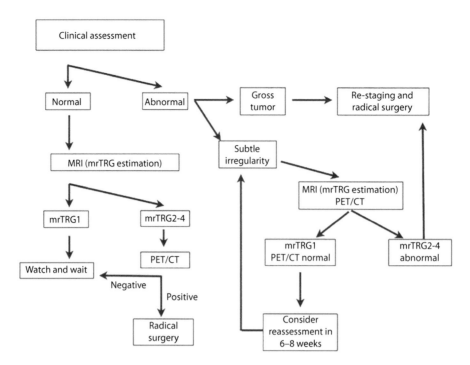

**Figure 30.5** Flow chart summarizes the Watch & Wait Strategy and assessment of tumor response following neoadjuvant chemoradiation.

required. Patients should be encouraged to adhere to this strict follow-up program in order to allow early recognition of any local or systemic recurrence and, therefore, increasing the chance of a successful salvage treatment (Figure 30.5). After initial assessment of response confirming a cCR, visits should be performed every 1–2 months during the first year, every 3 months during the second year, and every 6 months thereafter. DRE, proctoscopy, and carcinoembryonic antigen level determination are recommended for all visits. Timing for radiological assessment during follow-up has not yet been standardized. Routine MR for the assessment of the rectal wall, mesorectum, and pelvic nodes every 6 months for the first 2 years and yearly thereafter has been our practice (6).

## Outcomes

Patients managed nonoperatively under the WW strategy after a cCR following neoadjuvant chemoradiation were originally reported to have similar long-term oncological outcomes to patients with complete pathological response after radical surgery (9). Additional retrospective studies reported by others have consistently shown similar oncological outcomes between these subgroups of patients (31,58–63). These findings further support the idea that patients with a cCR may be spared from the surgical morbidity and mortality of radical surgery with no oncological compromise (5). In addition, functional outcomes of patients managed nonoperatively not only appear to be better than radical surgery but also better than other organ-preserving strategies (transanal local excision) (3,60).

Local recurrences after this treatment strategy are still a concern and may develop at any time during follow-up. The majority of local recurrences appear to develop within the first 12 months of follow-up and may represent limitations in the precise identification of microscopic residual disease among "apparent" complete clinical responders. For these reasons, these "early recurrences" developing within the initial 12 months of follow-up have been called "early regrowths" instead (4,63,64). Still, close and strict follow-up may allow early detection of regrowths leading to identical oncological outcomes to patients with incomplete clinical response immediately after 8–12 weeks from CRT completion (65). In addition, local recurrences (late and early regrowths) are usually amenable to salvage therapies, often allowing sphincter preservation and being associated with excellent long-term local disease control (4).

Considering that the rate of complete clinical or pathological response was historically <30% of patients across most of the studies, one could assume that this treatment strategy could benefit a rather limited proportion of patients with rectal cancer. However, the observation of increased rates of complete response (clinical or pathological) using regimens with consolidation chemotherapy and with the inclusion of earlier stages of disease (cT2N0 otherwise candidates for ultra-low resections or abdominoperineal resections) may result in nearly 50% that ultimately avoid surgical resection (25,42). This has been further confirmed in a prospective trial including patients with T2 and T3 rectal cancers managed by CRT and an additional endorectal high-dose brachytherapy boost (total 65 Gy) that showed a 58% cCR rate at 2 years of follow-up without surgical resection (31).

Finally, in the era of evidence-based medicine, a randomized prospective trial is still lacking to definitively demonstrate the oncological equivalence of WW and radical surgery in the setting of a cCR following nCRT (66). Even though such a trial is not likely to be performed, a recent study using a propensity-score matched cohort analysis comparing WW and radical surgery has been designed to demonstrate noninferiority of the WW approach. Curiously, however, the comparison between groups demonstrated a slight superiority of the nonoperative management of these patients in terms of survival and a clear benefit in colostomy-free survival even when accounting for the development of local recurrences (63).

## ADJUVANT TREATMENT

The use of adjuvant systemic chemotherapy following a cCR managed nonoperatively is still a matter of controversy. Most studies have not offered adjuvant chemotherapy to these patients even though several guidelines may recommend the use of adjuvant therapy based on pretreatment staging features rather than on response to nCRT. This means that a baseline cT3N1 would require adjuvant therapy, whereas a baseline cT2N0 would not, even though both patients develop cCR. However logical this may seem, there are insufficient data to support either strategy (based on pretreatment or posttreatment status).

In a pooled analysis of patients undergoing nCRT followed by radical surgery, patients with pCR showed an 11% distant metastases rate (67). Curiously, nearly 40% of these patients had received adjuvant 5FU-based chemotherapy. This compares to a 14% distant metastases rate among patients undergoing standard CRT with cCR managed nonoperatively without the use of adjuvant chemotherapy (4).

Finally, with the use of consolidation CRT regimens, the dose of adjuvant systemic therapy may ultimately have been shifted to the neoadjuvant period, rendering the discussion of adjuvant chemotherapy meaningless. However, there are still insufficient data to fully support this.

## LOCAL EXCISION

### LOCAL EXCISION AFTER NCRT AS A DIAGNOSTIC APPROACH

In the presence of an incomplete clinical response and in patients who are resistant to radical resection or who are medically unfit, the least we would offer is a full-thickness excisional biopsy, preferably with the use of transanal endoscopic microsurgery. This "excisional biopsy," otherwise referred to as a local excision, is primarily considered as a diagnostic procedure and may be appropriate for patients with small (≤3 cm) lesions that are restricted to the bowel wall (ycT0-2N0). However, we would restrict this to patients with low residual lesions that would otherwise require an abdominal-perineal excision or a coloanal intersphincteric resection as a definitive procedure (64). Appropriate pathological information regarding ypT classification, tumor regression grade, lymphovascular/perineural invasion, and resection margins may allow for a final decision regarding the need for total mesorectal excision and protectomy.

It has been our policy to offer strict follow-up to patients with a final pathological specimen showing ypT0 after this "diagnostic" transanal local excision. This is due to the fact that the risk of lymph node metastases among these patients has been shown to be very low in the setting of neoadjuvant CRT and long (≥8 weeks) intervals. This is already true for unselected patients with ypT0, where the risk of nodal metastases are well under 10%, and in most cases less than 5% (73,75,76). However, with significant improvements in radiological imaging, particularly with high-resolution MR with the use of a diffusion-weighted series and other lymphotropic agents, the selection of patients with ycT0N0 is expected to further improve (68).

There are at least three main drawbacks to this treatment strategy. First, healing of the rectal defects determined by local excision after neoadjuvant CRT is quite challenging and painful, particularly those closer to the anal verge (69,77). Healing problems are much more frequent, and it may take as long as 8 weeks to completely heal. Even though severe complications are not frequent, pain may be quite significant requiring readmission to the hospital. The second drawback is that sphincter preservation may be compromised after performance of full-thickness local excision in this setting. A few studies have addressed this issue and reported that patients requiring radical resection after full-thickness local excision frequently ended up with an abdominal perineal resection, even though they originally were considered candidates for a sphincter-preserving procedure (70,78). Finally, completion of TME in this setting may provide an imperfect mesorectal specimen for the pathologist. A recent review of patients undergoing completion TME indicated that previous transanal endoscopic microsurgery (TEM) was a risk factor for poor quality of the TME specimen (71). All of these issues should be kept in mind when offering patients "diagnostic" or "therapeutic" local excision after partial response.

### LOCAL EXCISION OR WATCH AND WAIT FOR cCR?

As mentioned previously, healing of local excision defects following neoadjuvant CRT is not as simple as after local excision alone. The rates of wound dehiscence may be significant (69,72,73). In this setting, not only is pain an issue, but also significant scarring following delayed healing may develop, which will make patient follow-up even more difficult. Even though ypT0 may be associated with a lower risk of local failures, the risk is not zero, and the patient still requires appropriate follow-up. Distinction between local recurrence in a rectal wall following wound dehiscence after a local excision with or without rectal stenosis may be quite challenging. Therefore, we believe that follow-up is considerably facilitated by preservation of rectal wall integrity with the WW approach allowing for earlier detection of possible recurrences.

Finally, considering that the ultimate goal of organ preservation is also function preservation, one has to compare functional outcomes between local excision and WW in the setting of neoadjuvant CRT. When patients with cCR managed by WW were compared to patients with "near-complete" response following nCRT by Wexner incontinence scores, manometric findings, and quality of life questionnaires, functional outcomes were significantly better among patients managed nonoperatively, suggesting that local excision may also risk function preservation despite providing organ preservation to these patients (3).

## CONCLUSIONS

Organ preservation in the management of rectal cancer has become a valid option for select patients after significant response to neoadjuvant CRT. Patients who develop complete tumor regression with no clinical, endoscopic, or radiological evidence of residual cancer may be offered no immediate surgery and enrolled in a strict surveillance program (WW) with excellent functional and acceptable oncological outcomes. Good responders to nCRT (ypT0 or ypTis) despite incomplete clinical response may warrant local excision as a diagnostic and therapeutic tool, also with good oncological outcomes but at the cost of slightly worse functional outcomes and significant postoperative morbidity.

## REFERENCES

1. Kosinski L et al. *CA Cancer J Clin.* 2012;62(3): 173–202.
2. Sanghera P et al. *Clin Oncol (R Coll Radiol).* 2008; 20(2):176–83.
3. Habr-Gama A et al. *Dis Colon Rectum.* 2016;59(4): 264–9.
4. Habr-Gama A et al. *Int J Radiat Oncol Biol Phys.* 2014;88(4):822–8.
5. Smith FM et al. *Dis Colon Rectum.* 2015;58(2): 159–71.
6. Habr-Gama A et al. *Hematol Oncol Clin North Am.* 2015;29(1):135–51.
7. Smith FM et al. *Br J Surg.* 2010;97(12):1752–64.
8. Habr-Gama A et al. *Dis Colon Rectum.* 2010;53(12): 1692–8.
9. Habr-Gama A et al. *Ann Surg.* 2004;240:711–7; discussion 7–8.
10. Lopes-Ramos C et al. *Cancer Genet.* 2015;208(6): 319–26.
11. Brettingham-Moore KH et al. *Clin Cancer Res.* 2011; 17(9):3039–47.
12. Watanabe T et al. *Cancer Res.* 2006;66(7):3370–4.
13. Rimkus C et al. *Clin Gastroenterol Hepatol.* 2008;6(1): 53–61.
14. Hardiman KM et al. *Lab Invest.* 2016;96(1):4–15.
15. Bettoni F et al. *Ann Surg.* 2017;265(1):e4–6.
16. Perez RO et al. *Dis Colon Rectum.* 2016;59(9):895–7.
17. Sauer R et al. *N Engl J Med.* 2004;351:1731–40.
18. Sauer R et al. *J Clin Oncol.* 2012;30:1926–33.
19. Taylor FG et al. *Ann Surg.* 2011;253:711–9.
20. Peeters KCMJ et al. *J Clin Oncol.* 2005;23(25): 6199–206.
21. Loos M et al. *Ann Surg Oncol.* 2013;20:1816–28.
22. Perez RO et al. *Tech Coloproctol* 2014;18:699–708.
23. Garcia-Aguilar J et al. *Ann Surg Oncol.* 2011;19(2): 384–91.
24. Habr-Gama A et al. *Dis Colon Rectum.* 2017;60: 586–94.
25. Habr-Gama A et al. *Dis Colon Rectum.* 2013;56: 264–6.
26. Bosset J-F et al. *J Clin Oncol.* 2005;23(24):5620–7.
27. Radu C et al. *Radiother Oncol.* 2008;87(3):343–9.
28. Wiltshire KL et al. *Radiat Oncol Biol.* 2006;64(3): 709–16.
29. Jakobsen A et al. *Int J Radiat Oncol Biol Phys.* 2012; 84(4):949–54.
30. Gerard J-P et al. *Acta Oncol.* 2015;54(4):545–51.
31. Appelt AL et al. *Lancet Oncol.* 2015;16(8):919–27.
32. Vuong T et al. *Clin Oncol (R Coll Radiol).* 2007;19(9): 701–5.
33. Schrag D et al. *J Clin Oncol.* 2014;32(6):513–8.
34. Habr-Gama A et al. *Colorectal Cancer.* 2015;4(1):1–4.
35. Habr-Gama A et al. *Dis Colon Rectum.* 2009;52(12): 1927–34.
36. Patel UB et al. *Ann Surg Oncol.* 2012;19:2842–52.
37. Francois Y et al. *J Clin Oncol.* 1999;17(8):2396.
38. Tulchinsky H et al. *Ann Surg Oncol.* 2008;15(10): 2661–7.
39. Kalady MF et al. *Ann Surg.* 2009;250:582–9.
40. Evans J et al. *Dis Colon Rectum.* 2011;54(10):1251–9.
41. Wolthuis AM et al. *Ann Surg Oncol.* 2012;19(9): 2833–41.
42. Garcia-Aguilar J et al. *Lancet Oncol.* 2015;16(8): 957–66.
43. Lefevre JH et al. *J Clin Oncol.* 2016;34(31):3773–80.
44. Perez RO et al. *Int J Radiat Oncol Biol Phys.* 2012; 84(5):1159–65.
45. Perez RO et al. *Colorect Dis.* 2012;14(6):714–20.
46. Lambregts DMJ et al. *Dis Colon Rectum.* 2011; 54(12):1521–8.
47. Patel UB et al. *J Clin Oncol.* 2011;29(28):3753–60.
48. Patel UB et al. *Ann Surg Oncol.* 2012;19(9):2842–52.
49. Nahas SC et al. *Dis Colon Rectum.* 2016;59(4): 255–63.
50. Smith FM et al. *Dis Colon Rectum.* 2014;57(3):311–5.

51. Bhoday J et al. *Dis Colon Rectum.* 2016;59(10): 925–33.
52. Lambregts DMJ et al. *Ann Surg Oncol.* 2011;18(8): 2224–31.
53. Curvo-Semedo L et al. *Radiology.* 2011;260(3):734–43.
54. Anjos Dos DA et al. *Ann Nucl Med.* 2016;30(8): 513–7.
55. Cascini GL et al. *J Nucl Med.* 2006;47(8):1241–8.
56. Kristiansen C et al. *Dis Colon Rectum.* 2008;51(1): 21–5.
57. Anjos Dos DA et al. *Dis Colon Rectum.* 2016;59(9): 805–12.
58. Vaccaro CA et al. *Cirugía Española.* 2016;94(5): 274–9.
59. Araujo ROC et al. *Eur J Surg Oncol.* 2015;41(11): 1456–63.
60. Maas M et al. *J Clin Oncol.* 2011;29(35):4633–40.
61. Dalton RSJ et al. *Colorect Dis.* 2012;14(5):567–71.
62. Smith RK et al. *Int J Colorectal Dis.* 2015;30(6):769–74.
63. Renehan AG et al. *Lancet Oncol.* 2016;17(2):174–83.
64. Perez RO et al. *Dis Colon Rectum.* 2013;56:6–13.
65. Habr-Gama A et al. *Rad Oncol Biol Phys.* 2008;71(4): 1181–8.
66. Perez RO. *Lancet Oncol.* 2016;17(2):125–6.
67. Maas M et al. *Lancet Oncol.* 2010;11(9):835–44.
68. Bach SP et al. *Br J Surg.* 2009;96(3):280–90.
69. Marks JH et al. *Surg Endosc.* 2009;23:1081–7.
70. Morino M et al. *Surg Endosc.* 2013;27:3315–21.
71. Hompes R et al. *Colorectal Dis.* 2013;15:e576–81.
72. Perez RO et al. *Dis Colon Rectum.* 2013;56(1):6–13.
73. Smith FM et al. *Dis Colon Rectum.* 2017;60(2):228–39.
74. Garcia-Aguilar J et al. *Ann Surg.* 2011;254:97–102.
75. Park IJ et al. *Dis Colon Rectum.* 2013;56:135–41.
76. Mignanelli ED et al. *Dis Colon Rectum.* 2010;53:251–6.
77. Perez RO et al. *Dis Colon Rectum.* 2011;54:545–51.
78. Bujko K et al. *Radiother Oncol.* 2013;106:198–205.

# 31

# Indications and outcomes for treatment of recurrent rectal cancer and colorectal liver/lung metastases

LUANNE M. FORCE AND DAVID J. MARON

## CHALLENGING CASE

An 85-year-old female patient presents a previous history of T3N1M0 rectal cancer 1 cm from the dentate line invasive into the internal and external anal sphincters. She underwent neoadjuvant chemoradiation therapy followed by an abdominoperineal resection two years prior to presentation, followed by adjuvant chemotherapy. On surveillance imaging she was found to have a pelvic mass with a PET avid lesion in the presacral area, consistent with local recurrence. MRI of the pelvis demonstrates a pelvic recurrence invasive into the posterior wall of the vagina and possibly the uterus, as well as the lower coccygeal segment. Metastatic work-up demonstrates no distant metastatic disease.

## CASE MANAGEMENT

The patient's case was discussed at the multidisciplinary tumor board. After reviewing the radiology images, the margins of resection along the pelvic sidewall were deemed to be free from tumor. As she has had previous radiation therapy, she was not a candidate for additional radiation treatment. The patient was brought to the operating room for a complete pelvic exenteration, with en bloc resection of the pelvic mass, uterus, posterior vagina and distal sacrum in combination with gynecology and neurosurgery. Once the pelvic mass was removed, the pelvis was reconstructed with a vertical rectus abdominis myocutaneous (VRAM) flap by plastic surgery. Pathology showed an invasive rectal adenocarcinoma into the vagina and distal sacrum, with margins completely free of tumor and no positive lymphadenopathy. The postoperative course was uneventful. Subsequent surveillance PET scan and CEA levels did not show any further recurrence.

## RECURRENT RECTAL CANCER

The management of rectal cancer has changed dramatically over the past 40 years, resulting in a significant reduction in the incidence of locally recurrent rectal cancer. Local recurrence rates historically were 20%–40%, but with the use of improved adjuvant, neoadjuvant, and surgical strategies, the local recurrence rate has been reduced to 4%–8% (1). The majority of patients with recurrent rectal cancer will present within 3 years; 70% will present within 2 years and 85% within 3 years (1). The management of locally recurrent rectal cancer is complex, and management needs to be tailored to the individual patient.

The risk of local recurrence increases with margin positivity, including distal and radial margins. A margin of 5 mm has been correlated with a reduced local recurrence rate; however, no additional benefit for margins greater than 5 mm has been reported (2). Pathologic characteristics of the tumor, specifically lymphovascular invasion and poor differentiation, also increase the risk of local recurrence (3). Surgeon experience and caseload have also been associated with rectal cancer outcomes; higher-volume surgeons (>10–12 cases per year) have better local recurrence rates when compared to surgeons who perform these operations less often (4). Abdominoperineal resection, compared to low anterior resection, has also been shown to have a higher recurrence rate, likely related to a higher rate of circumferential margin positivity (5). There is some evidence that colon perforation during resection for rectal cancer also significantly increases the risk for local recurrence (6).

## INITIAL EVALUATION

Most patients with local recurrence will present within 3 years after treatment rectal cancer. About 25% of these patients will be asymptomatic, with the recurrence detected by surveillance imaging or carcinoembryonic antigen (CEA) levels (7). Patients may present with bleeding, likely related to an intraluminal recurrence at the anastomosis. Recurrence may also manifest itself as a change of bowel habits or complete bowel obstruction. Pain as a presenting symptom is more worrisome and may indicate invasion or compression of surrounding structures such as nerves or bone (1). Significant pain on presentation has been correlated with worse survival outcomes when compared to those patients who do not have pain as a presenting symptom (8).

The first step in evaluation of a patient with recurrent rectal cancer is a thorough review of the patient's medical record and treatment history. Operative reports, treatment history, and comorbidities are all essential to plan further intervention. Physical examination may reveal lymphadenopathy or hepatomegaly. Rectal exam, when possible, is also important to characterize the extent and fixity of the tumor. It has been reported that tumor fixity in more than one area is correlated with significantly lower survival rates (8). Vaginal exam should be performed in women to determine if the vaginal wall is involved. If the patient is too uncomfortable to permit an exam in the office, the patient should undergo an examination under anesthesia before any intervention is planned (1). Laboratory values should be obtained, including a CEA level. A high CEA level at time of diagnosis may indicate distant metastatic disease and a poorer prognosis (9). Other laboratory values, including hemoglobin, nutritional parameters, and kidney function should also be investigated prior to any planned intervention (1). An elevated creatinine level may suggest ureteral compression or involvement by the tumor and should be evaluated preoperatively. Full endoscopic evaluation of the colon should be performed to detect any intraluminal recurrence, obtain tissue biopsy, and assess for other colonic lesions prior to intervention.

Imaging studies are essential in the evaluation and management of recurrent rectal cancer. It is imperative to perform a metastatic workup, as up to 50% of these patients will present with systemic metastasis (2). Computed tomography (CT) scan of the chest, abdomen, and pelvis should be performed to diagnose systemic metastasis, as the presence of distant metastasis may change management. A positron emission tomography (PET) scan should also be performed, which will give information about distant metastasis and will also characterize the recurrence (10,11). CT scan and magnetic resonance imaging (MRI) may provide anatomic information regarding local recurrence; however, these methods are not able to identify scar versus a new recurrence. PET scan may help differentiate these two processes, with an accuracy of 87% in previous studies (12). PET scan when combined with CT of the chest, abdomen, and pelvis have a combined sensitivity and specificity of 100% and 96%, respectively (9).

Local staging should also be performed with preoperative imaging. This step is essential to delineate the patient's anatomy, involvement of surrounding structures, and potential resectability. CT scan of the abdomen and pelvis is inferior for local staging when compared to MRI (12). CT scan does not accurately define invasion into surrounding structures likely due to the inability to differentiate scar from tumor (13). MRI is more accurate when determining local invasion, with a specificity of 70%–100%. Signal intensity on MRI provides a more detailed image, allowing better differentiation between normal tissue, scar, and tumor on T1- and T2-weighted images. Recurrent tumor will typically have a higher signal intensity on T2-weighted images (14). Invasion into surrounding structures can be reliably detected with reasonable sensitivity and specificity for most surrounding structures. An exception is invasion into the pelvic sidewall, which has a higher false-positive rate (14). Accuracy has been shown to improve when these images are enhanced with gadolinium (15).

Confirmation of the recurrence should be performed with tissue biopsy whenever possible (1,13,12). Prior to resection, the presence of a recurrence should be differentiated from other processes such as fibrosis. If the recurrence is intraluminal, tissue biopsy may be performed by endoscopy. If there is an extraluminal recurrence, CT-guided biopsy of the mass should be performed prior to undergoing resection (1). In some cases, tissue biopsy may be inconclusive or not possible. In these situations, PET/CT in combination with CEA levels and MRI can accurately detect local recurrence with a sensitivity of 84%–100% and specificity of 80%–100% (11).

Evaluation of each patient with recurrent rectal cancer should include a multidisciplinary team review (12). Evaluation by a team of specialists including colorectal surgeons, oncologists, radiation oncologists, radiologists, and pathologists has been shown to provide superior outcomes in the management of these highly complex patients. A recent study by Kontovousnisios et al. showed that the use of a multidisciplinary team can improve the outcomes of patients treated with recurrent rectal cancer, with the ability to achieve an R0 resection in 90% of patients (16).

Recurrences should be classified based on their location. Axial recurrences are those centrally located, which do not involve the anterior, posterior, or lateral walls of the pelvis; this includes anastomotic recurrences. Anterior recurrences invade the bladder, prostate, seminal vesicles in males, and the vagina in female patients. Posterior recurrences invade the sacrum or coccyx. Lateral recurrences involve the lateral sidewalls of the pelvis, which may involve structures such as the ureters, iliac vessels, and pelvic nerves. Classifying the tumor based on its anatomic location will help plan operative intervention, as well as determine resectability (17).

## MANAGEMENT

Management of recurrent rectal cancer is best achieved by a multimodal approach. Combined radiotherapy, chemotherapy, and surgery offers the best chance to achieve a curative resection. In addition, multiple surgical specialties are required to manage these complex patients. The ultimate goal is to achieve an R0 surgical resection, which will provide the patient the best chance for cure. Many factors must be taken into account, including the functional status of the patient, the feasibility of resection, as well as expected quality of life with or without the resection.

Neoadjuvant treatment should be initiated in suitable patients who are being considered for resection. Chemotherapy and radiation may downstage the tumor, increasing the likelihood for an R0 resection. If the patient has not undergone previous radiation treatment, pelvic radiation for a total of 50 Gy should be administered in conjunction with chemotherapy. Surgery can then be performed 6–8 weeks following completion of the radiotherapy. If the patient previously received radiation to the pelvis, there is evidence that an additional dose of radiation could be beneficial (18). Acute toxicity has been shown to be relatively low, up to 7% in some series. The incidence of delayed toxicity could be up to 17% (8,18). Reirradiation is associated with a greater chance at achieving an R0 resection, which will impact local control as well as disease-free survival at 42%–60% at 5 years (18). There is limited data regarding timing and dosing of additional radiation treatments, so treatment should be tailored to each individual patient.

Surgical intervention is the cornerstone of treatment for recurrent rectal cancer. The ability to achieve an R0 resection will confer the best survival benefit to the patient (19). Planning is key, and imaging should be reviewed to determine resectability and the involvement of adjacent structures. Care must be taken to avoid R2 resections, which confer no survival benefit to the patient and have a high complication rate (19). Anterior recurrences are more amenable to curative resection when compared to posterior and lateral recurrences due to lack of involved bone and vascular structures. The ability to achieve a complete resection in anterior recurrences ranges from 70% to 90%. This is compared to 6%–36% when the pelvic sidewall is involved (20). Resection is contraindicated in patients who are medically unfit to undergo a major operation. Sacral invasion above S2 is also a contraindication due to the involvement of neurovascular structures (21). Resection at this level is often incomplete and has significant morbidity. Similarly, encasement of the external iliac arteries, fixity in multiple locations, and circumferential involvement are all indications that a complete resection cannot be achieved without causing significant morbidity to the patient. There are several reports of concurrent vascular resection and reconstruction for rectal cancer, which have been performed in specialized centers with reasonable results (22). Unresectable distant metastasis such as lung and liver metastases are also a relative contraindication to curative resection.

The location of the recurrence will determine the operative approach and strategy. These operations often require multiple specialties including urology, gynecology, and plastic surgery. Cystoscopy with bilateral ureteral stents is often beneficial in assessing bladder involvement and to facilitate intraoperative identification of the ureters. All operations should begin with exploration of the abdomen and determination of the extent of disease or peritoneal carcinomatosis if present. Laparoscopy in this situation can be helpful in avoiding a laparotomy if resection is aborted due to the presence of carcinomatosis. Identification of major structures including vessels and ureters should also be carried out. Resection of the bladder may be performed en bloc with reconstruction by an experienced urologist. The survival rate after en bloc resection of recurrent cancer and bladder is 61% with negative margins, compared with 17% of patients with positive margins (11). In women, invasion of the uterus or vaginal structures must be assessed. Hysterectomy should be performed if there is invasion into the uterus (23). Low recurrences in women may necessitate partial or complete vaginectomy. In cases where <50% of the vagina is resected, the vagina can be closed primarily (23). If a more extensive resection is performed, flap closure by a plastic surgeon may be required. One report showed that anterior exenteration along with en bloc resection of the pubic bone may also be feasible if an R0 resection is achieved (24).

Posterior resections often involve sacrectomy if the lesion is located below S2. Identification and protection of the ureters and major vessels is important when performing a sacrectomy. Depending on the level of resection, the approach may be a combined abdominal and perineal approach. Bilateral internal iliac arteries may be ligated and resected to decrease blood loss during these procedures. Involvement of the ureter will require resection and reimplantation or reconstruction by an experienced urologist. These resections will often leave a large perineal defect requiring muscle flap closure by plastic surgery. Once involvement of the sacrum is identified in the operating room, an examination of the nerve roots should be performed to determine resectability. The ability to achieve R0 resection at a level above S2 is highly unlikely (23), but there have been several small series at specialized centers that demonstrate that it may be feasible (25). If a high sacrectomy is performed, sacral bony stabilization may be required (25). Once the tumor is completely mobilized and all adjacent surrounding organs resected en bloc, the patient will need to be placed in the prone position so sacrectomy can be completed (23), as this allows better exposure and a wider excision than what can be done in lithotomy. The colostomy may be matured, as well as harvesting of muscle flaps prior to turning the patient prone. Once prone, the perineal dissection is begun, and the sacrotuberous and sacrospinous ligaments are taken down. The level of resection may be confirmed by fluoroscopy. Care must be taken to ensure that the dural sac is closed, usually done in conjunction with an orthopedic or neurosurgeon (9,23). As a large tissue defect may be left behind, the space may be filled with a pedicled omental flap, biologic mesh, or muscle flap performed by a plastic surgeon (23). The complication rate for resections with combined sacrectomy is high, 82% in some series (26).

Lateral recurrences have the lowest chance of achieving an R0 resection (23). Tumors that invade the lateral walls of the pelvis have a high incidence of invading structures such as the ureters and iliac vessels. More recently, en bloc resection of one or more iliac vessels has been shown to have an R0 resection rate of 40%–53% in experienced centers (22,27). These studies are based on a relatively small subset of patients, and care must therefore be taken to choose appropriate patients prior to undertaking resection.

Intraoperative radiotherapy may be beneficial for the treatment of recurrent rectal cancer. Multiple series have demonstrated a survival benefit, as well as locoregional control at specialized centers (28). Directed radiation therapy minimizes the radiation effect to the surrounding structures and provides concentrated radiation directly to the area of treatment. The largest benefit has been shown in patients who have close margins, <5 mm (1,29). Intraoperative frozen section is performed to determine the margin of resection. Intraoperative doses of 1000–2000 cGy can be administered, depending on the amount of residual disease. Radiation can be administered via external-beam or high-dose brachytherapy, which is dependent on the location of the treatment area and positioning of the beam. In some cases, intraoperative radiotherapy cannot be performed due to logistical reasons. The brachytherapy applicator may conform better to the patient's anatomy (1).

Perineal reconstruction is often required after curative resection for recurrent rectal cancer. The incidence of wound complications is high, up to 40% of patients. Reasons for perineal wound failure are multiple, including large defects, irradiated tissue, and patient comorbidities. A large defect that cannot be closed primarily will require a muscle flap closure. The most common flap performed is a vertical rectus abdominus myocutaneous (VRAM) flap (23). This flap will provide a bulky flap to fill in large defects, such as after a vaginectomy. The location of any stomas must be considered when using a VRAM flap, especially in patients who will require both a colostomy and a urostomy (30). Other flaps include gracilis and gluteus flaps, which may be used to fill in smaller defects. In patients with bilateral stomas and large tissue defects, a free flap may be required; the most common free flap is a latissimus dorsi flap (9). Another attractive option for perineal reconstruction is the placement of a biologic mesh (1,23). This is most feasible when there is sufficient tissue to close the perineal defect but a large defect exists in the pelvic floor. The mesh may be placed circumferentially in the pelvis, with an omental flap if available, to prevent a perineal hernia (31).

Complication rates for recurrent rectal cancer resection are high, up to 80% in some series (26). The 30-day mortality rate ranges among reported series. A recent systematic review showed a wide range of mortality and complication rates, 0%–25% and 37%–100%, respectively (32). The median 30-day survival rate was 2.2% (32). Perineal wound complications are the most frequent postoperative complication among this population. These include perineal wound breakdown, dehiscence, and flap necrosis or failure. Wound infection is relatively common. Pelvic accesses and fluid collections may also occur, which can often be treated with CT-guided drainage. Concomitant sacrectomy increases the complication rate significantly (26). Urologic complications are also common, including ureteric injury or stenosis. This is often best treated with ureteral stents. Bladder dysfunction is also common.

## PALLIATIVE TREATMENT

Palliative operations may be performed for symptomatic patients who are not candidates for curative resection. The goal of palliative treatment is to alleviate some of the patient's symptoms related to the recurrent cancer. Most commonly, this is pain related to invasion of bone or nerves, bowel obstruction, or bleeding. Palliative radiation may help alleviate pain and bleeding (33,34). Intraluminal metallic stents can be used to alleviate obstruction (33). These can be used when the obstruction is at least 5 cm above the dentate line (35), as patients may experience significant complications with stent placement below that level, including pain, tenesmus, and migration (1,36). In cases where stent placement is not possible or has failed, diverting colostomy may be performed. Ureteral stents may be placed if there is significant ureteral obstruction. Pelvic exenteration for palliation should be avoided, as symptoms are rarely improved by this technique (37). There is some evidence that an R1 resection may provide some benefit to quality of life, but there was deleterious effect on quality of life if an R2 resection is performed (38).

## OUTCOMES

Survival rates for treatment of recurrent rectal cancer vary between 25% and 36% at 5 years for patients undergoing multimodal treatment (9). Ability to achieve negative margins will improve survival significantly, with reported survival rates of 37%–60% at 5 years (5,8,19,39). If macroscopic disease is left behind, survival rates drop to 10%–16% (5,8). Neoadjuvant chemotherapy and radiation treatment has also been shown to confer a survival benefit in these patients.

A large series from the Mayo Clinic demonstrated an R0 resection was able to be achieved in 45% of patients and that survival was significantly decreased for patients with residual macroscopic disease (8). Nielsen et al. reported outcomes for 213 patients, with a R0 resection rate of 61%. The authors demonstrated a 5-year survival rate of 40% for R0 resections, and survival was significantly lower for patients with previous abdominoperineal resections (40). A meta-analysis of 22 studies also confirmed a significant survival advantage for those patients who were able to undergo R0 resections (41). Overall, R0 resection was obtained in 53% of patients, which correlated with a survival benefit of an additional 37 months compared to patients who underwent an R2 resection (41). Quality of life for patients undergoing resections for recurrent rectal cancer is an important consideration. One study noted a significant decrease in quality of life for patients undergoing R1/2 resections when compared to R0 resections (42).

Extensive resection requiring major vascular resection for recurrent rectal cancer has been reported in some small series. En bloc iliac resection with reconstruction has been shown to be feasible and safe in specialized centers. One study by Brown et al. reported a morbidity rate of 52% with a median survival of 26–24 months (27). Another study by Abdelsattar et al. also demonstrated that an R0 resection can be achieved with en bloc resection of tumors involving the aortoiliac axis (22). The authors demonstrated a survival rate of 45% at 4 years. These small series show that vascular resection and reconstruction can achieve an R0 resection with acceptable results in highly selected patients.

Outcomes after sacral resection have also been reported. Milne et al. reported outcomes for sacrectomy for recurrent rectal cancer, with a R0 resection rate of 74% (26). Patients with an R0 resection were shown to have a survival rate of 45 months, versus 19 months for R1 and 8 months for R2 resections. The authors reported a complication rate of 80% (26). Another series of 30 patients undergoing sacral resections for recurrent rectal cancer demonstrated a R0 resection rate of 93%, with a 5-year survival rate of 46% for R0 resections (43). Another small series of nine patients assessed survival for patients undergoing high sacrectomy. Patients had an average survival of 31 months, with all deaths occurring secondary to metastatic disease (25).

Intraoperative radiation treatment (IORT) has also been shown to be beneficial, with an increase in survival of 15% in some series (23). The survival rate at 5 years has been reported as 30%–70% for patients treated with IORT with an R0 resection. This benefit decreases significantly for R1 or R2 resections, with a survival rate at 5 years of 7%–20%. However, these survival rates are improved over reported rates in patients who underwent R2 resections without IORT. Most authors debate the utility of intraoperative radiotherapy for resection margins >5 mm, advocating for treatment when microscopic margins are close intraoperatively (1,29). A recent meta-analysis performed showed that there is significant heterogeneity of studies for IORT, but that overall there is a survival benefit for these patients (28).

A French multi-institutional randomized trial, however, failed to show any benefit for intraoperative radiotherapy compared to radical resection (44).

Recurrent rectal cancer is a complex clinical problem. Extensive workup evaluating for distant metastasis and local invasion is extremely important when planning surgical intervention. Multimodal treatment with chemotherapy, radiation, and surgery, possibly combined with intraoperative radiation therapy, is the cornerstone of treatment for recurrent rectal cancer. A multidisciplinary treatment team is essential to evaluate and plan the treatment of these complex patients. Surgery is the mainstay of curative resection, with significantly better outcomes if an R0 resection can be achieved. When possible, all invaded organs and structures should be resected en bloc, and collaboration with multiple surgical subspecialists is often required. If an R0 or R1 resection cannot be performed, palliative options may be undertaken. Palliative chemotherapy, radiation, and endoluminal stents may help alleviate some symptoms.

## COLORECTAL LIVER METASTASIS

Despite improved screening programs, approximately 20% of all patients presenting with a new diagnosis of colorectal cancer will have synchronous liver metastasis (45). The survival of these patients is dependent on the ability to treat the primary as well as metastatic lesions. Several treatment options exist to manage the outcomes of these patients. The conventional approach involved resection of the primary tumor followed by adjuvant chemotherapy and resection or ablation of liver lesions. A second option is simultaneous resection of both the primary and the metastatic lesions. The third algorithm involves a liver first approach, where the liver metastases are resected and the primary tumor is left until after adjuvant chemotherapy is completed. This option may involve neoadjuvant chemotherapy or resection followed by chemotherapy (46). In addition, there are several other techniques employed to ablate liver metastases that are not amenable to surgical resection (47). Unfortunately, very few patients meet the criteria for curative resection, about 20% of those presenting with liver metastases (48,49).

## LIVER RESECTION

### PRIMARY FIRST APPROACH

The traditional, primary first, approach involves resection of the primary tumor followed by chemotherapy and management of the metastatic disease (50). Advocates of the primary first strategy seek to avoid complications related to the primary tumor during adjuvant chemotherapy. Complications such as obstruction or perforation often cause increased morbidity in patients undergoing active chemotherapy regimens. Another purported advantage of this approach is to rid the patient of the primary tumor, likely a source for subsequent metastases (46,45). The problem with this strategy is that complications related to the resection of the primary tumor often delay initiation of chemotherapy in these patients, decreasing overall survival (51). Furthermore, several studies have shown that primary chemotherapy for patients with unresectable metastatic disease can have direct benefits on the primary tumor (decreased bleeding or obstruction) without surgical intervention (52).

## SIMULTANEOUS APPROACH

The simultaneous approach aims at resecting the primary tumor as well as the liver metastases at the same operation. Justification for this strategy is to perform the curative resection in one operation, followed by adjuvant chemotherapy (53–55). Outcomes for this approach have been variable in the literature. Several studies have shown that there may be an increased morbidity rate from performing simultaneous bowel and liver resections. Most notably, increases in infectious complications and anastomotic leaks have been reported (50,53,56). A study by Broquet et al. demonstrated a similar complication and survival rate for simultaneous, combined, and reverse liver strategies. All of the strategies employed had a mortality rate of 3%–5%, with a morbidity rate of 30%–50%. The authors demonstrated a 5-year survival rate of 39%–55% for all three strategies (50). A recent systematic review by Lykoudis et al. also demonstrated that all three strategies had similar outcomes (57). Several other large studies, including a large meta-analysis and a multi-institutional analysis also found similar outcomes comparing simultaneous versus staged resections (54,58,59). Many of the studies on simultaneous resection have a selection bias toward smaller lesions. A study by Tanaka et al. demonstrated that the volume of liver resected had an impact on overall complication rates (53). The authors found that if more than a section of liver was resected or a patient's age was over 70 years, worse outcomes were seen (53). Another study demonstrated a cost benefit in those undergoing simultaneous resection, with 6 days fewer in the hospital (60). In general, simultaneous resections should be performed for a highly select group of patients, preferably those with small resectable liver metastasis and good functional status (46,58,61).

## LIVER FIRST APPROACH

The liver first approach is a more recent strategy that has been employed to manage colorectal liver metastasis (62). The major determinant of overall survival is the control of the metastatic disease (50,63). With this approach, the liver is managed first with subsequent intervention for the primary tumor later (46); however, neoadjuvant chemotherapy may be employed prior to the liver resection, particularly if the tumor is large. If the primary tumor is relatively asymptomatic, delaying the resection of the primary tumor can be done safely while the patient undergoes chemotherapy (51). There is some debate in the literature as to whether neoadjuvant chemotherapy is required prior to resection of the liver metastasis. If the lesion is resectable at initial presentation, there are several studies that show neoadjuvant chemotherapy may not have a survival benefit for the patient (64,65). If the tumor is unresectable at initial presentation, neoadjuvant chemotherapy followed by restaging and liver resection is appropriate (64). A recent systematic review of published studies showed that the liver first approach was feasible and safe, and had an overall median survival of 40 months (66). An international consensus group in 2012 noted that the liver first strategy is as good as other methods for the treatment of synchronous colorectal liver metastases (67). The group advocated for preoperative chemotherapy for as short a duration as possible, followed by liver resection in select cases. In general, the liver first approach is good for patients with large metastatic disease burden in the liver and a relatively asymptomatic primary tumor. The goal is to initiate systemic treatment as soon as possible and achieve an R0 resection (46,67).

Overall, multiple systematic reviews have been performed comparing the traditional, simultaneous, and liver first approaches. These reviews have all failed to demonstrate that one method is superior over the other in terms of overall survival for the patient (46,53,54,57,59), and therefore, treatment of synchronous liver metastasis must be tailored to the individual patient. A multidisciplinary evaluation is essential in determining the optimal treatment plan for each patient. A traditional primary first approach may be the most beneficial for patients with a symptomatic primary tumor—those who are at high risk for obstruction, perforation, or those continuing to have gastrointestinal bleeding. A simultaneous approach seems to work best for those patients with small disease burden in the liver that require only minor hepatic resections. A liver first approach may be best for those patients with a large burden of metastatic disease in the liver, with a relatively asymptomatic primary tumor (46,49,50,53,54,59).

## LIVER ABLATION

There are multiple liver ablation techniques employed to treat liver metastases, including radiofrequency ablation (RFA), ethanol ablation, as well as chemoembolization with hepatic intra-arterial embolization (HAI). These strategies are all employed to treat lesions that may not be amenable to surgical resection, such as those that will result insufficient liver function, those that have hepatic dysfunction, or those not suitable to undergo hepatic resection secondary to comorbidities (68). Ablation may be performed open, laparoscopically or percutaneously, with the open technique having the best results (69). However, these results are also dependent on the experience of the physician performing the ablation (69).

RFA is the most widely utilized of these techniques. Results for RFA as a primary treatment for liver metastases have been shown to be inferior to curative resection (70,71) and survival outcomes for those undergoing RFA when compared to surgical resection are significantly lower. One study compared outcomes for resection, RFA, or a combined approach. The authors found a survival rate of 65% at 4 years for those undergoing resection versus 36% for combined therapy and 22% for those undergoing RFA alone (70). While the survival for RFA alone is low, it still represents a significant improvement over no intervention for the metastatic disease. Another study by Siperstein et al. showed a similar outcome. The authors found that the number and size of metastases as well as CEA levels were strong prognostic factors. They demonstrated an overall survival rate of 18.4% for patients undergoing RFA, which was improved over nonsurgical therapies (72). RFA as a first-line treatment compared to surgical resection has also been evaluated. One study found a significantly higher local recurrence rate for patients undergoing RFA, however, very little difference in terms of overall survival (47). A systematic review done in 2010 as well as a Cochrane Review in 2012 concluded that the research done on RFA is limited to small, mostly retrospective data. The reviews found that survival rates in the literature are highly variable, 14%–55%, and most studies had highly variable patient selection criteria. These studies conclude that more research should be done to recommend RFA over resection (73,74). Overall, RFA is a good treatment technique for those not amenable to resection and can offer a survival benefit compared to no intervention (68).

Hepatic chemoembolization techniques are employed for patients who are not amenable to surgical resection or RFA techniques (75). This method directly delivers chemotherapy to the metastatic lesion via the hepatic artery, which has been shown to minimize systemic effects of the chemotherapy (76). Overall, the results in the literature have been highly variable. One multi-institutional trial showed HAI had some survival benefit in those failing systemic chemotherapy, with a median survival rate of 19 months (77). A Cochrane Review in 2009 showed a modest survival benefit for this treatment (78).

Survival of patients with metastatic colorectal disease to the liver is directly dependent on the ability to treat the metastatic disease. Many techniques have been employed to achieve the best survival rate for these patients. Overall, resection provides the best chance for curative treatment. The timing and method of resection is highly variable, and should be determined on a case-by-case basis in conjunction with a multidisciplinary team. If a curative resection is not possible, ablative techniques should be employed to improve the overall survival for the patient.

## PULMONARY METASTASIS

While the liver is the most common site of metastatic disease, lung metastases are seen in approximately 10%–15% of patients with metastatic disease (79). Rectal cancer patients are more likely to have lung metastasis than colon cancer patients, a finding that is likely related to the systemic venous drainage of the rectum via the inferior and middle rectal veins. The incidence of lung metastasis without liver metastasis is relatively low, reported to be around 1.7%–7% (79). In patients undergoing curative resection for rectal cancer, greater than four lateral pelvic lymph nodes involved or the presence of lateral pelvic lymph nodes bilaterally were shown to be risk factors for pulmonary metastases (80). In cases where there is metastatic disease to the lung, only 10% of those patients will be amenable to surgical resection (81).

Resection of the metastatic disease, when feasible, is the best chance for curative treatment. In one population-based study, survival improved for patients undergoing metastectomy for pulmonary metastasis from 11% to 53% over 3 years for synchronous metastases and from 13% to 59% for metachronous metastases (82). However, only 4% of synchronous and 14% of metachronous metastases were resected for cure. The authors of this study also confirmed that rectal cancer patients have a higher incidence of lung metastasis compared to colon cancer patients (82). Another study by Kim et al. demonstrated a 3- and 5-year survival rate of 54% and 30%, respectively, for patients undergoing curative metastectomy. The authors also determined that the absence of adjuvant chemotherapy, extrapulmonary metastases, elevated CEA level, and absence of pulmonary resection were all indicators of a poor prognosis (83). Suzuki et al. reported a 5-year survival rate of 45% for patients undergoing surgical resection of pulmonary metastases. This study also found that an elevated CEA level was a prognostic factor; patients with a normal CEA had a 5-year survival of 57%, compared to 30% of those with an elevated CEA level (84). Many of these studies are small and retrospective; however, there is currently a randomized control trial underway (85).

Metastectomy for synchronous liver and lung metastases has been evaluated in some small series. These series show the greatest benefit for patients undergoing both liver and lung resection, if the lesions are detected sequentially. Patients who underwent pulmonary and liver metastectomy had a survival rate of 44% if the lesions were detected sequentially, compared to 0% when they were detected simultaneously (86). Another retrospective study also confirmed this observation. The authors found that patients undergoing pulmonary metastectomy had better outcomes for metachronous lesions with a survival rate of 60%, compared to 0% for synchronous lesions (87). The studies on concurrent liver and lung metastases are limited to small, retrospective series.

Pulmonary metastases, although relatively rare when compared to liver metastases, also benefit from curative resection if the patient is a surgical candidate. Unfortunately, very few patients will meet the criteria for surgical intervention. For those who do meet criteria, there is a relatively good survival rate of 40%–50% in the literature for patients undergoing pulmonary metastectomy.

# REFERENCES

1. Bouchard P, Efron J. *Ann Surg Oncol.* 2010;17: 1343–56.
2. Kim YW et al. *J Surg Oncol.* 2009;99:58–64.
3. Ogiwara H et al. *Ann Surg Oncol.* 1994;1:99–104.
4. Stocchi L et al. *J Clin Oncol.* 2001;19:3895–902.
5. Heriot AG et al. *Dis Colon Rectum.* 2008;51:284–91.
6. Bulow S et al. *Colorectal Dis.* 2011;13:1256–64.
7. Palmer G et al. *Ann Surg Oncol.* 2007;14:447–54.
8. Hanloser D et al. *Ann Surg.* 2002;237(4):502–8.
9. Troja A et al. *Int J Colorectal Dis.* 2015;30:1157–63.
10. Watson AJ et al. *Dis Colon Rectum.* 2007;50:102–14.
11. Chessin DB et al. *J Am Coll Surg.* 2005;201:948–56.
12. Tekkis P. *Br J Surg.* 2013;100:1009–14.
13. Beets-Tan, RG et al. *Abd Imaging.* 2000;25:533–41.
14. Messiou C et al. *Br J Radiol.* 2008;81(966):468–73.
15. Colosio A et al. *J M Res Imag.* 2014;40:306–13.
16. Kontovounisios C et al. *Colorectal Dis.* 2017; 331–338.
17. Courtney D et al. *Langenbecks Arch Surg.* 2014;399: 33–40.
18. VanderMeji W et al. *Dis Colon Rectum.* 2016;59: 148–56.
19. Alberda WJ et al. *Dis Colon Rectum.* 2015;58:677–85.
20. Moore HG et al. *Dis Colon Rectum.* 2006;49:1257–75.
21. Kanemitsu Y et al. *Dis Colon Rectum.* 2010;53:779–89.
22. Abdelsattar ZM et al. *Dis Colon Rectum.* 2013;56: 711–6.
23. Mirnezami AH et al. *Dis Colon Rectum.* 2010;53: 1248–57.
24. Austin KKS et al. *Dis Colon Rectum.* 2016;59(9): 831–5.
25. Dozois EJ et al. *J Surg Oncol.* 2011;103(2):105–9.
26. Milne T et al. *Ann Surg.* 2013;258(6):1007–13.
27. Brown KGM et al. *Dis Colon Rectum.* 2015;58:850–6.
28. Mirnezami R et al. *Surg Oncol.* 2013;22:22–35.
29. Ferenschild FTJ et al. *Dis Colon Rectum.* 2006;49: 1257–65.
30. Moriya Y. *Jpn J Clin Oncol.* 2006;36(3):127–31.
31. Jensen KK et al. *Colorectal Dis.* 2014;16(3):192–7.
32. Yang TX et al. *Dis Colon Rectum.* 2013;56:519–31.
33. Willett CG, Gunderson LL. *J Gastrointest Surg.* 2004; 8(3):277–9.
34. Saltz LB. *J Gastroint Surg.* 2004;8(3):274–6.
35. Song HY et al. *Gastrointest Endosc.* 2008;68(4):713–20.
36. Kim EJ, Kim YJ. *World J Gastroenterol.* 2016;22(2): 842–52.
37. Quyn AJ et al. *Dis Colon Rectum.* 2016;59:1005–10.
38. Pacelli F et al. *Ann Surg Oncol.* 2010;17:152–62.
39. Rahbari NN et al. *Ann Surg.* 2011;253(3):522–33.
40. Nielson M et al. *Ann Surg Oncol.* 2015;22:2677–84.
41. Bhangu A et al. *Colorectal Dis.* 2012;14(12):1457–66.
42. Pellino G et al. *Dis Colon Rectum.* 2015;58:753–61.
43. Colibaseuanu DT et al. *Dis Colon Rectum.* 2014;57: 47–55.
44. Dubois JB et al. *Radiother Oncol.* 2011;98(3): 298–303.
45. Manfredi S et al. *Ann Surg.* 2006;244:254–9.
46. Inhat p et al. *World J Gastroenterol.* 2015;21: 7014–21.
47. Otto G et al. *Ann Surg.* 2010;251:796–803.
48. O'Connell JB et al. *J Natl Cancer Inst.* 2004;96: 1420–5.
49. Simmonds PC et al. *Br J Cancer.* 2006;94:982–99.
50. Brouquet A et al. *J Am Coll Surg.* 2010;210:934–41.
51. Tevis SE et al. *Dis Colon Rectum.* 2013;56(12): 1339–48.
52. Matsumo T et al. *Dis Colon Rectum.* 2014;57: 679–86.
53. Tanaka K et al. *Surgery.* 2004;136:950–9.
54. Mayo SC et al. *J Am Coll Surg.* 2013;216:707–18.
55. Thelen A et al. *Int J Colorectal Dis.* 2007;22: 1269–76.
56. McKenzie SP et al. *Int J Colorectal Dis.* 2014;29: 729–35.
57. Lykoudis PM et al. *Br J Surg.* 2014;101:605–12.
58. Yin Z et al. *Hepatology.* 2013;57:2346–57.
59. Kelly ME et al. *J Surg Oncol.* 2015;111:341–51.
60. Ejaz A et al. *HPB.* 2014;16:1117–26.
61. Weber JC et al. *Br J Surg.* 2003;90:956–62.
62. Mentha G et al. *Dig Surg.* 2008;25:430–5.
63. Ayez N et al. *Dis Colon Rectum.* 2013;56:281–7.
64. Lehman K et al. *Ann Surg.* 2012;255(2):237–47.
65. Lam V et al. *HPB.* 2014;16:101–8.
66. Verhoef C et al. *Dis Colon Rectum.* 2009;52:23–30.
67. Adam R et al. *Oncologist.* 2012;17:1225–39.
68. Amersi FF et al. *Arch Surg.* 2006;141:581–8.
69. Hildebrand P et al. *Eur J Surg Oncol.* 2006;32: 430–4.
70. Abdalla EK et al. *Ann Surg.* 2004;239:818–27.
71. Gleisner AL et al. *Arch Surg.* 2008;143(12):1204–12.
72. Siperstein AE et al. *Ann Surg.* 2007;246:559–67.
73. Wong SL et al. *J Clin Oncol.* 2010;28:493–508.
74. Cirocchi R et al. *Cochrane Database Syst Rev.* 2012; 6:1–63.
75. deGroote K, Prenen H. *World J Gastroinest Oncol.* 2015;7:148–52.
76. Boige V et al. *Ann Surg Oncol.* 2008;15:219–26.
77. Martin RC et al. *Ann Surg Oncol.* 2011;18:192–8.
78. Mocellin S et al. *Cochrane Database Syst Rev.* 2009;8.
79. Tan KK et al. *J Gastrointest Surg.* 2009;13:642–8.
80. Watanabe K et al. *Dis Colon Rectum.* 2011;54: 989–98.
81. Dahabre J et al. *Anticancer Res.* 2007;27:4387–90.
82. Mitry E et al. *Gut.* 2010;59:1383–8.
83. Kim CH et al. *Dis Colon Rectum.* 2012;55:459–64.
84. Suzuki H et al. *Ann Thorac Surg.* 2015;99:435–40.
85. Treasure T et al. *Thorax.* 2012;67:185–7.
86. Nagakura S et al. *J Am Coll Surg.* 2001;193:153–6.
87. Marudanayagam R et al. *HPB.* 2009;11:671–6.

# 32

# Evaluation and management of peritoneal metastatic disease

JAMES FLESHMAN AND KATERINA O. WELLS

## CHALLENGING CASE

A 56-year-old woman presents with a cecal cancer and four 1 cm nodules on the right peritoneum on computed tomography (CT) scan. Additional metastatic workup is negative.

## CASE MANAGEMENT

An R0 resection is possible with a right colectomy and en bloc resection of the right peritoneum.

## INTRODUCTION

It is estimated that 10%–13% of patients with colorectal cancer (CRC) present with synchronous or metachronous peritoneal carcinomatosis and these patients have traditionally a poor prognosis (1–4).

In the case of peritoneal carcinomatosis secondary to CRC (PCCRC) secondary to appendiceal carcinoma, peritoneal spread can occur without lymphatic involvement as even fairly small and early tumors can incur appendiceal perforation with local seeding. In retrospective comparison of appendiceal versus colon cancer, appendiceal cancer had higher rates of perforation at 44.7% versus 1.1% in colon cancer with a higher rate of peritoneal seeding, 25.5% versus 2.5% ($p = 0.001$) (5). PCCRC represents a more advanced stage of disease, often with lymphatic invasion preceding peritoneal involvement. This pattern of disease portends a uniformly poor prognosis with a median survival of 5–9 months (1). Though the presence of carcinomatosis represents stage IV disease, PCCRC can represent a distinct pathology more as a regionally disseminated disease rather than a systemic process (6). In a population-based cohort study of CRC patients from Stockholm County, of the 8% of patients identified as having PCCRC, half presented with isolated peritoneal disease without other solid organ metastases, suggesting that a discrete pathogenesis exists for this pattern of disease (7). As such, surgical therapies have proven to offer some survival benefit over standard systemic chemotherapy regimens.

## ETIOLOGY

The pathogenesis of PCCRC follows a series of steps called the "peritoneal metastatic cascade" initiated by destabilization of tumor cells from the primary lesion. Exfoliation of surface tumor cells from a T4 lesion can occur via downregulation of the intercellular adhesion molecule, E-cadherin (8). In addition to spontaneous exfoliation, tumor dissemination is thought to occur via interstitial hypertension, wherein increased intratumoral oncotic pressure results in tumor shedding (9). Iatrogenic trauma can also result in peritoneal seeding (10).

As free tumor cells gain access to the peritoneal cavity, the pathways of physiologic peritoneal transport distribute cells throughout the space and across the serosal linings (9). These epithelial cells undergo epithelial to mesenchyme transition (EMT), where they employ developmental processes to gain migratory and invasive properties, such as reorganization of the actin cytoskeleton with formation of membrane protrusions, filopodia, and lamellipodia, that allow for invasion to the mesothelium (11). Epithelial cells that lose sufficient cell-matrix interactions undergo a unique apoptotic pathway termed *anoikis* (12). Resistance to anoikis is critical for free tumor cells to maintain metabolism within the bloodless peritoneal environment. These phenotypic changes are mediated by a number of growth factors and molecular pathways (13). This pattern of integration is described in leukocyte migration during peritoneal inflammation and is "believed to be exploited by tumor cells" during peritoneal invasion (11). Once tumor cells invade the subperitoneal layer, production of growth factors and angiogenic factors stimulates proliferation and neovascularization (13).

## DIAGNOSIS

## IMAGING

CT imaging has significant diagnostic import in the staging of metastatic CRC. CT imaging is useful for the detection of both extraabdominal and solid organ metastatic disease. However, its accuracy is limited in quantifying the extent and nature of carcinomatosis, as adenocarcinoma tends to progress along the peritoneal surface in thin layers that outline the normal contours of intraabdominal structures. CT imaging can quantify mucinous adenocarcinoma with the presence of free colloid within the peritoneal cavity. Tumor nodules can sometimes be visualized as solid tissue mass if they are large enough in size or disrupt the usual contours of the abdominal cavity. Studding of surfaces may be seen (10) (Figure 32.1).

Due to these limitations, the role of CT in providing accurate preoperative prognostic data for success of cytoreductive surgery (CRS) is poor. The sensitivity of detecting individual peritoneal lesions larger than 5 cm is acceptable at 59%–67%; however, this decreases to 9%–24% for nodules smaller than 1 cm (14). In retrospective review of 25 patients who underwent CRS and heated intraperitoneal chemotherapy (HIPEC), preoperative imaging was analyzed using a simplified peritoneal cancer index (SPCI) and correlated to operative findings and postoperative outcomes. There were statistically significant interobserver differences

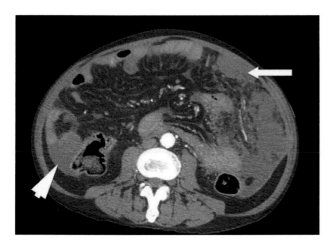

Figure 32.1 CT imaging of peritoneal carcinomatosis. Evidence of carcinomatosis on cross-sectional imaging can include peritoneal implants (thin arrow) and caking of the omentum in the left mid-abdomen, and the presence of ascites in dependent areas of the peritoneal cavity (thick arrowhead).

in scoring of lesions measuring less than 5 cm ($p = 0.007$) as well as determining the extent of regional involvement (14). In general preoperative CT, SPCI scoring considerably underidentified regions with peritoneal involvement with median SPCI scores of 1–2 correlating with median intraoperative peritoneal cancer index (PCI) scores of 6. High SPCI scores were associated with poor outcomes with SPCI >6 predicting an 83% likelihood of incomplete cytoreduction. Involvement of the ileocecal region on CT was unfavorable, and this correlated with poor prognosis when ileocecal involvement was also noted intraoperatively (HR 3.4, $p = 0.041$) (15). Similarly, in a multi-institutional study, Esquivel et al. (16) observed that CT scan underestimated a true PCI score of >20 in 12% of patients, therefore incorrectly qualifying patients for CRS intraperitoneal chemotherapy (IPC) not truly amenable for complete cytoreduction (16). These findings suggest that the extent of peritoneal involvement is often underappreciated on preoperative CT, and accuracy of findings is operator dependent; however, extensive disease on CT may be prognostic.

Based on the prognostic impact of PCI, a novel TNM staging classification for PCCRC was developed to practically stratify survival. T-staging refers to the value of PCI with T1 (PCI 1–10) to T4 (PCI 30–39). The presence of positive lymph nodes is classified as N1, and the presence of extraabdominal metastases is classified as M1. The 5-year survival rates for stage I (T1N0M), stage II (T2-3N0M0), and stage III (T4N0-1M0-1) are 87%, 53%, and 29%, respectively (17).

Positron emission tomography (PET)/CT has a reported sensitivity of 58%–100% for the detection of peritoneal metastasis. Most commonly, abnormally intense fluorodeoxyglucose (FDG) uptake is seen along the abdominal wall. An SUV (Standardised Uptake Value = concentration/dose/weight) maximum threshold of >5.1 is 78% accurate in identifying metastatic foci (18). In a prospective single-center study, PET/CT was able to stratify the extent of carcinomatosis with a sensitivity of 90% and specificity of 77%. In patients with PCCRC and negative PET/CT, the probability of complete cytoreduction was 80% (19). However, detection of FDG avidity is poor in lesions <1 cm in size and in mucinous tumors, limiting its accuracy in these cases.

The sensitivity of magnetic resonance imaging in detecting peritoneal involvement is 87% with a negative predictive value of 73% per segment of the abdominal cavity (20). As a limitation, magnetic resonance imaging is not readily available or cost effective for routine imaging. In addition, the quality of magnetic resonance imaging is highly operator dependent and thus subject to variation.

## DIAGNOSTIC LAPAROSCOPY

Due to the limitations of conventional imaging, direct visualization is the most accurate way of determining resectability. Unfortunately, 20%–40% of patients in whom CRS IPC is attempted are ultimately deemed not amenable for complete cytoreduction (2,21). Staging laparoscopy has been considered as a diagnostic measure to assess for resectability prior to undertaking laparotomy; however, its role as a standard preoperative measure is controversial. The benefits of preoperative laparoscopy include the ability to assess for negative prognostic factors such as small bowel and mesenteric involvement, to determine PCI and plan for anticipated multivisceral resection. In a review by Seshadri et al. (22), staging laparoscopy excluded 7%–41% of unnecessary laparotomies not amenable to complete cytoreduction. The feasibility of laparoscopy in the setting of PCCRC is limited, as most patients have undergone prior laparotomy. Thickness of the abdominal wall with tumor as well as significant adhesions are significant contributors to unsuccessful laparoscopy. A 37% rate of understaging was reported. This was primarily due to involvement of carcinomatosis within the lesser sac and pancreas (2) and along the ureters, and deep diaphragmatic invasion (21) that could not be thoroughly assessed by laparoscopy.

## TREATMENT

NCCN guidelines support the use of systemic chemotherapy in the management of PCCRC and consider more aggressive treatment, specifically CRS IPC, as controversial. CRS IPC can be considered in experienced centers for selected patients with limited peritoneal metastases for whom R0 resection can be achieved (23). A consensus statement on the management of such patients within major peritoneal surface malignancy centers offers a clinical pathway to optimize clinical outcomes (24). Patients with PCCRC and distant sites of dissemination should be considered for best systemic therapy. Those without distant disease should undergo a completeness of cytoreduction assessment at an established peritoneal surface malignancy center. This may involve diagnostic laparotomy or laparoscopy. At the time of surgery, if complete cytoreduction is possible, CRS IPC is performed followed by best systemic therapy. If complete cytoreduction is not possible, palliative surgery can be considered followed by best systemic therapy. Neoadjuvant systemic chemotherapy is supported in initially unresectable patients with reassessment for resectability performed at 2–3 months. If a substantial improvement is seen, CRS IPC is a reasonable consideration. However, if minimal response or progression is noted, the patient will not benefit from CRS IPC, and this therapy is associated with a higher morbidity and mortality in this subset of patients (25,26).

## CHEMOTHERAPY ALONE

PCCRC has a uniformly worse prognosis compared to metastatic colorectal cancer confined to the liver or lung. In the era of 5-FU/leucovorin monotherapy, median survival with PCCRC ranged from 5.2 to 7 months (1,4,27). A disease-free interval of less than 1 year, the presence of ascites and lung metastasis, and the stage of carcinomatosis are poor prognostic features (1,4).

In a 2002 retrospective analysis of 3,019 CRC patients, no significant improvement in patient outcomes had been achieved, with median survival approximating 7 months in patients with PCCRC (1). In comparative analysis of three trials of the North Central Cancer Treatment Group using different chemotherapy regimens for metastatic CRC, 2,095 patients with PCCRC were considered with 2.1% (44) of patients having isolated PC. Treatment with modern regimens such as FOLFOX afforded a median overall survival of 15.7 months with 5- and 8-year survival 4.1% and 1.1%, respectively, among patients with PCCRC. This is a significantly worse prognosis compared to non-PCCRC patients having other sites of metastatic disease with median overall survival 17.6 months and 5- and 8-year survival 6% and 3.2%, respectively (28). Patients with PCCRC also fared worse than non-PCCRC patients with second-line treatment following 5-FU treatment, after adjusting for treatment regimens (HR 1.37, $p = 0.006$). PCCRC also had shorter median progression-free survival at 5.8 months versus 7.2 months, $p = 0.002$, and higher rates of death from all causes compared to non-PCCRC (28). Over the last two decades, despite improvements to chemotherapy agents and other novel therapies, median survival for PCCRC remains dismal. The poor outcomes afforded by systemic chemotherapy and palliative surgery alone have stimulated interest in surgical options to more proactively manage PCCRC and improve survival.

## CYTOREDUCTIVE SURGERY AND INTRAPERITONEAL CHEMOTHERAPY

Several institutional studies have demonstrated a benefit of CRS and IPC in selected patients. The reported median survival ranges from 19.2 to 47 months with 1- and 5-year survival of 72%–90% and 19%–51%, respectively (29–34).

In 2004, a multicenter study of 506 patients from 28 centers treated with CRS HIPEC and/or early postoperative IPC, the overall median survival was 19.2 months with overall survival at 1 and 5 years of 72% and 19%, respectively (30). Elias et al. reported an improved median survival rate of 62.7 months and 2- and 5-year overall survival rates of 81% and 51%, respectively, using oxaliplatin perfusate (35).

Complete cytoreduction (CC) is the most consistent positive prognostic indicator across all reported studies with those patients <CC-1 achieving significantly better median survivals of 32.4–62 months versus 5–17.4 months among patients with residual disease (29,30,35). Other positive prognostic features include age younger than 65 years, and use of adjuvant chemotherapy (30,33). Poor prognostic features include high PCI and poor histologic features, specifically signet ring cell features, M1 liver disease, and N+ disease (30,33). Involvement of small bowel and small bowel mesentery are poor prognostic features owing to the inability to completely clear these surfaces of macroscopic disease and ensure adequate and uniform exposure of HIPEC to small bowel surfaces (29).

As evidenced by these predictive factors, the success of HIPEC is predicated on stringent patient selection and largely favorable pathologies. To address this bias, a randomized controlled study by Veerwal et al. (36) reported on 105 patients (54 CRS and HIPEC versus 51 systemic 5-FU/leucovorin with or without palliative surgery). Those treated with CRS and HIPEC achieved an overall survival 22.3 months versus 12.6 months, following systemic therapy (HR 0.55, $p = 0.32$). In 6-year long-term follow-up, those with complete cytoreduction achieved a median survival of 48 months and 5-year survival of 45% (37). Completeness of cytoreduction was also associated with improved survival with the majority of patients who had extensive tumor burden (more than five regions) seeing a median survival of only 5.4 months and contributing to the majority of significant postoperative complications (36).

## Complications

Early reporting of complications following the investigational phase of CRS and HIPEC reported significant major morbidity of 27%, including fistula 4.7%, leak 3%, bleeding 4.5%, peripancreatitis 7.1%, and hematological toxicity 4%. Duration of operation, extent of peritonectomy, and number of suture lines created were closely associated with postoperative morbidity. Treatment-related mortality was 1.8% largely due to neutropenic sepsis (38). In more recent review of CRS HIPEC-related morbidity and mortality, grade III/IV morbidity rates range from 12% to 52% and mortality from 0.9% to 5.8% in tertiary high volume centers. Sepsis and multiorgan failure secondary to surgical complications were the most common causes of mortality. Unique to IPC, hematological toxicity was reported as 0%–28%. Common postoperative complications include sepsis (0%–14%), fistula (0%–23%), abscess (0%–37%), ileus (0%–86%), perforation (0%–10%), anastomotic leak (0%–9%), venous thromboembolism (0%–9%), and renal insufficiency (0%–7%). These rates approach those seen with other major abdominal surgery suggesting that CRS IPC can be performed with acceptable morbidity in tertiary high-volume centers (39). Metabolic and hemostatic "derailment" is common following HIPEC and should only be performed in a setting with intensive care unit support and physicians experienced with this higher level of care.

## Indications

Patient selection is the basis for success to CRS IPC. Those who stand to benefit most from CRS IPC must have minimal residual disease to <CC-1 that is isolated to peritoneal surfaces that can be completely accessed by topical chemotherapy to allow for complete eradication. Tumor biology largely dictates long-term response with noninvasive tumors such as pseudomyxoma peritonei secondary to appendiceal neoplasm of low malignant potential and low-grade sarcomas responding best (10). Additional variables associated with complete cytoreduction include Eastern Cooperative Oncology Group (ECOG) performance status of two or less, absence of extraabdominal disease, absence of biliary or ureteral obstruction, one or less foci of intestinal obstruction, absence of gross small bowel or small bowel mesentery involvement, and no more than small volume disease in the gastrohepatic ligament (24). Lack of involvement of the cardia of the diaphragm or the pericardial sac is also important as peritoneal stripping of these areas is technically challenging. Approximately 8% of patients with PCCRC have concomitant liver metastases (LM). Historically, the presence of more than three LM was a relative contraindication for CRS IPC (40). CRS IPC for PCCRC and LM remains controversial. However, a growing body of literature supports the feasibility of cytoreductive surgery and liver metastectomy followed by HIPEC with better survival outcomes compared to chemotherapy alone (41–43).

## PCI staging and prognostic impact

The PCI is a scoring tool used in the intraoperative setting to grade the extent of carcinomatosis and guide operative decision-making (Figure 32.2). The PCI is a composite of both implant size and distribution. The lesions size score (LS) considers the size of visible nodules. In the case that nodules of varying sizes are seen, the sizes of the largest nodules are scored with LS-0 designating no visible tumor deposits, LS-1 designating nodules less than 0.5 cm in size, LS-2 designating nodules between 0.5 and 5 cm in size, and LS-3 for any nodule >5 cm or for tumor confluence. Distribution is divided into 13 abdomino-pelvic regions with each region designated an LS score. The sum of scores for each region is then calculated with a maximum available score of 39 ($13 \times 3$) (44).

A number of studies have supported the PCI as a prognostic indicator of postoperative outcomes. In a retrospective review of 168 patients by Huang et al. (45), patients with PCI <15 and treated with CRS IPC, overall major morbidity was 33.9%, and these patients had shortened intensive care unit lengths of stay. Median overall survival was 42.1 months with 1-, 3-, and 5-year overall survival 90%, 55.8%, and 34.5%, respectively. These rates of survival varied considerably by PCI score with 5-year survival for patients with PCI <5 at 58.1% and median DFS 11 months versus 8.6 months for PCI >15 ($p = 0.04$). On multivariate analysis, PCI was an independent prognostic factor for poor survival adjusting for other high-risk features. Sugarbaker (10) reports a significant decrement in 5-year survival as PCI increases with PCI <10 associated with a 5-year survival of 50% versus 20% for PCI 11–20 and 0% for PCI >20, $p < 0.0001$.

In review of patients undergoing second-look cytoreductive surgery for PCCRC, PCI was also useful in predicting long-term survival with PCI <12 associated with 2-year survival of 64% versus 14% for PCI >12, $p = 0.066$ (3). As such, some centers limit the option of CRS IPC to patients with PCI <12 (46). The PCI does have prognostic limitations as this scoring system does not take into account tumor histology with extensive burden of low-grade or noninvasive tumors still allowing for complete cytoreduction with good

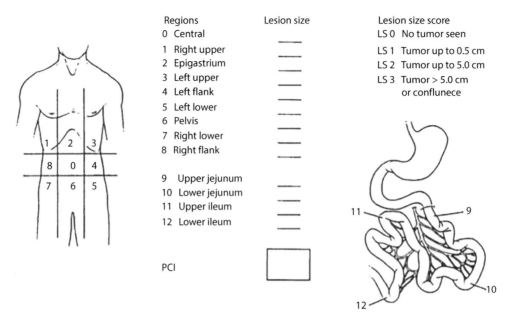

| Regions | Lesion size | Lesion size score |
|---|---|---|
| 0 Central | | LS 0 No tumor seen |
| 1 Right upper | | LS 1 Tumor up to 0.5 cm |
| 2 Epigastrium | | LS 2 Tumor up to 5.0 cm |
| 3 Left upper | | LS 3 Tumor > 5.0 cm |
| 4 Left flank | | or conflunece |
| 5 Left lower | | |
| 6 Pelvis | | |
| 7 Right lower | | |
| 8 Right flank | | |
| 9 Upper jejunum | | |
| 10 Lower jejunum | | |
| 11 Upper ileum | | |
| 12 Lower ileum | | |

PCI

**Figure 32.2** Peritoneal cancer index (PCI). PCI is a composite of both lesion size (LS) and distribution across abdomino-pelvic regions. The sum of scores for each region is then calculated with a maximum available score of 39 (13 × 3). (Reprinted with permission from Sugarbaker PH. *Langenbecks Arch Surg.* 1999;384[6]:576–87.)

long-term outcomes. Conversely, limited carcinomatosis in anatomically complex areas such as the porta hepatis may incur low PCI scores but high morbidity due to the inability to achieve complete cytoreduction in these areas (10). In a recent study by Faron et al. (47), overall survival followed a linear relationship to PCI, suggesting that no discrete cutoff in PCI score can independently contraindicate CRS IPC. Ultimately, the decision to proceed with CRS IPC must weigh a number of prognostic factors.

## Second-look surgery

Enthusiasts of CRS IPC would argue that patients with early, regionalized peritoneal involvement benefit most from CRS IPC. As such, selective second-look protocols with subsequent CRS IPC as part of routine follow-up of patients following primary resections at high risk for metachronous PCCRC have been supported as an early intervention. In retrospective review by Leung et al. (48) of patients with metachronous PCCRC, patients at high risk for peritoneal involvement included those with T4 lesions, macroscopic synchronous peritoneal or ovarian metastatic involvement at time of initial operation, perforated primary, and mucinous or signet ring pathology. The presence of any high-risk factor is 85.6% sensitive in identifying patients who go on to develop PCCRC. Such a protocol would include a planned second-look surgery at 12 months postoperatively and CRS IPC should PCCRC be present. The detection rate of second-look surgery is reported at 55% for patients deemed high risk despite no clinical evidence of disease recurrence at 12 months (49). The rate of conversion to long-term disease-free status following positive second-look surgery in asymptomatic patients is 17%. The rate of conversion to long-term

survival in symptomatic patients with positive second-look surgery is reported at 15%. Critics of this approach question the benefit of negative second look with its attendant morbidity and mortality (50).

Second-look CRS IPC is also supported for patients with PCCRC following initial CRS IPC. This is a planned reexploration scheduled 6–9 months after the initial CRS, wherein an attempt is made to visualize all peritoneal surfaces, perform repeat cytoreduction and/or visceral resection to achieve a score of CC-1 or less. If this is achieved and the patient had a fairly good response to the original cytoreductive surgery, HIPEC is repeated. If a poor response is noted, then the chemotherapy agent is changed (10).

## Palliation

CRS and IPC is also reported as a palliative treatment for malignant ascites as peritoneal fibrosis induced by HIPEC obliterates surface tumor and decrease potential space in the peritoneum (26,51). However, use of CRS with IPC is not routinely supported as a palliative measure owing to its morbidity.

Regardless of indication, candidates for cytoreduction and IPC must also be physiologically fit to undergo major abdominal surgery. In a retrospective observation cohort study by Malfroy et al. (52), the mean number of organs resected CRS was 4.3 (52). Hepatectomy was performed in 19% of patients. Diaphragmatic peritonectomy correlated with higher likelihood of ICU admission, $p = 0.013$. Heated IPC induces a second physiologic stress to the patient. An acute compartment syndrome is induced with instillation resulting in reduced venous return and cardiac index. The subsequent response to hyperthermia induces a systemic inflammatory response syndrome. In the 24-hour postoperative period, substantial fluid shifts occur with 24-hour postoperative peritoneal drain output approaching 2 L (52). Hypovolemia and vasopressor requirements can contribute to end organ hypoperfusion. Delayed IPC delivery through the use of abdominal Port-a-Cath does not induce a profound systemic inflammatory response syndrome response and is better tolerated by less physiologically robust patients (53).

## CYTOREDUCTION

### Goal of cytoreduction

Completeness of cytoreduction to R0 resection is a consistent and significant prognostic factor that is paramount to successful long-term outcomes (10,31,35,36). The primary goal of CRS is to remove all visible tumor to a residual tumor of 2.5 mm or less. The CC score is a clinical tool that objectively describes the extent of cytoreduction achieved at the time of surgery (44). CC-0 indicates no macroscopic residual cancer; CC-1 indicates less than 2.5 mm of residual tumor. Achieving a CC score of CC-1 or less is desired as this burden represents the level of residual disease for which complete extirpation with IPC would be feasible. CC-2 is defined as more than 2.5 mm but less than 2.5 cm of residual tumor, and CC-3 is defined as more than 2.5 cm of residual tumor. A CC score of CC-2 or CC-3 is considered incomplete. Complete cytoreduction should be done with the simultaneous goal of preserving as much viscera as possible (26).

### Technique of cytoreduction

The Sugarbaker technique was first described in 1995 (54). One or all procedures are employed depending on the extent of peritoneal involvement. Use of laser electrosurgery is recommended to both dissect viscera and ablate tumor nodules from surfaces of small bowel and mesentery where peritoneal resection is not feasible. The heat necrosis created at the line of dissection creates a tumor-free margin of resection (55). Sharp dissection of tumor nodules is not recommended as margins of resection can retain residual tumor, and cut surfaces serve as sites of bleeding during IPC instillation (44).

### Novel methods of cytoreduction

The presence of residual carcinoma following cytoreduction is a major contributor to treatment failure, disease progression, and mortality, as such novel therapies to identity residual tumor and aid in complete cytoreduction are of interest. In a pilot study by Liberale et al. (56), fluorescence of tumor nodules following indocyanine green injection was used to identify and resect peritoneal nodules. Of the nodules resected as a result of this technique, 84% were malignant. Nonmucinous tumors demonstrated a clear hyperfluorescence compared to benign nodules. This application served to improve the extent of resection in 29% of cases

by identifying peritoneal metastases not visible by conventional methods. Nanoprobe technology directed specifically toward tumor tissue similarly serves to accurately identify residual tumor tissue at the time of cytoreduction and is currently in development (57).

## HEATED INTRAPERITONEAL CHEMOTHERAPY

### Surgical principles

The argument against cytoreductive surgery alone and the rationale to explain the rapid progression of peritoneal-surface recurrence following cytoreductive surgery stems from the "tumor cell entrapment" theory wherein the surgeon acts as the promoter through the dissemination of malignant cells from surgical trauma (10). As inflammatory cells migrate to peritonectomized surfaces, free tumor emboli become entrapped in fibrin and adhere to stripped surfaces. Growth factors stimulated by the postsurgical healing process promote proliferation of entrapped tumor cells. By this theory, the addition of IPC at the time of cytoreduction is necessary to both extirpate free tumor emboli as well as reduce the burden of inflammatory cells that would contribute to postoperative healing. The procedure for application of HIPEC following cytoreduction has evolved over time to optimize tissue delivery and decrease complications related to this therapy. The principles of HIPEC are outlined in the following sections.

### Tissue penetration

The major limitation to HIPEC is the very superficial penetration of cytotoxic drugs into tumor tissue. Based on experimental animal models of tissue penetration, this is estimated to be a maximal depth of 1–2 mm (58,59).

Despite this superficial level of action, local tissue absorption is rapid based on pharmacokinetics testing (60,61). Thus, a 2.5 mm diameter nodule for residual tumor remnants is the cutoff at which adequate tissue penetration can occur (59).

### Hyperthermia

Application of heat at 41°C–43.5°C induces a profound and selective tumor necrosis (62). Heat also optimizes the intensity of tissue chemotherapy dose delivered by decreasing the interstitial pressure of tissues and increasing tumor cell membrane permeability and transport. Heat may also alter cellular metabolism of specific agents (63). This synergistic effect of heated chemotherapy varies by chemotherapy agent with the highest "thermal enhancement" seen with selected alkylating agents (64).

### Closed versus open technique

Original protocols of HIPEC involved the administration of heated chemotherapy via a closed circuit of catheters placed into the peritoneal cavity following cytoreduction (Figure 32.3a).

By this technique, inflow and outflow catheters are placed, and the laparotomy incision is sutured closed. A large volume of perfusate and heated chemotherapy is introduced via inflow catheters at high pressure. The abdomen is manually agitated externally to distribute the chemotherapy. Once the instillation is complete, the laparotomy incision is reopened and surgical anastomoses are completed. This approach keeps chemotherapy within a closed circuit without theoretical exposure to health-care personnel while maintaining hyperthermia and intraabdominal pressure to aid with tissue penetration. The major reported disadvantage of this approach is the nonuniform distribution of chemotherapy to peritonectomized surfaces. Gravity also leads to pooling and greater exposure of chemotherapy agents to dependent areas within the peritoneum (63). Early experience also reports small bowel thermal injury and fistula secondary to focal high temperatures of perfusate entering at the inflow catheter tip (65).

The open "coliseum" technique (Figure 32.3b) is the currently accepted technique for HIPEC delivery (44).

Following cytoreduction, inflow and outflow catheters are placed through the abdominal wall. The abdominal walls are sutured to a self-retaining retractor incorporating a plastic sheet into the suture to cover the abdominal cavity. A slit is made over the plastic sheet to allow for the introduction of a hand. Once the instillation is complete, the chemotherapy agent is drained from the abdomen, and reconstruction is undertaken. Limitations in drug distribution by the closed technique are addressed by this open technique, allowing for gentle manipulation of the viscera during the instillation to ensure uniform contact of chemotherapy agent to all surfaces. The theoretical risk of chemotherapy agent exposure to health-care personnel is negligible with the use of appropriate protective equipment (66). Other methods of delivery that are essentially hybrid open-closed techniques have been described to address the shortcomings of each of these approaches (67).

## Choice of chemotherapy agents

The peritoneal-plasma barrier allows for retention of large molecular weight chemotherapy agents into the peritoneal

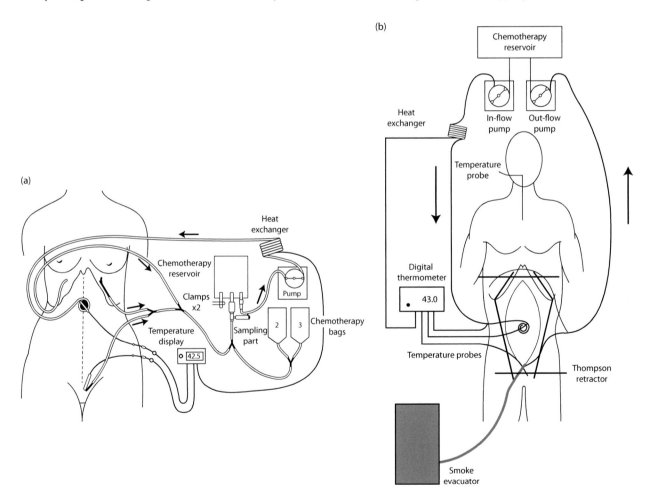

Figure 32.3 (a) HIPEC closed technique. In the closed approach, the laparotomy incision is closed and three intraperitoneal catheters are used to instill and drain heated chemotherapy in a closed circuit. (b) HIPEC open "coliseum" technique. In the open approach the abdominal wall is sutured to a self-retaining retractor incorporating a plastic sheet as a cover. Inflow and outflow catheters circulate heated chemotherapy with manual visceral manipulation.

cavity and dose-intensive therapy with significantly more potent concentration of agent to surface tumor cells (68). Systemic toxicity is reduced as the peritoneal cavity serves as a barrier against systemic absorption with the majority of drug that enters circulation cleared via first pass hepatic metabolism (69). The choice of chemotherapeutic agent for IPC varies across centers with selection based largely on institutional preference and experience. Chemotherapy agents most commonly used for PCCRC are mitomycin C and oxaliplatin. Mitomycin C was the earliest agent used in HIPEC for CRC and has been shown to be effective in randomized controlled trial when used at a rate of 10–12.5 mg/$m^2$ heated to 42°C with a dwell time of 90 minutes (37,70).

The efficacy of oxaliplatin as a HIPEC agent is also well supported in phase II trials with favorable rates of median overall survival and disease-free survival (35). This regimen, termed the Elias protocol, is most commonly employed and consists of oxaliplatin 460 mg/$m^2$ in 2 L/$m^2$ of dextrose at a temperature of 43°C over 30 minutes. In a retrospective analysis by Leung et al. (46) comparing mitomycin C versus oxaliplatin efficacy, oxaliplatin is associated with a greater unadjusted median survival compared to mitomycin C (56 versus 29 months) with oxaliplatin HR 0.59, $p = 0.0017$. This survival advantage was most pronounced in patients PCI >10 (HR 0.47, $p = 0.014$) and in well-differentiated and non-signet-ring pathologies in subgroup analysis compared to mitomycin C. As a limitation, oxaliplatin is associated with higher rates of surgical complications and higher morbidity of grade III and grade IV complications compared to mitomycin C (71).

Many specialized centers employ the use of bidirectional, or HIPEC-plus, chemotherapy protocols wherein simultaneous intraoperative systemic and intraperitoneal chemotherapy infusions are performed to obtain a bidirectional fluid gradient across the surface tumor cell. This was first employed by Elias et al. (35) with the use of IV 5-FU and leucovorin with intraperitoneal oxaliplatin due to pH incompatibility of delivering both agents intraperitoneally. In a pharmacologic study by Speeten et al. (72), intraoperative systemic infusion of 5-FU results in rapid circulation and equilibration throughout body compartments including peritoneal fluid. Circulating and intraperitoneal levels of 5-FU work synergistically with instilled intraperitoneal chemotherapy agents to enhance tumor toxicity.

## DELAYED INTRAPERITONEAL CHEMOTHERAPY

Delayed recurrent IPC via transperitoneal catheters is an alternative method of IPC delivery. The rationale for this approach is to provide high concentrations of chemotherapy to peritoneal surfaces repeatedly over time. Delayed IPC also offers shorter operating room times (243 minutes versus 440 minutes), less estimated blood loss (770 mL versus 4000 mL), shorter hospital lengths of stay (11 days versus 21 days), and less morbidity with fewer grade III–IV complications compared to HIPEC (53). As a limitation, nonuniform

distribution of IPC occurs when delivered in a delayed fashion due to the presence of intraabdominal adhesions and dependent distribution of perfusate. In retrospective case series of 31 patients treated with CRS followed by delayed IPC via abdominal Port-a-Cath, peritoneal scintigraphy performed prior to chemotherapy administration demonstrated free diffusion of tracer as intended in 58% of patients. Limited diffusion due to postoperative adhesions was noted in 35.5% of patients (53).

Regardless, limited experience with delayed IPC suggests long-term outcomes comparable to HIPEC can be achieved. In a case-controlled study of 18 PCCRC patients undergoing CRS and delayed IPC, Mahteme et al. (73) demonstrated a median survival of 32 months versus 14 months, $p = 0.01$ in matched controls treated with 5-FU/leucovorin. Two- and 5-year survival was 60% and 28%, respectively. In this experience, IPC was initiated via transabdominal catheters on postoperative day 1 and daily for 6 days; this was repeated at 4–6 week intervals. In 7/18 patients, treatment was discontinued due to catheter-related problems, with drain leakage being a source of morbidity. Culliford et al. (74) reports similarly favorable outcomes following delayed IPC with median survival 34 months and 5-year survival 28%. Morbidity was 26% with few grade III–IV complications; however, port malfunction and/or infection requiring revision and/or removal was the most common late complication. In a more recent randomized controlled trial by Cashin et al. (75) comparing CRS HIPEC to oxaliplatin/5-FU systemic chemotherapy, patients treated with delayed IPC achieved a median overall survival of 25 months versus 18 months (HR 0.51, $p = 0.04$) suggesting this treatment modality remains superior to modern systemic chemotherapy regimens. However, this study was terminated early due to low accrual. These benefits suggest that delayed IPC is an oncologically acceptable and perhaps better-tolerated therapeutic option in centers where HIPEC is not offered.

## SUMMARY

PCCRC carries a uniformly poor prognosis with a median survival of 5–9 months (1). A discrete pathogenesis exists for this pattern of metastatic disease, wherein local peritoneal seeding from perforated appendiceal carcinoma can occur in the absence of nodal or systemic disease. Defects in the e-cadherin pathway and cell interactions seem to play a role in the ability of cells to establish in a bloodless environment. Shedding or iatrogenic dissemination of tumor surface cells from locally advanced colon carcinoma also results in peritoneal seeding; however, peritoneal carcinomatosis from colon and rectal primary lesions represents a more advanced disease, often with lymphatic invasion preceding peritoneal involvement. Though the presence of carcinomatosis represents stage IV disease, PCCRC can represent a distinct pathology more as a regionally disseminated process rather than a systemic disease. Systemic chemotherapy is virtually ineffective. As such, local therapies targeted at cytoreduction of the peritoneum have proven to offer some survival benefit over standard systemic chemotherapy regimens. The most important positive prognostic indicator is completeness of cytoreduction, aiming for less than 2.5 mm of residual disease. Stringent selection of patients amenable to complete cytoreduction is paramount to long-term success; therefore, emphasis is placed on accurate preoperative staging of peritoneal tumor burden. Preoperative imaging has limited sensitivity for determining the extent of peritoneal tumor burden. CT imaging with IV contrast has been shown to have the best chance for accurate staging. PET/CT is of no use in mucinous tumors. Staging laparoscopy is supported in some centers to accurately stage the peritoneum and prevent unnecessary laparotomy in patients who would ultimately be determined unresectable. However, laparoscopy has been found to understage peritoneal involvement in 37% of cases due to limitations in accurately exploring the retroperitoneum (2). The PCI determined at the time of laparotomy is the most accurate method of staging. This intraoperative tool is used to guide decision-making and is well supported as a prognostic tool, with PCI >12 having significantly higher major morbidity and shorter overall survival compared to PCI <12 (3). Several reported experiences from established peritoneal malignancy centers have served to optimize the systematic approach of CRS as well as the method of delivery and choice of agent for IPC. Immediate IPC and delayed IPC techniques are described with similar rates in overall survival that far exceed survival rates achieved with systemic chemotherapy alone. Ultimately, effective surgical management of PCCRC prolongs median survival in appropriately selected patients.

## CONCLUSION

PCCRC carries a uniformly poor prognosis with a median survival of 5–9 months. A discrete pathogenesis exists for this pattern of metastases, as in the case of appendiceal carcinoma where high rates of perforation contribute to peritoneal seeding. In locally advanced colon tumors, shedding from the tumor surface due to increased oncotic pressure and/or iatrogenic trauma similarly seed the peritoneum. As such, local therapies targeted at cytoreduction of the peritoneum have proven to offer some survival benefit over standard systemic chemotherapy alone. With the experience of several established peritoneal malignancy centers, the management of PCCRC has evolved significantly over the past two decades to include a systematic approach of cytoreduction and optimized intraperitoneal chemotherapy agent and method of delivery. The most important positive prognostic indicator is completeness of cytoreduction, aiming for less than 2.5 mm of residual disease. Completeness of cytoreduction is most likely in patients with low burden of disease and favorable tumor biology. Stringent patient selection to achieve complete cytoreduction is the cornerstone

to long-term success. Preoperative imaging has limited sensitivity for determining the extent of peritoneal disease. Staging laparoscopy is supported in some centers to accurately stage the peritoneum and prevent unnecessary laparotomy; however, this approach is also limited in the ability to accurately survey the retroperitoneum and may understage peritoneal involvement. Ultimately the definitive cytoreductive laparotomy is the most accurate method of staging. Following systematic exploration and cytoreduction, IPC in an immediate fashion effective extirpates remaining surface and free tumor cells. CRS and HIPEC is a complex abdominal procedure with major morbidity and mortality rivaling other major multivisceral resections. Alternative methods of delayed IPC are described that offer similar rates of median survival in small series with the added benefit of less short-term morbidity compared to HIPEC. Ultimately the surgical management of PCCRC is effective at prolonging the median survival of patients compared to palliative chemotherapy and should be considered in patients eligible for complete cytoreduction.

## REFERENCES

1. Jayne DG et al. *Br J Surg.* 2002;89(12):1545–50.
2. Pomel C et al. *Eur J Surg Oncol (EJSO).* 2005;31(5): 540–3.
3. Portilla AG et al. *World J Surg.* 1998;23(1):23–9.
4. Chu DZ et al. *Cancer.* 1989;63(2):364–7.
5. Tae Son Il et al. *Surg Oncol.* 2016;25(1):37–43.
6. Spiliotis J et al. *Curr Oncol.* 2016;23(3):266.
7. Segelman J et al. *Br J Surg.* 2012;99(5):699–705.
8. Hirohashi S. *Am J Pathol.* 1998;153(2):333–9.
9. Hayashi K et al. *Cancer Res.* 2007;67(17):8223–8.
10. Sugarbaker PH. *Langenbecks Arch Surg.* 1999;384(6): 576–87.
11. Yilmaz M, Christofori G. *Cancer Metastasis Rev.* 2009; 28(1–2):15–33.
12. Cao Z et al. *Crit Rev Oncog.* 2016;21(3–4):155–68.
13. Lemoine L et al. *WJG.* 2016;22(34):7692.
14. de Bree E et al. *J Surg Oncol.* 2004;86(2):64–73.
15. De Bree E et al. *Eur J Surg Oncol.* 2006;32(1):65–71.
16. Esquivel J et al. *J Surg Oncol.* 2010;102(6):565–70.
17. Yan TD et al. *Cancer.* 2010;117(9):1855–63.
18. Suzuki A et al. *Eur J Nucl Med Mol Imaging.* 2004; 31(10):1413–1420.
19. Passot G et al. *Eur J Surg Oncol.* 2010;36(3):315–23.
20. Klumpp BD et al. *Abdom Imaging.* 2012;38(1):64–71.
21. Iversen LH et al. *Br J Surg.* 2012;100(2):285–92.
22. Seshadri RA, Hemanth Raj E. *Indian J Surg Oncol.* 2016;7(2):230–5.
23. Benson AB et al. *J Natl Compr Canc Netw.* 2015; 12:1028–59.
24. Esquivel J et al. *Ann Surg Oncol.* 2006;14(1):128–33.
25. Esquivel J. *J Gastrointest Oncol.* 2016;7(1):72–8.
26. Bhagwandin SB et al. *Oncology.* 2016;30(11): 1002–1007.
27. Sadeghi B et al. *Cancer.* 2000;88(2):358–63.

28. Franko J et al. *J Clin Oncol.* 2012;30(3):263–7.
29. Verwaal VJ et al. *Ann Surg Oncol.* 2005;12(1):65–71.
30. Glehen O. *J Clin Oncol.* 2004;22(16):3284–92.
31. Franko J et al. *Cancer.* 2010;116(16):3756–62.
32. Esquivel J et al. *Ann Surg Oncol.* 2014;21(13): 4195–201.
33. Huang Y et al. *Anticancer Res.* 2016;36(3):1033–40.
34. Alzahrani N et al. *ANZ J Surg.* 2016;86(11):937–41.
35. Elias D et al. *J Clin Oncol.* 2009;27(5):681–5.
36. Verwaal VJ. *J Clin Oncol.* 2003;21(20):3737–43.
37. Verwaal VJ et al. *Ann Surg Oncol.* 2008;15(9): 2426–32.
38. Stephens AD et al. *Ann Surg Oncol.* 1999;6(8): 790–6.
39. Chua TC et al. *Ann Surg.* 2009;249(6):900–7.
40. Elias D et al. *Eur J Surg Oncol.* 2006;32(6):632–6.
41. Lorimier G et al. *Eur J Surg* 2017;43:150–158.
42. Varban O et al. *Cancer.* 2009;115(15):3427–36.
43. de Cuba EMV et al. *Cancer Treat Rev.* 2013;39(4): 321–7.
44. Sugarbaker PH. *Cancer Chemother Pharmacol.* 1999; 43(Suppl):S15–25.
45. Huang Y et al. *Int J Surg.* 2016;32(c):65–70.
46. Leung V et al. *Eur J Surg Oncol.* 2017;43:141–149.
47. Faron M et al. *Ann Surg Oncol.* 2015;23(1):114–9.
48. Leung V et al. *Eur J Surg Oncol.* 2016;42(6):836–40.
49. Elias D et al. *Ann Surg.* 2008;247(3):445–50.
50. Sugarbaker P. *Surgl Oncol Clin N Am.* 2012;21(4): 689–703.
51. Graziosi L et al. *Ann Ital Chir.* 2016;87:312–20.
52. Malfroy S et al. *Surgical Oncology.* 2016;25(1):6–15.
53. Fajardo AD et al. *Dis Colon Rectum.* 2012;55(10): 1044–52.
54. Sugarbaker PH. *Ann Surg.* 1995;221(1):29–42.
55. Sugarbaker PH. *Cancer Treat Res.* 1996;82:375–85.
56. Liberale G et al. *Ann Surg.* 2016;264(6):1110–5.
57. Xi L et al. *Ann Surg Oncol.* 2014;21(5):1602–9.
58. Ozols RF et al. *Cancer Res.* 1979;39(8):3209–14.
59. Van der Speeten K et al. *Cancer J.* 2009;15(3): 216–24.
60. Panteix G et al. *Oncology.* 1993;50(5):366–70.
61. Elias D et al. *Ann Oncol.* 2002;13(2):267–72.
62. Cavaliere R et al. *Cancer.* 1967;20(9):1351–81.
63. González-Moreno S. *WJGO.* 2010;2(2):68.
64. Takemoto M et al. *Int J Hyperthermia.* 2009;19(2): 193–203.
65. Jacquet P et al. *Cancer.* 1996;77(12):2622–9.
66. Kyriazanos I et al. *Surg Oncol.* 2016;25(3):308–14.
67. Lotti M et al. *J Minim Access Surg.* 2016;12(1):86–9.
68. Jacquet P, Sugarbaker PH. *Cancer Treat Res.* 1996;82: 53–63.
69. de Bree E, Tsiftsis DD. *Recent Results Cancer Res.* 2007;169:39–51.
70. Esquivel J et al. *Ann Surg Oncol.* 2007;14(1):128–33.
71. Rouers A et al. *Acta Chir Belg.* 2006;106(3):302–6.
72. Van der Speeten K et al. *J Surg Oncol.* 2010;102(7): 730–5.
73. Mahteme H et al. *Br J Cancer.* 2004;90(2):403–7.
74. Culliford AT et al. *Ann Surg Oncol.* 2001;8(10):787–95.
75. Cashin PH et al. *Eur J Cancer.* 2016;53:155–62.

# 33

# Chemotherapy for colon and rectal cancer

JONATHAN LU AND MARC R. MATRANA

## CHALLENGING CASE

A 53-year-old man undergoes a left colectomy for a T3N1M0 adenocarcinoma.

## CASE MANAGEMENT

It is recommended by the Multidisciplinary Tumor Committee that he receive postoperative chemotherapy with FOLFOX.

## INTRODUCTION

Colorectal cancer is among the most common and deadliest malignancies in the United States. There is estimated to be over 130,000 new cases of colorectal cancer in the United States in 2016 with nearly 50,000 expected deaths (1). However, the annual incidence of colorectal cancer has been declining over the past few decades as a result of improved screening, risk factor modifications, and improved treatment modalities (2). Increased screening has led to increased removal of precancerous lesions, thus reducing colorectal cancer rates (2–4). Despite the declines in incidence and mortality, colorectal cancer remains the third most common cause of cancer death in both men and women (1). Management of colorectal cancer is dependent on staging and differs greatly between localized disease compared to metastatic disease. Surgical resection is the mainstay of therapy for localized disease and is further discussed in other chapters of this textbook. Adjuvant chemotherapy is often given postoperatively with the intent to eliminate any microscopic residual disease.

## ADJUVANT CHEMOTHERAPY IN RESECTABLE COLON CANCER

The administration of adjuvant chemotherapy in the setting of localized colon cancer is aimed at eradicating any micrometastases in order to reduce the chance of disease recurrence (5). Patients with AJCC (American Joint Committee on Cancer) stage 1 disease who have undergone surgical resection have an excellent prognosis. The overall 10-year survival for stage 1 colorectal cancer patients is 90% compared to 5% for stage 4 patients (6). Given the lack of data supporting the use of chemotherapy in stage 1 disease and overall excellent prognosis, patients with stage 1 disease do not require any adjuvant therapy (5). While patients with stage 3 disease have a clear benefit with adjuvant chemotherapy, the role of adjuvant chemotherapy for patients with stage 2 disease is more controversial. The QUASAR trial looked at 2,291 patients with stage 2 colon cancer who were randomized to chemotherapy with 5-FU (5-fluorouracil) and leucovorin (folinic acid) in comparison to observation alone (7). The results of the QUASAR trial showed that adjuvant chemotherapy can increase survival in patients with stage 2 colon cancer, albeit only a modest 3.6% absolute improvement (7). With regard to stage 3 disease, metastatic and/or local relapse can occur up to 50% of the time (8). Adjuvant chemotherapy should always be considered in stage 3 colon cancer. The MOSAIC trial looked at 2,246 patients with both stage 2 and stage 3 colon cancer and showed improved overall survival in stage 3 colon cancer patients given FOLFOX (leucovorin, 5-FU, and oxaliplatin) (9,10). In addition, data suggest a decreased recurrence rate in high-risk stage 2 patients, defined as those with T4 tumors, less than 12 lymph nodes examined after surgery, poorly differentiated histology, lymphatic invasion, vascular invasion, bowel obstruction/perforation, or microsatellite instability, who were treated with FOLFOX, even though there was no statistically significant increase in overall survival or disease-free survival (9,10). Therefore, patients with high-risk stage 2 disease in particular, should undergo serious consideration for adjuvant chemotherapy (11). Given the debatable nature of adjuvant chemotherapy for stage 2 colon cancer, patients should be encouraged to participate in clinical trials (11).

There have been many studies looking at the optimal chemotherapy regimen in the adjuvant setting. Most of the evidence is in the setting of patients with stage 3 disease, but the data are often extrapolated for the management of stage 2 colon cancer patients. Standard adjuvant chemotherapy is based on 6 months of a 5-FU–based chemotherapy regimen (8). Current recommendations for chemotherapy include FOLFOX, CapeOx (capecitabine and oxaliplatin), or FLOX (bolus 5-FU, leucovorin, and oxaliplatin) (9,10,12–14). In addition, capecitabine alone or 5-FU/LV (5-FU and leucovorin) are alternative treatments if oxaliplatin is not an appropriate option for the patient (15,16). The elderly population, for instance, had no benefit in overall survival or disease-free survival from the addition of oxaliplatin to 5-FU/LV based on subgroup analysis (17). However, FOLFOX and CapeOx are the preferred, especially in the setting of stage 3 disease. Studies comparing 3 months of FOLFOX versus 6 months of FOLFOX in this setting are being conducted with no data yet reported.

## CHEMOTHERAPY IN RESECTABLE RECTAL CANCER

As with colon cancer, stage 1 rectal cancer is managed with surgical excision alone given its good overall prognosis (6). However, in contrast to colon cancer, the administration of chemotherapy in the setting of locally advanced rectal cancer is often paired with radiation therapy. Specifically, chemotherapy is often given in the neoadjuvant setting in conjunction with radiation therapy to stage 2 and 3 rectal cancer patients. The combination of neoadjuvant chemotherapy with infusional 5-FU and radiation has been showed to improve local control of disease when compared to radiation alone (18). In addition, when looking at combined chemotherapy and radiation, there is evidence from the German Rectal Cancer Study Group supporting that neoadjuvant chemotherapy and radiation is superior with regard to local recurrence when compared to adjuvant chemotherapy and radiation (19). Moreover, neoadjuvant chemotherapy and radiation were tolerated better than the combination of adjuvant chemotherapy and radiation (19). Given the parallels between colon and rectal cancer, investigators have looked at the role of oxaliplatin in order to improve outcomes. However, several trials have shown that the addition of oxaliplatin did not improve clinical outcomes (20–22). Therefore, current guidelines recommend a 5-FU–based chemotherapy regimen to be given concurrently with radiation therapy. Infusional 5-FU or capecitabine are the chemotherapeutic agents of choice for concurrent chemoradiation (18,19,23).

The addition of adjuvant chemotherapy in the postoperative setting after undergoing neoadjuvant chemotherapy and radiation has also been investigated. Initial studies looking at adjuvant chemotherapy with 5-FU after neoadjuvant chemotherapy and radiation followed by surgery were not promising and showed no improvement to overall survival and no benefit to the rate of local recurrence (18,24). However, further investigations revealed an improvement in disease-free survival in patients who received adjuvant FOLFOX in addition to neoadjuvant chemotherapy and radiation (22). Even though there is no conclusive evidence for adjuvant chemotherapy, a 6-month treatment regimen of FOLFOX or CapeOx remains the standard chemotherapy of choice in the postoperative setting and should be considered for stage 2 and 3 rectal cancer patients. In addition, adjuvant chemotherapy should be started as soon as the patient is medically able after surgery, as delays can worsen survival (25).

## CHEMOTHERAPY IN METASTATIC COLORECTAL CANCER

Greater than 50% of all patients diagnosed with colorectal cancer will develop hepatic metastases, many of which are deemed unresectable (26). However, with the advances made in therapeutic options, the median survival has improved from 1 year to more than 30 months (27). The treatments for metastatic colon cancer and metastatic rectal cancer are approached in the same manner. Currently, initial management of metastatic colorectal cancer involves one of five chemotherapy regimens: FOLFOX, FOLFIRI (leucovorin, 5-FU, and irinotecan), CapeOx, infusional 5-FU or capecitabine, or FOLFOXIRI (leucovorin, 5-FU, oxaliplatin, and irinotecan). The timing and sequencing of these therapies have been investigated in a limited manner without a clearly defined preferred order of administration (28–30). In general, however, FOLFOX and FOLFIRI are comparable in efficacy and often the preferred regimen for initial management of metastatic colorectal cancer (31,32).

In addition to 5-FU–based chemotherapy regimens, the antivascular endothelial growth factor antibody bevacizumab are often added in the first-line setting to the various 5-FU–based options, including both FOLFOX and FOLFIRI (33). When added to FOLFOX, bevacizumab improves progression-free survival in patients with metastatic colorectal cancer (34). Similarly, the addition of bevacizumab to FOLFIRI significantly increases clinical improvement with regard to overall survival, progression-free survival, response rate, and duration of response (35). Moreover, cetuximab and panitumumab are monoclonal antibodies against epidermal growth factor receptor (EGFR) that are also utilized in the treatment of metastatic colorectal cancer. EGFR overexpression can be found in 50% of colorectal tumors (36). Multiple trials have found improved overall survival, progression-free survival, and response rate in metastatic colon cancer with the use of EGFR inhibitors in addition to traditional 5-FU chemotherapy regimens, specifically in the RAS wild-type population (37). Furthermore, cetuximab has been shown to have provided clinical benefit in overall survival and progression-free survival when utilized alone (38). Therefore, cetuximab and panitumumab are options for patient unable to undergo more intensive chemotherapy. Despite their benefits, when studies evaluated EGFR inhibitors added to combination 5-FU–based chemotherapy and the vascular endothelial growth factor antibody bevacizumab, the results were not as favorable. The results showed a shorter progression-free survival and worse quality of life (39); therefore, the addition of EGFR inhibitors to 5-FU–based chemotherapy and bevacizumab is not recommended.

After induction therapy, maintenance therapy has now become a mainstay of therapy. The phase 3 AIO 0207 trial looked at 472 patients who underwent induction with FOLFOX and bevacizumab or CapeOx and bevacizumab (40). After induction, the study compared standard maintenance with 5-FU plus bevacizumab, bevacizumab alone, and observation alone. Treatment with bevacizumab alone was shown to be noninferior to the group receiving both 5-FU and bevacizumab (40).

Treatment choices after disease progression are based on previous regimens used. In general, patients who have received FOLFOX or CapeOx for initial therapy will transition to FOLFIRI. Likewise, patients who received FOLFIRI for initial treatment should undergo FOLFOX or CapeOx therapy, which are comparable in efficacy (41). EGFR inhibitors such as cetuximab or panitumumab are viable options in the non-first-line setting for patients who have wild-type KRAS (42,43) and have progressed while on intensive 5-FU–based chemotherapy.

Regorafenib and combination trifluridine and tipiracil are two additional agents that should be considered for use as subsequent therapy options. The CORRECT trial looked at 760 patients who were noted to have disease progression after standard therapy and found that patients who received regorafenib had improved overall survival and progression-free survival when compared to placebo (44). Looking at the oral combination trifluridine and tipiracil, the RECOURSE trial examined 800 patients with metastatic colorectal cancer who had progressed on two lines of therapy and found improved overall survival and disease-free survival (45). As a result of these studies, both regorafenib and combination trifluridine and tipiracil can be utilized in the third- and fourth-line setting. However, there are no direct comparisons between the two regimens, so sequencing is deferred to the clinician and patient.

## HYPERTHERMIC INTRAPERITONEAL CHEMOTHERAPY IN METASTATIC COLORECTAL CANCER

There have been several studies looking at cytoreductive surgery in combination with hyperthermic intraperitoneal chemotherapy (HIPEC) for patients with peritoneal carcinomatosis from colorectal cancer with favorable results (46,47). When compared to systemic chemotherapy alone, cytoreductive surgery followed by HIPEC and adjuvant chemotherapy showed increased survival (47,48). However, the study utilized 5-FU and leucovorin as opposed to the standard combination therapy with FOLFOX or FOLFIRI. In addition, disease recurrence after cytoreductive surgery and HIPEC is common, ranging from 22.5% to 82%, and perioperative morbidity is high ranging from 19% to 49% (49,50). Therefore, cytoreductive surgery in combination with HIPEC should be limited to select patients (see Chapter 32).

## FUTURE DIRECTION IN COLORECTAL CANCER

Immunotherapy has quickly become a widely used therapy in many malignancies given its success. The therapy is based on the theory that many tumor cells upregulate PD-L1 (programmed death ligand 1) in order to escape the host's immune system (51). There have been limited studies looking at immunotherapy in the setting of colorectal cancer. A phase 2 study investigated the relationship between mismatch-repair status and possible clinical benefit of immune checkpoint blockade, specifically with pembrolizumab (52). Although overall survival and progression-free survival endpoints were not reached, the study did show that mismatch-repair status can predict benefit from such agents (52). There are several ongoing trials in this space, the results of which may help define the role of immunotherapy for colorectal cancers.

## CONCLUSION

Even with the advances made in therapeutic options and improvements in median survival from 1 year to more than 30 months, colorectal cancer remains the third leading cause of cancer-related death (1,27). There are still many areas of research that need to be investigated in order to help guide the management of colorectal cancer. Overall, it will undoubtedly rely on a multidisciplinary approach to obtain the best outcomes for patients.

## REFERENCES

1. Siegel RL et al. *CA Cancer J Clin.* 2016;66(1):7–30.
2. Edwards BK et al. *Cancer.* 2010;116(3):544–73.
3. Cress RD et al. *Cancer.* 2006;107(5 Suppl.):1142–52.
4. Siegel RL et al. *Cancer Epidemiol Biomarkers Prev.* 2012;21(3):411–6.
5. Saltz LB. *Surg Oncol Clin N Am.* 2010;19(4):819–27.
6. Patrlj L et al. *Hepatobiliary Surg Nutr.* 2014;3(5): 324–9.

7. Quasar Collaborative G et al. *Lancet*. 2007;370(9604): 2020–9.

8. Des Guetz G et al. *Cochrane Database Syst Rev*. 2010; (1):CD007046.

9. Andre T et al. *N Engl J Med*. 2004;350(23):2343–51.

10. Andre T et al. *J Clin Oncol*. 2009;27(19):3109–16.

11. Benson 3rd AB et al. *J Clin Oncol*. 2004;22(16): 3408–19.

12. Schmoll HJ et al. *J Clin Oncol*. 2007;25(1):102–9.

13. Haller DG et al. *J Clin Oncol*. 2011;29(11):1465–71.

14. Kuebler JP et al. *J Clin Oncol*. 2007;25(16):2198–204.

15. Twelves C et al. *N Engl J Med*. 2005;352(26): 2696–704.

16. Marsoni S et al. *Lancet*. 1995;345(8955):939–44.

17. Tournigand C et al. *J Clin Oncol*. 2012;30(27): 3353–60.

18. Bosset JF et al. *N Engl J Med*. 2006;355(11):1114–23.

19. Sauer R et al. *N Engl J Med*. 2004;351(17):1731–40.

20. Aschele C et al. *J Clin Oncol*. 2011;29(20):2773–80.

21. Gerard JP et al. *J Clin Oncol*. 2012;30(36):4558–65.

22. Rodel C et al. *Lancet Oncol*. 2015;16(8):979–89.

23. Hofheinz RD et al. *Lancet Oncol*. 2012;13(6):579–88.

24. Bosset JF et al. *Lancet Oncol*. 2014;15(2):184–90.

25. Biagi JJ et al. *JAMA*. 2011;305(22):2335–42.

26. Yoo PS et al. *Clin Colorectal Cancer*. 2006;6(3):202–7.

27. Heinemann V et al. *Lancet Oncol*. 2014;15(10): 1065–75.

28. Koopman M et al. *Lancet*. 2007;370(9582):135–42.

29. Ducreux M et al. *Lancet Oncol*. 2011;12(11):1032–44.

30. Seymour MT et al. *Lancet*. 2007;370(9582):143–52.

31. Tournigand C et al. *J Clin Oncol*. 2004;22(2):229–37.

32. Goldberg RM et al. *J Clin Oncol*. 2004;22(1):23–30.

33. Kabbinavar FF et al. *J Clin Oncol*. 2005;23(16): 3706–12.

34. Saltz LB et al. *J Clin Oncol*. 2008;26(12):2013–9.

35. Hurwitz H et al. *N Engl J Med*. 2004;350(23): 2335–42.

36. McKay JA et al. *Eur J Cancer*. 2002;38(17):2258–64.

37. Pietrantonio F et al. *Crit Rev Oncol Hematol*. 2015; 96(1):156–66.

38. Jonker DJ et al. *N Engl J Med*. 2007;357(20):2040–8.

39. Tol J et al. *N Engl J Med*. 2009;360(6):563–72.

40. Hegewisch-Becker S et al. *Lancet Oncol*. 2015;16(13): 1355–69.

41. Cassidy J et al. *Br J Cancer*. 2011;105(1):58–64.

42. Karapetis CS et al. *N Engl J Med*. 2008;359(17): 1757–65.

43. Van Cutsem E et al. *J Clin Oncol*. 2007;25(13): 1658–64.

44. Grothey A et al. *Lancet*. 2013;381(9863):303–12.

45. Mayer RJ et al. *N Engl J Med*. 2015;372(20):1909–19.

46. Elias D et al. *J Clin Oncol*. 2010;28(1):63–8.

47. Verwaal VJ et al. *J Clin Oncol*. 2003;21(20):3737–43.

48. Hendlisz A et al. *J Clin Oncol*. 2010;28(23):3687–94.

49. van Oudheusden TR et al. *Eur J Surg Oncol*. 2015; 41(10):1269–77.

50. McRee AJ et al. *Oncology*. 2015;29(7):523–4, C3.

51. Topalian SL et al. *N Engl J Med*. 2012;366(26):2443–54.

52. Le DT et al. *N Engl J Med*. 2015;372(26):2509–20.

# 34

# Adjunctive treatment of rectal cancer with radiation and the adverse effects of radiation exposure of the rectum

ROLAND HAWKINS

## CHALLENGING CASE

A 62-year-old man presents with blood per rectum. He has mild rectal discomfort with bowel movements and a feeling of incomplete evacuation. Two years previously he received external beam radiotherapy for prostate cancer. His rectal examination is normal except for some blood on the gloved finger. A flexible sigmoidoscopy demonstrates friable mucosa with neovascularity of the distal 4 cm of rectum. The mucosa is friable with telangiectasia.

## CASE MANAGEMENT

The history and endoscopic exam are suggestive of radiation proctitis. Management includes fiber and topical therapy. The friable areas of the rectum can be treated with topical application of a large swab soaked with 10% formalin passed through an anoscope or proctoscope. Argon plasma coagulation is also effective treatment.

## INTRODUCTION

Apart from a few exceptional circumstances, radiation treatment is used as an adjunct to surgical resection in the potentially curative treatment of adenocarcinoma of the rectum. The benefits and adverse effects of the adjunctive use of radiation in the surgical treatment of rectal cancer are the principal topics addressed in this chapter.

Radiation therapy is also used for the nonsurgical, potentially curative treatment of cancers of the cervix, uterus, bladder, prostate, and anus. To achieve cure of these pelvic cancers without surgical resection, a relatively high dose of radiation is necessary, for instance 70–90 Gy compared to the 40–54 Gy used for adjunctive treatment and for the nonsurgical treatment of squamous cell carcinoma of the anal canal. The rectal injury that sometimes results from exposure of the rectum in the course of treating pelvic cancers is occasionally referred to the rectal surgeon for treatment. Treatment of rectal injury from radiation exposure is addressed in the section "Rectal Injury and Its Treatment."

Adjunctive radiation treatment is employed to eradicate deposits of cancer in soft tissue beyond the margins of resection and in pelvic lymph nodes not removed at surgery. It is administered either before or following en bloc resection of the involved length of large bowel by low anterior resection (LAR) or abdominal perineal resection (APR). Preoperative treatment is referred to as neoadjuvant and postoperative treatment as adjuvant. Radiation treatment is usually administered to patients with locally advanced but resectable stage II or III disease (Table 34.1). Radiation treatment is also administered as an adjunct to local excision of less advanced rectal cancer.

Recurrence after apparently curative surgery for rectal cancer may develop in structures adjacent to the margin of resection, in regional lymph nodes in the pelvis, or as metastasis to the peritoneum or distant organs. Treatment with radiation and/or chemotherapy is judged as beneficial insofar as it increases patient survival or reduces the incidence of local, regional, or distant recurrence. Long-term survival is the most important outcome in judging benefit. It is unambiguously evaluable and reflects the balance of benefit and potentially life-threatening adverse effects of treatment. Local and regional recurrence is often not salvageable. Its

Table 34.1 Staging of rectal carcinoma

| Dukes | TNM group | TNM | Description |
|---|---|---|---|
| A | I | T1 N0 M0 | Tumor limited to submucosa |
|  |  | T2 N0 M0 | Tumor into, not through, muscularis propria |
| B | II | T3 N0 M0 | Tumor through muscularis propria |
|  |  | T4 N0 M0 | Tumor invades other organs or through peritoneal serosa |
| C | III | N1 or N2 | N1 (1–3 nodes +) |
|  |  | Any T, M0 | N2 (>3 nodes +) |
| D | IV | M1, any T or N | Distant metastasis |

prevention is important, if not a requirement, for achieving cure of the disease. It may itself be life threatening and may act as a source of distant metastasis. Furthermore, uncontrolled recurrence in the pelvis is detrimental to the quality of life of patients who are not cured. It may cause pain, bleeding, infection, obstruction, and incontinence affecting bowel and urogenital organs. Distant recurrence is important because it is usually an unsalvageable life-threatening form of treatment failure.

Evolution of the method of adjunctive radiation treatment of rectal cancer over the past 30 years has produced what are now two standard treatment regimens, referred to here as the short and long treatment courses. The short course has been used only for preoperative treatment. It typically consists of a dose of 25 Gy in fractions of 5 Gy each over a period of 5–7 days with surgery following within a week. A variant of the short course has been reported to give improved disease-free survival (1,2). It consists of short-course radiation followed by chemotherapy and then total mesorectal excision.

The long course has been used for both pre- and postoperative treatment. It typically consists of 45–54 Gy in fractions of 1.8–2 Gy over a period of 5–6 weeks and includes concurrent chemotherapy with 5-fluorouricil. When used preoperatively, surgical resection is usually 6–12 weeks after completing the long-course radiation treatment.

The cell killing effectiveness of a course of radiation treatment is expressed by a biologically effective dose with symbol $BED_{\alpha/\beta}$. The value of $BED_{\alpha/\beta}$ is defined so that fractionated treatment courses that have the same $BED_{\alpha/\beta}$ may be expected to kill the same fraction of the population of cells of a treated cancer or of an exposed normal tissue or organ (3,4). As such, it is used to quantitatively compare the level of effect of different fractionated radiation treatment courses with regard to their likelihood of curing a cancer or causing a specific organ injury. The value of $BED_{\alpha/\beta}$ for a course of radiation consisting of $n$ treatments (fractions) of dose $d$ Gy is calculated as

$$BED_{\alpha/\beta} = nd\left(1 + \frac{d}{\alpha/\beta}\right) - \frac{T \ln 2}{\alpha \tau_2} \qquad (34.1)$$

In which $T$ is the time between the first and last radiation treatments. The value of $\tau_2$ is the volume doubling time of the irradiated population of cells in the absence of radiation exposure. It includes the effect of the time from mitosis to mitosis of cycling cells, the presence of a subpopulation of cells that are not cycling, and cell death from causes other than radiation. The range of values of $\tau_2$ for clinically evident rectal cancer is from about 20 to 100 days. The values of $\alpha$ and $\beta$ are constants of the linear quadratic relation between dose and the fraction of cells that survive irradiation with the ability to reproduce enough times to form a visible colony. As shown in Equation 34.1, the ratio $\alpha/\beta$ determines the influence of variation of the fractional dose $d$ on the cell killing effect of the radiation course. The term that depends on $T$ represents the increase in the fraction of cells that survive because of cell replication during the course. The fraction of cells that survive a course of radiation is defined as the number of viable cells present immediately after the last exposure divided by the number present immediately prior to the first.

The value of the $\alpha/\beta$ ratio has been measured and tabulated for an array of experimental animal tumors, human cancers, and the cells upon which the function of various normal tissues and organs depends (5,6). For malignant tumors, $\alpha/\beta$ is usually estimated to be about 10 Gy. The value of $\alpha$ is estimated to be about 0.15 Gy$^{-1}$ for rectal and other carcinomas. With these values and assuming $\tau_2$ is about 30 days, the $BED_{\alpha/\beta}$ of the short course of radiation treatment consisting of five treatments of 5 Gy each over 7 days is 37.5–1.1 = 36.4 Gy. With these same values, the $BED_{\alpha/\beta}$ of the long course consisting of 28 treatments of 1.8 Gy each over 37 days is 59.5−4.3 = 55.2 Gy. This indicates the long course provides a biologically effective dose that is 52% greater than the short course.

However, consider that when given as a neoadjuvant preoperative treatment, the cancer cells that survive the long course are expected to continue replicating during the time between the last radiation exposure and the day of surgery. Therefore, to include the effect of cell replication on the fraction of the cells that survive at the time of surgery, the value of $T$ in Equation 34.1 should be the time from the day of the first radiation exposure to the day of surgery. For the long course this is about 90 days. With $T$ equal to 90 and the other constants the same as for the short course, $BED_{\alpha/\beta}$ of the long course is 59.5−13.9 = 45.6 Gy. Doing the same thing for the short course and making $T$ equal to about 12 days gives $BED_{\alpha/\beta}$ for the short course equal to 35.6 Gy. That is, the long course is a biologically effective dose that is about 28% greater than the short course with respect to fraction of the cancer cells present at the start of the radiation course that are still viable at the time of the surgery. The addition of concurrent chemotherapy to the long course is expected to make the differential between long and short courses even greater.

With the exception of some lymphocyte subsets that die within hours of exposure to radiation, the physiologic death, disintegration, and disappearance of nearly all cells lethally injured by ionizing radiation takes place only after they and/or their descendants go through one or more, often aberrant cell divisions. As a result, there is a time lag between exposure of a cancer and the physiological death and disappearance of the irradiated carcinoma cells that is variable and dependent on their mitotic activity. This lag ranges from a few days to a year or more. A typical time to manifest the maximal response of a carcinoma or sarcoma to radiation is the order of a few weeks to a month or two. The same phenomenon is in part responsible for the delay of 6 months to a year or more in the development of some forms of radiation injury to normal organs.

With short-course preoperative radiation, there is little time for tumor response before surgery. There is evidence that at surgery after short-course irradiation, the average tumor size and average number of lymph nodes with metastatic carcinoma have decreased slightly, but this is not enough to produce a change in the distribution of tumor or nodal stage in a study population (7). With long-course preoperative irradiation, more time is allowed for response of the disease and downstaging to occur. This is evident in some of the trials listed in Tables 34.3 and 34.4. This was demonstrated in a trial in which all patients were treated with 13 daily fractions of 3 Gy each and randomly assigned to surgery within 2 weeks after the end of radiation or surgery 6–8 weeks after radiation (8).

With both long and short courses, radiation is directed at the pelvis with the superior border placed at about the L5-S1 interspace. The inferior border is placed at least 3–5 cm below the distal-most extent of tumor or at the inferior margin of the obdurator foramen. For distal tumors, it may include all or part of the anal canal. In earlier studies, treatment was restricted to anterior-posterior directed beams (9). More recently, laterally directed beams that exclude some bladder and bowel in the anterior part of the pelvis are a standard part of the beam arrangement referred to as a three-dimensional (3D) conformal plan. Only the volume that is exposed to all the beams gets the full prescribed dose. This includes, in addition to the rectum and mesorectum, small and large bowel in the posterior pelvis, the posterior part of the bladder and prostate, the presacral area, the sacrum and sacral canal nerves, the lymph nodes of the internal iliac, and the most distal part of the common iliac chains. If there is extension to urogenital organs, the lymph nodes of the external iliac chains are sometimes included. After APR, the perineal incision, which tends to be a site of recurrence, is included in the treatment volume (10,11).

With the availability of intensity modulated radiation therapy, the clinical treatment volume can sometimes be encompassed with less dose to bowel, bladder, and perineal skin than with the 3D conformal plan. When given as a rotational arc (volumetric-modulated arc therapy [VMAT]) the intensity modulated treatment has been reported to have efficacy equivalent to the 3D conformal treatment. There were similar acute and long-term side effects except that the VMAT treatment was associated with significantly less high-grade anal incontinence, 4% compared to 16% with *p*-value of 0.032 (12).

## BENEFIT OF ADJUVANT AND NEOADJUVANT RADIATION TREATMENT

Tables 34.2, 34.3, and 34.4 summarize several trials in which patients were randomly assigned to treatment consisting of various combinations of pre- and postoperative radiation and chemotherapy. The radiation treatment plans of each assignment are similar to either the short or long course previously described and can be gleaned from the table by noting the dose shown. When the dose is about 25 Gy, it is a short course and when 40–60 Gy it is similar to the long course. Benefits and adverse effects of pre- and post-operative radiation treatment reported in these studies will be examined and compared. Adjuvant treatment after local excision is also discussed.

Several randomized trials of postoperative adjuvant therapy in the late 1970s and 1980s listed in Table 34.2 indicate that postoperative radiation and chemotherapy can lead to statistically significant improvement in overall survival and the incidence of local recurrence when compared to surgery alone. Based on gastrointestinal tumor study group (13), North Central Cancer Treatment Group (NCCTG) (14), and National surgical adjuvant breast and bowel program (NSABP) (15) studies, a U.S. National Institutes of Health consensus development conference in 1990 recommended that postoperative radiation and chemotherapy be standard treatment for stages II and III rectal cancer (16). An advantage of postoperative treatment is that selection for adjuvant treatment can be based on pathologic staging, whereas with preoperative treatment selection is based on necessarily imperfect clinical staging.

The use of preoperative radiation has been extensively evaluated in Europe. From inspection of the randomized trials in Table 34.3, it is evident that preoperative radiation treatment reliably produces a clinically and statistically significant reduction in the incidence of local recurrence by about 50%–60%. This remains true even in the Dutch colorectal cancer trial, which was designed to minimize the need for pelvic irradiation by mandating surgery to include a total mesorectal excision (TME) (17). Note that the results for the surgery-only arms shown in Table 34.3 indicate that TME is more rigorously extirpated than the surgery of historical practice. Its use reduced the total recurrence at 5 years after surgery alone to 10.4% compared to the 25%–28% found in the Stockholm I and II and Swedish rectal trials that did not require TME (9,18,19).

About 35% of the patients in the Dutch study had disease found in pelvic nodes making them stage III. Among this subgroup, 20.6% of those who did not have radiation treatment and 10.6% of those who did suffered a local recurrence

Table 34.2 Postoperative adjuvant radiation studies

| Study | Number of patients | Therapy arms | Pelvic recurrence %, 5 years | Survival %, 5 years | Comments |
|---|---|---|---|---|---|
| GITSG (13) | 202 | S | 24 | 46 | T3, T4, or N+ |
| | | S-C | 27 | 56 | Semustine + 5-FU |
| | | S-44 Gy | 20 | 52 | |
| | | S-44 Gy + C | 11 | 59 ($p = 0.07$) | |
| NCCTG (14) | 204 | S-50.4 Gy | 25 | 47 | Semustine + 5-FU |
| | | S-50.4 Gy + C | 13 ($p = 0.036$) | 57 ($p = 0.02$) | |
| NSABP (15) R-01 | 555 | S | 25 | 43 | Semustine + 5-FU |
| | | S-46 Gy | 16 ($p = 0.06$) | 41 | +Vincristine |
| | | S-C | 21.4 | 53 ($p = 0.01$) | |
| Norway (63) | 144 | S | 30 | 50 | Bolus 5-FU on 6 days |
| | | S-46 Gy + C | 12 ($p = 0.01$) | 64 ($p = 0.05$) | During radiation |
| NSABP (64) R-02 | 694 | S-C | 14 | 58 | Semustine + 5-FU |
| | | S-50.4 Gy + C | 8 ($p = 0.02$) | 58 | +Vincristine or 5-FU + leukovorin |
| MGH and Emory (31) | 99 | LE (T1) | 11 | | Chemotherapy for some patients |
| | | LE-xrt (T1) | None | | |
| | | LE (T2) | 67 | | |
| | | LE-xrt (T2) | 15 ($p = 0.004$) | | |
| RTOG (30) 89-02 | 65 | LE, T1 (fav) | 14.3 | 86 | Fav = favorable |
| | | LE-xrt (T1,T2,T3) | 17.6 | 72 | Features, see text |

Table 34.3 Preoperative neoadjuvant radiation studies

| Study | Number of patients | Therapy arms | Pelvic recurrence %, 5 years | Survival %, 5 years | Comments |
|---|---|---|---|---|---|
| Stockholm I (9) | 849 | S | 28 | 36 | No lateral beam |
| | | 25 Gy-S | 14 ($p < 0.001$) | 36 | |
| Stockholm II (18) | 557 | S | 25 | 39[a] | Patients ≤80 |
| | | 25 Gy-S | 12 ($p < 0.001$) | 46[a] ($p = 0.03$) | |
| Swedish (19) Rectal | 1,168 | S | 27 | 48 | Patients ≤80 |
| | | 25 Gy-S | 11 ($p < 0.001$) | 58 ($p < 0.001$) | |
| Dutch TME (17) | 1,861 | S | 10.4 | 64 | Patients ≤80 |
| | | 25 Gy-S | 5.6 ($p < 0.001$) | 64 | |
| Manchester (20) | 284 | S | 36 | 39[a] | |
| | | 20 Gy-S (5 Gy x 4) | 13 ($p < 0.001$) | 46[a] ($p = 0.03$) | |
| MRC II (21) | 289 | S | 48 | 19 | S 4 weeks |
| | | 40 Gy-S (2 Gy x20) | 32 ($p = 0.04$) | 26 ($p = 0.09$) | After external radiation therapy |
| Polish (22) | 312 | 25 Gy-S | 9 | 67.2 | Mostly TME (T3/T4) |
| | | 50.4 Gy + C-S | 14 | 66.2 | Patients ≤75 |
| EORTC (23) | 1,011 | 45 Gy-S | 17.1 | 63.2 two arms | Patients ≤80 |
| | | 45 Gy + C-S | 9.6 | Without post-op C | |
| | | 45 Gy-S-C | 8.7 | 67.2 two arms | |
| | | 45 Gy + C-S-C | 7.6 | With post-op C ($p = 0.12$) | |
| FFCD (24) | 762 | 45 Gy-S-C | 16.5 | 67.2 | Patients ≤75 |
| | | 45 Gy + C-S-C | 8.1 ($p = 0.004$) | 66.2 | |

[a] Surviving percent is for patients who underwent a potentially curative resection.

Table 34.4 Pre- versus postoperative radiation studies

| Study | Number of patients | Therapy arms | Pelvic recurrence %, 5 years | Survival %, 5 years | Comments |
|---|---|---|---|---|---|
| Uppsala (25) | 471 | 25.5 Gy-S | 12 | 44 | 5.1 Gy × 5 |
| | | S-60 Gy | 21 ($p = 0.02$) | 39 ($p = 0.49$) | 2 Gy × 30 |
| German (26) | 823 | 50.4 Gy + C-S-C | 6 | 74 | TME |
| | | S-50.4 Gy + C-C | 13 ($p = 0.006$) | 76 ($p = 0.8$) | Patients <75 |

($p < 0.001$). About 28% had stage II disease. Among these, the local recurrence rate without radiation was 7.2% and with radiation 5.3% ($p = 0.331$). About 28% had stage I disease. Among these a local recurrence rate was 1.7% without radiation and 0.4% with ($p = 0.091$). Among 7% of patients with distant metastasis found at surgery (stage IV) there was local recurrence in 26.9% without radiation and with 15.9 with ($p = 0.207$). Thus, for all four stages there was less local recurrence in patients who had radiation, but the differential only reach statistical significance for the node-positive (stage III) subgroup and the entire randomized population. Similarly, it was found that the difference reached statistical significance in the subgroup that had LAR but not in subgroups that had APR or Hartmann pouch surgery and in the subgroup for which the distal tumor edge was between 5 and 10 cm from the anal verge, but not those more proximal or distal.

The Swedish rectal study differs from the Dutch study in that TME was not required (19). The proportion of patients in each stage was similar, but the differential in rate of local recurrence between arms of the trial was greater and statistically significant for all stages. In the stage III subgroup of the Swedish study, local recurrence was 40% without preoperative radiation and 20% with ($p < 0.001$). For stage II it was 23% without and 10% with radiation ($p = 0.002$). For stage I it was 4% without and 2% with radiation ($p = 0.02$).

Comparison of these two studies suggests that benefit from preoperative radiation in preventing local recurrence is maximal if given to patients likely to have node-positive (stage III) disease, expected to have LAR as opposed to APR, and with lowest tumor extent in the middle to distal rectum. However, some reduction in risk of local recurrence may be expected for all patients.

As shown in Table 34.3, overall survival rate was not affected by the short-course preoperative radiation treatment in the Dutch TME trial and in the earlier Stockholm I trial. In the Swedish rectal trial, the short-course preoperative radiation treatment produced a statistically significant gain in overall survival. Two other short-course preoperative radiation trials, Stockholm II and Manchester, showed statistically significant improvement in overall survival among the subgroup that actually underwent curative resection but not in all randomized patients (18,20).

Failure to improve overall survival even though local recurrence rate is significantly reduced can occur in two important ways. First, the dominant cause of death may be from development of distant metastatic disease to such

an extent that a small incidence of local recurrence in the surgery-only arm and its reduction by radiation treatment has no statistically significant, or even discernible, impact on survival. This may be the principal explanation in the Dutch TME trial.

The other way impact on survival of a local recurrence advantage may be reduced, or lost, is if excess nonrectal cancer death is produced in the radiation treatment arm. This is likely the explanation for limitation of statistically significant survival benefit to the subgroup that had curative surgery in the Stockholm II trial (18). At median follow-up of 8.8 years for this trial, 19% of the radiation arm and 12% of the surgery-only arm had died of noncancer causes ($p = 0.1$). There was cardiovascular death in 13% of the radiation arm and 7% in the surgery-only arm ($p = 0.07$). This differential was established within the first 6 months after surgery during which 5% of radiated patients and 1% of the surgery-only patients died from cardiovascular causes ($p = 0.02$). The excess cardiovascular death was predominantly in patients older than 68 years. It is suggested this is due to change in the coagulation properties of blood during the several months of recovery from pelvic surgery that has followed radiation treatment. This leads to increased thrombotic events in the irradiated patients.

The only randomized study of preoperative radiation with a surgery-only control arm that used a radiation treatment regimen resembling the long course described above is the MRC II trial (21). Patients were eligible if they had a partially or totally fixed rectal tumor on physical examination. The population likely consisted mostly of T3 and T4 tumors. There were likely more locally advanced cancers than in the short-course trials. As shown in Table 34.3, there was a significant decrease in local recurrence in the radiation arm and a tendency toward increased survival, though not statistically significant, similar to the findings in several short-course trials.

The Polish trial compares short-course preoperative radiation with long-course preoperative radiation plus concurrent chemotherapy (22). Most of the surgery was with TME. Patients were clinically staged with physical examination, transrectal ultrasound, and/or magnetic resonance imaging. Only those with evidence of T3 or T4 tumors that were palpable on digital examination and had no anal sphincter involvement were included. Patients found to have involved nodes at surgery usually received postoperative chemotherapy. More in the short-course arm were node positive, suggesting downstaging by the long-course treatment. There was no difference in survival between the two arms. There is a suggestive difference in local recurrence favoring the short course, but it did not reach statistical significance. There was no statistically significant difference in the fraction that received a permanent stoma with a tendency to favor the long-course arm for sphincter preservation.

The EORTC trial examined the effect of adding chemotherapy to long-course preoperative radiation with a finding that if chemotherapy is given concurrently with preoperative radiation, postoperatively, or both, the rate of local recurrence is reduced significantly relative to the preoperative long-course radiation with no chemotherapy (23). This suggests concurrent radiochemotherapy does not contribute much if postoperative chemotherapy is given. Alternatively, the FFCD trial in which both arms got postoperative chemotherapy reports a significant decrease in local recurrence if concurrent chemotherapy is given with preoperative radiation (24). There was no survival difference.

Two randomized trials listed in Table 34.4 have directly compared pre- and postoperative radiation treatment arms. In the earlier Uppsala trial, the preoperative arm had the short course of radiation (25). Those randomized to the postoperative arm and found to have stage II or III disease were treated with long course to a higher dose of 60 Gy in 2 Gy fractions. In the recent German trial, the surgery was mandated to be with TME, and clinical staging was intended to exclude stage I patients from the study (26). Those randomized to the long-course preoperative arm and the subset of those randomized to the postoperative arm who were proved to have stage II or III disease at surgery, received similar regimens of chemotherapy. The radiation courses were concurrent with 5-FU chemotherapy and consisted of 50.4 Gy in fractions of 1.8 Gy except that an additional 5.4 Gy to a reduced volume was included in the postoperative treatment. Both of these trials showed statistically significant difference in local recurrence rate favoring the preoperative arm and no significant difference in survival when grouped by intention to treat at randomization. It is of note that 28% of the postoperative arm of the German trial received no radiation treatment. Of these, in 18% the cause was finding pathologic stage I disease, and in 10% the cause was postoperative death or complications, or the finding of stage IV disease at surgery. Patient selection and the treatment regimen of the preoperative arm of the German trial are now standard treatment in many institutions.

Several reviews and meta-analyses of neoadjuvant and adjuvant radiation treatment of resectable, locally advanced rectal cancer have been compiled (27–29). They indicate that radiation approximately halves the rate of recurrence in the pelvis when given either preoperatively or postoperatively and gives a small increase in overall survival.

Preoperative irradiation has become the favored way to include radiation in rectal cancer treatment. It is informative to examine the most recent of these meta-analyses, which compares preoperative irradiation, with and without concurrent chemotherapy, with surgery alone (29). It is compiled from a database of 41,121 patients. Patients

from randomized trials and other comparative studies are included. Overall survival, disease-free survival, cancer-specific survival, local recurrence-free survival, and metastasis-free survival are tabulated for the whole population and for subgroups defined by follow-up time, patient age, $BED_{\alpha/\beta}$, study time period, pathologic stage, radiation regimen, anatomic location in rectum, surgical procedure, and geographic origin of the included population. The hazard ratio (HR) of death is less than or equal to one favoring better overall survival with neoadjuvant treatment over surgery alone for all patients and subgroups. However, it reaches statistical significance or near significance only for treatment with long-course radiation with concurrent combination chemotherapy (HR = 0.54, $p < 0.06$) and for the American patient population treated with long-course radiation and concurrent 5-fluorouricil chemotherapy (HR = 0.39, $p < 0.01$). Local recurrence-free survival favors neoadjuvant treatment and reaches statistical significance for the population as a whole (HR = 0.63, $p < 0.04$) and for all the subgroups.

In all of the above trials, surgery consisted of LAR or APR. For patients with evidence of stage T1 or T2 rectal cancer distal to the peritoneal reflection, usually within 10 cm from the anal verge, smaller than about 4 cm and occupying a limited fraction of the circumference of the rectal wall, local excision via transanal, transsphincteric (York-Mason), or posterior proctotomy (Kraske) procedure may be able to achieve en bloc full-thickness excision of the tumor with negative margins. This limited surgery may be elected in lieu of APR or LAR to preserve sphincter function or to avoid major surgery in those not fit or not willing to undergo it. Comparison of local excision (LE) with APR or LAR as to the ability to remove all the carcinoma has not been established by the randomized trial. Nevertheless, it is expected that limited local excision will not as reliably prevent local recurrence as the more radical surgery, particularly TME. This is confirmed by the local recurrence rates reported in the retrospective series shown in Table 34.2, particularly for T2 disease (30,31). The decrease in local recurrence with adjuvant radiation, with or without concurrent chemotherapy, suggests that the local excision with adjuvant treatment is efficacious enough to be considered as an option under some circumstances. Bias in the retrospective studies would be to select for radiation treatment those patients with unfavorable features in the pathology, such as positive or close margins, lymphovascular invasion, or high histologic grade. Thus, the benefit from adjuvant treatment may be more than indicated by the results shown.

The RTOG protocol 89-02 study enrolled patients with tumors judged by the surgeon to be distal enough to not allow clearance by LAR and who underwent local excision via transanal, transsacral, or transcoccygeal approach (30). To be eligible the tumor had to be mobile, less than 4 cm in size and occupy less than 40% of the rectal circumference. Those patients with cancer found to be pathologic stage TI, with histologic grade 1 or 2, excised with at least 3 mm margin in all directions, absent any lymphatic or vascular invasion and with normal CEA received no postoperative treatment. Patients lacking any one of these favorable features were treated with radiation to the pelvis with boost to the tumor site to a total dose of 50–56 Gy in 1.8–2 Gy fractions with concurrent 5-FU chemotherapy. If the margin was microscopically positive or closer than 3 mm, the dose to the tumor bed was increased to give a total dose of 59.4–66 Gy. The local recurrence rate for T2 tumors, all of which received adjuvant treatment, was 4 of 25 (16%) that for T3 tumors was 3 of 13 (23%). It is not clear what the chance of salvage for local failure with APR is, but it may be as much as 50% (32). The results for local excision shown in Table 34.2 support the view that local excision with postoperative adjuvant treatment with radiation and chemotherapy, although not as likely to be curative as radical surgery, is an acceptable option for tumors of the size and position that permit it, when there is sufficient reason to avoid radical surgery. The treatment of early rectal cancers has recently been reviewed (33).

## ACUTE ADVERSE EFFECTS

By acute adverse effect is meant one that develops during a radiation course, or in the 1 or 2 weeks following it, and which resolves within a month or two after the completion of the course, without treatment, other than that to relieve the temporary symptoms. The acute adverse effects that most often require a break from treatment are the perianal skin reaction and diarrhea. A scale adopted by the RTOG and EORTC for reporting acute effects of radiation of the lower GI tract is representative and in use in current trials (34). Grade 1 is given for increased frequency or change in bowel habits not requiring medication or rectal discomfort not requiring analgesics. A score of grade 2 implies diarrhea requiring Imodium or Lomotil medication, or mucus or bloody discharge not requiring sanitary pads, or rectal or abdominal pain requiring analgesic medication. A score of grade 3 is given for diarrhea requiring parenteral support, mucous or bloody discharge requiring sanitary pads, or abdominal distention with distended bowel loops on radiograph. Grade 4 implies acute or subacute bowel obstruction, or fistula or perforation or GI bleeding requiring transfusion, or abdominal pain or tenesmus requiring tube decompression or bowel diversion. Grades 3 and 4 are often combined and reported as severe adverse effects.

In the EORTC trial, 1,011 patients were treated with preoperative irradiation to a dose of 45 Gy in 25 fractions over 5 weeks (23). Half were randomly assigned to also have concurrent preoperative chemotherapy, and half had none. Acute grade 2 toxicity was reported in 38.4% of those who received the concurrent preoperative chemotherapy and 29.7% of those who did not ($p < 0.001$). Grade 3 or 4 acute adverse effects were reported in 13.9% of those whose treatment included preoperative chemotherapy and 7.4% of those who had only preoperative for irradiation ($p < 0.001$). The

rate of local recurrence as the first event was approximately 9% at 5 years among those who received chemotherapy preoperatively, postoperatively, or both, and 17% in those who had no chemotherapy ($p < 0.002$). There was no statistically significant difference in overall survival. This suggests the additional acute toxicity of preoperative concurrent radiation and chemotherapy over that of preoperative radiation alone may not be necessary if postoperative chemotherapy is to be given. This is contradicted by the FFCD trial (24).

The incidence of severe diarrhea during postoperative radiation treatment following LAR or APR depends on the specific concurrent chemotherapy regimen. For 656 patients treated on the phase III NCCTG trial, it was found to be 13% for bolus infusion of 5-FU at a dose of 500 mg/m$^2$ on each of 3 days of the first and fifth weeks. It was 23% for infusion of 5-FU at the rate of 225 mg/m$^2$ per day given continuously for the entire length of the course of radiation (35). Improvement in survival at 4 years of 70% with a continuous regimen compared to 60% with bolus infusion was felt to justify the definite, though modest, increase in toxicity.

The type of surgery was also a significant determinant of the risk of severe diarrhea. In those who had undergone LAR, there was a 31% rate of severe diarrhea compared to 13% in those who had an APR ($p < 0.001$). This differential is not unexpected as there is a significant rate of diarrhea after LAR in the absence of radiation. In this regard, it is of note that the frequency of bowel movements at the time of discharge after LAR via total mesorectal excision in 81 patients who were not treated with radiation averaged about 8 per day (36).

In the trial that randomized patients to pre- versus postoperative long-course chemoradiotherapy conducted by the German rectal cancer study group, the incidence of severe diarrhea among 399 patients randomized to preoperative treatment was 12%. Among the 237 patients actually treated with postoperative radiation, the rate of severe diarrhea was 18% ($p = 0.04$) (26). The postoperative arm included some 23% that had APR. Thus, among those who had a LAR, and are most comparable to patient's preoperative arm with respect to bowel function, the rate of severe diarrhea must have been greater than 18% and the differential in favor of the preoperative treatment even greater. But if the 110 patients in the postoperative arm who, for one reason or another, had no radiation treatment are included in the toxicity score, there was no difference in rate of severe acute grade 3 or grade 4 toxicity.

Other grade 3 or 4 acute side effects reported in the German study were hematologic and dermatologic. The percent of grade 3 and 4 hematologic toxicity was 6% in the preoperative and 8% in the postoperative arms ($p = 0.27$). Dermatological toxicity refers to radiation dermatitis in the perianal skin or perianal crease suture line (Figure 34.1). Grade 3 or 4 radiation dermatitis is reported for 11% of preoperative and 15% of the postoperative patients who had radiation ($p = 0.09$). The rate of grade 3 or 4 acute toxicity of any kind was 27% in the preoperative and 40% in the postoperative patients who had radiation ($p = 0.001$).

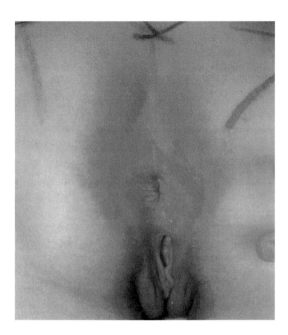

Figure 34.1 **(See color insert.)** Radiation dermatitis.

These results from two randomized studies support the conclusion that preoperative standard fractionated 5–6 week radiation treatment with chemotherapy produces less diarrhea and other acute adverse effects than in comparable patients who have had the same treatment after surgery. The differential is definitely present. However, it is a modest difference so that, in itself, it does not provide a compelling reason for preferring preoperative neoadjuvant treatment over postoperative treatment. Furthermore, 28% of patients in the postoperative arm of the German study were spared radiation treatment because of the finding of stage I disease (18%) or distant metastasis (10%) at surgery, and thus had zero adverse radiation effects.

The short preoperative radiation treatment course of five fractions of 5 Gy each in 1 week does not usually produce significant adverse effects in the 2–3 weeks during the radiation treatment and before surgical resection. In the Dutch TME trial, grade 1 acute gastrointestinal side effects were reported in 12%, grade 2 was reported in 2.3%, and grade 3 in 1 of 605 patients (17). Acute neurologic effects of radiation were reported as grade 1 (requiring no intervention) in 7.5%, as grade 2 (requiring narcotic pain medicine or adjustment of treatment) in 1%, and grade 3 (intractable severe pain or causing treatment interruption) in 2.8%. This has been attributed to radiation-induced lumbosacral plexopathy. It was first reported in patients treated with a short course in the Uppsala and Swedish rectal trial (19,25). It consists of pain in the lower extremities and buttocks and in a minority of the patients was associated with other lower extremity neurologic signs. In a few patients, the effect persisted or recurred for months to years. Acute neurologic effects have not been reported with the lower fractional doses of the long-course preoperative radiation treatment. Acute effects on the genitourinary and other

systems were less frequent than those in the gastrointestinal and neurologic systems.

## SURGICAL COMPLICATIONS AFTER PREOPERATIVE IRRADIATION

Patients treated preoperatively with short-course radiotherapy in the Stockholm I trial had surgical mortality of 8% compared with 2% in the surgery-only arm ($p < 0.01$) (9). Among patients over 75 years of age, the mortality in the preoperative arm was 16% and again only 2% in the surgery-only arm. The dominant cause of the increase in postoperative death was cardiovascular. The radiation treatment in Stockholm I was specified to be anterior-posterior and posterior-anterior directed beams only, and encompassed, in addition to the pelvis, the para-aortic nodes cephalad to the L2 vertebral level. With the inclusion of laterally directed beams and restriction of the radiated volume to the pelvis as well as exclusion of elderly patients in the subsequent Stockholm II, Swedish rectal, and Dutch TME trials, the surgical mortality was not statistically different between pre-op radiation and surgery-only arms (17–19). For instance, in the Dutch TME trial the surgical mortality was 3.5% in the preoperative radiation arm and 2.6% in the surgery-only arm ($p = 0.38$) (17). The in-hospital death rate was 4% in the pre-op radiation arm and 3.3% in the surgery-only arm ($p = 0.49$) and very strongly correlated with age in both arms. There was no exclusion for age in the Dutch TME trial with the oldest patient age 92 years.

In the Dutch TME trial, there was no significant difference between the two arms in operating time (180 minutes) or length of hospital stay (15 or 14 days median) (37). Median blood loss in the pre-op radiation arm was 1,100 mL and in the surgery-only arm was 1,000 mL. The percent of LAR patients with a diverting stoma increased from 60% to 67% in the 60 days following surgery. In the surgery-only arm it increased from 54% to 63% ($p = 0.17$). A statistically significant difference in postoperative complications between the arms was found for cardiac events, 5% with pre-op radiation and 3% surgery only ($p < 0.05$); psychologic disorders, 4% with pre-op radiation and 1% surgery only ($p < 0.01$); and for any complication, 48% in pre-op radiation arm and 41% surgery only ($p < 0.01$). Complications in the APR patients occurred in 29% of the radiated patients and 18% of surgery-only patients ($p < 0.01$). There was no significant difference in complication rate among LAR patients, 11% and 12%, respectively, in the radiation and surgery-only arms. These results indicate that there is the potential for short-course preoperative radiation to complicate the ensuing surgery and recovery particularly manifest in patients over the age of 70 and even more so in those over the age of 80. This is minimized but not eliminated by adherence to the now standard radiation treatment planning specifications noted in the introduction.

The German trial required TME surgery and excluded patients over the age of 75. The radiation treatment was the long course (50.4 Gy in 28 fractions of 1.8 Gy each) with concurrent chemotherapy and was given either preoperatively or postoperatively (26,38). There was 0.8% surgical mortality in the preoperative arm and 1% in the postoperative arm indicating no increase attributable to the preoperative radiochemotherapy. The incidence of any postoperative complication was 34.5% in the preoperative arm and 34% in the postoperative arm. Anastomotic leak occurred in 13% and 12%, delayed wound healing in 5% and 6% of, respectively, pre- and postoperative arms. All other complications occurred in less than 3% of each arm with no significant difference.

The Polish trial randomized patients between preoperative short-course radiation and long-course radiation with chemotherapy (22,39). Surgery was by TME for the more distal tumors, and patients over age 75 were excluded. The overall rate of complication events was 31% in the short-course arm and 22% in the long-course arm ($p = 0.06$) showing a near significant trend. The overall number of patients suffering a complication was 27% of the short-course and 21% in the long-course arm ($p = 0.27$). Postoperative death occurred in 0.7% of the long-course and 1.3% of the short-course arms ($p = 1.0$). Reoperation was needed in 8.2% of the short-course and 9.5% of the long-course patients ($p = 0.85$). No statistically significant difference and no suggestive trend were found to favor one or the other arm with respect to other less severe complications.

Postoperative complications after preoperative irradiation examined in the meta-analysis (29) include wound complications, anastomotic leakage, bowel obstruction, and mortality. Notable findings expressed as a hazard ratio are as follows. Preoperative short-course radiation versus surgery alone had statistically significant unfavorable outcome for wound complications (HR = 1.65, $p < 0.01$), over all postoperative morbidity (HR = 1.45, $p < 0.01$) and postoperative mortality (HR = 2.15, $p < 0.01$). The mortality increase was predominantly from thrombotic vascular events such as pulmonary embolus, myocardial infarction, and stroke. The long-course preoperative treatment with concurrent chemotherapy showed statistically significant increase in wound complications (HR = 1.52, $p < 0.02$) and anastomotic leakage (HR = 1.22, $p < 0.05$). For patient populations with median age less than 65 years, none of the post-op complications showed a statistically significant increase for either long- or short-course radiation treatment.

In conclusion, the studies shown in Tables 34.2, 34.3, and 34.4, and the meta-analysis indicate that inclusion of radiation in preoperative neoadjuvant treatment of rectal cancer is associated with a statistically significant increase in postoperative complications in elderly patients but not in younger patients. The dividing age between the elderly and the young is somewhere in the 70s. The most important increase is in postoperative mortality, which is found following the short-course preoperative treatment. It does not reach statistical significance with the long course.

## CHRONIC LATE ADVERSE EFFECTS OF ADJUVANT AND NEOADJUVANT IRRADIATION

By late adverse effect is meant one that persists or develops 4–6 months or more after the last radiation treatment and becomes a chronic injury. Examples are frequent bowel movements, rectal bleeding, incontinence, constipation, and bowel obstruction. The total dose, fractional dose, and time span of the long and short courses of adjuvant and neoadjuvant radiation treatment have been established so that chronic injury that significantly affects quality of life is unusual, and one that is life altering is rare. Chronic injury may be more likely in patients who have had severe acute reactions to radiation, termed *consequential chronic injury*, but may also occur in those who experienced little or no acute effect. It also may have increased likelihood in patients with diabetes.

Chronic injury occurs as a result of depletion of the population of stem cells responsible for maintenance of tissue integrity and organ function due to radiation-induced cell reproductive death. For instance, the death of the stem cells responsible for maintaining the microvascular circulation leads to occlusion of arterioles that is the distinguishing feature of the histology of irradiated tissue examined more than a few months after radiation exposure. Over ensuing years, the impaired microcirculation may cause progressive ischemic injury to the exposed tissue manifest principally as telangectasia, fibrosis, and defective healing. These effects may be associated with bleeding; incontinence; stenosis of bowel, ureter, or urethra; and bowel obstruction. They may complicate surgery on irradiated tissue several months to many years after the radiation treatment.

Several long-term quality of life outcomes are reported in the meta-analysis (29). These are expressed as an odds ratio (OR) of having the unfavorable complication with preoperative radiation treatment compared to surgery alone. The OR reached statistical significance for use of an absorbent pad (OR = 2.4, $p < 0.01$), incontinence of gas (OR = 1.62, $p < 0.04$), incontinence of stool (OR = 1.81, $p < 0.01$), fecal urgency (OR = 2.4, $p < 0.03$), and male erectile dysfunction (OR = 2.25, $p < 0.01$). It did not reach statistical significance for constipation, diarrhea, or urinary incontinence.

Patients enrolled in the Dutch TME preoperative short-course radiation trial who are alive with no evident disease were sent a questionnaire by mail to assess bowel, stoma, and urinary function (40). A response was obtained from 597 (84% of those mailed). Among these the median time since surgery was 5.09 years. The mean number of bowel movements during the day among the 362 patients who had no stoma was 3.69 in the irradiated patients and 3.02 in the surgery-only patients ($p = 0.011$). The mean number of nocturnal movements was 0.48 in the irradiated patients and 0.35 in the surgery-only patients ($p = 0.207$). Daytime fecal incontinence was reported as 62% of those irradiated and

38% of the surgery-only patients ($p < 0.001$), and nocturnal incontinence in, respectively, 32% and 17% ($p = 0.001$). The incontinence also occurred more often and was more troublesome in the irradiated compared to surgery-only patients. Pads were in use for incontinence and anal mucous and blood loss in 56% irradiated and in 33% of surgery-only patients ($p < 0.001$). Among 235 responding patients with a stoma, there was no significant difference between irradiated and surgery-only patients with respect to stoma function.

A review of the patients treated on the Dutch TME trial was conducted to determine risk factors for development of fecal incontinence (41). Potential risk factors examined included age, gender, childbirth, body mass index, cancer stage, tumor distance from anal verge, anastomosis distance from anal verge, duration of surgery, blood loss at surgery, presence of a pouch, temporary stoma, and an anastomotic leak. No risk factors emerged as statistically significant among the surgery-only patients. Among the preoperative radiation patients, only blood loss at surgery and distal tumor margin distance from the anal verge were statistically significant risk factors. Blood loss of surgery greater than 1,400 mL had relative risk (RR) of incontinence of 3.24 ($p = 0.005$) compared to those with less blood loss. Compared to patients with distance of distal tumor margin less than 5 cm from the anal verge, a distance between 5 and 10 cm had RR of 0.21 ($p = 0.016$), and a distance greater than 10 cm had RR of 0.13 ($p < 0.003$). The location of distal tumor extent determines the inferior extent of the radiation treatment port. Among those few respondents who had the perineum and consequently the entire anal sphincter included in the radiation field compared to those who did not, the RR for fecal incontinence at 2 years after surgery was 2.64 ($p = 0.085$) and at 5 years after surgery the RR was 7.45 ($p = 0.059$). It was also noted that the fraction of patients reporting fecal incontinence increased after reaching a minimum at 2 years postsurgery, whereas that in surgery-only patients increased only slightly. This time course is consistent with a late effect of radiation on pelvic nerves and fibrosis.

Urinary function was not significantly different in irradiated and surgery-only patients. About 39% of patients in each group reported incontinence of urine. Back and buttock pain, hip stiffness, and difficulty walking were not significantly different in the two groups, suggesting an absence of chronic radiation-induced lumbosacral plexopathy in this trial.

The rate of hospital admission was significantly increased in the irradiated patients compared with surgery-only patients in the first 6 months after surgery. Admissions were for infection, endocrine, cardiovascular, and gastrointestinal diagnoses. Of note among gastrointestinal admissions, those for constipation and abdominal pain are significantly increased in the radiated patients, but those for bowel obstruction were not. The rate of hospital admission more than 6 months after surgery was not significantly different for patients in the two groups, including for myocardial infarction or stroke.

A comparative study by phone interview of patients 2 or more years after they had undergone LAR for rectal cancer at Mayo Clinic reports significantly more bowel symptoms in the 41 who had also had postoperative long-course pelvic irradiation and chemotherapy than in the 59 who had only surgery (42). The fraction having more than five bowel movements a day was 37% in the irradiated group and 14% in the surgery-only group ($p < 0.001$). The fraction of patients who reported incontinence was 66% in the irradiated group and 7% in the surgery-only group ($p < 0.001$). In the irradiated group 41% wore a pad, and in the surgery-only group, 10% ($p < 0.001$). Urgency with the inability to defer defecation for 15 minutes was reported in 78% of the irradiated and 19% of the surgery-only patients ($p < 0.001$).

A retrospective study of 192 patients who had LAR with coloanal anastomosis at the Mayo Clinic and had preoperative long-course radiation, postoperative radiation, or no radiation reports an anastomotic stricture was the most common effect requiring surgical intervention. This occurred with nearly the same frequency in all three groups: 16% no radiation, 14% pre-op radiation, and 15% post-op radiation. It was usually managed with dilation and was not a significant cause of permanent fecal diversion. Permanent fecal diversion resulted from recurrence, bowel obstruction, incontinence, fistula, stricture, abscess/leak, and patient preference. The 5-year survival without colostomy was 92% in patients who had no radiation treatment and 72% in those who did ($p < 0.001$). There was no significant difference between the rates in pre- and postoperative irradiated patients.

A scale adopted by the RTOG and EROTC for reporting late chronic effects of radiation on the bowel is as follows (34). Grade 1 implies mild diarrhea, mild cramping, less than five movements per day, and slight rectal discharge or bleeding. Grade 2 implies moderate diarrhea and colic, more than five bowel movements per day, excessive mucus, or intermittent bleeding. Grade 3 implies obstruction or bleeding requiring surgery. Grade 4 implies necrosis perforation or fistula. Fecal incontinence was not explicitly included in the grading criteria.

The German trial reports grades 3 and 4 long-term gastrointestinal effects, for example, diarrhea and small bowel obstruction, in 9% of the pre-op group and 15% of the post-op group ($p = 0.07$); anastomotic stricture in 4% of the pre-op and 12% of the post-op arms ($p = 0.003$) (26,38). Bladder dysfunction of grade 3 or 4 occurred in 2% of the pre-op and 4% of the post-op arms ($p = 0.21$). Any grade 3 or 4 effect occurred in 14% of the pre-op and 24% of the post-op patients ($p = 0.01$). With the long-course fractionation of pelvic chemoradiotherapy for adjunctive treatment of rectal cancer, the preoperative irradiation appeared significantly less likely to produce severe, chronic, long-term sequelae then postoperative radiation.

The Polish trial comparing short-course preoperative radiation with long-course preoperative radiochemotherapy at median follow-up of 48 months reports the overall incidence of late toxicity is 28.3% in the short-course and 27% in the long-course arms ($p = 0.81$)(43). The incidence of severe late toxicity, presumably grade 3 or 4, was 10.1% in the short-course and 7.1% in the long-course arms ($p = 0.36$). Severe gastrointestinal toxicity occurred in 5.1% of the short-course and 1.4% of the long-course patients, no $P$ value given. Quality of life questionnaire on anorectal function including questions on bowel function, incontinence, and urgency reports no significant difference between short- and long-course arms (43). For instance, 39% and 41% of, respectively, the short-course and long-course patients reported use of pads. In answering the question, "did your health status and/or treatment cause your sexual life to decline," there also was no significant difference in the two arms. This direct comparison with long- and short-course preoperative treatment shows no statistically significant difference in late toxicity.

The evidence from several trials summarized here indicates that both preoperative and postoperative radiation treatment are associated with increased chance of chronic adverse effect on bowel function. The direct comparison of pre- and postoperative long-course radiochemotherapy in the German trial indicates there is less likelihood of this with the preoperative treatment. The Polish trial comparing long- and short-course preoperative radiation finds no clear difference.

## RECTAL INJURY AND ITS TREATMENT

A part of the rectum or the nearby sigmoid colon is sometimes exposed to radiation dose as great as 70–80 Gy with $BED_{\alpha/\beta}$ greater than 100 Gy in the nonsurgical radiation treatment of cervical, endometrial, or prostate cancer. As many as 20% of these patients may develop symptoms of chronic proctitis with rectal bleeding, urgency, pain, and tenesmus. Some may develop fistulas, strictures, and incontinence (44). It should not be assumed that these symptoms and findings represent radiation proctitis without a thorough evaluation, as recurrent cancer may cause the same symptoms.

Endoscopy reveals friability, pallor, erythema, or prominent mucosal telangiectasias (Figure 34.2) (45). Histologic findings in the chronic phase include vascular changes such as the telangiectatic capillaries, platelet thrombi formation, and lumen of arterioles filled in with fibrin. These changes are accompanied by fibrosis in the lamina propria and crypt distortion (46).

Numerous therapeutic agents have been evaluated and are currently utilized against radiation-induced proctitis. In many cases, patients presenting initially with symptoms suggestive of radiation proctitis will first be offered treatment with anti-inflammatory medications. This most commonly involves either oral or enema-delivered steroids or various 5-amino salicylic acid preparations. Though often utilized in both acute and chronic settings, evidence is lacking for the use of steroid preparations in the treatment of radiation proctitis. A prospective randomized trial compared

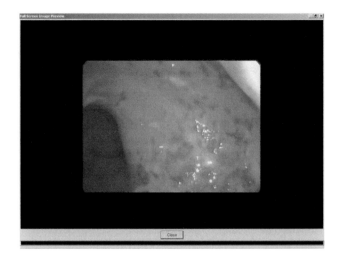

Figure 34.2 **(See color insert.)** Radiation proctitis.

oral sulfasalazine plus rectal steroids to rectal sucralfate and oral placebo. The sulfasalazine regimen demonstrated a significant improvement in both clinical symptoms and endoscopic findings; however, by comparison clinically this was less effective than sucralfate (47). One randomized, controlled trial found that oral sucralfate decreased diarrhea symptoms in both the acute and chronic phases (48). Short-chain fatty acids act as a major fuel source for rectal mucosa. Two small randomized placebo controlled trials using short-chain fatty acid enemas noted improvement in symptoms and endoscopic findings (49,50).

Various endoscopic ablation therapies have been applied to the treatment of colonic proctitis–related bleeding due to local telangiectasias. The two most commonly utilized approaches are the laser and the argon plasma coagulator. There are no prospective randomized trials assessing either of these approaches, only several retrospective case series. The largest series reporting on the use of Nd:YAG laser found excellent response rates and a significant decrease in rectal bleeding (51). Rare complications include mucus discharge, ulcers, or stricture. Similar results were obtained using an argon plasma coagulator in three treatment sessions (52). However, over 70% required maintenance treatment over the long term (53).

For treatment of bleeding related to chronic proctitis, 4% and 10% formalin have been utilized. Two approaches are commonly utilized: rectal formalin irrigation and dab technique utilizing topical application of formalin with swabs or soaked gauze (54,55). De Paradies et al. reported a prospective case series using the formalin gauze application and noted a beneficial result in 70% (56). However, significant rates of stricturing and incontinence were reported. Numerous other retrospective series have reported good success with formalin. Of those using of gauze or pledget-mediated application, at least a 75% success rate for cessation or improvement in bleeding was reported (57). Many required multiple treatments, though complications were minimal. Due to the small volume used, 10% formalin is often used. Of those reporting use of formalin rectal irrigations, 50 cc aliquots of 4% formalin were utilized up to a total volume of 400–500 cc. Again, >75% success rate was noted with this approach, with the most common reported complication being anal or pelvic pain occurring in 25% of those treated (58).

There is low-level evidence supporting the use of hyperbaric oxygen treatments for chronic radiation proctitis and a single prospective series, which reported significant improvement of bleeding, diarrhea, and urgency, but no change in rectal pain with oral vitamins E and C (59,60). Metronidazole along with anti-inflammatory agents (oral mesalazine and betamethasone enema) produced a significantly lower incidence of rectal bleeding and diarrhea in chronic radiation proctitis (61).

Despite the numerous medical approaches available for the treatment of radiation proctitis, surgical therapy remains an option for refractory cases. The indications for surgery are most commonly rectum or rectosigmoid stenosis and rectovaginal fistula, while the most common presenting symptoms are rectal bleeding, diarrhea, or tenesmus (61). The majority of patients undergo diversionary procedures (proctectomy with colostomy, with or without a Hartmann rectal stump) with resection performed less commonly. When continuity is restorative, coloanal anastomosis (with or without colonic J-pouch) with proximal covering stoma is the procedure of choice in selected cases. Successful outcomes with diversion alone are reported in the range of 70%–73% (62). In refractory rectal bleeding, this option has less morbidity. Overall, morbidity with surgical intervention is extremely high, ranging from 30% to 65% with mortality rates in the postoperative period reported at 6.7%–25% (62).

## CONCLUSION

Chemotherapy and radiation treatment to the pelvis as an adjuvant to surgical resection, either individually or when both are administered, reduces the chance of pelvic recurrence and increases by a small increment the chance of the patient surviving the disease. This has been demonstrated in several randomized trials for both the pre- and postoperative treatment sequences, as noted in the tables and in meta-analyses (27–29).

That preoperative treatment with radiation can complicate ensuing surgery and postoperative recovery is illustrated in the occurrence of additional noncancer, mostly cardiovascular, death among irradiated patients in the immediate postoperative period and in the first 6 months postsurgery in the Stockholm trials. A similar adverse effect was not evident in the later Swedish and Dutch TME trials that also used the short-course radiation regimen, and it was not evident in the studies that used the long-course preoperative treatment regimens. These later trials were with better radiation therapy technique, and all but the Dutch TME trial excluded the most elderly patients. The potential for serious adverse effect of preoperative irradiation on the surgery is eliminated or minimized by restricting the irradiated volume to those parts of the pelvis at risk for harboring disease, possibly by using intensity modulated radiation therapy, and by avoiding the short-course treatment for patients with age greater than about 70.

The Polish trial, which directly compared short-course with long-course preoperative irradiation, was inconclusive (22). The German trial has provided evidence that preoperative long-course chemoradiation is in balance preferable to the similar treatment postoperatively (26,38). The selection criteria and preoperative treatment arm of the German trial have become the standard in many treatment centers. The long course can be expected to produce some downstaging and facilitate R0 resection.

For younger patients, the short-course preoperative radiation treatment may be considered for several reasons. It has a theoretical advantage of more timely removal of all evident disease than the long course. It has better compliance and is more economical. The surgical staging is undistorted by downstaging from the long course of treatment, and this may affect the recommendation for adjuvant chemotherapy. For instance, patients found to have no lymph node metastases may be spared adjuvant chemotherapy. But chemotherapy with the full adjuvant regimen, as opposed to 5-FU alone, can begin earlier with the short course than with the long course. The high fractional dose of the short course has the theoretical disadvantage of greater risk of chronic injury, particularly that related to pelvic nerves that is associated with neuropathic pain, bowel and bladder continence, and sexual function.

## REFERENCES

1. Markovina S et al. *Int J Radiat Oncol Biol Phys* 2017; 99:417–26.
2. Bisscchop C et al. *Ann Surg Oncol.* 2017;24:2632–8.
3. Barendsen GW. *Int J Radiat Oncol Biol Phys.* 1982; 8:1981–97.
4. Jones B et al. *Clin. Oncol.* 2001;13:71–81.
5. Bentzen SM, Joiner MC. 2009. The linear quadratic approach in clinical practice. In: Joiner M, van der Kogel A (eds) *Basic Clinical Radiobiology*, 4th edition, Hodder Arnold. London, 120–134.
6. Kian Ang K et al. Altered fractionation schedules. In: Brady LW and Perez CA (eds) *Principles and Practice of Radiation Oncology* 2nd edition. Lipincott-Raven, Philadelphia New York, 119–142. 1998.
7. Marijnen CAM et al. *J Clin Oncol.* 2001;19:1976–84.
8. Francois Y et al. *J Clin Oncol.* 1991;17:2396.
9. Cedarmark B et al. *Cancer.* 1995;75:2269–75.
10. Walz BJ et al. *Int J Radiat Oncol Biol Phys.* 1981; 7: 477–84.
11. Rich T et al. *Cancer* 1983;52:1317–29.
12. Regnier A et al. *Frontiers Oncol* 2017;7:225.
13. Gastrointestinal Tumor Study Group. *New Engl J Med.* 1985;312:1465–72.
14. Krook JE et al. *New Engl J Med.* 1991;324:709–15.

15. Fisher B et al. *J Natl Cancer Inst.* 1988;80:21–9.
16. NIH consensus conference. *JAMA.* 1990;264: 1444–50.
17. Koen CMJ et al. *Ann Surg.* 2007;246:693–701.
18. Martling A et al. *Cancer* 2001;92:896–902.
19. *New Engl J Med.* 1997;336:980–7.
20. Marsh PJ et al. *Dis Colon Rectum.* 1994;37:1205–14.
21. *Lancet* 1996;348:1605–10.
22. Bujko K et al. *Brit J Surg.* 2006;93:1215–23.
23. Bosset J et al. *New Engl J Med.* 2006;355:1114–23.
24. Gerard J et al. *J Clin Oncol* 2006;24:4620–5.
25. Fyrkholn GJ et al. *Dis Colon Rectum.* 1993;36: 564–72.
26. Saur R et al. *New Engl J Med.* 2004;351:1731–40.
27. Colorectal Cancer Collaborative Group. *Lancet.* 2001; 358:1291–1304.
28. Glimeliius B J et al. *Acta Oncologica.* 2003;42: 476–92.
29. Bin Ma et al. *Int J Cancer.* 141:1052–65.
30. Russell AH et al. *Int J Radiat Oncol Biol Phys.* 2000; 46:313–22.
31. Chakravarti A et al. *Ann Surg.* 1999;230:49–54.
32. Sharma A, Hartley, Monson JR. *Surg Oncol.* 2003;12: 51–61.
33. Tytherleigh MG et al. *Brit J Surg.* 2008;95:409–23.
34. Cox JD et al. *Int J Radiat Oncol Biol Phys.* 1995;31: 1341–6.
35. Miller RC et al. *Int J Radiat Oncol Biol Phys.* 2002;54: 409–13.
36. McAnena OJ et al. *Surg Gynoecol Obstet.* 1990;170: 517–21.
37. Marijnen CAM et al. *J Clin Oncol.* 2002;20:817–24.
38. Sauer R et al. *Strahlentherapie Oncol.* 2001;177: 173–81.
39. Bujko K et al. *Colorectal Dis.* 2005;7:410–6.
40. Peeters KCMJ et al. *J Clin Oncol.* 2005;23:6199–206.
41. Lange MM et al. *Br J Surg.* 2007;94:1278–84.
42. Kollmorgen CF et al. *Ann Surg.* 1994;220:676–82.
43. Pietrzak L et al. *Radiother Oncol.* 2007;84:217–25.
44. Hayne D et al. *Br J Surg.* 2001;88:1037–48.
45. Reichelderfer M, Morrissey JF. *Gastrointest Endosc.* 1980;26:41–3.
46. Haboubi NY et al. *Am J Gastroenterol.* 1988;83: 1140–4.
47. Kochlar R et al. *Dig Dis Sci.* 1991;36:103–7.
48. Henriksson R et al. *Scand J Gastroenterol.* 1992;191: 7–11.
49. Pinto A et al. *Dis Colon Rectum.* 1999;42:788–95.
50. Kennedy GD, Heise CP. *Clin Colon Rectal Surg.* 2007; 20:64–72.
51. Vigiano TR et al. *Gastrointest Endosc.* 1993;39:513–7.
52. Tam W et al. *Endoscopy.* 2000;32:667–72.
53. Taylor JG et al. *Gastrointest Endosc.* 1993;39:641–4.
54. de PV et al. *Dis Colon Rectum.* 2005;48:1535–41.
55. Parik S et al. *Dis Colon Rectum.* 2003;46:596–600.
56. Luna-Perez P, Rodriguez-Ramirez SE. *J Surg Oncol.* 2002;80:41–4.
57. Dall'era MA et al. *J Urol.* 2006;176:87–90.
58. Kennedy M et al. *Am J Gastroenterol.* 2001;96: 1080–4.
59. Cavcic J et al. *Croat Med J.* 2000;41:314–8.
60. Pricolo VE, Shellito PC. *Dis Colon Rectum.* 1994;37: 675–84.
61. Anseline PF et al. *Ann Surg.* 1981;194:716–24.
62. Camma C et al. *JAMA.* 2000;284:1008–15.
63. Tveit KM et al. *Br J Surg.* 1997;84:1130–5.
64. Wolmark N et al. *J Natl Cancer Inst.* 2000;92: 388–96.

# 35

# Surgical management of ulcerative colitis

SHANNON McCHESNEY AND BRIAN R. KANN

---

## CHALLENGING CASE

A 45-year-old man with a 20-year history of ulcerative colitis (UC) is presenting with perineal pain, tenesmus, bloody stools, and incontinence. He has a history of restorative proctocolectomy with ileal pouch anal anastomosis (IPAA) performed 10 years prior.

## CASE MANAGEMENT

Pouchitis is a complication frequently seen in UC patients following restorative proctocolectomy with IPAA. Diagnosis of this condition involved clinical assessment, as well as endoscopic examination via pouchoscopy, to confirm mucosal inflammation, and biopsy. Treatment is primarily medical, consisting of antibiotics, probiotics, and steroids; however, in refractory cases surgical intervention may be required. Surgical options include pouch excision with diverting ileostomy or redo IPAA.

## INTRODUCTION

UC is a chronic inflammatory condition predominantly involving the colon and rectum, characterized by recurrent inflammatory episodes. This inflammatory bowel disease may present with abdominal pain, rectal bleeding, diarrhea, and weight loss. Bowel involvement can vary, from isolated rectal disease to pancolitis. Extraintestinal manifestations may present as well. Diagnosis is most common in late adolescence or early adulthood but occurs at all ages (1). An estimated 3 million U.S. adults have ever received a diagnosis of inflammatory bowel disease (2), with up to 1.4 million people in the United States currently living with the disease (1). The prevalence of UC is higher in adults than children; 238 versus 28 per 100,000, respectively (3).

Of these patients, up to 40% will require colectomy at some point in their lifetime, despite current medical therapies (4). This chapter explores the indications, methods, and outcomes of surgery in UC.

## INDICATIONS FOR SURGERY

### URGENT/EMERGENT

The timing of surgery is dependent on severity of disease. Truelove and Witts classification system is commonly used to categorize mild, severe, and fulminant disease, with the latter described as greater than 10 continuously bloody stools per day, fever, pulse greater than 90, anemia requiring transfusion, erythrocyte sedimentation rate greater than 30, colonic dilatation, and abdominal distension and tenderness (5) (Table 35.1). Since the classification was published in 1955, describing the benefit of steroids for acute colitis, corticosteroids have been implemented for controlling active disease, which has resulted in reduced mortality (6).

Urgent or emergent surgery is indicated for patients with acute toxic colitis and associated complications thereof, including perforation, hemorrhage, and obstruction. It is also indicated in patients with toxic megacolon, sepsis, or fulminant disease unresponsive to maximum medical therapy.

Urgent or emergent colectomy for acute colitis is associated with considerable morbidity and mortality. A systemic review of 29 studies comprising 2,714 patients demonstrated 50.8% morbidity and 8% in-hospital mortality (7).

Total abdominal colectomy with end ileostomy is most commonly performed in emergent surgery, and recommended (8). The colon is divided at the level of the sacral promontory, leaving the rectum in place to safely avoid pelvic dissection during the period of acute inflammation. The rectal stump should be kept long and may be left in place as a Hartmann's pouch, exteriorized as a mucous fistula, or placed in an extrafascial position. Completion proctectomy can be planned for a later date following resolution of acute inflammation.

Table 35.1 Truelove and witts classification system

|  | Mild | Severe | Fulminant |
| --- | --- | --- | --- |
| Bowel movements/day | <4 | >6 | >10 |
| Rectal bleeding | Intermittent | Frequent | Continuous |
| Hemoglobin | Normal | <75% of normal | Requiring transfusion |
| Erythrocyte sedimentation rate (mm/h) | <30 | >30 | >30 |
| Temperature (C) | Normal | >37.5 | >37.5 |
| Heart rate | Normal | >90 | >90 |
| Colonic features on x-ray |  | Thumbprinting, edema | Dilatation |
| Clinical signs |  | Abdominal tenderness | Abdominal tenderness and distension |

## ELECTIVE

There are several indications for elective colectomy in UC, including failure of medical management, which is most common, as well as intolerable medication complication or side effects, stricturing disease, dysplasia, invasive cancer, and growth retardation, the latter more frequently seen in the pediatric population. Severe extraintestinal manifestations may be an indication for colectomy; uveitis, monoarticular arthritis, and iritis are observed to improve following colon resection (9).

Colonic strictures develop in 5%–10% of UC patients and can pose a risk of large bowel obstruction. While the majority are benign, as many as 25% will be malignant, with 30% of cancers occurring in UC presenting as such (8). For this reason, all UC patients with strictures should undergo oncologic resection (8). Strictures developing in long-standing disease, causing obstruction, or located proximal to the splenic flexure are more likely to be malignant (10).

Patients with UC are at increased risk of developing colorectal cancer: 2% at 10 years, 8% at 20 years, and 18% at 30 years in patients with long-standing disease (11), with risk factors for malignancy including disease duration and extent, family history of colon cancer, and concurrent primary sclerosing cholangitis (12). Surveillance colonoscopy and biopsy are recommended. Patients with extensive disease should undergo colonoscopy after 8 years of disease, with surveillance colonoscopy every 1–2 years thereafter (8).

A finding of high-grade dysplasia, dyplasia-associated lesion or mass, or invasive cancer on colonoscopy is an absolute indication for surgery (8). The indication for surgery in low-grade dysplasia is debated, as studies are conflicting. The current practice parameters recommend either total proctocolectomy or surveillance endoscopy (8).

## SURGICAL OPTIONS

Surgical options for UC include a proctocolectomy with Brooke ileostomy, proctocolectomy with continent ileostomy, total abdominal colectomy (TAC) with ileorectal anastomosis, and restorative proctocolectomy (RP) with IPAA.

## PROCTOCOLECTOMY WITH BROOKE ILEOSTOMY

The proctocolectomy option followed by Brooke ileostomy is a one-stage operation that was originated by Brooke in 1952. This technique was previously considered the "gold standard" and involves removal of colon and rectum and formation of end ileostomy. The procedure is considered safe, effective, and curative of UC. While this option may avoid certain complications associated with anastomoses or pouch formation, it does entail a permanent ostomy, which may be undesirable to patients.

### Indications

Proctocolectomy with Brooke ileostomy is indicated in patients with UC requiring colectomy who are poor candidates for a more extensive restorative procedure, such as those with preoperative incontinence or perianal disease, those with a distal rectal cancer, or for those desiring a single-stage operation.

### Technique

Prior to operation, it is essential that the patient meet preoperatively with an enterostomal therapist to select the ideal ostomy placement. The patient should be assessed in different positions, and the site selected should be away from any folds, scars, or bony prominences. The patient should also be prepared for the operation with mechanical bowel preparation.

Preoperative antibiotics should be administered in the operating room and the patient placed in lithotomy position. The proctocolectomy may be performed via open or laparoscopic approach. Full mobilization from terminal ileum to rectosigmoid junction is performed, followed by pelvic dissection to elevate the rectum along a total mesorectal excision plane, taking care to identify and avoid the ureters and the hypogastric nerves. The dissection is carried down to the levators, at which time attention may be turned to the perineum. For the perineal approach, the skin is incised circumferentially around the anus, and dissection carried down until the peritoneum is entered.

Following removal of the colon and rectum, the ileostomy is created. The ileostomy should be placed within the rectus muscle over a relatively flat area, and everted to minimize effluent contacting the skin and optimizing the fit of ostomy bag appliance.

## Complications/outcomes

While ileostomy may avoid complications related to pouch creation, proctocolectomy has associated complications to be anticipated.

Perineal wound complications may arise, which should alert the surgeon to ascertain the presence of retained mucosa, foreign body, or Crohn disease. Management of this issue ranges from simple wound care to debridement and flap closure. Additional complications include sexual dysfunction such as impotence, retrograde ejaculation arising from autonomic nerve injury, and dyspareunia and infertility due to scar tissue formation (13). Overall, the most common long-term complications are ostomy related, such as skin excoriations, parastomal hernia, stomal prolapse, necrosis, retraction, or stenosis, all of which have potential to require ileostomy revision. Considering that patients with ileostomy are more prone to dehydration and related sequelae such as electrolyte derangements and kidney stone formation, it is important to educate patients on the importance of maintaining adequate hydration.

## PROCTOCOLECTOMY WITH CONTINENT ILEOSTOMY

Another single-stage operation for UC is proctocolectomy with continent ileostomy, first introduced by Nils Kock in 1969 (14). While initially met with enthusiasm, it became less utilized with the advent of IPAA.

## Indications

The continent ileostomy is an elaborate construction involving a reservoir with internal nipple valve. It is more commonly reserved for patients who have failed previous Brooke ileostomy or IPAA, those who are not pouch candidates, or those with poor sphincter tone, who wish to avoid a conventional ileostomy (15,16). Important contraindications include Crohn disease, obesity, and physical limitations or psychological disabilities that would prevent successful self-catheterization.

## Technique

Following the initial proctocolectomy, a continent ileostomy, or Kock pouch, is constructed from the terminal 50 cm of ileum. There are two main components: a reservoir and an outlet valve. A nipple valve is fashioned by the intussuscepting efferent loop of ileum. The opposing intussuscepted intestinal walls must adhere to each other to prevent dessusception, which would result in incontinence. There are several variable techniques for construction, including the S-pouch (Figure 35.1), the Barnett continent ileal reservoir, and the T-pouch, the latter of which lacks an intussuscepting valve, but was shown to have acceptable outcomes (13,17).

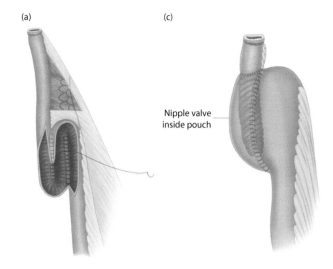

(a)

(c)

Nipple valve inside pouch

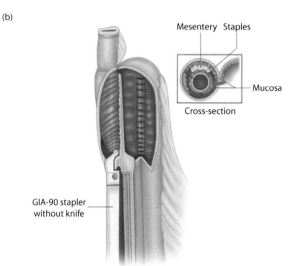

(b)

Mesentery  Staples

Mucosa

Cross-section

GIA-90 stapler without knife

Figure 35.1 Continent ileostomy. **(a)** S-shaped pouch created first with inner posterior suture line, **(b)** Nipple valve is created with three firings of a non-cutting GIA stapler, **(c)** Anterior layer of pouch is closed. (From Krane MK, Lange EO, Fichera A. Ulcerative colitis: Surgical management. In Steele SR, Hull TL, Read TE, Saclarides TJ, Sebagore AJ, Whitloe CB. (eds). *The ASCRS Textbook of Colon and Rectal Surgery*, 3rd Edition, 2016, Figures 50–5 and 6, p.876.)

## Complications/outcome

Due to the complexity of the procedure, continent ileostomies have been associated with a considerable rate of complication and reoperation. The continent ileostomy is vulnerable to both early and late complications. Common early complications include valve necrosis, hemorrhage, and leakage. Late complications range from valve malfunction (including slippage, prolapse, and stenosis) to herniation, perforation, fistula, and pouchitis. A retrospective review demonstrated valve slippage to be the most common complication, occurring in 29.7% (18). The main causes for reoperation are cited as slipped nipple valve, fistula, and stenosis (16).

An evaluation of quality of life after continent ileostomy of 330 patients reported higher scores when compared to patients who had conversion of Kock pouch to Brooke ileostomy (18). Likewise, an evaluation following patients who underwent continent ileostomy creation following failed IPAA reported good quality of life, despite a 60.9% complication rate (15).

Overall, while associated with significant complications, a continent ileostomy may allow patients freedom from traditional ileostomy and remains a viable option for selected patients.

## TOTAL ABDOMINAL COLECTOMY WITH ILEORECTAL ANASTOMOSIS

### Indications

Considering that the majority of patients with UC will have rectal involvement, this surgical option is selected for patients with indeterminate colitis, rectal sparing, and satisfactory rectal compliance and adequate sphincter function, or in high-risk patients who are poor candidates for IPAA. Advantages of this option include avoidance of both a pelvic dissection and permanent stoma, and a single-stage operation.

Pursuing TAC with ileorectal anastomosis obligates continued rectal surveillance. Endoscopy with rectal biopsies every 6–12 months is recommended.

### Technique

The patient is similarly prepared as described for proctocolectomy placed in lithotomy position. The colon is fully mobilized from the terminal ileum to the rectosigmoid junction and removed via laparoscopic or open approach. The ileorectal anastomosis may be performed in a side-to-side or side-to-end via stapled or hand-sewn fashion. Leak test confirms integrity.

### Complications/outcomes

In comparison to proctocolectomy, TAC is associated with less infertility and fewer functional complications due to the avoidance of pelvic dissection (19–21). The main concern for UC patients undergoing TAC is retained rectum and potential for persistent inflammation and development of dysplasia or cancer, resulting in ileorectal anastomosis (IRA) failures, shown to be 27% and 40% at 10 and 20 years, respectively (22). A retrospective study out of the Cleveland Clinic demonstrated rectal dysplasia and rectal cancer to occur in 17% and 8%, respectively, over a 9-year period. The reported cumulative probability of rectal dysplasia at 5, 10, 15, and 20 years was reported to be 7%, 9%, 20%, and 25%, respectively. For rectal cancer along the same time interval, it was reported to be 0%, 2%, 5%, and 14%, respectively. Proctectomy was necessary in 53% of patients (23). The most common indication for proctectomy after TAC is refractory proctitis, followed by dysplasia and cancer (23).

## RESTORATIVE PROCTOCOLECTOMY (PROCTOCOLECTOMY WITH IPAA)

Considered the most appealing option for patients with UC requiring surgery, restorative proctocolectomy with IPAA, introduced in 1978 (24,25), effectively removes all diseased bowel while preserving continence and avoiding a permanent stoma.

### Indications

Restorative proctocolectomy with IPAA is indicated in UC patients with adequate sphincter function requiring surgery. Preoperatively, sphincter function should be thoroughly evaluated using digital rectal exam. Endoanal ultrasound and anal manometry may also be utilized. The presence of preoperative incontinence is considered a contraindication to IPAA. IPAA is typically avoided in low or mid-rectal cancers due to the need for adjuvant radiotherapy and the potential effects on the pouch. Neoadjuvant therapy has also been shown to have adverse effects on pouch function, and significantly contributes to pouch failure (26). Morbid obesity is considered a relative contraindication to IPAA. In a retrospective review of patients categorized by body mass index (BMI), obese patients were found to have an increased risk of pouch-related complications after IPAA (61% versus 26%) (27), and a retrospective review comprising 1,046 patients evaluated the association of BMI and ability to technically perform IPAA and found that increasing BMI was associated with not being able to perform IPAA, with chance of unsuccessful pouch rising from 2% at BMI 30, to 15% at 40 (28).

### Technique

The patient is prepared as described above for proctocolectomy with mechanical bowel preparation, perioperative antibiotics, and placed in lithotomy. Full mobilization to free the colon from retroperitoneal attachments is carried out from the terminal ileum to the rectosigmoid junction. Dissection is carried along a total mesorectal excision plane, elevating and then dividing the rectum, leaving a short rectal cuff, and taking care to preserve the sphincter muscle complex.

The pouch may be configured as a J-pouch, S-pouch, or W-pouch, by either a double-stapled or hand-sewn anastomosis (Figure 35.2). The most commonly used variety is the J-pouch, which is constructed from the terminal 30–40 cm of ileum. The apex of the pouch is selected after identifying the longest mesentery. The segment of small intestine is folded into two 15 to 20 cm segments, and the two limbs are approximated using stay sutures. A longitudinal enterotomy is made at the apex, and a side-to-side anastomosis of the two segments is done using a linear stapler, taking care not to involve the mesentery, thus creating a reservoir. An end-to-end anastomosis stapler is used to create the pouch-anal anastomosis. The anvil is secured in the apex of

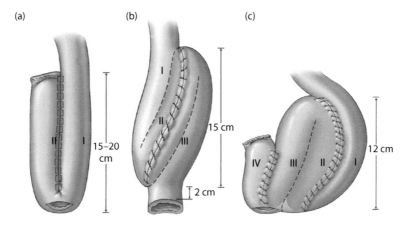

Figure 35.2 Ileal pouch configurations. **(a)** J-pouch, **(b)** S-pouch, **(c)** W-pouch.

the pouch with purse-string suture, and the stapler is introduced transanally. The suture line is inspected endoscopically, and a leak test is performed to ensure integrity.

The S-pouch involves three limbs of ileum, each 12–15 cm in length, anastomosed side-to-side, with a 2 cm exit conduit. This variation allows additional length and may be used when a J-pouch will not reach without tension. The W-pouch consists of a quadruplicated reservoir with increased capacity and compliance. A meta-analysis comprising 18 studies compared the three pouches and demonstrated increased bowel frequency associated with J-pouch, increased need for pouch intubation with S-pouch, and no difference otherwise in regard to early postoperative complications (29). Comparison of S- and W-pouch demonstrated decreased bowel frequency, as well as greater efficiency of evacuation in W-pouch (30). In a prospective comparison of the J-pouch and the W-pouch, however, no significant difference was identified in regard to bowel frequency (31).

## Mucosectomy and hand-sewn anastomosis versus double-stapled anastomosis

The type of anastomosis used for IPAA, hand-sewn or stapled, is a controversial issue.

Mucosectomy with hand-sewn anastomosis is included in the original description of IPAA and involves complete removal of anorectal mucosa up the dentate line, including the anal transition zone (ATZ) (24). Proponents of mucosectomy and hand-sewn anastomosis maintain that complete removal of mucosa more effectively eliminates the risk of malignant degeneration.

Alternatively, performing a double-stapled anastomosis leaves a short rectal cuff and preserves the ATZ, which thus preserves specialized anoderm and results in improved sensation and function. Together with the rectoanal inhibitory complex, the ATZ allows sampling of rectal contents, contributing to continence. Moreover, a double-stapled anastomosis avoids the extensive manipulation and dilation required for a complete mucosectomy, which avoids undue trauma to the sphincter complex (13,32).

Long-term studies comparing mucosectomy with hand-sewn anastomosis and double-stapled anastomosis have found the latter to be safe and with better functional outcome (33–35). Fichera et al. demonstrated excellent functional results long term without new-onset dysplasia, suggesting that preserving the ATZ is oncologically safe (33). Ziv et al. likewise described significantly more septic complications and subsequent pouch excisions after hand-sewn anastomosis in their retrospective review (34).

Prospective randomized trials comparing mucosectomy and hand-sewn anastomosis and double-stapled anastomosis have found either no difference or improved outcomes with double-stapled anastomosis (36–39).

The Cleveland Clinic prospectively evaluated 3,382 patients undergoing IPAA and compared hand-sewn and stapled anastomosis and found significantly greater use of ileostomy, longer length of stay, anastomotic stricture, septic complications, bowel obstruction, and pouch failure with hand-sewn anastomosis. Additionally, a significantly larger portion of patients in the hand-sewn group described incontinence, seepage, and worse quality of life (26).

Overall, a stapled anastomosis is preferred, as it is not only easier to perform, but is also associated with better functional outcomes and quality of life.

## One versus two versus three stages

The RP with IPAA can be achieved in one, two, or three stages.

One-stage procedure consists of proctocolectomy followed by IPAA without ileostomy.

Two-stage procedure consists of proctocolectomy, IPAA, and ileostomy during the initial operation, followed by ileostomy closure. Modified two-stage procedure consists of subtotal colectomy with end ileostomy during the initial operation, followed by proctectomy and pouch creation.

Three-stage procedure consists of subtotal colectomy and end ileostomy, followed by proctectomy and pouch creation with diverting loop ileostomy, and finally ileostomy closure (40). Unlike the modified two-stage, the three-stage procedure has a diverting loop ileostomy with interval closure after pouch creation. The three-stage procedure is typically recommended for patients with active colitis, malnutrition, or taking high-dose steroids.

A retrospective review of over 2,000 patients undergoing RP IPAA observed that while patients who underwent ileostomy had an older mean age, were taking greater doses of preoperative steroids, and required more blood transfusions, there were no differences in the ileostomy and nonileostomy groups in regard to septic complications, quality of life, or functional outcomes. Early postoperative ileus was found to be more common in the one-stage group. They concluded that in selected patients, such as those with a stapled, tension-free anastomosis, with intact tissue rings, adequate hemostasis, and without air leak, anemia, toxicity, malnutrition, or prolonged steroid course, ileostomy can be avoided (41).

A retrospective database review of 17 studies including 1,486 patients undergoing RP IPAA from 1978 to 2005 demonstrated single-stage IPAA to have similar outcomes to those with ileostomy but was associated with a significant increased risk of anastomotic leak (42).

Proponents of the ileostomy maintain that diversion prevents morbidity and mortality associated with anastomotic leakage, and that ileostomy closure itself is associated with minimal morbidity.

A retrospective review of 190 patients undergoing IPAA at a single institution from 1995 to 2003 compared modified two-stage IPAA to traditional three-stage IPAA, and found no anastomotic complications among the modified two-stage group, and also concluded the modified two-stage IPAA to be more cost effective (43). A retrospective comparison of the traditional two-stage and the modified two-stage found that the modified group had a significantly lower rate of anastomotic leak (44).

In a 5-year review of national trends of restorative proctocolectomy for UC, it was concluded that use of two-stage and three-stage has remained stable. It was observed that patients undergoing three-stage were less likely to have preoperative steroid therapy, hypoalbuminemia, preoperative sepsis, and weight loss at the time of initial pouch creation. It was also found that superficial surgical site infections are more common following three-stage surgery (45).

## Reach

A tension-free IPAA is critical to avoid adverse sequelae. Certain maneuvers may be performed to achieve adequate length, such as complete mobilization of the small bowel mesentery, exposure of the inferior portion of the head of the pancreas, scoring the peritoneum of the small bowel mesentery on anterior and posterior surfaces, and relaxing transverse incisions along the SMA mesentery. Specific arcades under tension can be identified within the mesentery and ligated, as can the ileocolic vessels. Goes et al. describes a technical procedure, performed in cadavers, in which the marginal vascular arcade of the right colon is preserved, while the distal third of the superior mesenteric artery, the ileocolic artery, and right colic artery are ligated,

to allow complete division on the terminal ileum mesentery and subsequent additional length (46).

If adequate length cannot be obtained despite implementation of each maneuver, the patient can be diverted proximally, leaving the pouch in the pelvis to revisit at another operation. Gravity, along with the weight of the pouch, may allow anastomosis at a later date.

## Complications/outcomes

Pouch-related complications range from pouchitis to pelvic sepsis and pouch failure, requiring intervention spanning from medical management to redo IPAA.

Aiming to identify risk factors for pouch failure, a single institution retrospectively reviewed 3,754 patients who underwent ileoanal pouch between 1983 and 2008, and found the strongest predictors of pouch failure to be completion proctectomy, hand-sewn anastomosis, diabetes, Crohn disease, and age at surgery (47).

A review of outcomes, complications, and quality of life in 3,707 patients after IPAA from 1984 to 2010 reported that 33.5% of patients had early perioperative complications, with a 0.1% mortality rate, 29.1% had late complications (excluding pouchitis) with a 5.3% pouch failure rate overall, and declared IPAA to be a safe procedure with favorable outcomes and high levels of satisfaction. Pelvic sepsis occurred in 6.5% of patients, early anastomotic leak in 4.8%, late anastomotic leak in 1.7%, pouch bleeding in 3.4%, early anastomotic stricture in 5.2%, and late stricture in 11.2% (48).

## Functional results: Bowel, urinary, gynecologic, sexual

A meta-analysis of 96 studies comprising 14,966 patients investigated outcomes observed in pre-2000 studies, and post-2000 studies. Incidence of pouch failure significantly decreased from 8.5% to 4.7%. Other functional outcomes were not significantly different from pre-2000 findings. Review of studies since 2000 reflected pelvic sepsis occurring in 7.5%, fistula in 4.5%, stricture in 10.7%, pouchitis in 26.8%, sexual dysfunction in 3%, small bowel obstruction in 11.4%, mild daytime incontinence in 14.3%, severe daytime incontinence in 6.1%, mild nighttime incontinence in 17.3%, and severe nighttime incontinence in 7.6% (49).

In regard to IPAA in the elderly, studies demonstrate worse outcomes but maintain that IPAA can be offered to select patients (50–53). Retrospective review of 1,454 patients who underwent IPAA for UC observed worse functional outcomes in older patients compared to younger patients, finding nocturnal stooling, fecal incontinence, pad, and constipating medication usage to be higher in patients undergoing surgery after age 45. Moreover, these issues become more common as follow-up duration increases. These outcomes were similar among both men and women (50). Delaney et al. likewise observed improved functional outcomes in patients under 45, while describing an overall high percentage of patients reporting satisfaction with the surgery (54). Moreover, a survey of 154 patients after IPAA echoed that functional outcomes worsened the further out from surgery, finding that daytime and nighttime incontinence became significantly more common 12 years or more after surgery (51).

Women and men are at risk of developing sexual dysfunction after IPAA. Men are at risk of developing erectile dysfunction and retrograde ejaculation, while women can experience dyspareunia and infertility. Considering that the majority of women undergoing IPAA are at childbearing age, this is an important consideration (55). The cause of sexual dysfunction is multifactorial; hypogastric or pelvic nerve injury during surgery can result in vaginal dryness, contributing to dyspareunia, while adhesions can cause occlusion of the fallopian tubes (55). Diagnostic laparoscopy performed at the time of ileostomy closure in IPAA patients demonstrated fewer adnexal adhesions in the laparoscopic group compared to open, using the American Fertility Society adhesion score (56).

Meta-analysis of 22 studies comprising 1,852 women investigated the effect of RP on urinary, sexual, and gynecologic function, and found incidence of infertility to increase from 12% pre-RP to 26% after. Dyspareunia likewise increased following RP, from 8% preoperatively to 25%. No association was found between sexual dysfunction and pouch function. No significant difference in urinary function was found after RP, nor was an increase in pregnancy complications observed (57).

In spite of the pouch-related complications, patients report improvement in quality of life and satisfaction with IPAA (58).

## Other complications

### SEPTIC COMPLICATIONS: LEAK AND SEQUELAE

Presentation of pelvic sepsis typically manifests as fever, leukocytosis, pelvic and perineal pain, ileus, and purulent drainage, but may be more conspicuous, characterized only by vague complaints and failure to progress along the expected clinical course. The incidence of pelvic sepsis after IPAA by meta-analysis is reported to be 7.5% (49). Pouch-related septic complications include anastomotic leak, pouch abscess, and pouch anal fistula.

A single institution study of 3,707 patients identified a 7.5% incidence of anastomotic leak among IPAA patients (48), whereas meta-analysis reported 7.1% (42). A leak may occur at the pouch anal anastomosis, as well as any suture or staple line, including the tip of the J-portion of the pouch. A leak at this location may be difficult to diagnose, and suture or staple repair may salvage the pouch.

Risk factors for anastomotic leak include anastomosis under tension and compromised blood supply. Additionally, a review of 3,233 patients found factors significantly associated with septic complications to include BMI >30, pathology consistent with inflammatory bowel disease, and intraoperative and postoperative blood transfusion (51).

Presentation of pelvic sepsis typically manifests in fever, leukocytosis, pelvic and perineal pain, ileus, and purulent drainage, but may be less conspicuous, characterized only by vague complaints, and failure to progress along clinical course. Beyond clinical findings, cross-sectional imaging is of utility in defining pathology, as is pouchogram and examination under anesthesia.

Patient management depends on source and severity of septic complications. In additional to broad-spectrum IV antibiotics and close observation, computed tomography-guided or open drainage may be required. Any patient demonstrating hemodynamic instability should be explored, the anatomy examined, and washout performed, leaving drains in place. Intestinal diversion may be required.

### SMALL BOWEL OBSTRUCTION

Small bowel obstruction is a frequently seen complication after IPAA, occurring in up to 25% of patients (48,59), and may be the foremost cause for hospitalization. A systematic review of 28 studies describes early small bowel obstruction occurring in 2%–12% of patients, with late small bowel obstruction occurring more frequently at 17% (60). Small bowel obstruction may occur due to adhesions, stenosis, volvulus, or internal hernia. Several studies have found use of diverting ileostomy to be associated with an increased risk of bowel obstruction (61–63), and increased risk of requiring surgery for small bowel obstruction (59). A prospective randomized study determined the use of an adhesion barrier, Seprafilm® (Sanofi, Bridgewater, NJ), reduced the incidence of small bowel obstructions requiring surgery; however, it did not reduce the incidence of small bowel obstruction overall (64).

A retrospective review of patients with medically treated small bowel obstruction after IPAA demonstrated an increased total number of bowel movements per day in the first postoperative year compared to patients without small bowel obstruction, as well as more daytime seepage at 10 years postoperative. Quality of life, however, was comparable among groups (65).

The majority of small bowel obstructions resolve without surgery, with the need for surgery ranging from 3% to 19% (59); however, if no progression is observed, operative intervention should be pursued.

### HEMORRHAGE

Bleeding from the pouch is a less common complication of IPAA and may present from ostomy or anus. Incidence of bleeding was shown to be 1.5% in a study of 3,194 patients (66). Intervention, while frequently required, is typically nonsurgical. Endoscopy with clot evacuation and cautery or epinephrine enemas has been shown to be effective (66).

### STRICTURE

Pouch stricture is a common complication of IPAA. Risk factors for stricture include use of small stapling gun, use of defunctioning ileostomy, anastomotic dehiscence, and pelvic sepsis (67). Two locations prone to stricture formation include the pouch-anal anastomosis and the junction of the neoterminal ileum and pouch. Endoscopic dilation of strictures has proven efficacious (66,67).

# Fistula

## POUCH VAGINAL FISTULA

Pouch vaginal fistula (PVF) is a major cause of morbidity and pouch failure after IPAA, with an incidence between 4% and 16% (68). Pouch failure occurs in 21%–30% of patients with PVF, with excision required in 26% (69). Major risk factors for PVF include pelvic sepsis, anastomotic separation and stricture, small bowel obstruction, hemorrhage, and pouchitis (69), as well as a diagnosis of indeterminate colitis or Crohn disease (70).

Patients with diagnosis of indeterminate colitis or Crohn disease have a higher incidence of PVF, as well as a higher rate of morbidity with PVF compared to UC (71). A delayed diagnosis of Crohn disease after IPAA is associated with worse outcomes and higher rates of pouch failure after treatment (72).

The type of anastomosis employed at the time of surgery has been investigated as a possible cause of PVF. Lee et al. described an association between PVF and hand-sewn anastomosis (73), as did Mallick et al., whereas Groom et al. observed an insignificant increased incidence among stapled anastomoses (74).

PVF were found located above the anastomosis in 24%–26%, at the anastomosis in 26%–28%, and below the anastomosis in 48% of cases in two separate retrospective reviews (68,75).

Surgical repair is varied and includes local repair via a transanal approach with either advancement flap or direct repair in layers, transvaginal repair with advancement flap, fistulectomy, interposition flap, transabdominal approach, and redo IPAA. The choice of repair is dependent on location and character of the fistula. It is imperative to treat pelvic sepsis prior to definitive repair, and to attempt the simplest approach first. Diverting ileostomy is frequently employed in surgical treatment (70). A retrospective review by Tsujinaka et al. reported a mean number of 2.2 surgical treatments, with Crohn patients requiring a mean of 3 (75).

An algorithm suggested by Lolohea et al. outlines management of PVF, with surgical intervention ranging from local procedure and interposition flap to pouch excision, depending on location of fistula (70).

## POUCHITIS AND CUFFITIS

Pouchitis and cuffitis are two similar complications unique to IPAA. Cuffitis, referring to the remnant rectal cuff, and pouchitis, referring to the pouch itself, are characterized by inflammation, bleeding, abdominopelvic pain, anal discharge, incontinence, tenesmus, urgency, and increased stool frequency, in the setting of mucosal inflammation. Pouchitis is the most common complication in patients with UC following IPAA, reported to occur in 14%–59% (48,76).

Diagnosis involves pouchoscopy and biopsy. Frequently used parameters comprising the pouchitis disease activity index (PDAI) include stool frequency, rectal bleeding, fecal urgency/cramping, fever, endoscopic inflammation, histologic findings, and degree of ulceration (77).

Treatment consists primarily of oral or topical medications: antibiotics, probiotics, and steroids (76). Should surgical treatment be required for symptomatic, refractory pouchitis, diversion, pouch excision, or redo IPAA can be performed.

## CROHN DISEASE

Crohn disease of the pouch is an unfortunate complication that may occur after IPAA and is a leading cause of pouch failure (78). Presentation is similar to that of pouchitis, characterized by abdominopelvic pain and diarrhea. Perianal disease and fistula are also suggestive of Crohn disease, especially if occurring greater than 12 months after IPAA, especially in the absence of postoperative complications such as sepsis, abscess, or leak (79).

Patients found to have Crohn disease after IPAA experience significant complications. A 93% complication rate was observed in a series of 31 patients with subsequent Crohn diagnosis after IPAA. The complications included perineal abscess/fistula, pouchitis, and anal stricture. Pouch excision was necessary in 29% (80). In another series, patients with a subsequent diagnosis of Crohn disease had a 47.8% pouch excision rate, compared to a 10.9% rate for those diagnosed with UC (81).

Management of Crohn disease of the pouch depends on phenotype—inflammatory, fibrostenotic, or fistulizing—and consists of combined medical, endoscopic, and surgical treatment. Inflammatory Crohn disease may be difficult to distinguish from pouchitis or cuffitis and is treated with oral and topical agents. Fibrostenotic frequently presents with ulcerated strictures in the distal small bowel, afferent limb, pouch inlet or outlet, or mid-pouch (78); management consists of medication, endoscopic balloon dilation (82), and bowel-preserving strictureplasty. Of the Crohn disease phenotypes, fistulizing disease may be associated with higher risk of pouch failure (79). Fistulas suggestive of Crohn disease present in areas outside the anastomosis, tip of the "J" suture line, or dentate line (78). Infliximab has been shown to be effective in short- and long-term treatment of Crohn disease of the pouch, with 62% of patients demonstrating a complete short-term response in a case series of 26 patients (83).

Due to the associated morbidity, IPAA is not routinely recommended for patients with known Crohn disease.

## POUCH FAILURE AND SALVAGE

Pouch failure is defined as a nonfunctioning pouch or pouch excision within 12 months of IPAA, and occurs in 5.3% (48,84). Risk factors contributing to pouch failure include Crohn disease, and chronic pouch-related issues, with pelvic sepsis and pouch fistula reported as the most common causes (50,84–87).

Evaluation of pouch dysfunction should include digital and endoscopic examination, as well as cross-sectional imaging and anal manometry (88).

Salvage procedures can be performed locally at the perineum, with an abdominal approach, or via a combined abdominoperineal approach. Pouch revision, augmentation, resection, mobilization, repair, or new construction, with or without ileostomy, are all options for reoperative pouch surgery (87).

A retrospective series of 51 patients who underwent reoperative pouch surgery, either via abdominal or perineal approach, reported a 69.5% or 75% success rate, respectively (85).

Meta-analysis demonstrated salvage procedures to be performed an average of 24 months after initial RP, with an overall successful healing rate of 73.5%, 82.2%, 79.6%, and 68.4% for overall, redo, revisional, and local perineal procedures, respectively. Overall functional success was reported in 71.9% (89).

Following salvage surgery, patients are found to have significantly higher daytime and nighttime seepage, as well as daytime pad usage. Quality of life, dietary, work, social, sexual restrictions, incontinence, and total bowel movements were not significantly different compared with those undergoing primary restorative proctocolectomy and IPAA (87,89).

## BIOLOGICS—IMPACT ON SURGICAL PROCEDURE AND TIMING

Classically treated medically with corticosteroids, 5-aminosalicylates, and immunosuppressants, UC entered the era of biologic treatment with advent of tumor necrosis factor-alpha (TNF-$\alpha$) inhibitors such as infliximab in 2005. Since then, additional biologics, such as adalimumab, golimumab, and certolizumab, have been introduced and have helped, as monotherapy or in combination with other drugs, to induce and maintain remission in UC patients (90,91).

Despite the medical therapy available, surgery is still ultimately required in 30%–40% of patients with UC (4). The data regarding surgical complications after treatment with anti-TNF-$\alpha$ therapy are mixed.

When retrospectively reviewing postoperative complications after IPAA, the risk of early and late complications, as well as need for three-stage operation, is increased in patients treated with infliximab (91). Systemic review of 162 patients receiving biologics echoed this finding, demonstrating an increased risk of pouch-related complications with preoperative infliximab (92).

Likewise, meta-analysis comprising five studies and 132 patients treated with infliximab demonstrates an increased risk of short-term complications with preoperative infliximab including abdominal wound infection, anastomotic leak, pelvic sepsis, and small bowel obstruction. Considering that patients with UC receiving systemic corticosteroids >40 mg/day have significantly increased risk of pouch-related complications after IPAA (93), and that the majority of patients with UC taking infliximab are also taking additional medications, it is unclear whether infliximab alone is culpable (94).

Conversely, retrospective analysis of 142 patients treated with infliximab prior to surgery did not demonstrate any increased risk in regard to morbidity or mortality, including anastomotic leak and infections (95).

When examining the preoperative serum level of anti-TNF-$\alpha$ medication levels in UC patients, no significant increase in postoperative complications was observed between the patients with detectable and undetectable serum levels (96).

In regard to timing of surgery, Waterman et al. compared postoperative complications between patients taking either infliximab or adalimumab within different time intervals prior to surgery: 14 days, 15–31 days, and 31–180 days. The study declared that biologic agents alone were not associated with an increased risk of postoperative complications, but rather that combination therapy of biologic agents and thiopurines was associated with increased postoperative complications. Moreover, shorter time interval did not increase postoperative complications, suggesting that surgery should not be delayed based on use of biologic agents alone (97).

## REFERENCES

1. Loftus EV Jr. *Gastroenterology*. 2004;126(6):1504–17.
2. Dahlhamer JM et al. *Morb Mortal Wkly Rep*. 2016; 65(42):1166–9.
3. Kappelman MD et al. *Clin Gastroenterol Hepatol*. 2007;5(12):1424–9.
4. Hancock L, Mortensen NJ. *Inflamm Bowel Dis*. 2008; 14 Suppl 2:S68–9.
5. Truelove SC, Witts LJ. *Br Med J*. 1955;2(4947):1041–8.
6. Sobrado CW, Sobrado LF. *Arq Bras Cir Dig*. 2016; 29(3):201–5.
7. Teeuwen PH et al. *J Gastrointest Surg*. 2009;13(4): 676–86.
8. Ross H et al. Standards Practice Task Force of the American Society of Colon and Rectal Surgeons. *Dis Colon Rectum*. 2014;57(1):5–22.
9. Beck DE et al. *The ASCRS Manual of Colon and Rectal Surgery*. New York, NY: Springer 2014.
10. Gumaste V et al. *Gut*. 1992;33(7):938–41.
11. Eaden JA et al. *Gut*. 2001;48(4):526–35.
12. Bernstein CN. *Curr Gastroenterol Rep*. 1999;1(6): 496–504.
13. Steele SR et al. *The ASCRS Textbook of Colon and Rectal Surgery*. New York, NY: Springer Science + Business Media 2016.
14. Kock NG. *Dis Colon Rectum*. 1994;37(3):278–85; discussion 285–7.
15. Lian L et al. *Dis Colon Rectum*. 2009;52(8):1409–14; discussion 4414–6.
16. Wasmuth HH et al. *Colorectal Dis*. 2007;9(8):713–7.
17. Kaiser AM. *Dis Colon Rectum*. 2012;55(2):155–62.
18. Nessar G et al. *Dis Colon Rectum*. 2006;49(3):336–44.
19. Mortier PE et al. *Gastroenterol Clin Biol*. 2006;30(4): 594–7.
20. Saito Y et al. *J Gastroenterol*. 1995;30(Suppl 8):131–4.
21. Khubchandani IT, Kontostolis SB. *Arch Surg*. 1994; 129(8):866–9.

22. Uzzan M et al. *Ann Surg.* 2017;266(6):1029–34.
23. da Luz Moreira A et al. *Br J Surg.* 2010;97(1):65–9.
24. Utsunomiya J et al. *Dis Colon Rectum.* 1980;23(7): 459–66.
25. Parks AG, Nicholls RJ. *Dis Colon Rectum.* 1988;31(10): 826–30.
26. Wu XR et al. *J Crohns Colitis.* 2013;7(10):e419–26.
27. Klos CL et al. *J Gastrointest Surg.* 2014;18(3):573–9.
28. Khasawneh MA et al. *Dis Colon Rectum.* 2016;59(11): 1034–8.
29. Lovegrove RE et al. *Colorectal Dis.* 2007;9(4):310–20.
30. Sagar PM et al. *Gastroenterology.* 1992;102(2):520–8.
31. Johnston D et al. *Gut.* 1996;39(2):242–7.
32. Miller R et al. *Dis Colon Rectum.* 1990;33(5):414–8.
33. Fichera A et al. *J Gastrointest Surg.* 2007;11(12): 1647–52; discussion 1652–3.
34. Ziv Y et al. *Am J Surg.* 1996;171(3):320–3.
35. Gemlo BT et al. *Am J Surg.* 1995;169(1):137–41; discussion 141–2.
36. Choen S et al. *Br J Surg.* 1991;78(4):430–4.
37. Luukkonen P, Järvinen H. *Arch Surg.* 1993;128(4): 437–40.
38. Reilly WT et al. *Ann Surg.* 1997;225(6):666–76; discussion 676–7.
39. Kirat HT et al. *Surgery.* 2009;146(4):723–9; discussion 729–30.
40. Sofo L et al. *World J Gastrointest Surg.* 2016;8(8): 556–63.
41. Remzi FH et al. *Dis Colon Rectum.* 2006;49(4):470–7.
42. Weston-Petrides GK et al. *Arch Surg.* 2007;143(4): 406–12.
43. Swenson BR et al. *Dis Colon Rectum.* 2005;48(2): 256–61.
44. Zittan E et al. *J Crohns Colitis.* 2016;10(7):766–72.
45. Bikhchandani J et al. *Dis Colon Rectum.* 2015;58(2): 199–204.
46. Goes RN et al. *Dis Colon Rectum.* 1995;38(8):893–5.
47. Manilich E et al. *Dis Colon Rectum.* 2012;55(4):393–9.
48. Fazio VW et al. *Ann Surg.* 2013;257(4):679–85.
49. de Zeeuw S et al. *Int J Colorectal Dis.* 2012;27(7): 843–53.
50. Farouk R et al. *Ann Surg.* 2000;231(6):919–26.
51. Bullard KM et al. *Dis Colon Rectum.* 2002;45(3): 299–304.
52. Kiran RP et al. *Ann Surg.* 2010;251(3):436–40.
53. Pellino G et al. *BMC Surg.* 2013;13(Suppl 2):S9.
54. Delaney CP et al. *Ann Surg.* 2003;238(2):221–8.
55. Bharadwaj S et al. *Inflamm Bowel Dis.* 2014;20(12): 2470–82.
56. Hull TL et al. *Br J Surg.* 2012;99(2):270–5.
57. Cornish JA et al. *Dis Colon Rectum.* 2007;50(8): 1128–38.
58. Hueting WE et al. *Int J Colorectal Dis.* 2004;19(3): 215–8.
59. Aberg H et al. *Int J Colorectal Dis.* 2007;22(6):637–42.
60. Peyrin-Biroulet L et al. *Aliment Pharmacol Ther.* 2016;44(8):807–16.

61. MacLean AR et al. *Ann Surg.* 2002;235(2):200–6.
62. Marcello PW et al. *Dis Colon Rectum.* 1993;36: 1105–11.
63. Francois Y et al. *Ann Surg.* 1989;209:46–50.
64. Fazio VW et al. *Dis Colon Rectum.* 2006;49(1):1–11.
65. Erkek AB et al. *J Gastroenterol Hepatol.* 2008;23(1): 119–25.
66. Lian L et al. *J Gastrointest Surg.* 2008;12(11):1991–4.
67. Lewis WG et al. *Dis Colon Rectum.* 1994;37(2):120–5.
68. Mallick IH et al. *Dis Colon Rectum.* 2014;57:490–6.
69. Heriot AG et al. *Dis Colon Rectum.* 2005;48(3): 451–8.
70. Lolohea S et al. *Dis Colon Rectum.* 2005;48(9): 1802–10.
71. Koltun WA et al. *Dis Colon Rectum.* 1991;34(10): 857–60.
72. Shah NS et al. *Dis Colon Rectum.* 2003;46(7):911–7.
73. Lee PY et al. *Dis Colon Rectum.* 1997;40(7):752–9.
74. Groom JS et al. *Br J Surg.* 1993;80(7):936–40.
75. Tsujinaka S et al. *J Am Coll Surg.* 2006;202(6):912–8.
76. Hata K et al. *Dig Endosc.* 2017;29(1):26–34.
77. Sandborn WJ et al. *Mayo Clin Proc.* 1994;69(5):409–15.
78. Shen B. *Inflamm Bowel Dis.* 2009;15:284–94.
79. Shen B et al. *Dis Colon Rectum.* 2007;50(9):1450–9.
80. Braveman JM et al. *Dis Colon Rectum.* 2004;47(10): 1613–9.
81. Keighley MR. *Acta Chir Iugol.* 2000;47(4 Suppl 1): 27–31.
82. Shen B et al. *Am J Gastroenterol.* 2004;99(12):2340–7.
83. Colombel J-F et al. *Am J Gastroenterol.* 2003;98: 2239–44.
84. Lepistö A et al. *Dis Colon Rectum.* 2002;45(10): 1289–94.
85. Shawki S et al. *Dis Colon Rectum.* 2009;52(5):884–90.
86. Körsgen S, Keighley MR. *Int J Colorectal Dis.* 1997; 12(1):4–8.
87. Remzi FH et al. *Dis Colon Rectum.* 2009;52(2):198–204.
88. Sagar PM, Pemberton JH. *Br J Surg.* 2012;99(4): 454–68.
89. Theodoropoulos GE et al. *J Am Coll Surg.* 2015;220(2): 225–42.e1.
90. Biondi A et al. *World J Gastroenterol.* 2012;18(16): 1861–70.
91. Mor IJ et al. *Dis Colon Rectum.* 2008;51(8):1202–7; discussion 1207–10.
92. Selvaggi F et al. *Inflamm Bowel Dis.* 2015;21(1):79–92.
93. Heuschen UA et al. *Ann Surg.* 2002;235(2):207–16.
94. Yang Z et al. *Aliment Pharmacol Ther.* 2010;31(4): 486–92.
95. Krane MK et al. *Dis Colon Rectum.* 2013;56(4):449–57.
96. Lau C et al. *Ann Surg.* 2015;261(3):487–96.
97. Waterman M et al. *Gut.* 2013;62(3):387–94.
98. Krane MK, Lange EO, Fichera A. Ulcerative colitis: Surgical management. In Steele SR, Hull TL, Read TE, Saclarides TJ, Sebagore AJ, Whitloe CB. (eds). *The ASCRS Textbook of Colon and Rectal Surgery*, 3rd Edition, 2016. Figures 50–5 and 6, p.876.

# 36

# Surgery for Crohn disease

EMILY STEINHAGEN AND SHARON L. STEIN

## CHALLENGING CASE

A 29 year-old man, with a 10 year history of Crohn's disease, has been maintained on biologics. He previously had two ileocolic resections. He recently developed postparandial pain (1 hour after eating) with bloating. On MR enterography, a long fibrotic stricture is found in mid jejunum.

## CASE MANAGEMENT

A fibrotic stricture will rarely respond to medical management. Therefore, the patient is offered a stricturoplasty.

## INTRODUCTION

Crohn disease (CD) is a chronic inflammatory disease of the intestinal tract. It is hypothesized to be an overreaction of the immune system to the bacterial biome found within the intestines, although the precise etiology has not been elucidated. While CD affects the entire intestinal tract, the terminal ileum and colon are the most frequent sites of disease.

CD most commonly affects adults, with onset of symptoms generally between the second and fifth decades of life. The incidence of CD has been increasing worldwide. While it was historically diagnosed in patients in North America, Western Europe, and Australia, cases are increasingly diagnosed in Asia and South America as well (1). Women and urbanites are more likely to develop CD. In the United States, prevalence may be as high as in 330 per 100,000 Americans (2).

Symptoms of CD are heterogeneous, based on the severity and location of disease. Abdominal pain, weight loss, and diarrhea are common symptoms, but patients may also initially present with perianal fistulization or with extraintestinal manifestations such as joint pain, eye problems, or skin lesions. Symptoms of CD are generally relapsing and remitting.

Surgery does not cure CD. Therefore, the goals of surgery in a patient are to treat symptoms and complications of the disease that are not adequately managed with medication. The most common indications for surgery are obstruction, neoplasia, fistulization, or failure to respond to medical management. Approximately 70% of patients with CD will require surgical intervention during their lifetime. Of patients requiring an initial surgery, 50% will require a second surgery.

## NONSURGICAL MANAGEMENT OF CROHN DISEASE

### BIOLOGICS AND SURGERY FOR CROHN DISEASE

The majority of patients are initially and chronically treated with medical management. Medical management is a complex process involving a combination of antibiotics, aminosalicylates, and immunosuppressants, including steroids, immunomodulators, and biologics, to achieve a clinical and endoscopic remission. Medical management is generally considered to be lifelong, with the goal of preventing disease progression. Increasingly, biologics are being used in the hope of maintaining a durable remission for patients with CD.

However, whether the increased use of biologics will decrease the risks of surgical intervention is unclear. Initial data demonstrated lower rates of surgery for patients who received biologic therapy. The ACCENT I trial demonstrated a twofold lower rate of surgery at 54 weeks, and the CHARM trial demonstrated a nine times lower rate of surgery at 56 weeks (3,4). Surgical rates during both trials were lower than historical data, with a reduction from 7.5% to 3% in ACCENT I, and 3.8% to 0.6% in the CHARM trial. A longitudinal study of patients with CD from 1991 to 2014 noted that the use of biologics increased from 3.1% to 41.2% during the study period; during the same period, the frequency of surgical intervention decreased from 42.9% to 17.4% (5).

However, subsequent studies have not maintained these conclusions. A review of data from the National Inpatient Sample did not support decreasing surgical rates in the biologic era; in this study the frequency of surgical interventions was unchanged, and patients who did undergo surgery were more likely to be malnourished (6). A study of 195 patients with CD noted that patients on biologics appeared to have a longer lead time from initial diagnosis of CD to operation (29 to 61 months, $p = 0.005$) but did not demonstrate a decreased amount of bowel resected when surgery was required (7).

The longer duration of medical management and the finding of malnourished patients suggests an additional concern in patients on biologic therapies who do require surgery: they may be sicker and at increased risks of perioperative complications both from the disease and the significant immunosuppression that may also impact healing. A single-center study from St. Marks recently demonstrated a hazard ratio of 24.6 for septic complications in CD patients on preoperative biologics (8). A meta-analysis including over 5,700 patients noted that patients on infliximab had an increased risk of total complications (odds ratio [OR] 1.45, confidence interval [CI] 1.04–2.02), infectious complications (1.47, CI 1.08–1.99), and other complications (2.29, CI 1.14–4.61) (9). Similar results were noted in several additional studies; Kopylov et al. found a trend toward increased rate of total complications, infectious complications, and noninfectious complications (10). A second meta-analysis by El Hussana noted that patients with exposure to biologics within 3 months of surgery were more likely to have anastomotic complications, particularly in trials with lower risk of bias (OR 1.63, CI 1.03–2.60) (11). However, the data are still not definitive: a recent multinational, multicenter trial recently demonstrated no increased rate of complications, intraabdominal sepsis, or anastomotic leak in patients on immunologics or biologics (12). Notably, this trial did note that subsets of patients including those who required transfusions, those with perforating disease, and patients with prior surgery were at increased risk for complications when they were on biologics at the time of surgery. This supports the concern that at least for some patients, biologics increase their surgical risk.

Most biologics function as antagonists to tumor necrosis factor-alpha (TNF-$\alpha$); these include medications such as infliximab and adalimumab. Vedolizumab has an alternative mechanism of action and is an anti-integrin that inhibits leukocyte migration into the gut. A recent study of vedolizumab demonstrated a significant increase in the rate of postoperative infections and superficial site infections, even when compared to other biologics (13). Although this represents a small cohort, as new biologics are available to patients, data need to be reevaluated, rather than assuming all treatments are the same.

## MULTIDISCIPLINARY MANAGEMENT OF CROHN DISEASE

Given the concern regarding increasing risks of perioperative complications as well as the need for perioperative optimization of patients, the use of multidisciplinary decision-making has become increasingly common in the treatment of CD. Similar to the care of patients with cancer, patients with benign complications of CD are best treated by a multidisciplinary group of physicians. The goals of therapy, preoperative patient optimization, and timing of surgical intervention can be optimized through a coordinated care process. Gastroenterology, dietary, psychology, radiology, and surgical services should discuss complex cases of CD with respect to whether continued medical management, endoscopic evaluation and treatment, or surgical intervention is optimal. Several papers discussing the psychosocial benefits of multidisciplinary care, health-care cost benefits, and improved medical outcomes secondary to unified care plan have been published (14,15). Multidisciplinary decision-making can also help surgeons optimize patients prior to surgery.

## PREOPERATIVE EVALUATION OF PATIENTS WITH CROHN DISEASE

Prior to surgery for Crohn disease, a full assessment of the gastrointestinal tract is strongly preferred. Endoscopic evaluation is generally a first step. This allows for visualization of affected portions of the stomach and duodenum as well as the colon and terminal ileum. Although a colonoscopy report is useful, a surgeon should examine the colon directly if an anastomosis is planned; visualization of the quality of the mucosa for the "landing" zone of the anastomosis is important to ensuring the integrity of the anastomosis and preoperative planning. Not surprisingly, inflamed tissue increases the risk of anastomotic leak (16).

Since upper endoscopic evaluation is limited in its ability to identify disease in the jejunum and proximal ileum, video capsule endoscopy has added to the field by allowing imaging of the small bowel mucosa and determination of existence, location, and extent of small bowel disease. In capsule endoscopy, a criterion of three or more ulcers is used as diagnostic for CD, and sensitivity ranges around 77%, with a negative predictive value of 96% (17). Compared with magnetic resonance imaging (MRI), capsule endoscopy has better sensitivity for proximal disease identification (18,19). However, capsule endoscopy is limited by its inability to pass through severely strictured areas, which occurs with some frequency. In early studies, retention rates of up to 13% have been reported (20). If the capsule is retained within the small intestines, it necessitates surgical intervention for retrieval. A patency capsule, which dissolves over time, can exclude significant stenosis prior to giving the true capsule.

Cross-sectional imaging is used with increasing frequency in CD patients. A recent study noted a 1.9-fold increase in imaging (computed tomography and MRI) for CD over the last decade (21). These imaging modalities have the advantage of demonstrating both intraluminal and extraluminal disease and offer information about spatial relationships that are unable to be demonstrated with traditional barium techniques. However, dynamic imaging studies such as contrast enema can be quite helpful in distinguishing intermittent spasm or peristaltic contraction from CD.

For acute evaluation of patients, CT scans are almost always performed. They provide relatively low cost, highly reliable data for rapid diagnosis and are widely available in most medical centers. CT is extremely helpful for identifying obstruction, perforation, and abscess. However, standard imaging techniques fail to provide optimized distension of the bowel or dynamic imaging. Therefore, in the nonemergent setting, enterography is preferred for a more detailed examination and the ability to identify mucosal abnormalities.

CT enterography (CTE) is generally also widely available, cost effective, and has good sensitivity for CD lesions. However, it does require an experienced radiologist to interpret the study accurately. Compared to magnetic resonance enterography (MRE), CTE generally has superior interobserver agreement (22). However, other studies have demonstrated improved sensitivity of diagnosis of fistula, stenosis, and abscess with MRE compared to CTE (23). In addition, MRE may include the ability to predict response to treatment for CD in the future (24). Both modalities have the ability to discern whether strictures are inflammatory or fibrotic in nature, which can help drive surgical decision-making. Because of the chronic nature of CD, and repeat imaging requirements for patients over their lifetime, there is concern about the increased exposure to ionizing radiation (25). For this reason, MRE has become a diagnostic test of choice.

When surgery is planned for CD, imaging is crucial. An appropriate evaluation will define the extent and location of disease, determine the existence of fistulizing disease, demonstrate the presence and extent of stenotic disease, identify abscess or phlegmon, and prepare the surgeon and patient with respect to extent of resection and need for stoma.

## Intraabdominal abscess

As opposed to other types of intestinal perforations, disease progression in CD is generally slow—therefore, patients are more likely to present with a contained perforation or abscess than free intraabdominal perforation. When patients present with intraabdominal abscess, the first-line treatment is generally antibiotics with or without radiologic-guided placement of drainage tube, rather than immediate surgical intervention. This enables surgical planning as well as patient optimization. Even if it is clear that a patient will require surgery to address the problem, controlling active inflammation can decrease surgical risks. One review demonstrated successful temporizing treatment in 74% of cases (26). Patients who were more likely to require surgery included those with stenotic disease, enterocutaneous disease, or refractory active disease. A meta-analysis also demonstrated a reduction in the rate of complications via initial percutaneous abscess drainage compared with initial surgery (OR 0.44) (27). However, a different meta-analysis demonstrated that 70% of patients who presented with an abscess still ultimately required surgery and did not find a reduction in complication, stoma rates, or length of stay with delayed surgical intervention (28).

## Strictures

For some patients with intestinal stricture, balloon dilation has been utilized effectively. This is particularly common for short-segment ileocolic disease. A systematic review of endoscopic balloon dilation in CD that included over 1,000 patients demonstrated that symptomatic response was achieved in 70% of patients, and technical response (ability to pass the scope following procedure) was achieved in 90% of cases. Complications occurred in 6.4% and perforation occurred in 3% of patients. However, the cumulative rate of surgery at 5 years was still 75%. Outcomes were not different in de novo versus anastomotic strictures (29).

Recent data indicate that salvage after failed endoscopic dilation may be associated with increased risk of diversion as well as deep space and superficial infections (30). However, it is unclear if this is directly correlated with the dilation, or if it is because patients are clinically worse at the time of surgery.

## Thromboembolic disease

Active inflammation is a risk factor for thromboembolic disease. Studies demonstrate that patients with inflammatory bowel disease (IBD) have an increased rate of thromboembolic disease when compared to the general population. Thromboembolic events are 1.5–3.5 times more likely to occur in patients with IBD, with a 2.5-fold increase in mortality following a venous thromboembolism (VTE) event (31). Within this patient population, patients with malnutrition, reduced preoperative functional status, chronic steroid use, and anemia are all at even higher risk of VTE. Emergency surgery and prolonged anesthesia time also increased this risk. Patients who experience a VTE are more likely to have prolonged hospital stays, experience a greater risk of additional complications, and have a higher mortality rate (32). After discharge, VTE events may be as high as 3.3% for these patients. Patients with increased risks include those who have a new stoma, are on steroids, and have a longer postoperative hospital stay (33). Based on this evidence, surgeons should consider extended postoperative prophylactic anticoagulation for patients with IBD at the time of discharge.

## SURGICAL MANAGEMENT OF SMALL BOWEL DISEASE

Some patients with CD are at higher risk of requiring surgery than others. While inflammatory disease is most likely to respond to medical management, fibrostenotic disease is least likely to respond. Additional risk factors for surgical intervention include terminal ileal disease, proximal small bowel disease, and prior appendectomy (34). There are several specific technical issues that merit detailed discussion when considering surgery for CD.

## STRICTUREPLASTY

The idea of revision of a segment of CD rather than resection was first popularized by Lee in the 1970s. Success after increasing luminal diameter had previously been reported in patients with tuberculosis in India, and this experience was extrapolated to CD patients with multifocal disease.

The most commonly used strictureplasty is the Heineke-Mikulicz (Figure 36.1). This is used for short-segment disease without signs of fistulization, cancer, or abscess. It allows for revision and luminal restructuring without resection of intestinal mucosal absorptive surface. Generally,

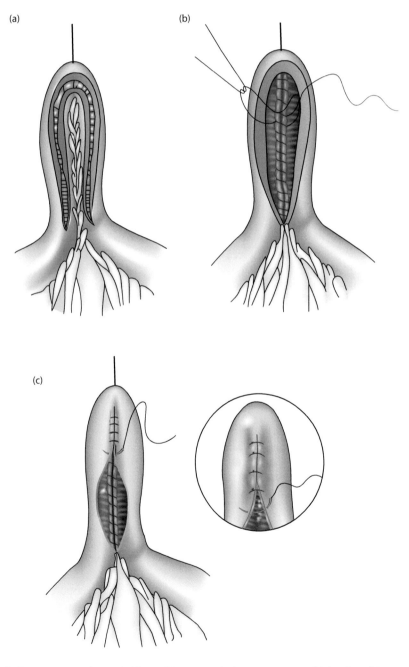

Figure 36.1 Heineke-Mikulicz strictureplasty. **(a)** Bowel is opened along stricture, **(b)** backwall is sutured together, **(c)** Anterior edges are approximated. Insert demonstrates correct suture placement. (Reproduced with permission from the Cleveland Clinic.)

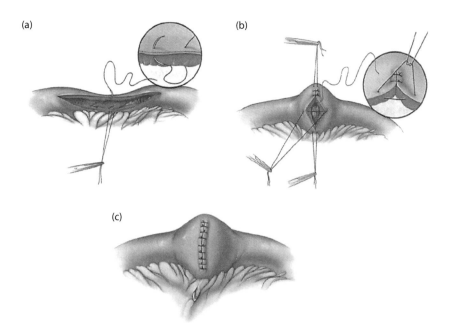

Figure 36.2 Finney stricturoplasties. **(a)** Stricture is opened on antimesenteric border, **(b)** Traction on sutures approximates edges of opened stricture and enterotomy is closed with interupted sutures. Insert demonstrates correct suture placement. **(c)** Completed one layer anastomosis. (Reproduced with permission from the Cleveland Clinic.)

segments less than 10 cm are ideal for Heineke-Mikulicz strictureplasty. Longer segments of disease can be treated with Finney or Michelassi strictureplasty techniques. Finney stricturoplasties (Figure 36.2) are generally preferred for single long segment of strictured bowel; although a low-flow diverticulum is created, which may be an area of stasis within the small intestines. Michelassi, or side-to-side isoperistaltic strictureplasty (Figure 36.3), can be used for lengths of up to 150 cm. The strictured segment of bowel is married to a dilated area of bowel, causing widening of the entire length of bowel. This allows for restoration of flow

through diseased segments, while maintaining an absorptive surface within the bowel.

Recent data of the recurrence rates for long-segment side-to-side isoperistaltic strictureplasties has been favorable: 90% of patients were shown to have resolution of symptoms, though 45% had recurrence at a mean of 55 months after surgery, with 15 of 83 requiring surgery for their recurrence (35). A recent examination of stricturoplasty that utilized the National Surgical Quality Improvement Program (NSQIP) database demonstrated decreasing use of strictureplasty from 5.1% in 2005 to 1.7% of surgeries for

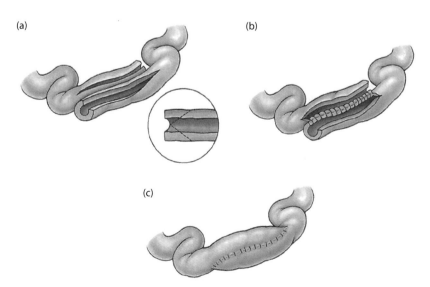

Figure 36.3 Michelassi, or side-to-side isoperistaltic strictureplasty. **(a)** Stricture is divided, opened on anti-mesenteric border and overlapped. Insert demonstrates tapering ends of opened bowel **(b)** Back wall sutured together. **(c)** Anterior layer is sutured together. (Reproduced with permission from the Cleveland Clinic.)

CD in 2012. Over 9,000 patients underwent strictureplasty with an average albumin of 3.6%. During the study period, risk of complications and reoperation rate remained low (36). A second review of the literature demonstrated early complication rates of 15% in patients undergoing "conventional strictureplasty" (Heinicke Mikulicz, or Finney) with long-term complication rates of 29%. Patients undergoing "unconventional strictureplastly" such as isoperistaltic strictureplasty had even lower complication rates: 8% short term and 17% long term (37).

## ILEOCOLIC RESECTION

The most common location of CD is the terminal ileum. Approximately 40% of patients present with isolated terminal ileal disease. Multiple options exist for treatment, depending on severity of disease as well as presence of structuring disease. When disease is fibrotic and strictured, dilation and medical management are less likely to be effective. A recent randomized controlled study demonstrated that resection is a reasonable alternative to biologics for patients with disease segments less than 40 cm. In this study, 37% of patients undergoing treatment with biologics required surgery within 4 years, while only 26% of patients undergoing surgery required escalation to biologics in the same time period (38). Surgical resection of an isolated segment of terminal ileal disease may be the best option and may leave the patient with no visible disease in these cases.

The resection generally includes the terminal ileum and the cecum. Even if the disease does not abut the colon, placing an anastomosis in close proximity to the ileocecal valve is generally discouraged. This may increase the risk of dilation of the new anastomosis, just upstream from a physiologic sphincter. The ascending colon should be maintained as much as possible, as patients will often require reoperation for recurrence of disease in the same location. Equally important is resection back to the area of healthy appearing bowel, without external signs of CD (corkscrew vessels and creeping fat), and without internal signs of CD (aphthous ulcers, or cobblestoning). The small bowel should be soft and pliable at the transection location.

Resection of repeated segments of the terminal ileum may lead to issues with malabsorption such as wasting of bile salts, fat-soluble vitamins (A, D, E, K), and B-12 related anemia (39). Generally, patients with greater than 20 cm of terminal ileal disease are at greater risk of deficiencies. In cases of repeat resection, consideration of strictureplasty may be reasonable. Generally, this will be an isoperistaltic anastomosis with the longitudinal opening on the diseased small intestine to the normal ascending colon.

Disease segments in the terminal ileum may be noted to have fistulized to healthy appearing adjacent bowel. This may include proximal segments of small intestine, or frequently as segment of sigmoid colon. Prior colonoscopy, or if needed intraoperative colonoscopy, can assess the segment of colon to rule out primary disease. In this case, a wedge resection can be performed, rather than segmental resection, of the bystander bowel. If the secondary segment appears to have primary CD, it should be resected as well.

## LAPAROSCOPIC VERSUS OPEN INTERVENTION

Following the overall rise of minimally invasive surgical techniques, laparoscopy has been increasingly applied to CD cases. A small trial found that endoscopic recurrence was more common after laparoscopic surgery than open surgery (58.3% versus 22.7% at 1 year, and clinical recurrence rates were 28.6% versus 11.8%) (40). Other studies demonstrate equivalence between groups (41), and a meta-analysis of data found that there was no evidence of increased rate of surgical recurrence (relative risk [RR] 0.78, CI 0.54–1.11, $p = 0.17$) but did show reduced preoperative complications (RR 0.71, CI 0.58–0.86) and decreased rate of incisional hernia (0.24, 0.07–0.82) (42). A 2011 Cochrane Review evaluating laparoscopic resection for small bowel disease demonstrated trends toward decreased wound infection rates and reoperation rates, but these differences were not statistically significant (43).

An advanced laparoscopic skill set is needed to approach CD. It is important to run the bowel to evaluate for distant disease. The surgeon should be comfortable handling inflamed bowel and mesentery, adhesions, and possibly fistulizing disease or abscess. Often, the mesentery will be significantly thickened in the area of CD. Energy devices may be inadequate in the treatment of this mesentery, and the surgeon should be prepared to assess this intraoperatively, and vary approaches as appropriate.

## TYPE OF ANASTOMOSIS

The type of anastomosis used to restore intestinal continuity may be important both in terms of perioperative risks and long-term disease recurrence. Data from Simillis et al. demonstrated that end-to-end anastomosis had increased risk of anastomotic leaks in CD as well as increased recurrence rates (44). However, they also noted a decreased rate of other postoperative complications and a shorter hospital stay. The explanation for this is unclear. However, a meta-analysis demonstrated no change in anastomotic leak rate but a decreased rate of recurrence with *stapled* side-to-side anastomosis when compared to other anastomotic configurations (45). Conversely, a second meta-analysis found statistically reduced rates of postoperative complications (0.54, 0.32–0.93), anastomotic leak (0.45, CI 0.20–1.00), and recurrence rates (OR 0.20, CI 0.07–0.55). Perioperative morbidity and hospital stay were similar (46). Other data have suggested that the length of anastomosis may be a key to decreasing clinically significant recurrence rates, and this can be achieved by utilizing a longer stapler or multiple firings. A more recent technique,

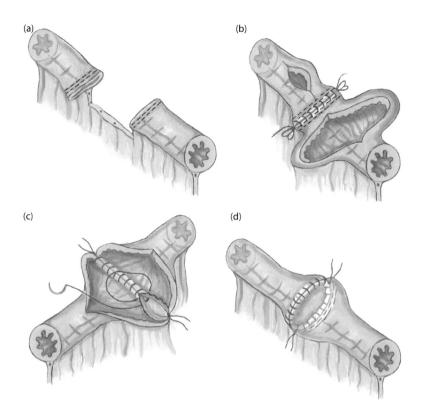

Figure 36.4 Kono side-to-side anastomosis. **(a)** The intestinal segments are divided with the staple lines perpendicular to the axis of the mesentery. **(b)** The supporting column is constructed by suturing the two staple lines together and a longitudinal enterotomy and colotomy are performed. They start no more than 1 cm away from the supporting column, extending proximally and distally to allow a transverse lumen of 7 cm on the small intestine and close to 8 cm on the large intestine. **(c)** The longitudinal enterotomy and colotomy are closed transversely with an outer layer of 4/0 silk Lembert interrupted sutures, and an inner layer of running 3/0 absorbable suture starting on the posterior wall. **(d)** The complete anastomosis is shown.

popularized by Japanese surgeon T. Kono, has impressive early results regarding recurrence (Figure 36.4). The current data evaluating 187 patients undergoing Kono-S antimesenteric anastomosis demonstrated 98.6% freedom from recurrence requiring surgery at 5 and 10 years after surgery (47).

## CROHN COLITIS

CD affects the colon in approximately 30% of patients. It may affect the entire colon or be segmental, and it may occur in conjunction with other disease distributions. Perianal disease, in particular, suggests a more aggressive phenotype for Crohn colitis. Indications for surgery for Crohn colitis include strictures, perforation, hemorrhage, severe or fulminant colitis, medically refractory disease, and neoplasia.

## COLONIC STRICTURES

Colonic strictures may be inflammatory or fibrotic in nature, and both mechanisms often coexist. Obstructive

strictures occur in approximately 17% of cases of colonic CD (48). Endoscopic balloon dilation has been used to manage strictures with a 90% success rate; 28% required surgery for recurrence at approximately 4 years of follow-up (49). Endoscopic dilation is most suitable for isolated, short strictures. Risks include bleeding and perforation, and the major benefit is potentially avoiding a resection. Colonic stricturoplasty for CD can be used for short strictures and has equivalent outcomes to resection, but there is about a 7% chance that a stricture harbors a malignancy (48,50). Shorter strictures and longer duration of disease are both associated with a higher risk. Colonic strictures, then, should be carefully surveyed and biopsied based on the cancer risk. Resection is the preferred management strategy for strictures in Crohn colitis (51).

## COLECTOMY

When CD affects only a segment of the colon and surgery is required, segmental resection may be performed when indicated without any alteration in complications, incidence of recurrence, or need for a permanent stoma when compared to subtotal or total colectomy (52). However, many authors believe that because of the high recurrence rate, when operating on the colon for CD, a subtotal colectomy or total proctocolectomy should be performed regardless. When two or more segments of colon are affected, it appears that subtotal or total colectomy is beneficial. Laparoscopic colectomy for CD can be performed safely with a reported conversion rate of 16%–26% and the benefit of quicker return of bowel function and shorter hospital stay (53–55). An urgent or emergent operation for colonic CD does not change the beneficial impact of laparoscopy (56).

There is a subset of patients who have Crohn colitis with relative rectal sparing and no perianal disease who are candidates for colectomy with ileorectal anastomosis. These patients should first be evaluated to make sure their rectal compliance is normal, either by distending it via proctoscopy or with manometry. Those with a tolerated rectal volume of less than 150 cc do not have good function with ileorectal anastomosis (57). Some of these patients, or those with isolated disease in the colon only above the distal rectum, may be candidates for an ileal pouch, which can be attached to the mid- to distal rectum (58), and while they have a relatively high incidence of disease recurrence and pouch loss (10%–52%), some are able to avoid a permanent stoma (59–62).

Most patients with Crohn colitis require total proctocolectomy with end ileostomy. These patients may have proctitis, sphincter dysfunction, or severe perianal disease. There is a significant risk of cancer in the residual rectum, so even if it is done as a staged procedure, the entirety of the rectum should ideally be removed (63). It is also feasible in some cases to perform an ultra-low Hatrmann procedure leaving only a few centimeters of rectum so there is less residual rectum, and it also enables the surgeon to perform the completion proctectomy from the perineal approach. This is preferable as it avoids another abdominal operation and its associated morbidity for the patient.

## TOXIC COLITIS

Severe colitis is a serious and potentially fatal manifestation of Crohn colitis. A flare accompanied by six or more bloody stools per day with evidence of systemic toxicity including anemia, elevated erythrocyte sedimentation rate (ESR), fever, or tachycardia can be a strong indication for surgery if it does not respond to initial medical management. Those with more than 10 bloody bowel movements per day, continuous daily bleeding, transfusion requirements, elevated fever, tachycardia, tenderness and distention, and colonic dilation on imaging are labeled as having fulminant colitis (51). When there is dilation greater than 5.5 cm on imaging in association with systemic symptoms, toxic megacolon should be considered, and the risk of perforation is heightened.

Patients should be evaluated for concomitant *Clostridium difficile* and cytomegalovirus infection. Endoscopy can be carefully performed to evaluate the mucosa. Medical therapy includes high-dose steroids, antibiotics to minimize sepsis from microperforation, and close serial abdominal examinations with x-rays as necessary to evaluate colonic distention. Any worsening of the patient's condition should prompt operative intervention. Severe colitis may progress to perforation, toxic megacolon, hemorrhage, or peritonitis.

When surgery is undertaken for severe, medically refractory disease, a staged approach is logical because of the added operative risk of proctectomy and the possibility of a nonhealing perineal wound. The rectal stump may be left closed either with staples or sutures in the pelvis, or tacked above the anterior abdominal wall fascia to avoid the risk of stump disruption and pelvic abscess. There are no data on the use of rectal tubes in the setting of subtotal colectomy for Crohn colitis, but some routinely use this approach. Occasionally it is necessary to form a mucous fistula when the residual rectosigmoid is too inflamed to hold sutures or staples. Completion proctectomy can be performed at a later date when the patient is medically and nutritionally optimized. Patients should be counseled about the options of completion proctectomy or leaving the residual rectum with surveillance endoscopy due to the risk of neoplasia and the possibility of disease-related symptoms (64,65).

## COLON CANCER

The relative risk of colon cancer in CD is 2.4 times that of the general population (66). Patients with Crohn colitis have up to a 25% chance of dysplasia by their 10th surveillance colonoscopy (67,68). Patients who have CD that does not affect their colon are not at particularly increased risk of colon cancer (69). When low- or high-grade dysplasia is biopsied, it should be confirmed by a pathologist experienced in IBD, as interobserver variability is high. Additionally, when dysplasia is found incidentally using standard endoscopy techniques, the examination should be repeated with high-definition and/or chromoendoscopy techniques (70). Dysplasia often, but not always, precedes colorectal cancer, and dysplasia does not always progress from low to high before manifesting as invasive carcinoma in CD. Patients with high-grade dysplasia on random biopsies have a 73% chance of cancer in the final specimen, and with low-grade dysplasia the risk is 36% (71). When dysplasia is present in a visible lesion that can be completely resected endoscopically, close surveillance is appropriate. Multifocal high-grade dysplasia should be a consideration for colectomy, and obviously invasive cancer warrants colectomy. In general, patients with CD undergoing surgery for neoplasia should have a complete proctocolectomy because of the high rate of synchronous lesions as well as the high rate of metachronous cancer (72).

## PERIANAL CROHN DISEASE

The incidence of perianal disease in CD patients ranges from 25% to 40% (73–75). It may represent the presenting symptom of CD for a subset of patients (76). Those patients with multiple abnormalities, atypical fissures located laterally, cavitating ulcers, complex fistulas, large fibrotic skin tags, and other unusual features of typical perianal problems should be suspected of CD. When there is isolated perianal disease at the time of diagnosis, most patients manifest intraluminal disease within 5 years.

## PERIANAL ABSCESS AND FISTULA

The incidence of perianal fistulas appears to correlate with the location of luminal disease: 15% of patients with isolated ileocolic disease develop fistulas, but more than 90% of those with Crohn colitis and proctitis are affected (73).

Abscess presents with pain, fever, erythema, and fluctuance in any of the potential spaces where a sporadic perianal abscess may develop. However, in CD, complex fistulas should always be suspected. In cases where it is not immediately apparent that there is a drainable collection, imaging may be helpful. Endorectal ultrasound increases the sensitivity of physical examination in this group of patients (77). CT is easily available and has excellent effectiveness in diagnosing abscesses. While MRI is usually beneficial for delineating fistulas, it is not typically necessary to identify an abscess.

An abscess should be treated first with simple incision and drainage. An attempt should be made to find the associated fistula, with care to avoid making false tracts. Long-term, continuous drainage can be facilitated by insertion of a mushroom or Malecot catheter or by the application of seton drainage. Antibiotics are often prescribed if there is associated cellulitis or signs of systemic illness. Most abscesses in CD patients eventually develop into fistulas. In addition, it is possible for a patient to present with a symptomatic fistula even without ever reporting an abscess.

A loose or noncutting seton, often made from silastic vessel loops and secured in a circular or tear-shaped loop, maintains the patency fistula tract and enables it to drain freely. The primary goal of the seton is to allow local sepsis and inflammation to resolve. In many cases, it will be a temporary solution until a suitable time for a more definitive procedure, but for some patients with complex, refractory disease, it can be a long-term solution. The combination of seton and anti-TNF agents has been very effective for the treatment of fistulae. Patients treated with infliximab and noncutting seton placement have better outcomes than patients treated with infliximab alone in terms of response rate, recurrence rate, and time to recurrence (78,79). The optimal timing for seton removal with this approach is not clearly defined, but initial studies reported that setons were removed after the second infusion with infliximab.

Medical management plays an important role in perianal fistula management. It has been suggested that metronidazole may produce symptomatic improvement in some patients with perianal disease, though it nearly always recurs after the antibiotics are stopped. Immunomodulators increase the rate of healing in approximately half of fistula patients (80). Furthermore, anti-TNF medications such as infliximab have altered the treatment paradigm for perianal

CD. While some have demonstrated a decreased need for surgical intervention with infliximab, others have shown no difference in fistula surgery rates since the introduction of these agents in population-based studies. However, the ACCENT II trial demonstrated that infliximab must be continued as maintenance therapy to increase the change of a sustained response (81). In cases refractory to infliximab, adalimumab can be used with long-term response rates of approximately 41% without surgical intervention (82,83). Currently, several sets of guidelines recommend anti-TNF agents as the standard for complex anorectal CD (84–87). In rectovaginal fistulas, the response to anti-TNF agents is decreased compared to other types of fistulas; 14%–38% versus 46%–78% (81,88).

## Surgical management

The goal of treatment of anal fistulas in CD patients should be the absence of symptoms rather than the absence of the fistula. Many individuals with fistulae are relatively asymptomatic. A single institution series with long-term follow-up determined that the overall cumulative probability of avoiding proctectomy was 91.6% at 10 years and 82.5% at 20 years in this patient group. Resection of all proximal CD did not ameliorate the anorectal condition, except in those with all proximal disease removed who did not have a recurrence (89).

It is important to determine if there is concomitant anal inflammation related to the CD. Those who do not have active CD in the anal canal are more likely to have success with any intervention. In those with anal canal disease, it may be more prudent to manage their symptoms with long-term seton placement until their anal canal is normal on examination and there are no signs of inflammation in their proximal bowel (90).

Definitive management of fistulas is based on location, complexity, the presence or absence of proctitis, and anal canal disease. Complexity is defined as the presence of an internal opening above the dentate line, traversing significant sphincter muscle, branching, or multiple openings. Rectovaginal fistulas are always considered to be complex fistulas (91).

It is often helpful to perform examination under anesthesia to fully delineate the fistula prior to determining a plan for surgical intervention. Proctosigmoidoscopy should be performed at the same time to evaluate the presence and activity of inflammatory changes in the rectum and distal colon. The presence of an anal stricture is a particularly poor prognostic indicator for both the success of any attempt at repairing the fistula and the possibility of preserving the rectum in the long term.

Imaging can increase the accuracy of the examination, either via endorectal ultrasound or pelvic MRI. Either of these modalities has been demonstrated to improve diagnostic accuracy (92,93). MRI can show the path of the fistula, the presence of deeper abscesses not apparent on clinical examination, and relationship to the sphincters, and can differentiate between inflammatory changes and fibrosis (94). Furthermore, MRI has been shown to substantially alter the operating plan with additional or more complex findings than were demonstrated on EUA in up to 40% of cases (95,96). MRI may also be helpful in assessing the persistence of fistulas after medical management that has resolved symptoms. Despite clinically appearing healed, inflammatory changes may persist on imaging and demonstrate that the fistula is still present. For patients who are considering a change in their therapy or who have been diverted to allow time to heal, this is of particular importance (97).

For simple, low-lying fistulas without associated proctitis, fistulotomy may be appropriate if there is no threat to continence. Success rates for this range from 80% to 100% (91). Timing for fistulotomy is important: there is no associated inflammation to increase the chance of healing. When performed in the setting of biologic therapy, the rate of healing significantly improves as well (98).

Both fibrin glue and collagen plugs have been described for treatment of CD-related fistulas. The advantage of these techniques is there is no risk to the sphincter complex. Fibrin glue is a mix of fibrinogen and thrombin with the goal of plugging the hole and promoting healing. The best reported results are from a study of highly selected CD patients who had a 38% success rate, with 15% of those recurring by 16 weeks and no longer-term follow-up, and most authors report significantly lower success rates (99,100). The fistula plug is made of porcine submucosa that is inserted into the tract. It acts as a scaffolding for healing. A meta-analysis of the small series that included CD patients found an overall success rate of 55%, but with varying follow-up and recurrence rates (101). While early results were encouraging, long-term results have been discouraging, particularly in CD patients, and these methods are generally not employed.

Endorectal advancement flaps can be used when there is no proctitis or anal stenosis. It is often the procedure of choice for rectovaginal fistulas. The technique is identical for treating non-CD-related fistulas; a broad flap is mobilized from mucosa and submucosa. The internal opening is excised. Some surgeons will close the internal opening. The flap is mobilized until it can be brought down below the opening and secured in a tension-free manner with interrupted sutures. Advancement flaps have a success rate of up to 71% in series with CD patients (102). There is a potential for alterations in continence with this procedure. While the success rates of this technique for sporadic cryptograndular fistulas are reportedly 81%, it was 64% in CD patients in a meta-analysis that specifically compared these groups (103).

Ligation of the intersphincteric tract (LIFT) is a more recently described procedure that poses minimal to no danger to the sphincter complex (104). A probe is placed into the fistula tract, and an incision is made in the intersphincteric groove. The fistula tract is then dissected out and tied off at the internal and external sphincter; it is then divided. The remainder of the external tract is curetted, and the external opening is widened. The skin incision is closed. This technique is relatively effective in comparison with other fistula repairs, healing up to 91% of fistulas (105). LIFT has not been well studied in the context of CD; one small series of 15 patients reported 53% healing at 12 months, but three patients developed a novel fistula (106). However, because it is performed entirely outside of the lumen and does utilize anal or rectal mucosa while also avoiding damage to the sphincter complex, some practitioners prefer it as an initial approach in CD-related fistulas.

## Rectovaginal fistula

Rectovaginal fistula (RVF) affects 9% of women with CD; they more commonly occur in conjunction with colonic disease than small bowel disease, following the same pattern as other manifestations of perianal CD (107). It has a substantial impact on quality of life and can be quite disabling for those who are affected. The presence of a RVF also increases the risk of requiring proctectomy for disease control (98). Common presenting symptoms are air or stool from the vagina, but patients may also report purulence from the vagina, dyspareunia, irritation, and urinary tract infection. Though on examination it may be possible to visualize the fistula, the diagnosis can be made with a high clinical suspicion based on symptoms even when it cannot be visualized in an outpatient setting. In these cases, examination under anesthesia is mandated prior to planning repair. It is also possible for fistulae to develop from the colon or small bowel to the vagina in CD.

There are numerous options for addressing RVFs in women with CD. The success of the repair depends on overall CD control, patient comorbidities, inflammation of the involved tissue, anal stricture, and the size of the fistula. As with perianal fistulas, prior to undertaking definitive repair, medical management should be optimized, all local inflammation and infection should be completely resolved, and a staged approach may be helpful. It is important to manage patient expectations, as there is a high rate of recurrence and need for multiple procedures, and for patients who are asymptomatic or minimally symptomatic, there is no mandate to treat the fistula. The surgical approach may be transanal, transvaginal, or transperineal. Tissue transfer may be used to treat RVF. The use of biologic mesh interposition has been reported with disappointing results; the failure rate was 80% (108). The overall healing rate for all techniques is 63%, and multiple procedures are often required (107). Consideration for diverting stoma should be given, either before the repair to aid in diminishing inflammation or at the time to allow the repair time to heal.

When there is no sphincter involvement, very low simple fistulas can be treated with fistulotomy. Transrectal approach usually involves an endorectal advancement flap. It is an option only when the anorectal mucosa is healthy. Initial healing rates are approximately 54%–71% (109,110). Transperineal repairs are particularly well suited for RVF with concomitant sphincter defects. The first method, episioproctotomy involves a linear incision over the perineum, in essence creating a fourth-degree tear. The fistula tract is debrided back to healthy tissue. The edges of the sphincter are mobilized, the rectal mucosa is repaired, and an overlapping sphincteroplasty is performed. The vagina is then repaired. The second option for transperineal repair is a transverse approach, which utilizes a transverse incision through the perineal body. The plane is dissected proximally, mobilizing the posterior vagina and anterior rectum until healthy tissue above the fistula is reached. The tract is debrided, and then all layers are reapproximated. Both of these transperineal approaches have success rates of approximately 70% (111). The vaginal approach may be beneficial when there is significant scarring or disease of the anal canal limiting the ability to manipulate the tissues. A vaginal flap is created similarly to an endoanal advancement flap. The layers are separated and repaired at the level of the fistula, and then the flap is tacked down. Levator muscles are closed between the layers as reinforcement.

Tissue transfer typically involves using a gracilis muscle flap or healthy tissue from the labia majora, a Martius flap. The gracilis flap is usually used as a second- or third-line intervention, after other techniques have failed (112). A Martius flap can be combined with transperineal repairs (113). A longitudinal incision is made in the labia majora, and the bulbocavernosus and its associated fat pad are dissected out; it remains attached inferiorly. They are passed through a subcutaneous tunnel and brought through to the fistula where they are tacked posterior to the vaginal wall, which is closed over it.

## Fecal diversion

Fecal diversion may be employed to allow fistula repairs time to heal, or to allow inflammation to subside. Diversion alone improves perianal disease in approximately 80% of patients, but about half will relapse once they are reversed (114). Diversion or proctectomy may be required when perianal disease is so severe that it cannot be salvaged through maximal medical and surgical options. Predictors of diversion include colonic disease, anal strictures, and multiple complex fistulas (115). Many patients are reluctant to commit to permanent stoma; for this group of patients, temporary diversion has the benefit of showing them the improvement in quality of life and makes it easier for them to accept permanent stoma. In patients with severe perianal disease, a multidisciplinary approach working with plastic and reconstructive surgeons for flaps is recommended. In patients with complex or nonhealing fistulas, fecal diversion may play a role. This generally improves quality of life, but fewer than 25% of these patients have intestinal continuity restored after a secondary procedure aimed at resolving the perianal problem (114,116). Proctectomy is required in 5% of CD patients for perianal disease alone.

## Carcinoma in a fistula

Cancer in a chronic perianal fistula is extremely rare in CD and typically occurs after years of active disease and long-standing fistulas in patients with severe perineal disease (117). The presentation can range from increasing pain to pelvic sepsis, or with typical fistula, symptoms such as chronic drainage unchanged from baseline. When a patient has a long-standing, quiescent fistula that suddenly becomes symptomatic, carcinoma should be suspected. Adenocarcinoma and squamous cell carcinoma are both described in this setting, and treatment ranges from chemoradiation to proctectomy with wide margins in the perianal region (118).

## FISSURES

Fissures in CD may be located in the anterior or posterior midline like idiopathic fissures, but can occur in any location around the anus. Atypical presentation of a fissure should always raise suspicion that it is the first clinical manifestation of CD. The etiology may be related to the inflammatory process, trauma from excessive diarrhea, or from the same etiology as sporadic fissures.

Many fissures in CD are painless unless they are associated with an abscess, and many respond to medical therapy. The same symptomatic therapies used for idiopathic fissures, i.e., nitroglycerin, calcium channel blockers, warm baths, pain medications, and bowel management, may be trialed, but their effectiveness in CD has not been evaluated. Topical mesalamine or hydrocortisone suppositories are often helpful to promote healing, and limiting the amount of diarrhea either with systemic medications or antidiarrheal agents is also beneficial. In general, surgical treatment for isolated fissures in patients with active CD should not be undertaken, as there is a real risk of nonhealing and incontinence.

## SKIN TAGS

Many patients with CD will have characteristic, large, atypically shaped skin tags. The etiology is thought to be from fissures and chronic inflammation leading to lymphedema. A conservative surgical approach is critically important in CD patients. Though these skin tags may be large and cause hygiene difficulties as well as pruritus, outcomes of any attempt to excise them may be worse than the initial complaint. Chronic, nonhealing anal or perianal ulcers can be painful and more difficult to manage.

## ANAL STENOSIS

Anal stenosis or strictures may present later than would be expected in CD patients due to softer stool consistency. In large series from major referral centers, the prevalence of anal strictures is up to 22% (89). Most often, they occur in the presence of perianal disease or represent consequences of long-term inflammation. Patients may report overflow diarrhea, perineal pain, constipation, and fecal incontinence. Medical management may be helpful for the inflammatory component of the stricture, but surgical intervention should be limited to patients who have difficulty with evacuation.

Dilation, either with digital dilation or Hegar dilators, is the most common management technique. This may need to be repeated at regular intervals. Many patients can be taught to maintain dilation performed in the office or operating room using a set of Hegar dilators at home on a regular basis. Balloon dilation has also been popular but is more expensive and must be done in an office or endoscopy setting (119). Use of a bougie dilator has also been successfully described (120). Potential risks associated with stricture dilation include bacteremia, worsening pain, and perforation. Fecal incontinence from chronic injury to the sphincter, both from the stenosis and the dilation procedure, is also a concern.

Historically, anorectal strictures in CD have been a poor prognostic indicator and often suggested the need for a stoma (115,121). Even with the use of biologic therapy, which is often effective for other perianal manifestations of CD, long-term outcomes in patients with anal strictures were not significantly improved (122).

## POSTOPERATIVE MEDICAL THERAPY

Since surgery for CD is not curative, there should be some consideration of empiric therapy to prevent endoscopic and clinical recurrence after resection. Up to 80% of CD patients will have an endoscopic recurrence at 1 year after surgery (123). Factors that should be weighed include both disease- and patient-specific factors to reach an individualized plan. Smoking (124,125), history of multiple resections (126,127), and a perforating phenotype (128,129) have all been identified as high risk for recurrent disease (130). Length of resection, perianal disease, and short duration from onset to surgery have also been proposed as high-risk features.

If the decision is made to treat prophylactically after surgery, the options for medications are the same as those in the preoperative setting. In several meta-analyses, mesalamine appears to decrease the risk of clinical recurrence but is less favorable in terms of endoscopic recurrence (131,132). Thiopurines are more efficacious in reducing endoscopic and clinical recurrences but have a higher likelihood of medication intolerance and side effects, leading to 22% cessation in one clinical trial of patients in the postoperative period (133,134). Metronidazole and other similar antibiotics have been explored in the postoperative period and found to be relatively well tolerated as a 3-month course but probably do not further reduce risk if used with another agent (135). Using metronidazole postoperatively but prior to introduction of a biologic agent has not been studied, but starting these agents is often delayed by weeks to months after surgery, and they can be used as a bridge in this setting. Notably, a decision analysis model found that antibiotics are the most cost effective for reducing clinical postoperative recurrence (136). Anti-TNF therapy is the most efficacious for reducing clinical and endoscopic recurrences (131,137). There are improved short- and long-term outcomes in terms

of endoscopic and clinical findings, and also less need for additional surgery (122,138). Adalimumab appears to be as effective as infliximab (139), but there is less data regarding other anti-TNF agents or other newer medications such as vedolizumab.

## REFERENCES

1. Kaplan GG. *Nat Rev Gastroenterol Hepatol* 2015; 12(12):720–7.
2. Molodecky NA et al. *Gastroenterology* 2012;142(1): 46–54.e42.
3. Hanauer SB et al. *Lancet* 2002;359(9317):1541–9.
4. Colombel J et al. *Gastroenterology* 2007;132(1): 52–65.
5. Jeuring SFG et al. *Am J Gastroenterol* 2017;112(2): 325–36.
6. Hatch QM et al. *J Gastrointest Surg* 2016;20(11): 1867–73.
7. de Groof EJ et al. *Colorectal Dis* 2017;19(6):551–8.
8. Morar PS et al. *J Crohns Colitis* 2015;9(6):483–91.
9. Yang Z-P et al. *Int J Surg* 2014;12(3):224–30.
10. Kopylov U et al. *Inflamm Bowel Dis* 2012;18(12): 2404–13.
11. El-Hussuna A et al. *Dis Colon Rectum* 2013;56(12): 1423–33.
12. Yamamoto T et al. *United Eur Gastroenterol J* 2016; 4(6):784–93.
13. Lightner AL et al. *J Crohns Colitis* 2017;11(2):185–90.
14. Mikocka-Walus AA et al. *Inflamm Bowel Dis* 2012; 18(8):1582–7.
15. Louis E et al. *J Crohn's Colitis* 2015;9(8):685–91.
16. Shental O et al. *Dis Colon Rectum* 2012;55(11): 1125–30.
17. Tukey M et al. *Am J Gastroenterol* 2009;104(11): 2734–9.
18. Kopylov U et al. *Dig Liver Dis* 2017;49(8):854–63.
19. Dionisio PM et al. *Am J Gastroenterol* 2010;105(6): 1240–8; quiz 1249.
20. Cheifetz AS et al. *Am J Gastroenterol* 2006;101(10): 2218–22.
21. Kordbacheh H et al. *Inflamm Bowel Dis* 2017;23(6): 1025–33.
22. Jensen MD et al. *Inflamm Bowel Dis* 2011;17(5): 1081–8.
23. Qiu Y et al. *Aliment Pharmacol Ther* 2014;40(2): 134–46.
24. Ordás I et al. *Gastroenterology* 2014;146(2):374–82.e1.
25. Kroeker KI et al. *J Clin Gastroenterol* 2011;45(1): 34–9.
26. de Groof EJ et al. *Dig Dis* 2014;32(s1):103–9.
27. He X et al. *J Clin Gastroenterol* 2015;49(9):e82–90.
28. Clancy C et al. *J Crohns Colitis* 2016;10(2):202–8.
29. Morar PS et al. *Aliment Pharmacol Ther* 2015;42(10): 1137–48.
30. Li Y et al. *Br J Surg* 2015;102(11):1418–25; discussion 1425.

31. Murthy SK, Nguyen GC. *Am J Gastroenterol* 2011; 106(4):713–8.

32. Wallaert JB et al. *Dis Colon Rectum* 2012;55(11): 1138–44.

33. Brady MT et al. *Dis Colon Rectum* 2017;60(1):61–7.

34. Liverani E et al. *World J Gastroenterol* 2016;22(3): 1017.

35. Fazi M et al. *JAMA Surg* 2016;151(5):452–60.

36. Geltzeiler CB et al. *J Gastrointest Surg* 2015;19(5): 905–10.

37. Campbell L et al. *Dis Colon Rectum* 2012;55(6):714–26.

38. Ponsioen CY et al. *Lancet Gastroenterol Hepatol* 2017;2(11):785–92.

39. Ward MG et al. *Inflamm Bowel Dis* 2015;21(12): 2839–47.

40. Bellinger J et al. *J Laparoendosc Adv Surg Tech* 2014;24(9):617–22.

41. Stocchi L et al. *Surgery* 2008;144(4):622–8.

42. Patel SV et al. *BMC Surg* 2013;13(1):14.

43. Dasari BV et al. Laparoscopic versus open surgery for small bowel Crohn's disease. *Cochrane Database Syst Rev* 2011;(1):CD006956.

44. Simillis C et al. *Dis Colon Rectum* 2007;50(10):1674–87.

45. Guo Z et al. *World J Surg* 2013;37(4):893–901.

46. He X et al. *Dig Dis Sci* 2014;59(7):1544–51.

47. Kono T et al. *J Gastrointest Surg* 2016;20(4):783–90.

48. Yamazaki Y et al. *Am J Gastroenterol* 1991;86(7):882–5. http://www.ncbi.nlm.nih.gov/ pubmed/2058631. Accessed January 4, 2017.

49. Wibmer AG et al. *Int J Colorectal Dis* 2010;25(10): 1149–57.

50. Broering DC et al. *Int J Colorectal Dis* 2001;16(2): 81–7. http://www.ncbi.nlm.nih.gov/pubmed/ 11355323. Accessed January 4, 2017.

51. Strong S et al. *Dis Colon Rectum* 2015;58(11): 1021–36.

52. Tekkis PP et al. *Colorectal Dis* 2006;8(2):82–90.

53. da Luz Moreira A et al. *J Gastrointest Surg* 2007; 11(11):1529–33.

54. Holubar SD et al. *Inflamm Bowel Dis* 2010;16(11): 1940–6.

55. Umanskiy K et al. *J Gastrointest Surg* 2010;14(4): 658–63.

56. Marceau C et al. *Surgery* 2007;141(5):640–4.

57. Keighley MR et al. *Gut* 1982;23(2):102–7. http://www. ncbi.nlm.nih.gov/pubmed/7068033. Accessed January 4, 2017.

58. Kariv Y et al. *J Am Coll Surg* 2009;208(3):390–9.

59. Melton GB et al. *Ann Surg* 2008;248(4):608–16.

60. Regimbeau JM et al. *Dis Colon Rectum* 2001;44(6): 769–78. http://www.ncbi.nlm.nih.gov/pubmed/ 11391134. Accessed January 4, 2017.

61. Sagar PM et al. *Dis Colon Rectum* 1996;39(8):893–8. http://www.ncbi.nlm.nih.gov/pubmed/8756845. Accessed January 4, 2017.

62. Braveman JM et al. *Dis Colon Rectum* 2004;47(10): 1613–9.

63. Cirincione E et al. *Dis Colon Rectum* 2000;43(4):544–7. http://www.ncbi.nlm.nih.gov/pubmed/10789755. Accessed January 4, 2017.

64. Lavery IC, Jagelman DG. *Dis Colon Rectum* 1982; 25(6):522–4. http://www.ncbi.nlm.nih.gov/pubmed/ 7117054. Accessed January 4, 2017.

65. Guillem JG et al. *Dis Colon Rectum* 1992;35(8): 768–72. http://www.ncbi.nlm.nih.gov/pubmed/ 1644001. Accessed January 4, 2017.

66. von Roon AC et al. *Dis Colon Rectum* 2007;50(6): 839–55.

67. Itzkowitz SH, Present DH, Crohn's and Colitis Foundation of America Colon Cancer in IBD Study Group. *Inflamm Bowel Dis* 2005;11(3):314–21. http:// www.ncbi.nlm.nih.gov/pubmed/15735438. Accessed January 4, 2017.

68. Friedman S et al. *Clin Gastroenterol Hepatol* 2008; 6(9):993–8.

69. van den Heuvel TRA et al. *Int J Cancer* 2016;139(6): 1270–80.

70. Laine L et al. *Gastrointest Endosc* 2015;81(3):489– 501.e26.

71. Kiran RP et al. *Ann Surg* 2012;256(2):221–6.

72. Maser E a et al. *Inflamm Bowel Dis* 2013;19(9): 1827–32.

73. Schwartz DA et al. *Gastroenterology* 2002;122(4) 875–80. http://www.ncbi.nlm.nih.gov/pubmed/ 11910338. Accessed January 4, 2017.

74. Beaugerie L et al. *Gastroenterology* 2006;130(3): 650–6.

75. Gelbmann CM et al. *Am J Gastroenterol* 2002;97(6): 1438–45.

76. Williams DR et al. *Dis Colon Rectum* 24(1):22–4. http://www.ncbi.nlm.nih.gov/pubmed/7472097. Accessed January 4, 2017.

77. el Mouaaouy A et al. *Z Gastroenterol* 1992;30(7): 486–94. http://www.ncbi.nlm.nih.gov/pubmed/ 1509788. Accessed January 4, 2017.

78. Regueiro M, Mardini H. *Inflamm Bowel Dis* 2003;9(2): 98–103. http://www.ncbi.nlm.nih.gov/pubmed/ 12769443. Accessed January 4, 2017.

79. Topstad DR et al. *Dis Colon Rectum* 2003;46(5): 577–83.

80. Pearson DC et al. *Ann Intern Med* 1995;123(2): 132–42.

81. Present DH et al. *N Engl J Med* 1999;340(18): 1398–405.

82. Fortea-Ormaechea JI et al. *Gastroenterol Hepatol* 2011;34(7):443–8.

83. Echarri A et al. *J Crohns Colitis* 2010;4(6):654–60.

84. Gecse KB et al. *Gut* 2014;63(9):1381–92.

85. Orlando A et al. *Dig Liver Dis* 2011;43(1):1–20.

86. Sciaudone G et al. *Can J Surg* 2010;53(5):299–304. http://www.ncbi.nlm.nih.gov/pubmed/20858373. Accessed January 4, 2017.

87. Hyder SA et al. *Dis Colon Rectum* 2006;49(12): 1837–41.

88. Parsi MA et al. *Am J Gastroenterol* 2004;99(3): 445–9.
89. Wolff BG et al. *Dis Colon Rectum* 1985;28(10):709–11. http://www.ncbi.nlm.nih.gov/pubmed/4053875. Accessed January 4, 2017.
90. Thornton M, Solomon MJ. *Dis Colon Rectum* 2005; 48(3):459–63.
91. Sandborn WJ et al. *Gastroenterology* 2003;125(5): 1508–30. http://www.ncbi.nlm.nih.gov/pubmed/14598268. Accessed January 4, 2017.
92. Schwartz DA et al. *Gastroenterology* 2001;121(5): 1064–72.
93. Villa C et al. *Eur J Radiol* 2012;81(4):616–22.
94. Haggett PJ et al. *Gut* 1995;36(3):407–10. http://www.ncbi.nlm.nih.gov/pubmed/7698701. Accessed January 4, 2017.
95. Buchanan GN et al. *Radiology* 2004;233(3):674–81.
96. Beets-Tan RG et al. *Radiology* 2001;218(1):75–84.
97. Van Assche G et al. *Am J Gastroenterol* 2003;98(2): 332–9.
98. El-Gazzaz G et al. *Color Dis* 2012;14(10):1217–23.
99. Grimaud J et al. *Gastroenterology* 2010;138(7): 2275–2281.e1.
100. Zmora O et al. *Dis Colon Rectum* 2003;46(5):584–9.
101. O'Riordan JM et al. *Dis Colon Rectum.* 2012;55(3): 351–8.
102. Joo JS et al. *Am Surg* 1998;64(2):147–50. http://www.ncbi.nlm.nih.gov/pubmed/9486887. Accessed January 5, 2017.
103. Soltani A, Kaiser AM. *Dis Colon Rectum* 2010;53(4): 486–95.
104. Rojanasakul A. *Tech Coloproctol* 2009;13(3):237–40.
105. Bleier JIS et al. *Dis Colon Rectum* 2010;53(1):43–6.
106. Gingold DS et al. *Ann Surg* 2014;260(6):1057–61.
107. Narang R et al. *Dis Colon Rectum* 2016;59(7):670–6.
108. Mege D et al. *Color Dis* 2016;18(2):O61–5.
109. Kodner IJ et al. *Surgery* 1993;114(4):682–9.
110. Hull TL, Fazio VW. *Am J Surg* 1997;173(2):95–8.
111. Valente MA. *World J Gastrointest Pathophysiol* 2014; 5(4):487.
112. Zmora O et al. *Dis Colon Rectum* 2006;49(9):1316–21.
113. McNevin MS et al. *Am J Surg* 2007;193(5 SPEC. ISS.): 597–9.
114. Yamamoto T et al. *World J Surg* 2000;24(10):1258–62. http://www.ncbi.nlm.nih.gov/pubmed/11071472. Accessed January 5, 2017.
115. Galandiuk S et al. *Ann Surg* 2005;241(5):796–801.
116. Kasparek MS et al. *Dis Colon Rectum* 2007;50(12): 2067–74.
117. Church JM et al. *Dis Colon Rectum* 1985;28(5):361–6. http://www.ncbi.nlm.nih.gov/pubmed/3158499. Accessed January 5, 2017.
118. Shwaartz C et al. *Dis Colon Rectum* 2016;59(12): 1168–73.
119. Singh VV et al. *J Clin Gastroenterol* 2005;39(4): 284–90. http://www.ncbi.nlm.nih.gov/pubmed/15758621. Accessed January 5, 2017.
120. Kashkooli SB et al. *Can J Surg* 2015;58(5):347–8.
121. Linares L et al. *Br J Surg* 1988;75(7):653–5. http://www.ncbi.nlm.nih.gov/pubmed/3416120. Accessed January 5, 2017.
122. Uchino M et al. *World J Gastroenterol* 2011;17(9): 1174.
123. Buisson A et al. *Dig Liver Dis* 2012;44(6):453–60.
124. Reese GE et al. *Int J Colorectal Dis* 2008;23(12): 1213–21.
125. Kane S V et al. *J Clin Gastroenterol* 2005;39(1): 32–5. http://www.ncbi.nlm.nih.gov/pubmed/15599207. Accessed January 5, 2017.
126. Fortinsky KJ et al. *Dig Dis Sci* 2017;62(1):188–96.
127. Riss S et al. *Dis Colon Rectum* 2013;56(7):881–7.
128. Simillis C et al. *Am J Gastroenterol* 2008;103(1): 196–205.
129. Sachar DB et al. *Inflamm Bowel Dis* 2009;15(7): 1071–5.
130. DeCruz P et al. *Lancet* 2015;385(9976):1406–17.
131. Singh S et al. *Gastroenterology* 2015;148(1):64–76. e2; quiz e14.
132. Doherty G et al. *Cochrane Database Syst Rev* 2009; (4):CD006873.
133. D'Haens GR et al. *Gastroenterology* 2008;135(4): 1123–9.
134. Reinisch W et al. *Gut* 2010;59(6):752–9.
135. Mañosa M et al. *Inflamm Bowel Dis* 2013;19(9): 1889–95.
136. Ananthakrishnan AN et al. *Am J Gastroenterol* 2011; 106(11):2009–17.
137. Zhao Y et al. *Clin Res Hepatol Gastroenterol* 2015; 39(5):637–49.
138. Regueiro M et al. *Clin Gastroenterol Hepatol* 2014; 12(9):1494–1502.e1.
139. Kotze PG et al. *J Crohns Colitis* 2015;9(7):541–7.

# 37

# Evaluation and management of lower gastrointestinal bleeding

ARJUN N. JEGANATHAN AND SKANDAN SHANMUGAN

## CHALLENGING CASE

A 78-year-old male on Coumadin for atrial fibrillation presents with massive hematochezia and associated hypotension. He has never had a colonoscopy.

## CASE MANAGEMENT

Large-bore IV access is obtained, labs, including a cross-match, are sent, and he is resuscitated with rapid infusion of lactated Ringer solution. He is given fresh frozen plasma to normalize his international normalized ratio (INR) and transfused 2 units of packed red blood cells for a hemoglobin of 6.2 g/dL. His vital signs normalize, and the bleeding appears to have slowed. A computed tomography (CT) angiography is done, which shows a blush of extravasation in the ascending colon, where there appears to be diverticular disease. He subsequently undergoes angiographic embolization of the bleeding vessel with cessation of hemorrhage.

## BACKGROUND

Lower gastrointestinal bleeding (LGIB) is classically defined as luminal hemorrhage arising distal to the ligament of Treitz. The incidence of LGIB has slightly declined, but recent estimates show that LGIB still accounts for 35 hospitalizations/year/100,000 adult patients, with a case fatality rate between 1% and 3% (1). An important consideration to remember when evaluating a patient with gastrointestinal (GI) bleeding is that upper gastrointestinal bleeding (UGIB) still remains the more common cause by at least twofold (2). Thus, paramount to the treatment of LGIB is the elimination of the stomach and/or duodenum as the source of

hemorrhage. Classically, the aspiration of nonbloody, bilious fluid on nasogastric lavage was considered to have effectively excluded an UGIB; however, due to low sensitivity and the invasive nature of the procedure, it is becoming less popular in favor of clinical scoring systems (3). For the purposes of this chapter, we assume UGIB has been effectively excluded, most commonly with an upper endoscopy.

The patient with acute lower GI bleeding traditionally presents with hematochezia, defined as passage of bright red blood or clots per rectum. A patient with an upper GI bleed traditionally presents with melanotic (i.e., black and tarry) stools due to enzymatic breakdown of blood during the period of intestinal transit. Hemorrhage from the small intestine distal to the ligament of Treitz is a difficult clinical entity to diagnose, and the investigational workup varies quite a bit from colonic etiologies (4). In general, the differential diagnosis is affected by age, but the more common causes include inflammatory bowel disease, neoplasia, Meckel diverticulum, angioectasia or other vascular malformations, and nonsteroidal anti-inflammatory drug ulcers. For this chapter, we have chosen to focus our discussion on colorectal etiologies of LGIB.

## ETIOLOGY

Table 37.1 lists the causes of lower GI bleeding in a retrospective series of 1,112 patients from 1998 to 2006 at an urban medical center (5). Each disease entity is briefly described in the following sections and is covered in-depth in prior chapters; herein, we focus on the management strategies of lower GI bleeding.

### DIVERTICULAR BLEEDING

Diverticular bleeding is the most common cause of hemorrhage from the lower GI tract in adults (5). Diverticulosis

Table 37.1 Etiologies of lower gastrointestinal bleeding from 1998 to 2006 in an Urban U.S. Medical Center

| Disease | Percentage (%) |
|---|---|
| Diverticulosis | 37.3 |
| Hemorrhoids | 21.1 |
| Neoplasia | 11.8 |
| Colitis (noninflammatory) | 10.7 |
| Inflammatory bowel disease | 5.4 |
| Vascular malformation | 2.3 |
| Other colonic disease | 6.6 |
| Small intestine disease | 1.3 |
| Unknown | 3.5 |

is widely prevalent, and its presence on screening colonoscopy increases with age. Diverticular bleeding results from thinning of the colonic wall with eventual erosion of the penetrating vasa recta. While the presence of diverticulosis is more common in the left side of the colon, diverticular bleeding occurs more commonly in the right side of the colon (6). In a cohort of 1,514 patients with colonoscopy-confirmed asymptomatic diverticulosis, the cumulative incidence of diverticular bleeding was 0.21% at 1 year, increasing to 9.5% at 10 years (6). Diverticular bleeding classically presents as painless hematochezia. The bleeding is generally self-limited, with 75% of cases stopping spontaneously without requiring transfusion (7). During endoscopy, an active bleeding vessel, a nonbleeding but visible vessel, or an adherent clot may be identified and necessitate endoscopic intervention (8). Current American College of Gastroenterology (ACG) clinical guidelines favor endoscopic clips as they are generally safer than contact thermal therapy and easier to apply than ligation bands (9). However, after a second episode of diverticular hemorrhage, the risk of a future occurrence is close to 50%; thus, elective segmental resection can be considered after localization (7).

## HEMORRHOIDS

Painless rectal bleeding in a patient younger than 40 years can most commonly be attributed to a hemorrhoidal source, while alternative diagnoses must be sought if clinical suspicion exists. Bright red blood will generally coat the stool at the end of a bowel movement, drip into the toilet bowl, and/or stain the toilet paper. Anoscopy with visualization of the hemorrhoidal cushions may identify active bleeding or any stigmata of recent bleeding. Treatment for indolent bleeding from hemorrhoids is often conservative with dietary and lifestyle changes, but office-based procedures such as rubber band ligation or surgical intervention may occasionally be required.

## NEOPLASIA

Colorectal neoplasms are a less common cause of LGIB, accounting for 11% of all cases (5). The bleeding tends to be more occult in nature and is caused by ulceration of the mucosa. Classically, right-sided lesions present with melanotic or maroon stools, while left-sided lesions tend to produce bright red blood. While endoscopic therapies are often limited for bleeding secondary to neoplasia, the diagnostic benefit is immense. Surgical treatment for colorectal neoplasms will be dictated by clinical staging, but recurrent bleeding can often be an indication for palliative resection even in locally advanced malignancies that would otherwise require neoadjuvant therapy.

## COLITIS (NONINFLAMMATORY)

Noninflammatory causes of colitis are extremely diverse but can include infectious, ischemic, and radiation-induced etiologies. On endoscopy, the mucosal lining appears erythematous, friable, and ulcerated. Since the treatment is dictated by the underlying disease, importance is placed on arriving at a diagnosis. Infectious colitis often presents with diarrhea and malaise. In the United States, the most common causes include *Salmonella*, *Shigella*, *Campylobacter*, and *Escherichia coli* (10). Diagnosis is best established by stool culture and/or toxin assay. Ischemic colitis is more common in the elderly population and often associated with abdominal pain. Fulminant presentation with bowel necrosis is a surgical emergency and requires resection of the nonviable segments. Alternatively, ischemic colitis from low flow states without infarction can be managed conservatively with fluid resuscitation and bowel rest. Last, radiation-induced colitis can occur early (within 6 weeks) from direct mucosal damage or as a late manifestation associated with obliterative endarteritis and chronic mucosal ischemia. Bleeding from radiation proctitis generally responds well to a trial of sucralfate enemas, with formalin instillation and/or endoscopic argon plasma coagulation reserved for refractory cases (11).

## INFLAMMATORY BOWEL DISEASE

Inflammatory causes of LGIB include Crohn disease and ulcerative colitis, with the latter more commonly causing hematochezia. Fortunately, less than 6% of patients have progression to massive LGIB requiring urgent surgical intervention (12). Differentiating Crohn disease from ulcerative colitis is important when considering the extent of surgical resection. Classically, subtotal colectomy with end ileostomy is indicated for refractory bleeding from ulcerative colitis, while limited resection of affected segments is preferred for Crohn disease (13).

## VASCULAR MALFORMATION

Vascular malformations of the GI tract encompass a myriad of clinical entities and are quite poorly described in the literature due to inconsistent nomenclature (14). Colonic lesions include vascular tumors/angiomas, anomalies associated with congenital/systemic disease (i.e., hereditary hemorrhagic telangiectasia), and acquired/sporadic disease, such as angiodysplasia and vascular ectasia. While rare, angiodysplasia remains the most common vascular malformation. Pathologically, angiodysplasia refers to dilated submucosal vessels, likely caused by degenerative changes of the colonic walls with aging (15). Bleeding most often originates from the cecum or ascending colon but is often episodic and self-limiting (16). Clinical guidelines favor the use of noncontact thermal therapy, namely, argon plasma coagulation, due to improved outcomes with decreased transfusion requirements (9).

## INITIAL EVALUATION

The chief complaint of lower GI bleeding is a very common clinical entity and mandates a systematic, stepwise approach. In general, LGIB can be categorized into acute (urgent or emergent) or chronic. Relevant past medical history should be elucidated so as to identify potential sources of bleeding, as well as any prior episodes of LGIB. Concurrent comorbidities could dramatically alter management strategies and must be included in relevant past medical history. Additionally, a careful review of medications must be conducted with emphasis on contributory pharmacologic drugs, such as anticoagulant, antiplatelet, and nonsteroidal anti-inflammatory agents.

General supportive measures must first be undertaken, including establishment of adequate IV access, supplemental oxygen via nasal cannula, and initiation of resuscitation. The first assessment must include a determination of the severity of bleeding, including an estimation of blood loss. In a comparison of a restrictive (Hgb <7 g/dL) versus liberal (Hgb <9 g/dL) transfusion strategy, a restrictive strategy significantly improved outcomes in patients with acute UGIB and LGIB (17). The probability of survival at 6 weeks was higher in the restrictive-strategy group than in the liberal-strategy group (95% versus 91%). As for management of coagulopathies, the risk of holding or reversing anticoagulation should be weighed against the indicated benefit. The decision must be individualized, but, in general, the transfusion of platelets and/or plasma is indicated for patients with large transfusion requirements, as well as coagulopathies (INR >1.5 or platelets <50,000/microL) with ongoing bleeding. When major bleeding was studied in the trauma population, early administration of plasma, platelets, and red blood cells in a 1:1:1 ratio compared with a 1:1:2 ratio resulted in increased hemostasis and fewer deaths due to exsanguination by 24 hours, but did not result in significant differences in mortality at 24 hours or at 30 days (18).

## MANAGEMENT

Upon completion of the initial evaluation, the management of acute LGIB can generally be approached in a stepwise fashion, as detailed by Figure 37.1.

## ENDOSCOPIC STRATEGIES

As supported by the 2016 ACG clinical guidelines, colonoscopy should be the initial diagnostic procedure for nearly all patients presenting with acute LGIB (9). Careful inspection of the colonic mucosa and intubation of the terminal ileum to rule out more proximal bleeding is generally recommended (19). Ideally, endoscopic examination should be conducted within 24 hours of presentation after a mechanical bowel preparation. A randomized trial of 100 consecutive patients presenting with LGIB found that urgent colonoscopy (<8 hours), when compared to standard colonoscopy (1–3 days), was more successful in identifying a source of bleeding, though a clear improvement in outcomes (namely, rebleeding, transfusion requirements, length of stay, and mortality) was not supported (20). Of note, a recent feasibility study of 12 patients demonstrated that urgent colonoscopy without the use of bowel preparation was found to be adequate for presumptive identification of the source of bleeding in all procedures, without the need to repeat colonoscopy because of inadequate preparation (21). However, the current ACG clinical guidelines recommend bowel preparation, consisting of a large volume (4–6 L) of polyethylene glycol–based solutions administered rapidly (over 3–4 hours) until effluent is clear (9).

## RADIOLOGIC STRATEGIES

One advantage of radiographic testing for acute GI bleed is the ability to assess the entirety of the GI tract, including small bowel sources. The two most commonly performed tests for luminal hemorrhage include nuclear scintigraphy (radionuclide scanning) and CT angiography. According to our treatment algorithm, radionuclide scanning is best applied for ongoing bleeding despite a negative colonoscopy, while CT angiography has applicability for the patient with severe bleeding who cannot be stabilized for colonoscopy or who cannot undergo a rapid bowel prep for colonoscopy.

The most sensitive radiographic test for GI bleeding is a radionuclide scan, capable of detecting bleeding at a rate of 0.04–0.1 mL/min (22). Scintigraphy for GI bleeding was first described in 1977 using Tc-99m sulfur colloid but mostly has been replaced by Tc-99m red blood cell (RBC) imaging to allow for longer periods of sequential imaging if needed. While very sensitive in its ability to detect active bleeding, the major limitation of radionuclide scanning is its ability to only localize bleeding to a general region of the abdomen and not to a specific anatomic structure. In fact, in a study of 203 patients, tagged RBC scan was positive in 26% of patients, but incorrectly localized the site of bleeding in 1 out of 4, resulting in 8 misguided surgical procedures (23).

CT angiography for the localization of GI bleeding has become increasingly popular due to widespread availability. However, when compared to scintigraphy, CT angiography lacks the ability to sequentially image over time without repeated radiation and contrast exposures. In swine models, researchers had success detecting bleeding

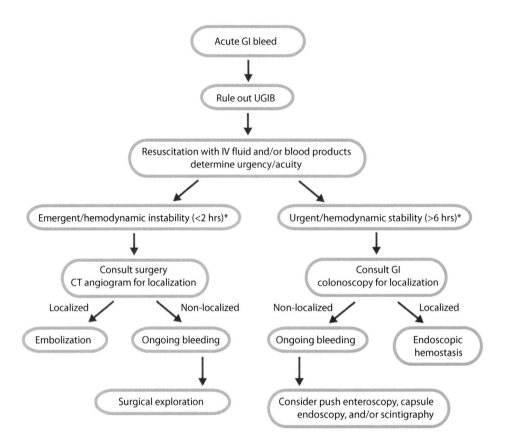

**Figure 37.1** Diagnosis and treatment algorithm for acute lower GI bleeding. *Determination of urgency/acuity is a difficult clinical decision but can generally be stratified into emergent cases who need intervention within 2 hours and cases who will require urgent colonoscopy but may wait at least 6 hours before intervention.

at a rate of 0.3–0.5 mL/min (24). CT angiography has excellent results when studied clinically, with a recent meta-analysis arriving at a sensitivity and specificity of 85% and 92%, respectively, for the detection of GI hemorrhage (25). A positive CT angiography is typically followed by a therapeutic angiographic procedure in patients who are hemodynamically stable. A study in 2015 concluded that preceding visceral angiography with a diagnostic study (i.e., CT angiography) improved localization of the site of lower GI hemorrhage when compared with visceral angiography alone (26).

Diagnostic visceral angiography is typically reserved for patients not favorable for endoscopy, namely, individuals with severe bleeding with hemodynamic instability and high operative risk. Detection as a contrast blush or extravasation generally requires blood loss of 0.5–1 mL/min (27). In the absence of prior localization, the superior mesenteric artery is generally examined first, followed by the inferior mesenteric artery, due to the predilection of bleeding to occur in the embryologic midgut distribution. The distinct advantage of visceral angiography is that, like colonoscopy, therapeutic interventions may occur. In patients with active bleeding, superselective embolization of distal vessels is successful in 80% with no episodes of rebleeding in 97% of cases (28). However, the major complication profile of visceral angiography includes arterial injury, thrombus

formation, and renal failure, with bowel infarction occurring in up to one-third of cases (29).

## SURGICAL STRATEGIES

Due to the significant associated morbidity and mortality, urgent operative exploration for LGIB is often reserved for massive hemorrhage with hemodynamic instability despite resuscitation. Additionally, patients who have failed repeated endoscopic or interventional approaches or cannot obtain these less invasive modalities are also surgical candidates. For ongoing hemorrhage, surgical procedures will occasionally be indicated as first-line treatment based on the pathology alone, including bleeding from early stage colorectal neoplasms or benign anorectal disease. The decision to operate on massive LGIB is a challenging one based on numerous clinical entities, but the literature would support that only a small percentage (4.7%) require urgent operative procedures (30). No single predictor can accurately dictate the need for surgical intervention, but ongoing bleeding with transfusion requirements upward of 4 units of RBCs within 24 hours has become a general benchmark (31). While our outcomes have likely improved, early data suggested that the overall mortality, while not statistically different, was not insignificant for urgent total abdominal colectomy versus limited colonic resection (6% versus 15%, respectively) (32).

In a retrospective study of 77 patients, recurrent bleeding was significantly more common in the segmental colectomy group than the total abdominal colectomy group (18% versus 4%), and morbidity and mortality were not significantly different (33). Consequently, total abdominal colectomy with end ileostomy should remain the procedure of choice for surgical treatment of massive LGIB without a clearly localized source. However, when the bleeding site has been localized and confirmed without control, a segmental colectomy with primary anastomosis can be undertaken with rebleeding and mortality rates of 4%–10% and 0%–40%, respectively. A "blind" segmental colectomy without localization should not be performed. Last, in a retrospective review of subtotal colectomies performed for LGIB, 55 of 58 patients were treated with a primary ileorectal anastomosis with an overall mortality of 17%, mainly resulting from sepsis due to anastomotic leak (34). The current data would strongly argue against reestablishment of GI continuity during the index emergent operation, while an elective ileorectal anastomosis at a later date has far fewer consequences.

## SUMMARY

Key points in the diagnosis and management of LGIB include stabilization with resuscitation, localization of the bleeding source, and cessation of ongoing hemorrhage via endoscopy, angiography, or surgery. Given the recent advances in nonsurgical strategies, fewer patients are undergoing subtotal colectomies for nonlocalized bleeding. Segmental colectomy should be reserved for patients with a localized bleeding site; subtotal colectomy with an ileorectal anastomosis should be reserved for elective patients and avoided in the emergent settings.

# REFERENCES

1. Laine L et al. *Am J Gastroenterol.* 2012;107(8):1190–5.
2. Rotando G. *Gastroenterol Clin North Am.* 2014;43(4): 643–63.
3. Srygley FD et al. *JAMA.* 2012;307(10):1072–9.
4. Gerson LB et al. *Am J Gastroenterol.* 2015;110(9): 1265–87.
5. Gayer C et al. *Surgery,* 2009;146:600–7.
6. Niikura R et al. *Aliment Pharmacol Ther.* 2015;41(9): 888–94.
7. McGuire HH. *Ann Surg.* 1994;220(5):653.
8. Jensen DM et al. *N Engl J Med.* 2000;342(2):78–82.
9. Strate LL, Gralnek IM. *Am J Gastroenterol.* 2016;111: 459–74.
10. DuPont HL. *Curr Opin Gastroenterol.* 2012;28(1): 39–46.
11. van de Wetering FT et al. *Cochrane Database Syst Rev.* 2016;4:CD003455.
12. Berg DF et al. *Am J Surg.* 2002;184(1):45–51.
13. Shanmugan S, Stein SL. Lower gastrointestinal bleeding. In Cameron JL, Cameron AM (eds). *Current Surgical Therapy,* 302–307, 11th Edition. 2014. Elsevier, Philadelphia, PA.
14. Regula J et al. *Best Pract Res Clin Gastroenterol.* 2008;22(2):313–28.
15. Boley SJ et al. *Gastroenterology.* 1977;72(4):650.
16. Diggs NG et al. *Clin Gastroenterol Hepatol.* 2011; 9(5):415–20.
17. Villanueva C et al. *N Engl J Med.* 2013;368(1):11–21.
18. Holcomb JB et al. *JAMA.* 2015;313(5):471–82.
19. Jensen DM. *Am J Gastroenterol.* 2005;100:2403–6.
20. Green BT et al. *Am J Gastroenterol.* 2005;100(11): 2395–402.
21. Repaka A et al. *Gastrointest Endosc.* 2012;76(2): 367–73.
22. Currie GM et al. *J Clin Gastroenterol.* 2011;45(2): 92–9.
23. Hunter JM, Pezim ME. *Am J Surg.* 1990;159(5):504.
24. Kuhle WG, Sheiman RG. *Radiology.* 2003;228(3): 743–52.
25. García-Blázquez V et al. *Eur Radiol.* 2013;23(5):1181.
26. Jacovides CL et al. *JAMA Surg.* 2015;150(7):650–6.
27. Walker TG. *Tech Vasc Interv Radiol.* 2009;12(2): 80–91.
28. Strate LL, Naumann CR. *Clin Gastroenterol Hepatol.* 2010;8(4):333–43.
29. Khanna A et al. *J Gastrointest Surg.* 2005;9(3): 343–52.
30. Newman J et al. *Colorectal Dis.* 2012;14(8):1020–6.
31. Bender JS et al. *Am Surg.* 1991;57:536–40.
32. Baker R, Senagore A. *Am Surg.* 1994;60(8):578–81.
33. Farner R et al. *Am J Surg.* 1999;178(6):587–91.
34. Plummer JM et al. *Int J Clin Pract.* 2009;63(6):865–8.

# 38

# Ostomies

DANIELLE PICKHAM AND SUPRIYA S. PATEL

## CHALLENGING CASE

A 55-year-old morbidly obese male undergoes a low anterior resection with concomitant loop ileostomy for a T2 rectal cancer. Six weeks postoperatively, he presents to the clinic with an easily reducible parastomal hernia. He complains of increasing pain, difficulty with application of his ostomy appliances, and symptoms of intermittent obstruction.

## CASE MANAGEMENT

The optimal management for a symptomatic parastomal hernia of temporary stoma includes reversal of the ostomy after ensuring that the distal anastomosis has healed. Anastomotic integrity is confirmed by a contrast study, often a Gastrografin enema or computed tomography scan with rectal contrast. An ostomy reversal ameliorates and addresses all of the symptoms including the hernia, obstruction, and pain. After reversal, the skin of the ostomy can be partially closed; however, extreme vigilance of the wound is necessary secondary to an increased rate of local wound infection. Depending on the size of the fascial defect and corresponding hernia, additional mesh may be needed for hernia repair. Due to increased risk of infection of most prosthetics, biologic materials should be considered as a first option. For patients who are not candidates for ostomy reversal, various options are available and include both open and laparoscopic approaches. These options include primary fascial repair, repair with biologic or prosthetic mesh, and finally, stoma relocation. The approach and the method of repair are dependent on the surgeon's preference and experience. Certainly, observation for minimally symptomatic parastomal hernias is the preferred option until stomal takedown is possible.

## INTRODUCTION

Stoma formation is a common procedure for colon and rectal surgeons. It is estimated that approximately 450,000 people in the United States are currently living with an intestinal stoma, and 120,000 new stomas are created each year (1). There are various types of intestinal stomas created for a broad spectrum of diseases and clinical situations. When successful, stomas are designed to save lives or ultimately enhance a patient's quality of life. However, they can be fraught with a number of complications, resulting in significant economic, physiologic, and psychological impact. The focus of this chapter is to review complications associated with stoma formation and discuss how to prevent or manage these adverse outcomes.

## HISTORICAL PERSPECTIVE

To botanists a "stoma" refers to a pore in the epidermis of a plant that participates in gas exchange. Similarly, in medicine, a stoma refers to a surgically created opening of the intestine through a patient's anterior abdominal wall. The first recorded stoma surgeries were in the 1700s (2). Based on the observation that patients were able to survive intestinal rupture due to formation of cutaneous fistulas, surgical techniques were devised to intentionally create those fistulas in similar, emergent settings (2). In the 1800s, the first elective stoma surgery was described by Freer, the loop colostomy was introduced, and the concept of a temporary stoma was devised (2). Since then, surgical techniques have evolved to include the Hartmann end colostomy (1923) and the Brooke ileostomy (1952) (2). Currently, there are a wide variety of stomas, and multiple techniques have been developed to assist in the prevention and management of stoma-related complications.

## CONSIDERATIONS

## SURGICAL DECISION-MAKING

Stomas are utilized over a broad range of clinical scenarios, including lower intestinal cancer, diverticulitis, inflammatory bowel disease, bowel perforation or obstruction, trauma, and fistulizing disease. There are two general indications for stoma creation: (1) to provide a solution for elimination when intestinal continuity is not feasible and (2) to provide fecal diversion in the setting of distal obstruction or to allow additional time for healing. Multiple different stoma options exist with respect to type (ileostomy/colostomy), duration (temporary/permanent), and configuration (end/looped). Individualizing the stoma to each patient and circumstance is critical to preventing or minimizing future complications.

The following case study illustrates the multitude of surgical options that may be present in any one clinical scenario.

### CASE STUDY

A 72-year-old female presents with an obstructing rectosigmoid mass. Colonoscopy is performed and confirms the diagnosis of adenocarcinoma. She has no prior surgical history but is obese with hypertension, diabetes, and coronary artery disease. Multiple surgical options can be considered:

a. Resection with primary anastomosis
b. Resection with primary anastomosis and diverting stoma
c. Resection with end colostomy or ileostomy
d. Diverting loop colostomy or ileostomy

After taking into account patient-related factors such as age, comorbidities, patient's functional status including mobility and continence, stage of the cancer, and overall prognosis, the surgeon should also consider what surgical options, including type of stoma, will offer the patient the lowest risk of complications and the best quality of life.

## PRIMARY ANASTOMOSIS

Primary anastomosis is always favored whenever feasible, but the risks of anastomotic leak and alterations in bowel function must be weighed against the potential complications and lifestyle modifications required with a stoma. In our clinical scenario, primary anastomosis may be avoided due to a variety of factors, such as concern for increased risk of infection due to unprepped bowel, concern for increased risk of anastomotic leak due to size discrepancy and poor viability of a chronically dilated proximal segment, and decreased healing potential due to nutritional or electrolyte deficiencies

that may exist in patients with cancer or chronic obstructions. However, endoscopic stenting, subtotal colectomy, or on-table colonic lavage are alternative options to achieve primary anastomosis and have been demonstrated to be safe, but discussion of them is beyond the scope of this chapter (3–6).

Perforated diverticulitis is another common clinical scenario in which a primary anastomosis has historically been avoided. However, in recent years this has been challenged, and primary anastomosis, with or without a temporary diverting ileostomy, is being utilized with no significant increase in morbidity or mortality, evidence of higher stoma reversal rates (7–10), and decreased cost and hospital stay (11). In-depth discussion of management in these emergent settings is beyond the scope of our chapter, but we encourage the reader to always consider the option of primary anastomosis when reasonable to do so.

## PRIMARY ANASTOMOSIS WITH DIVERSION

When an anastomosis is feasible, but the risk of an anastomotic leak is increased, a diverting stoma should be considered. Loop ileostomies are favored over loop colostomies due to an overall lower complication rate and ease of closure (12–14). Harris et al. demonstrated loop colostomies having the highest complication rate at 38% and end ileostomies the lowest (16%); however, skin-related issues (more common in ileostomies) were not taken into account in this study (13).

One of the most common settings for a diverting loop ileostomy is rectal cancer. Surgical resection results in the creation of a colorectal anastomosis, which is often diverted with an ileostomy, the benefit of which has recently been challenged. Multiple studies (15–17), including a recent meta-analysis by Gu including 13 publications and over 8,000 patients, demonstrated that diversion significantly reduced post-op anastomotic leakage and reoperation after low anterior resections (17). This was supported by a few other studies (14,18,19), but others have shown similar anastomotic leak rates and need for reoperations with and without stomas (20). It is also acknowledged that the addition of an ileostomy is not without risk of other adverse outcomes. Diverting ileostomies have been shown to be associated with increased hospital stays (15), increased risks of acute renal failure (18), and stoma-related complications (20), which will be outlined in more detail within this chapter.

While the benefit of a diverting ileostomy in this setting has been challenged and is clearly controversial, it may help to consider factors that increase the risk of anastomotic leak, thereby favoring the formation of a diverting stoma. These include technically challenging case, male gender, colorectal anastomosis <10 cm or coloanal anastomosis (14), musculoskeletal disorders, and high American Society of Anesthesiologists score (21). In our practice, we routinely use a diverting stoma in those patients who have received neoadjuvant chemoradiation and those with an anastomosis below 6 cm. We would encourage surgeons to weigh the established risk of an anastomotic leak with the potential increased mortality and hospital stay from a stoma to help individualize patient care. Furthermore, while a diverting loop ileostomy may not change the anastomotic leak rate, it may decrease the severity of an anastomotic leak, especially in low pelvic anastomosis having an impact on long-term function.

# END STOMA

When a primary anastomosis is determined to be technically impossible, too high risk, or the patient's function will be unacceptable, an end stoma is created. The colon or the small intestine can be utilized for this purpose, and either would be an option in our case study. A Hartmann procedure, resulting in an end colostomy with a rectal stump, may save operative time as well as preserve intestinal length and colon function for this patient. However, in the setting of chronic obstruction, some may find the proximal colon too dilated or unhealthy to bring up as a colostomy, and therefore, an abdominal colectomy with an end ileostomy may be preferred.

In regard to stoma complications, similar rates exist between end ileostomies and colostomies (22,23). However, there are clear advantages and disadvantages to each that may influence surgical choice. Common complications seen with ileostomies include high output resulting in dehydration, skin irritation, and requirement for nighttime emptying (22,23). Patients with colostomies have problems with odor and parastomal hernias, especially in the setting of obesity (22,23). It is important to note that approximately 50% of the time a temporary stoma will end up becoming permanent (24).

## STOMA COMPLICATIONS

The incidence of stoma complications varies widely in the literature, depending on the definition of the complication within the study and the length of follow-up, but many estimate an incidence of 50%–70% (15,21,25–27). These complications can be divided into two categories: early and late (Table 38.1). Early complications refer to those within the first 30 days of surgery, and late complications are defined as those thereafter, often observed between 6 and 10 weeks postoperatively (1). Risk factors associated with stoma complications include emergent operation, age >65 years, obesity, and diabetes (25). Stoma height and type can affect complications rates (28). The specialty of the surgeon creating the stoma has also been demonstrated to influence

Table 38.1 Stoma complications

| Early complications | Late complications |
| --- | --- |
| Dehydration | Stenosis |
| Skin complications | Parastomal hernia |
| Mucocutaneous separation | Prolapse |
| Retraction | Stomal varices |
| Ischemia/necrosis | |

Table 38.2 Risk factors for stoma-related complications

| Patient-related factors | Surgical-related factors |
| --- | --- |
| Obesity | Emergent surgery |
| Diabetes | Stoma type |
| Nutritional status | Stoma height |
| Emergent surgery | Surgeon specialty |
| Age >65 | |
| Gender | |
| Steroid use | |

complication rates, with one study showing colorectal specialists to have nearly half the number of stoma complications when compared with general surgeons (27) (Table 38.2). In the upcoming section, we review the most common complications associated with intestinal stomas, including their management and prevention.

# DEHYDRATION

More commonly seen after ileostomies than colostomies, dehydration remains a leading cause of postoperative readmissions following stoma creation. The magnitude of this complication cannot be overstated, as demonstrated in a study by Fish et al. (2017) in which postoperative readmissions were monitored in 407 patients following ileostomy creation. A 60-day readmission rate of 28% was noted, with the most frequent reason for readmission being dehydration (42%) (29). Additionally, patients readmitted with dehydration were noted to have increased morbidities, longer hospital lengths of stays, and repeat readmissions (29).

Electrolyte imbalances after ileostomy creation, including hyponatremia, hypokalemia, hypomagnesemia, and hypocalcemia, are most commonly observed between postoperative days 3–8 (24,30). These imbalances can lead to additional complications such as renal failure and cardiac arrhythmias. Careful monitoring in the postoperative period is critical to early recognition and management. Patients may present with stoma output exceeding 1–2 L/day, or more generalized signs, such as increased weakness, malaise, nausea, and vomiting. Higher risks of dehydration are noted in the setting of proximal stomas, short gut, small bowel obstruction, sepsis, and diuretic use (31,32).

Implementation of "ileostomy pathways" that emphasize patient education prior to stoma creation and active management and attention to intakes and outputs in the postoperative period have demonstrated great appeal; Nagle et al. (2012) reported that readmission rates secondary to dehydration dropped from 15.5% to 0% in their study population following the implementation of such a pathway at Best Israel Deaconess Medical Center. Central to this ileostomy pathway is active participation by the patient in his or her stoma care and output monitoring during the patient's hospital stay (33).

Management of dehydration involves fluid resuscitation and correction of electrolyte abnormalities. Patients should be counseled to consume electrolyte-enriched solutions, such as sports drinks, as opposed to hypotonic fluids such as water, fruit juices, and tea, which can augment hyponatremia (24). Dietary counseling regarding fiber supplementation and avoidance of foods that are likely to increase stoma output should be provided. Addition of pharmacologic therapies, such as loperamide, diphenoxylate, and opioid derivatives, may be required if outputs remain persistently high.

## SKIN COMPLICATIONS

Cutaneous complications following stoma creation may result from mechanical, chemical, allergic, or infectious causes, and are more frequently observed in the setting of ileostomies, as a consequence of the high volume, liquidlike, alkaline output associated with this type of stoma (24). Obesity and diabetes have been identified as independent risk factors for cutaneous complications (34). Poor siting, incorrect appliance application, and other stoma-related complications, such as prolapse and hernia, may further exacerbate local skin irritation, highlighting the importance of preoperative marking and postoperative education. Appliances should generally be changed no more frequently than every 3 days, to prevent excessive skin trauma. Following appliance removal, the skin should be gently cleaned with water and dried. Wafers should be cut to the appropriate size, and barrier creams, powders, and pastes should be applied to protect the skin from stoma effluent.

Allergic dermatitis can be treated with topical steroid creams and antihistamines, while antifungal creams or antibiotics may be required in the setting of infectious etiologies. *Candida albicans* is the most common infectious cause of peristomal skin irritation, as the warm, moist peristomal skin provides the perfect fungal environment; treatment with a light dusting of miconazole nitrate 2% powder is sufficient in most cases (34).

## PYODERMA GANGRENOSUM

Peristomal pyoderma gangrenosum is a rare and debilitating cutaneous complication associated with inflammatory bowel disease. The initial presentation is one of small pustules, which progress into large, painful, ulcers with necrotic edges (Figure 38.1). The diagnosis is frequently made only after other more common causes have been ruled out. Treatment frequently begins with topical or intralesional steroids, but response rates are variable, and other systemic treatments, including IV steroids, infliximab, dapsone, and immunomodulators, have been tried also with variable success. Conflicting reports exist with regard to the association between pyoderma gangrenosa and intestinal disease activity, but shorter healing times have been observed following the resection of actively diseased bowel (24,34). Stoma relocation is generally not advised, as the disease frequently recurs at the new stoma site.

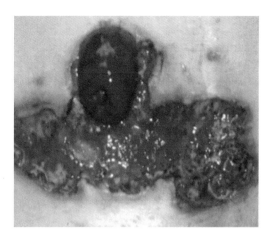

Figure 38.1 **(See color insert.)** Pyodermia gangrenosum.

## MUCOCUTANEOUS SEPARATION

Mucocutaneous separation refers to separation of the stoma from the surrounding skin, and may occur as a result of improper stoma maturation, excessive traction, or poor healing (24). Once identified, the extent of the detachment should be properly evaluated by an enterostomal nurse so that treatment can be initiated. Predisposing risk factors, including the presence of an immunocompromised state, diabetes, and smoking, should be optimized whenever possible. The space between the skin edge and stoma should be cleaned and filled with a paste or powder to promote healing. Long-term separation can result in stomal retraction and stenosis.

## STOMA RETRACTION

Stoma retraction is most often seen in the acute postoperative period and may ensue from inadequate mobilization of the bowel and/or mesentery, leading to undue tension, or from impaired wound healing. Retraction is most often seen with ileostomies, with rates of up to 17% observed (34). Treatment frequently involves repeat laparotomy with further mobilization of the bowel. Retracted ileostomies often require additional mobilization, and in selected cases suture fixation of proximal bowel to the fascia. Retracted colostomies often require high ligation of mesenteric vessels, relaxing incisions, flexure takedown, and mobilization along the peritoneal reflections. A final option is conversion to an end-loop stoma (24,34).

## ISCHEMIA/NECROSIS

Necrosis of the stoma is an uncommon complication, with incidence rates ranging between 1% and 34%, and is usually noted in the immediate postoperative period (30). Ischemic changes should be assessed in terms of both extent and depth; while small, superficial patches of mucosal ischemia can frequently be treated conservatively, larger areas or fullthickness involvement may require stomal revision and/or repeat laparotomy. It is important to differentiate whether or not the ischemia extends below the level of the fascia. In order to facilitate this assessment, a lubricated test tube or endoscope can be inserted into the stoma and transilluminated so that the color of the mucosa can be evaluated. Necrotic changes noted below the level of the fascia mandate reexploration and resection of any dead bowel. In some cases, evaluation with a flexible scope can further assist in evaluation. For ischemia/necrosis above the fascia, immediate surgery is not necessary, and in some cases, later stoma revision will be needed due to stenosis.

Predisposing factors to stomal ischemia and necrosis include arterial insufficiency, venous congestion, and mechanical factors, such as inadequate trephine size. Care should be taken to assess for ischemia, after division of the bowel and prior to the creation of the stoma. Excessive trimming of the mesentery or de-fatting of the bowel wall should be avoided, so as to avoid injury to the collateral vessels that are providing the blood supply to the stoma. When creating colostomies, at least a 1 cm segment of mesentery should be preserved at the edge of the bowel so that the marginal artery is not compromised (24). An adequate trephine should be created to avoid constriction of the mesenteric vessels as the bowel is brought out through the abdominal wall. In the setting of the obese patient, consideration should be given to bringing out the stoma in the upper abdomen or creation of an end-loop stoma, to avoid ischemic complications secondary to undue tension (24).

## STENOSIS

Stomal stenosis refers to a narrowing of the stomal lumen at the skin or fascial level. Symptomatic patients may present with symptoms of partial obstruction or decreased stool caliber. Although this complication is typically seen as a consequence of prior ischemia or stomal retraction, the differential diagnosis should include Crohn disease and malignancy. Initial management consists of dietary modification (i.e., low-residue diet), fluid hydration, and gentle catheter irrigation, in the setting of colostomies. The utility of serial dilation has been questioned, as repeated trauma can stimulate fibrosis, thus worsening the underlying stenosis (1). If conservative measures fail, surgical options, including stomal revision and Z- or W-plasty techniques (Figure 38.2), whereby the skin opening is enlarged using plastic surgery methods, can be considered (1,35). A A-plasty technique is particularly helpful when bowel length is limited, such as in continent ileostomies.

## PARASTOMAL HERNIA

Parastomal hernias are incisional hernias occurring near the site of a stoma that can result in symptoms ranging from an unsightly bulge and difficulty with pouching to bowel ischemia, obstruction, and perforation. Risk factors for parastomal hernias include obesity, pulmonary disease, malnutrition, steroid use, emergency surgery, and the

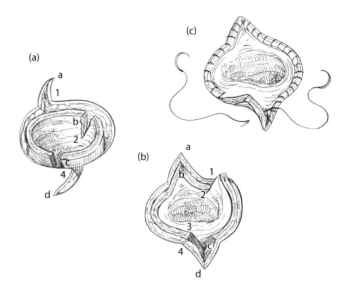

Figure 38.2 Z-plasty repair for stenosis: **(a)** the stoma is separated from the skin and underlying subcutaneous tissue, then incisions are made in the skin and bowel as depicted, **(b)** the bowel is realigned to fit within the new skin incisions, **(c)** stoma is matured to the skin.

presence of end stomas. Although transrectus stoma creation is thought to reduce the incidence of parastomal hernias, these hernias can occur even when stomas are brought out through the rectus musculature. It has been suggested that an increase in the stoma aperture size of even 1 mm can lead to a 10% increase in the risk of parastomal herniation (36). While uncommon in the immediate postoperative period, the incidence of these hernias correlates with the duration of the stoma, and ranges from 14% to 40% (24).

Evaluation of patients suspected to have parastomal hernias should include examination in the supine and upright positions, as well as during a Valsava maneuver. In some cases, additional imaging studies, such as computed tomography scans, may be required to further characterize the extent of the defect. Treatment options vary with degree of symptomology. Minimally symptomatic hernias can be treated using stoma belts and modified pouching systems, while more symptomatic hernias may require surgical intervention, ranging from primary and mesh repairs to stoma re-siting. Consideration of stoma reversal should be entertained before embarking upon repair, because rates of recurrence remain high, ranging from 7% to 100% depending on the technique of repair used (24,30,34).

Primary parastomal hernia repairs have largely been abandoned secondary to high recurrence rates. This type of repair is best suited for patients in whom a repeat laparotomy may be contraindicated or deemed high risk. The technique involves dissection through the subcutaneous tissues in the parastomal space, excision/reduction of the hernia sac, and primary repair of the fascial defect.

Mesh repairs involve the placement of a synthetic or biologic mesh in the overlay, underlay, or sublay positions, and can be performed using a laparoscopic or open approach

(a)

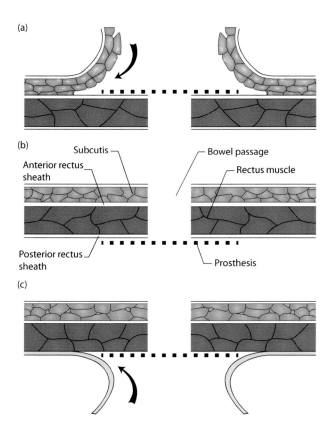

Figure 38.3 Mesh positions: **(a)** overlay, **(b)** underlay, and **(c)** sublay. (From Hansson BM et al. *Ann Surg* 2012;255(4):685–95.)

(Figure 38.3) (37). Overlay approaches refer to the placement of mesh above the level of the fascial closure, while sublay or retrorectus repairs involve the placement of mesh between the rectus abdominus muscle and posterior sheath. Recurrence rates have been observed to be higher with the onlay approach in comparison to the retromuscular technique (18.6% versus 6.9%) (37).

The two most common types of intraperitoneal repairs are the keyhole and Sugerbaker techniques (Figures 38.4 and 38.5) (37). Both intraperitoneal repairs start with identification and reduction of the hernia sac. In the keyhole technique, the stoma is brought out through a 2–3 cm "keyhole" within a mesh placed intraperitoneally, in such a manner that 4–5 cm of fascial overlap is achieved (34,38). The "Sugarbaker" technique, as originally conceived by Paul Sugarbaker in 1958, involves placement of mesh around the fascial defect and positioning the bowel such that it travels laterally between the mesh and abdominal wall for 5 cm, before it enters the peritoneal cavity (38). In a meta-analysis of 270 laparoscopic repairs involving the keyhole and Sugarbaker techniques, recurrence rates of 20.8% were observed with the keyhole method, compared to 11.6% with the Sugarbaker technique (37). A sandwich technique involving a combination of the keyhole and Sugarbaker methods has been described by Berger et al., in which one piece of mesh is fashioned as a keyhole around the stoma, while a second, larger piece of mesh is placed around the fascial defect, and the bowel is lateralized between the

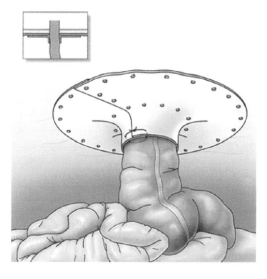

Figure 38.4 Keyhole technique. (From Hansson BM et al. *Ann Surg* 2012;255(4):685–95.)

two meshes (38). Using this method, only one recurrence was noted in 47 patients, resulting in a much lower overall recurrence rate of 2.1% (37,38).

Stoma re-siting is another option for repair. This technique may require a repeat laparotomy. A new site should be selected prior to the procedure and properly marked. A site on the contralateral site of the abdomen is generally advised, but a site on the same side (upper abdomen) is also an option. Unfortunately, this procedure is associated with a risk of incisional hernia formation at the site of fascial closure, as well as a risk of recurrent parastomal herniation, at the new stoma site. To avoid this problem, a technique called *translocation* is considered.

With translocation, the ostomy is mobilized locally. The mucocutaneous junction is divided, and the stoma is mobilized down and through the fascia in a manner similar to

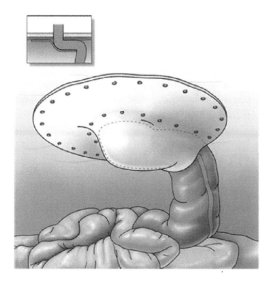

Figure 38.5 Sugarbaker technique. (From Hansson BM et al. *Ann Surg* 2012;255(4):685–95.)

closing a stoma. The presence of a parastomal hernia often eases this dissection. With retractors, the abdominal wall is elevated and through the ostomy opening and adhesions between the abdominal wall between the old and new stoma site are divided. With the surgeon's hand inside the abdomen, the new ostomy site is created. A clamp is inserted into the new site, and the end of the open bowel is grasped. The bowel is then maneuvered to the new site. Some mobilization of the bowel may be required to obtain adequate length. The bowel is then matured at the new site, and the old ostomy and hernia site is closed. This repair is often reinforced with mesh (Figure 38.6).

Given the prevalence and morbidities associated with parastomal hernias, increasing attention has been placed on the use of prophylactic mesh at the time of the original stoma creation. In a meta-analysis involving 649 patients, Cross et al. observed that prophylactic mesh placement reduced the rate of parastomal hernia repair by 65%, without an increase in mesh-related complications, including infection, stomal necrosis, and stenosis (39). Placement of sublay mesh in the setting of open surgery and use of a Sugarbaker technique with synthetic mesh in the laparoscopic setting have been shown in multiple studies, including randomized control trials, to prevent hernias (40–44). While this has not been adopted as standard practice for many colorectal surgeons, it should be considered, especially in patients at increased risk for hernia formation.

## PROLAPSE

Stomal prolapse is defined as a full-thickness protrusion of the bowel wall through the stomal orifice. It can be characterized as fixed, with a permanent length of protruding bowel, or sliding, wherein a variable length of bowel is noted to prolapse with increased abdominal pressure (Figure 38.7). Prolapse is more commonly noted with loop stoma, as compared to end stomas with transverse loop colostomies carrying a risk of prolapse of up to 30% (45), and frequently involves the distal stomal limb. The reasons for this are unclear but may be related to atrophy of the distal limb secondary to disuse or excessive mobility due to lack of fixation (24,34). It has been suggested that distal, as compared with proximal transverse loop stomas, may be associated with decreased rates of prolapse, secondary to partial fixation of the distal limb by the splenic flexure (24).

Management of stomal prolapse varies with symptomatology. Often, stomal prolapses are asymptomatic but may result in cosmetic concerns or difficulties with pouching. Intermittent prolapses can be manually reduced via application of gentle pressure, following the application of table sugar to help decrease the edema content of the bowel. Surgical intervention is merited in the setting of obstruction, ischemia, or perforation. Surgical options include stoma reversal, excision of redundant bowel and refashioning of the stoma, or Delorme or Altemeier-type procedures (1). In other cases, conversion of a loop stoma to an end or end-loop stoma or stoma re-siting may be required (34).

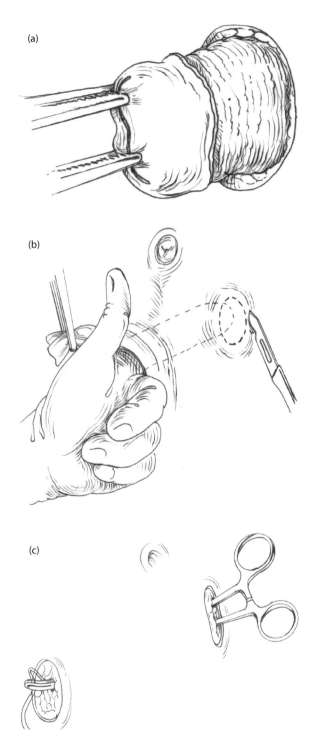

Figure 38.6 Translocation of stoma: **(a)** The stoma is mobilized off the abdominal wall, **(b)** abdominal wall defect created at the new, pre-chosen stoma site, **(c)** clamp is used to translocate the bowel from original site to the new location.

## STOMAL VARICES

Stomal varices present a potentially life-threatening complication in patients with portal hypertension. Making the diagnosis often requires a heightened level of suspicion; an

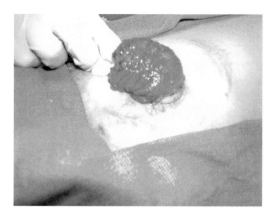

Figure 38.7 **(See color insert.)** Stomal prolapse.

understanding of the state of the patient's liver disease coupled with a careful examination of the stoma itself is critical. A bluish collection of vessels is seen in the subcutaneous tissue surrounding the ostomy (Figure 38.8). It is not uncommon for this diagnosis to be overlooked; in a case series presented by Spier et al. (2008) involving eight patients, the diagnosis was initially overlooked in six (46). If the stoma appears normal, and the level of clinical suspicion remains high, evaluation should include ultrasound, computed tomography, or magnetic resonance imaging studies.

Local treatment options for management of stomal variceal bleeding include compression, sclerotherapy, and suture ligation. These are frequently temporizing measures, as the bleeding commonly recurs. Mucocutaneous separation, stomal relocation, and percutaneous embolization are similarly associated with high recurrence rates. Pharmacologic therapy with ß-blockade has been proposed, but the efficacy of this therapy has been questioned (46). Definitive treatment options include surgical and percutaneous shunting (i.e., transjugular intrahepatic portosystemic shunt) and liver transplantation. In a literature review by Conte et al. (1990), no cases of rebleeding were observed in patients with ileostomies and colostomies following shunting; additionally, shunting was noted to have a low overall morbidity and was associated with improved patient mortality (47).

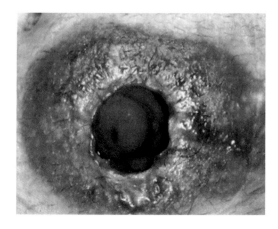

Figure 38.8 **(See color insert.)** Parastomal varices.

## PREVENTION

Due to the high incidence of stomal complications and substantial economic cost, a focus has been placed on prevention. For colorectal surgery patients, multiple steps can be taken in the perioperative and intraoperative setting to help reduce the incidence of complications and ultimately enhance the experience for the patient.

## PRE-OP PREPARATION

The management of a patient for colostomy or ileostomy starts before the operation.

*B.N. Brooke* (1954)

In the era of enhanced recovery after surgery (ERAS) pathways, and the Enhanced Recovery Program (ERP) in the United Kingdom, there has been an increased focus on pr-operative patient education. For the colorectal surgery patient, a large portion of this education focuses on stoma marking and education. The importance of this was recognized in the 2015 position statement (47), revised from the original in 2007 (48), published jointly by the American Society of Colon and Rectal Surgeons and Wound, Ostomy, and Continence Nurses Society stating that ostomy site selection and education should be performed preoperatively whenever possible.

There are multiple reasons for this. Preoperative site selection has been shown to reduce stoma-related complications and result in improved independent care of the stoma by the patient (21,49,51). The preoperative education allows time for the patient to psychologically prepare for the presence of a stoma, develop basic understanding of supplies used and general care, and answer common lifestyle-related questions (51–54). In a randomized study, Chaudhri et al. (2005) found that preoperative education resulted in significant difference in stoma proficiency (5.5 versus 9 days), decreased hospital stay (8 versus 10 days), and hospital anxiety depression scale tended lower (51).

To ensure appropriate site selection, patients should be evaluated standing and sitting, both fully clothed and with skirt lifted. During this process, observations of belt line, other stoma bags, scars, or skin creases can be made. The patient is then moved into the supine position with shirt off. By having the patient lift his or her head off the exam table, the rectus muscle can be identified and marked. The stoma site marking must be made overlying the rectus muscle and should be at least 5 cm away from surgical incision, centered in the quadrant of interest, and within the patient's visual field. Avoidance of bony prominences, scars, and skin folds (which often are not visible with the patient in supine position) is important. The most common stoma site is within the "ostomy triangle" bordered by the anterior superior iliac spine, pubic tubercle, and umbilicus (55) (Figure 38.9).

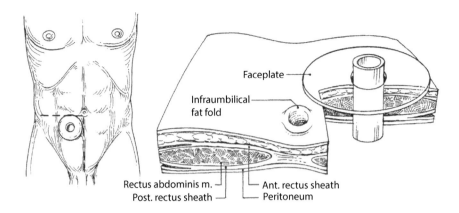

Figure 38.9 Stomal siting.

Special considerations should be made for patient with contractures or impaired mobility. Obese patients are at higher risk for stoma complications and can be more difficult to find an ideal stoma site. It is important to keep in mind that there may be a significant shift in subcutaneous tissue when an obese patient is moved from sitting to standing. It is typically recommended that an obese patient be marked at a higher site on the abdominal wall, as the upper quadrants are often more visible to the patient, thinner, and closer to the intended bowel. Once marked, it is important to have the patient reassess the site himself or herself to confirm visibility and access (Figure 38.10).

## INTRAOPERATIVE TECHNICAL TIPS

The closest attention must therefore be paid to the minutiae of technique and the subsequent care.

*BN Brooke (1952) (56)*

Stomas are created toward the end of what can typically be considered difficult and somewhat time-consuming operations. As such, exquisite care must be taken to continue to adhere to strong surgical principles and techniques, in

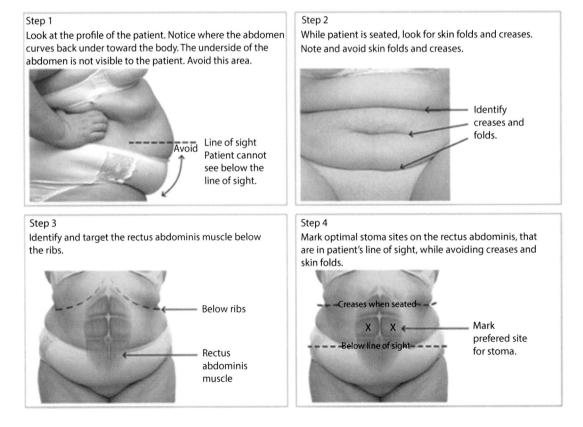

**Step 1**
Look at the profile of the patient. Notice where the abdomen curves back under toward the body. The underside of the abdomen is not visible to the patient. Avoid this area.

Avoid / Line of sight Patient cannot see below the line of sight.

**Step 2**
While patient is seated, look for skin folds and creases. Note and avoid skin folds and creases.

Identify creases and folds.

**Step 3**
Identify and target the rectus abdominis muscle below the ribs.

Below ribs

Rectus abdominis muscle

**Step 4**
Mark optimal stoma sites on the rectus abdominis, that are in patient's line of sight, while avoiding creases and skin folds.

Creases when seated

X  X — Mark prefered site for stoma.

Below line of sight

Figure 38.10 Marking the obese patient. (From Salvadalena G et al. *J Wound Ostomy Continence Nurse* 2015;42(3):249–52.)

order to prevent surgical-related complications. The standard of care for everting ileostomies was first established by Brooks in 1952 (56) and continues today. When creating an ileostomy, it is generally recommended that approximately 6–8 cm of small bowel be eviscerated for creation of an end ileostomy, and 3 cm at the apex of small bowel for an ileostomy. This allows for an eversion of at least 2 cm above the skin level. Persson et al. (2010) followed 180 patients with stomas over a 2-year period and found that all ileostomies less than 2 cm in height were associated with fewer complications (57). Hall (1995) has suggested making the inferior edge of a stoma approximately 1 cm shorter so as to tip the bowel and help prevent skin irritation (58).

Similar to Brooke's technique for the small bowel, surgeons have found that everting a colostomy, coined "spouted colostomy" by Marsh (2007), can result in decreased complications (59). It is generally recommended that 2–4 cm of colon be eviscerated for creation of an ideal colostomy to allow for appropriate eversion. The appropriate height of an everted colostomy has varied in research. All recommend a colostomy height over 1 cm to be associated with fewer complications (30,57), and some have suggested height over 1.5 cm (28).

Thick abdominal wall and a shortened and fat mesentery make ideal stoma creation particularly difficult in the obese patient. As previously mentioned, stoma siting higher on the abdominal wall can help. If the patient has not been marked preoperatively, consider intraoperative fluoroscopy to correctly identify the anterior-superior iliac spine to guide location (55), as traditional landmarks such as the umbilicus may be misleading. Once your site has been chosen, using a wound protector at the stoma site can aid in pulling the bowel and mesentery up. All attempts should be made to preserve the marginal artery at or above the level of the skin to ensure adequate blood supply.

An additional option is abdominal wall modification or contouring. The technique has been described by several authors and uses plastic surgery techniques to create an abdominal wall that supports a well-constructed stoma (54,60,61). In a manner similar to an abdominoplasty, the skin and subcutaneous tissue are mobilized off the fascia via a low transverse or midline incision. If a stoma is present, it is mobilized from the skin and subcutaneous tissue to the fascia. Excess subcutaneous fat is then excised from the skin (Figure 38.11). The flaps are not as thin as those produced by plastic surgeons to reduce the potential for flap loss. After removing the fat, the stoma is then brought through the skin at its original site or through a new location. If excess skin is present, it can be excised before the stoma is brought through the skin. Subcutaneous drains are usually placed to encourage adherence of the flaps and to reduce seromas.

For a colostomy that will not reach the skin, it is important to complete full mobilization of the bowel, medial, lateral, and around the flexure. The main blood supply can be taken to increase length (as one would for a low coloanal

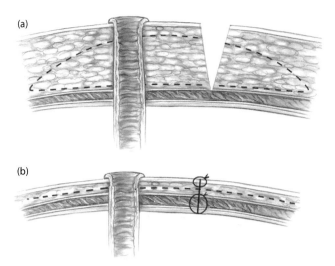

Figure 38.11 **(a)** Cross section demonstrating midline incision and areas of subcutaneous fat excision. **(b)** After removal of excess subcutaneous tissue, incision is closed, flaps attached to fascia, and stoma matured with adequate eversion.

anastomosis), but care must be taken to preserve the marginal artery. Scoring or creating a window in the mesentery may provide additional length. Excess subcutaneous fat can be removed as described previously. When these techniques do not work, creation of a loop end or "pseudo-loop colostomy," in which only the antimesenteric border of the colon is brought through the abdominal wall and matured to the skin without eversion, can be considered (62) (Figure 38.12).

Similar techniques can be used for an ileostomy that has difficulty reaching the skin surface, including mobilization up to the duodenum, sacrifice of the ileocolic artery, or creation of a pseudoloop without eversion (20).

A colon distended from a distal obstruction is another common clinical scenario that can make stoma creation difficult. In addition to being dilated, this bowel has a tendency toward ischemia and impaired mobility. The increased abdominal wall defect required to bring the bowel up to the skin can increase the risk of parastomal hernia. The most important intraoperative maneuver in this setting to make colostomy creation easier is to decompress the bowel ideally prior to bringing up through the abdominal wall or alternatively once it is up.

## POSTOPERATIVE SUPPORT

The introduction of ERAS protocols has resulted in a reduction in readmissions due to complications in the colorectal surgical population (63); however, complications associated with an ileostomy remain the most likely cause of readmission—emphasizing the importance of appropriate postoperative support. During hospitalization, a wound care nurse should follow the patient. Their role, during this time, is to reinforce education introduced preoperatively, provide hands-on teaching for stoma appliance changes and care, and provide initial supplies for the patient.

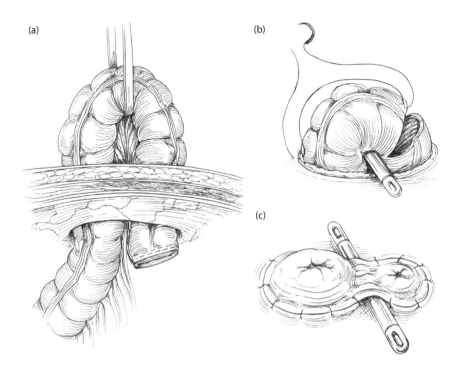

Figure 38.12 Loop-end (pseudo-loop) colostomy. **(a)** After the bowel is divided a loop of colon is brought up through the defect **(b)** An incision is made in the distal end of the loop and matured in standard brooke fashion over a stoma rod **(c)** Final appearance of loop-end colostomy.

It is recommended that upon discharge a patient has established follow-up with a wound care/stoma specialist. The frequency of postoperative visits will be individualized and dependent on patient needs. In addition to pouch changes, enterostomal nurses can cover topics related to physical, psychologic, and social issues that arise when living with a stoma. This type of support has been shown to improve a patient's quality of life with a stoma (64). Moreover, they can monitor for and begin early intervention for any complications that may arise (57).

## OSTOMY REVERSAL

Reversal of temporary stomas should be undertaken as soon as physiologically feasible to reestablish gastrointestinal continuity and for psychological improvement. This, of course, implies that the purpose of the stoma placement has been met, and the patient is capable and a candidate for another operative procedure. There are two main operative approaches to ostomy reversal: local or via a laparotomy. While both approaches are associated with inadvertent enterotomies, bleeding, wound infections, and anastomotic complications, the biggest advantages of the laparotomy approach are improved exposure and the ability to reexplore the abdomen. Certainly, the type of ostomy is important to consider when planning the operative approach as loop ileostomies are technically the least challenging to reverse and are often amenable to local reversal. Although a local approach is preferred, patients with a prior Hartmann procedure or those in which the distal remnant is not available via a local approach are obviously forced to undergo a repeat laparotomy. Surprisingly, there is a paucity of recent data that highlight the potential perils of this seemingly benign operation. The most recent study, published in 2005, was a retrospective review of 533 patients undergoing stoma closure at the University Hospital of Vienna (64). The majority of the patients (51%) underwent reversal of a colostomy, 44% had closure of an ileostomy, and 5% had combined reversals of both a colostomy and an ileostomy. All patients underwent a laparotomy using the intraperitoneal approach. Their 30-day mortality was 3% (15 patients) with rates similar for either ileostomy or colostomy reversal. Causes of death were multisystem organ failure after nonsurgical complications in nine patients, and anastomotic leakage, missed small bowel injury, and cecal perforation in the remaining six patients. Overall complications were 20%, with anastomotic leakage (5%), ileus (4%), postoperative bleeding (2%), and wound infection (2%). When analyzing patient-related factors between survivors and nonsurvivors, only advanced patient age was found to be statistically significant. This study, which highlights the potential morbidity of stoma reversal, also emphasizes the importance of meticulous surgical technique required in these challenging patients with reoperative abdomens.

Our approach to ostomy reversal begins with a thorough preoperative evaluation, which includes interrogation of the distal colon with either a barium enema or endoscopy. The primary reason for which sentinel procedure was performed

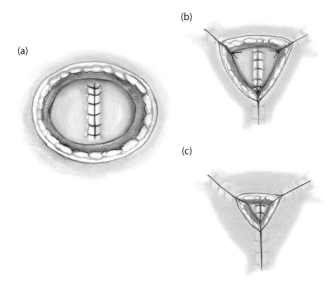

Figure 38.13 Mercedes or triangular closure. **(a)** Stoma site with fascia closed. **(b)** Initial approximation of skin and subcutaneous fat. **(c)** Completed closure with small area in center left open for drainage and secondary healing.

is important to consider, since it may reveal if the purposes of the ostomy have been met and may potentially alter the decision on reversal. An obvious but sometimes overlooked step should also be the evaluation of the patient's sphincter tone and ability to control fecal stream once continuity has been restored. This may require not only clinical evaluation, but formal documentation through anorectal physiology testing including manometry. Baseline poor sphincter tone or incontinence should be considered a contraindication for ostomy reversal in all but the rarest of cases. Finally, additional patient factors that can be altered, such as nutritional status, steroid use, and tobacco abuse, should be optimized prior to surgery. When planning the operative approach for end colostomy reversals, additional factors to consider prior to embarking on the operation should include the expected amount of adhesive disease likely to be encountered or previously encountered (i.e., review prior operative notes), whether there is a history of prior abdominal or pelvic radiation, concomitant pathology such as the presence of incisional hernias, and the type of ostomy. For instance, patients with multiple prior surgeries and a history of radiation will most likely benefit from a laparotomy approach that includes preoperative ureteral stent placement, while those patients with loop ostomies without any other comorbidities can be managed with a local approach. Whether a stapled or hand-sewn anastomosis is performed is up to the surgeon's discretion. Key technical points in each method, however, are to ensure adequate mobilization and visualization of the distal colonic or rectal stump with resection of the exteriorized bowel or end stump back to normal healthy bowel prior to the anastomosis. Finally, delayed primary closure or partial closure is performed for the area in which the stoma was placed, and drains are not routinely placed (Figure 38.13).

## SUMMARY

Creation of intestinal stomas is a common procedure, meant to ultimately enhance the patient's recovery and quality of life, but with complication rates of up to 70% with reoperations required in up to 20%, this can have significant impact both on patient's life and health-care economics. For this reason, thoughtful decision-making, meticulous surgical technique, and thorough perioperative education are imperative.

## REFERENCES

1. Husain SG, Cataldo TE. *Clin Colon Rectal Surg.* 2008; 21:31–40.
2. Lewis L. History and evolution of stomas and appliances. In: Taylor P (ed.) *Stoma Care in the Community: A Clinical Resource for Practitioners.* London: EMAP Healthcare. 1999, pp. 1–20.
3. Arezzo A et al. *Surg Endosc.* 2016 (epub).
4. Sasaki K et al. *Dis Colon Rectum.* 2012;55(1):72–8.
5. Lim JF et al. *Dis Colon Rectum.* 2005;48(2):205–9.
6. Lee, YM et al. *J Am Coll Surg.* 2001;192:719–25.
7. Steinermann DC et al. *Langenbecks Arch Surg.* 2015; 400(5):609–16.
8. Constantinides VA et al. *Dis Colon Rectum.* 2006; 49(7):966–81.
9. Di Saverio S et al. *Surg Endosc.* 2016;30(12): 5656–64.
10. Alizai PH et al. *Int J Colorectal Dis.* 2013;28(12): 1681–8.
11. Oberkolfer CE et al. *Ann Surg.* 2012;256(5):819–26.
12. Rullier E et al. *World J Surg.* 2001;25:274–7.
13. Harris DA et al. *Ann R Coll Surg Engl.* 2005;87: 427–31.
14. Hanna MH et al. *Langengecks Arch Surg.* 2015;400: 145–52.
15. Ihnat P et al. *Surg Endosc.* 2016;30(11):4809–16.
16. Wu S et al. *World J Gastroenterol.* 2014;20(47): 18031–7.
17. Gu W, Wu S. *World J Surg Oncol.* 2015;13(9).
18. Jafari MD et al. *Ann Surg.* 2013;79(10):1034–9.
19. Gastringer I et al. *Br J Surg.* 2005;92(9):1137–42.
20. Wong NY, Eu KW. *Dis Colon Rectum.* 2005;48(6): 2076–9.
21. Nastro P et al. *Br J Surg.* 2010;97(12):1885–9.
22. Robertson I et al. *Colorectal Dis.* 2005;7:279–85.
23. Leenen LP, Kuypers JH. *Dis Colon Rectum.* 1989;32: 500–4.
24. Kwiatt M, Kawata M. *Clin Colon Rectal Surg.* 2013; 26:112–21.
25. Arumugam PJ et al. *Colorectal Dis.* 2003;5(1):49–52.
26. Mahjoubi B et al. *Colorecal Dis.* 2005;7:582–7.
27. Saghir JH et al. *Eur J Surg.* 2001;167(7):531–4.

28. Cottam J et al. *Colorectal Dis.* 2007;9:834–8.
29. Fish DR et al. *Ann Surg.* 2017;265(2):379–87.
30. Velasco M et al. *Cir Esp.* 2014;92:149–56.
31. Hayden DM et al. *J Gastrointest Surg.* 2013;17(2): 298–303.
32. Messaris E et al. *Dis Colon Rectum.* 2012;55(2): 175–80.
33. Nagle D et al. *Dis Colon Rectum.* 2012;55(12): 1266–72.
34. Bafford A, Irani J. *Surg Clin North Am.* 2013;93(1): 145–66.
35. Beraldo S et al. *Colorectal Dis.* 2006;8(8):715–6.
36. Pilgrim CH et al. *Dis Colon Rectum.* 2010;53(1):71–6.
37. Hansson BM et al. *Ann Surg.* 2012;255(4):685–95.
38. Aquina CT et al. *Dig Surg.* 2014;31(4–5):366–76.
39. Cross AJ et al. *Br J Surg.* 2017;104(3):179–86.
40. Lopez-Cano M et al. *Hernia.* 2017;21(2):177–89.
41. Janes A et al. *World J Surg.* 2009;33(1):118–21.
42. Serra-Aracil X et al. *Ann Surg.* 2009;249(4):583–7.
43. Lambrecht JR et al. *Colorectal Dis.* 2015;17(10): O191–7.
44. Shellito PC. *Dis Colon Rectum.* 1998;41(12):1562–72.
45. Spier BJ et al. *Clin Gastroenterol Hepatol.* 2008;6(3): 346–52.
46. Conte JV et al. *Dis Colon Rectum.* 1990;33(4):308–14.
47. Salvadalena G et al. *J Wound Ostomy Continence Nurs.* 2015;42(3):249–52.
48. American Society of Colon and Rectal Surgeons Committee Members; Wound Ostomy Continence Nurses Society Committee Members. *J Wound Ostomy Continence Nurs.* 2007;34(6):627–8.
49. Park JJ et al. *Dis Colon Rectm.* 1999;42:1575–80.
50. Person B et al. *Dis Colon Rectum.* 2012;55(7):783–7.
51. Chaudhri S et al. *Dis Colon Rectum.* 2005;48(3):504–9.
52. Millan M et al. *Colorectal Dis.* 2010;12(7):e88–92.
53. Gulbiniene J et al. *Medicine (Kaunas.)* 2004;40(11): 1045–53.
54. Beck SJ. *Clin Colon Rectal Surg.* 2011;24(4):259–62.
55. Brooke BN. *Lancet.* 1952;2:102–4.
56. Persson E et al. *Colorectal Dis.* 2010;12:971–6.
57. Hall C et al. *Br J Surg.* 1995;82:1385.
58. Marsh P, Clark JS. *Ann R Coll Surg Eng.* 2007;89(1):78.
59. Cataldo, P. *Clin Colon Rectal Surg.* 2008;21(1):17–22.
60. Evans JP et al. *Dis Colon Rectum.* 2003;46(1):122–6.
61. Beck DE. *Clin Colon Rectal Surg.* 2008;21(1):71–5.
62. Shah PM et al. *Dis Colon Rectum.* 2017;60(2):219–27.
63. Karadag A et al. *Int J Colorectal Dis.* 2003;18:234–8.
64. Pokorny H et al. *Arch Surg.* 2005;140:956–60.

# 39

# Operative and nonoperative therapy for chronic constipation

ROBERT J. SINNOTT, MICHELLE C. JULIEN, AND DANIEL E. SARMIENTO

## CHALLENGING CASE

A 24-year-old female presents with a 2-year history of constipation. She stated that the symptoms started after surgery for perforated appendicitis. Medical management with fiber supplements, therapeutic enemas, and various forms of laxatives have failed. Her symptoms have had a significant impact in her daily activities.

## CASE MANAGEMENT

Colonoscopy revealed no stricture or stenosis. Sitzmarks study was positive and demonstrated markers distributed throughout her colon with a preponderance in the rectosigmoid junction. Anal manometry had a positive rectoanal inhibitory reflex, excluding Hirschsprung disease. Conventional defecography showed a partial outlet obstruction. Scintigraphy study showed decreased whole gut transit. Diagnosis of colonic inertia as well as pelvic outlet dysfunction was made. Because of her debilitating symptoms, she initially underwent loop ileostomy. Biofeedback therapy was started and continued for over a year. Repeat defecography showed improvement. She underwent total abdominal colectomy with takedown of her ileostomy and ileorectal anastomosis. She had a prolonged postoperative ileus but was discharged without further complication. Her bowel function has markedly improved. She continues with biofeedback and is under the care of a psychologist for behavioral issues but views her quality of life as an improvement to her preoperative state and does not regret having surgery.

## INTRODUCTION

Constipation is an extremely common complaint in North America with a prevalence between 2% and 27% of the population, estimating that about 63 million people are suffering from this diagnosis. Women report two- to threefold higher incidence in constipation than men. There is a higher incidence of constipation in non-Caucasians as well as individuals with less education and lower income. Additionally, age has played a role in constipation with multiple studies showing that older age leads to a higher prevalence of constipation (1). In an effort to standardize the definition of constipation to identify patients who might require further evaluation and treatment, a system-based classification was established by a panel of experts with specific parameters in 2006 by the Rome Committee and is termed the Rome III Criteria (Table 39.1) (2). For a diagnosis of functional constipation to be made, the listed criteria must be met for at least 3 months with the onset of symptoms initiating at least 6 months prior to diagnosis.

Normal defecation is a complex process that results from stool formation, colon motility, and pelvic floor function. It is a coordinated event that relies on the interaction of the autonomic, enteric, and somatic nervous systems stimulating the contraction of smooth muscle in the colon wall, resulting in the forward movement of stool and the ultimate relaxation of the anal sphincters allowing for evacuation. Disruption of any part of this pathway will lead to some form of constipation. Contributing factors may include diet, medications, neurologic or endocrine disorders, psychosocial issues, colonic disease, or pelvic floor abnormalities (Tables 39.2 and 39.3) (1–3). Often patients may have constipation with no identifiable cause.

Several subtypes of constipation have been identified, including slow transit constipation, pelvic outlet obstruction or pelvic constipation, and combined slow transit constipation with outlet obstruction. Slow-transit constipation,

Table 39.1 Rome III diagnostic criteria for constipation

Criteria must be fulfilled for the last 3 months
Symptom onset at least 6 months before diagnosis
1. Must include two or more of the following:
    a. Straining ≥25% of defecation
    b. Lumpy or hard bowel movements ≥25% of defecation
    c. Sensation of incomplete evacuation ≥25% of defecation
    d. Sensation of anorectal obstruction ≥25% of defecation
    e. Manual maneuvers to facilitate bowel movement ≥25% of defecation
    f. Fewer than three defecations per week
2. Loose stools are rarely present without the use of laxatives
3. Insufficient criteria for irritable bowel syndrome

Table 39.2 Drugs associated with constipation

| | |
|---|---|
| Anticholinergics | Antidepressants |
| | Antipsychotics |
| Cation-containing agents | Aluminum (antacids and sucralfate) |
| | Bismuth |
| | Calcium (antacids and supplements) |
| | Iron supplements |
| Neurally active agents | Opiates |
| | Antihypertensives |
| | Ganglionic blockers |
| | Vinca alkaloids |
| | Calcium channel blockers |
| Others | Antihistamines |
| | Antiparkinsonian drugs |
| | Diuretics |
| | Nonsteroidal anti-inflammatory drugs |

also referred to as colonic inertia, is a motility disorder in which stool moves through the colon at a slow rate. In some patients, only the colon is affected, and patients may not have bowel movements for days to weeks at a time. Pelvic constipation, a second subtype of constipation, is the lack of coordination of the pelvic floor during defecation. Examples of this include rectocele, enterocele, sigmoidocele, rectal prolapse, and rectal intussusception. Pelvic constipation results in excessive straining, the need for digital evacuation of stool, and incomplete evacuation (4,5).

## EVALUATION OF CONSTIPATION

The initial evaluation of a patient with constipation should always begin with a thorough history and physical examination to help distinguish constipation subtypes. Information collected during the history should include details regarding stool consistency, blood in the stool, caliber and frequency of bowel movements, as well as onset and duration of symptoms. In addition, questions specifically addressing defecatory habits including excessive straining, bloating, the ability to sense and completely evacuate, and maneuvers such as perineal pressure or digitalization of the vagina used to aid in evacuation should be asked. A stool diary kept by the patient, which details stool form and frequency, may also provide valuable information. Dietary intake, fluid consumption, exercise habits, medications including both prescription and over-the-counter supplements, and family history of colorectal cancer should be assessed. The number and type of laxatives used as well as their effect on bowel function should be documented. Finally, any associated or undiagnosed psychiatric, neurologic, or endocrine disorder such as diabetes or hypothyroidism or a history of sexual abuse should be identified in the initial assessment.

Once a detailed history has been obtained, a complete physical examination directed at the abdominal and anorectal regions is required. The abdominal examination in general will be unrevealing; however, any specific areas of tenderness on palpation or evidence of distention resulting from colonic dilatation should be noted. Anorectal

Table 39.3 Medical conditions causing constipation

| Endocrine and metabolic | Neurogenic | Collagen vascular and musculoskeletal |
|---|---|---|
| Chronic renal failure | Autonomic neuropathy | Amyloidosis |
| Diabetes mellitus | Cerebrovascular disease | Dermatomyositis |
| Hypothyroidism | Dementia | Myotonic dystrophy |
| Hypercalcemia | Depression | Systemic sclerosis |
| Hypokalemia | Multiple sclerosis | Scleroderma |
| Pregnancy | Muscular dystrophy | |
| Milk-alkali syndrome | Parkinson disease | |
| Porphyria | Spinal cord lesions | |
| Carcinomatosis | Hirschsprung disease | |
| | Chagas disease | |

examination should include a direct inspection for any associated anorectal pathology, such as hemorrhoids, fissures, fistulas, or prolapse. Digital rectal exam should be performed to exclude a mass, stricture, anal hypertonia, or fecal impaction that can be associated with constipation. In addition, a straining maneuver will assist in diagnosing a rectocele, internal or full-thickness rectal prolapse, cystocele, or pelvic floor descent.

## FUNCTIONAL EVALUATION AND DIAGNOSTIC STUDIES

The initial diagnostic workup for constipation should include an anatomic evaluation of the colon with colonoscopy, barium enema, or virtual colonoscopy to exclude a stricture or mass. A colonoscopy should be recommended if the patient meets guidelines for screening or if symptoms such as rectal bleeding, change in bowel habit, weight loss, or anemia are identified (6). A colonoscopy is considered in other patients as it provides a picture of the large intestine that more readily identifies strictures and volvulus and may provide better screening in patients who often achieve adequate cleansing required for an adequate colonoscopy. Blood tests used to identify anemia, hypothyroidism, diabetes, and other medical conditions can be helpful in assessing constipation. In patients with no other underlying cause for constipation and in those who do not respond to basic treatments including fiber supplements and laxatives, then further physiological testing is indicated, as discussed in the following text.

## ANAL MANOMETRY

The study and recording of pressures in the anal canal has been practiced for decades, offering valuable information regarding several aspects of anorectal function. It is one of the most commonly utilized diagnostic tests in the evaluation of pelvic floor function. The basic equipment needed for manometry consists of a probe to sense pressure, a recording device, a monitor, and a software system to aid in analysis. Manometry can assess the anal canal tone by measuring resting pressure (difference between the intrarectal pressure and the anal canal pressure), anal canal length, and squeeze pressure (contribution of the external anal sphincter and puborectalis muscles) (6). Rectoanal inhibitory reflex (RAIR) allows discrimination of solid, liquid, and gas. The presence of this reflex confirms a functioning myenteric plexus and, therefore, the absence of Hirschsprung disease (7). Rectal sensation can also be assessed by incrementally inflating a balloon in the rectum. The patient's first sensation and urge to defecate and maximum tolerated volumes are recorded. Alterations in rectal sensation are contributed to constipation. A systematic review has demonstrated that anorectal manometry shows that 20%–75% of patients suffer from anorectal dysfunction (8). Manometry is advantageous with respect to cost and the convenience of being able to perform the test in the colorectal surgeon's office. When utilizing manometry, the surgeon is able to interpret the analysis and discuss the findings with the patient after the procedure is completed.

## BALLOON EXPULSION TEST

The balloon expulsion test is an essential component of physiologic testing to assess evacuatory function with regard to constipation. There is no standardized method of performing the test. In general, the balloon is attached to a catheter and placed into the rectum and inflated. A typical balloon is inflated with 50 mL of warm water. In the seated position, the patient attempts to expel the balloon. In a normal person, expulsion time is usually within 1 minute (9). The time is recorded for the length of time required for expulsion. Variables in the technique include the type of balloon, the material used to fill, and the amount filled. Although this test has the convenience of being performed in the office with specificity ranging from 80% to 90%, its sensitivity is low at around 50% (10).

## RADIOPAQUE MARKERS

The ingestion of radiopaque markers to assess constipation has been utilized since the 1960s (11). In this test a capsule with multiple radiopaque rings is used, and serial radiographs are taken. There are several protocols for this type of study, but all require cessation of laxatives during the study. Contributing factors may include diet, medications, neurologic or endocrine disorders, psychosocial issues, colonic disease, or pelvic floor abnormalities (Tables 39.2 and 39.3) (1,3). Often patients may have constipation with no identifiable cause. Accurate documentation of the date and time of ingestion of the capsule is important so that plain radiographs are scheduled to be taken on days 1, 3, and 5 to monitor the passage of the markers. A normal study requires passage of 80% of the markers by day 5 (12). The number and distribution of the markers are noted at the end of the study. The segmental transit times are then calculated by the distribution of the markers. The diagnosis of colonic inertia can be made if greater than five markers are noted throughout the colon on day 5. Outlet obstruction should be considered when multiple markers have accumulated in the region of the rectosigmoid junction and have not progressed into the rectum or been evacuated on radiographic review (13). Radiopaque markers have the benefit of decreased cost; however, the patient is subjected to small amounts of ionizing radiation.

## SCINTIGRAPHY

Scintigraphic techniques have already been used successfully to characterize the propulsive or contractile activity, or both, of the esophagus, stomach, gallbladder, and small intestine. Colonic transit is evaluated by assessing the pattern of the tracer and percent excretion at 24, 48, and 72 hours (14). The use of $\gamma$-emitting radionuclide markers would seem to be ideal for the study of colonic motility because of low radiation exposure, noninvasive imaging, and patient comfort. Studies have shown the ability to delineate segmental colonic transit. However, despite attempts to simplify the techniques and make them more applicable for clinical use, measurement of colonic transit time by scintigraphy is not yet widely available (15).

## ANATOMICAL EVALUATION AND FUNCTIONAL STUDIES

## DEFECOGRAPHY

Conventional defecography, also referred to as evacuation proctography, is widely used to evaluate posterior pelvic floor dysfunction related to obstructed defecation syndrome (16). It assesses dynamic changes in the rectal wall, anal canal, vagina, and pelvic floor anatomy during the defecation process. Specific measurements of the anal rectal angle, extended perineal descent, and puborectalis length can be calculated. The rectal contrast is thickened to simulate stool weight and consistency. Images are obtained when the patient is asked to squeeze and contract the external anal sphincter and puborectalis at rest and with Valsalva. Patients with pelvic dyssynergy related to a nonrelaxing puborectalis muscle can be identified by failure of the anal rectal angle to open, persistence of the puborectalis compressing the rectum, and inadequate rectal emptying of the barium paste (17,18). If the patient digitates to facilitate or initiate evacuation, images during these maneuvers are performed (19). One of the advantages of defecography is that this can be performed in the upright sitting position allowing for the natural physiologic influence of gravity, abdominal wall muscles, and weight of the intestines to exert their effects on the patient's ability to evacuate. This type of imaging modality can also detect rectocele, rectal intussusception, rectal prolapse, enterocele and sigmoidocele, and descending perineum syndrome (19). Disadvantages of this method include the inability to evaluate soft tissues, provide information about sphincter defects, exposure to radiation, and an awkward and embarrassing experience for patients.

## ULTRASOUND

Current advancement in imaging technologies and the development of three-dimensional (3D) ultrasound equipment have enhanced the ability to study pelvic floor anatomy and dysfunction in different planes. Echodefecography, introduced by Murad-Regadas (20), is a dynamic 3D anal rectal ultrasonography technique using a 360° rotational transducer placed in the rectum with automatic scans in the axial, sagittal, and oblique planes. In a multicenter study of 86 women, a high degree of agreement was noted when comparing echodefecography and conventional defecography in the diagnosis of anal rectal disorders (13).

Dynamic 3D transvaginal and transrectal ultrasonography (TTUS) using a biplane transducer has been shown to be an acceptable alternative method in the evaluation of women with obstructed defecation syndrome. In a recent review, TTUS achieved high rates of concordance compared with echodefecography in the diagnosis of anismus, rectocele, enterocele/sigmoidocele, and intussusception (21). The benefits of ultrasound techniques compared to other imaging modalities such as defecography and dynamic magnetic resonance imaging (MRI) include the ability to visualize the anal sphincter looking for defects, atrophy, and scarring as well as identifying dynamic dysfunction. In addition, it does not expose patients to radiation, is readily available in the office making it cost effective, and involves less discomfort compared to conventional imaging. In a study by Vitton et al., patient tolerance was significantly better for anorectal endosonography compared to defecography and MRI, and the majority of patients would choose ultrasound over the other studies if a second imaging study was necessary (22). Available techniques include 2D/3D/4D, which allow for multiplanar reconstructions of the complex pelvic floor (23).

## PELVIC MAGNETIC RESONANCE IMAGING

In recent years, MRI has been used more often due to stronger gradients and shorter scanning time to help diagnosis pelvic pathology. Some of the pelvic pathologies that can be explored using MRI include rectocele, rectoanal intussusception, measurement of the anorectal angle, and perineal descent (24). In a study by Matsuoka and colleagues, pelvic MRI was compared to videoproctography (VP). They found that patients had no radiation exposure, and no rectal contrast was needed to evaluate the above-mentioned pathologies, making it an attractive imaging modality for patients. However, at the conclusion of their study, they found no difference between the use of MRI (which is 10 times more expensive) and VP. In fact MRI was not able to show small rectoceles and anorectal intussusception, and this was attributed to patients having to be in the prone position and not using rectal contrast (25).

## MEDICAL TREATMENT OF CONSTIPATION

Constipation is a common problem, and unfortunately its treatment has been far from satisfactory. A 2002 meta-analysis suggested that there was little credible evidence to support many of the drugs that are commonly used, especially the over-the-counter preparations (26). However, this analysis grouped all agents into a single "laxative group," which may have obscured any benefits of individual medications (27).

Patient education and dietary and lifestyle modifications play an essential role in the initial treatment of constipation, regardless of its etiology. Education should include proper sitting positions and an explanation of normal physiologic bowel patterns (28). It is also wise to advise the patient that a daily bowel movement is not a requisite to good health, and all providers should strive to decrease patient anxiety over the act of defecation. It is up to the physician to identify patients who need psychological support, since constipation may be aggravated by stress or depression and should communicate to the patient that his or her symptoms will not improve overnight, and modifications of the treatment regimen may be required.

General measures such as adequate hydration and regular exercise may improve overall health; however, there is no evidence to support success in the treatment of chronic constipation except in situations of dehydration (29,30). Nonetheless, diet modification to increase water and fiber consumption is considered an important, first-line component and is typically recommended before technical investigations of pelvic floor function and colon motility are performed or medications are started (31–35). Dietary fiber supplementation has been shown to allow discontinuation of laxatives in 59%–80% of elderly patients with chronic idiopathic constipation while improving body weight and well-being (36).

Fibers are bulking laxatives known to increase fecal mass/weight by absorbing and retaining fluid, which in turn stimulates motility and accelerates colonic transit time, resulting in an increase in bowel frequency (37,38). Its treatment relies heavily on the ingestion of an adequate amount of fluid to reach efficacy. They are also reasonably inexpensive, making an effective therapeutic intervention for addressing constipation-related bowel dysfunction (32,35). Fiber is found in grains, fruits, vegetables, nuts, seeds, and beans, and can be categorized as soluble or insoluble. Examples include psyllium (Metamucil and Kosyl), methylcellulose (Citrucel), and calcium polycarbophil (Fibercon). Dietary additives such as bran may cause abdominal bloating and discomfort, which in turn may decrease patient compliance. Gradual dose increase may minimize these symptoms. However, fiber may not be the most appropriate therapy for all causes of constipation. In a study published by Winfried et al., fiber was of limited value in 83% of patients with slow-transit constipation and 63% of patients with a disorder of defecation and outlet obstruction. Conversely, 85% of patients without a pathological finding or underlying motility disorder either improved or became asymptomatic with fiber therapy (35). These data suggest that a therapeutic trial of dietary fiber, in the range of 25–35 g/day, should be considered as initial treatment for patients with constipation, with the expectation of a more effective response in normal-transit or fiber-deficiency constipation patients as opposed to those patients with slow-transit constipation or pelvic floor dysfunction.

When nonpharmacologic management does not improve symptoms, laxative medications should be added for the management of constipation. A list of common medications used to treat constipation is shown in Table 39.4. There are many options available, and the choice of therapy should be subject to a consensus between the treating physician and patient preference (39).

Osmotic laxatives are poorly absorbed or nonabsorbed compounds that work by increasing water content within the large bowel; they include milk of magnesia, magnesium citrate, and sodium phosphate. These agents are not recommended in patients with cardiac and renal dysfunction given that excessive absorption may lead to electrolyte abnormalities and volume overload. When ingested as hypertonic solutions, rapid osmotic equilibration occurs, and overuse may result in significant dehydration (40).

Table 39.4 Medications commonly used for constipation

| Category | Example | Mechanism of action |
| --- | --- | --- |
| Bulking laxatives | • Psyllium<br>• Methylcellulose<br>• Calcium polycarbophil | Increase fecal mass to stimulate peristalsis |
| Osmotic laxatives | • Lactulose<br>• Sorbitol<br>• Magnesium salts<br>• Polyethylene glycol (PEG) | Increase water content in large bowel<br>Lactulose is fermented by colonic bacteria, which decrease gut pH, resulting in fecal volume expansion and accelerated transit |
| Stimulant laxatives | • Senna<br>• Cascara<br>• Bisacodyl | Increase intestinal motility |
| Softeners | • Mineral oil<br>• Docusate<br>• Glycerine | Change stool composition creating softer stools |
| Prosecretory agents | • Lubiprostone<br>• Linaclotide | Activate chloride channels to increase intestinal chloride secretion |
| Prokinetics | • Almovipan | Mµ-opioid receptor antagonist |
| Serotonin receptor agonist | • Prucalopride | Selective 5-HT$_4$ agonist |

Lactulose and sorbitol are nonabsorbable disaccharides. Lactulose is readily fermented by the colonic bacterial flora with the production of short-chain fatty acids and various gases, which act as osmotic agents that stimulate intestinal motility and secretion (41). Lactulose has been shown to increase stool frequency in chronically constipated patients (42); side effects may include abdominal bloating, discomfort, and flatulence, which may decrease patient compliance. Sorbitol is a poorly adsorbed sugar alcohol that produces similar effects. In a trial of constipated men over the age of 65, sorbitol administered as a 70% syrup (10.5 g/15 mL; 15–60 mL daily) was equivalent to lactulose in improving symptoms (43). Furthermore, it was cheaper and better tolerated during a 4-week trial.

High molecular weight polyethylene glycol (PEG) is a large polymer with substantial osmotic activity commonly used along with a balanced electrolyte solution for colon cleansing in preparation for colonoscopy and bowel surgery (44,45). A 2011 Cochrane Review evaluated relevant data to determine whether lactulose or polyethylene glycol was more effective in treating chronic constipation and fecal impaction. The meta-analysis included 10 randomized controlled trials; their findings indicated that polyethylene glycol is better than lactulose in outcomes of stool frequency per week, form of stool, relief of abdominal pain, and the need for additional products (46). PEG is a reliable treatment for chronic constipation because of its high efficacy, proven benefit when compared with other agents, and its long-term effectiveness. Other agents such as MiraLAX have been effectively used as osmotic laxatives for the treatment of chronic constipation. MiraLAX does not contain absorbable salts and generally does not alter measured levels of core electrolytes as well as calcium, glucose, blood urea nitrogen (BUN), creatinine, and serum osmolality (47–49).

Stimulant laxatives are not absorbed and exert their effects at the mucosal level, causing a reduction in the absorption of water and electrolytes and stimulating the production of secretions, which creates a prokinetic effect in the colon. Abdominal discomfort and cramping are common side effects of these agents. Bisacodyl produces defecation within 6–8 hours of taking the tablet, or 15–30 minutes after suppository. Its mechanism of action is the conversion into the active metabolite, bis-($p$-hydroxyphenyl)-pyridyl-2-methane (BHPM) which has a dual action as an antiabsorptive-secretory agent as well as inducing high-amplitude propagated contractions of the bowel resulting in a direct prokinetic effect (50). In a randomized, double-blind, placebo-controlled, multicenter trial in the United Kingdom, patients were randomly assigned, in a 2:1 ratio, to groups that were given 10 mg of bisacodyl or placebo, once daily, for 4 weeks. Patients used an electronic diary each day to record information relating to their constipation. The number of complete spontaneous bowel movements per week during the treatment period increased from $1 \pm 0.1$ in both groups to $5.2 \pm 0.3$ in the bisacodyl group and $1.9 \pm 0.3$ in the placebo group. Compared with baseline, there was a statistically significant improvement in the overall Patient Assessment of Constipation quality of life score, and all subscales in the hisacodyl-treated patients, compared with those who received placebo ($p \leq 0.70$), and treatment with bisacodyl was well tolerated (50).

Senna is a member of the anthraquinone family of laxatives that are common constituents of herbal and over-the-counter laxatives that are metabolized in the colon by bacteria into their active forms. In a trial of elderly nursing home residents ($n = 77$), a senna and fiber combination was reported to be better than lactulose in improving stool frequency, stool consistency, and ease of passage (51). Furthermore, the senna and fiber combination was 40% cheaper than lactulose therapy.

Side effects of stimulant laxatives may include allergic reactions, electrolyte imbalances, melanosis coli, and "cathartic colon." Melanosis coli is an abnormal pigmentation of the colonic mucosa caused by the accumulation of apoptotic epithelial cells being phagocytosed by macrophages (52). "Cathartic colon" is an alteration of the normal colon anatomy. It includes colonic dilatation, loss of haustra folds, strictures, colonic redundancy, and wide gaping of the ileocecal valve "fish mouth appearance" (53). Despite this common finding, current evidence supports the safety of currently available laxatives at recommended doses for long-term use.

Newer agents for constipation such as prosecretory agents (lubiprostone and linaclotide) and prokinetic agents (alvimopan) may be considered when dietary modifications, as well as osmotic and stimulant laxatives, have failed.

Lubiprostone (Amitiza) is an oral bicyclic functional fatty acid that activates the type 2 chloride channels located on the intestinal epithelial cell leading to an active secretion of chloride into the intestinal lumen (54,55), This drug has been shown to slow gastric emptying but accelerate small bowel and colonic transit time at 24 hours in healthy volunteers (56). In a multicenter, 4-week, double-blind, randomized, placebo-controled trial, lubiprostone produced a bowel movement in the majority of individuals within 24–48 hours of initial dosing and significantly increased the number of spontaneous bowel movements within the study period (57). These findings are similar to other well-developed studies (55). Lubiprostone is currently approved by the U.S. Food and Drug Administration for the treatment of chronic idiopathic constipation in adults, opioid-induced constipation in adults with chronic non-cancer pain, and irritable bowel syndrome with predominant constipation in women older than 18 years of age (58). Common side effects include nausea, headaches, and diarrhea.

Linaclotide (Linzess) is a minimally absorbed peptide agonist of the guanylate cyclase C receptor. It results in the generation of cyclic guanosine monophosphate (cGMP), which in turn, activates transmembrane channels inducing the secretion of chloride and bicarbonate into the intestinal lumen, increasing luminal fluid secretion and accelerating intestinal transit. In two randomized, controlled, double-blind multicenter studies, Lembo et al. attempted to determine the efficacy and safety of linaclotide in patients with chronic constipation. After randomization, patients received either 145 micrograms or 290 micrograms of linaclotide versus placebo daily for 12 weeks. The primary efficacy endpoint was three or more complete spontaneous bowel movements (CSBMs) per week and an increase of one or more CSBMs from baseline during at least 9 of the 12 weeks. This was reached in 16% and 21% of patients who received 145 micrograms of linaclotide and by 19.4% and 21.3% of patients who received 290 micrograms versus 3.3% and 6% of patients who received placebo ($p < 0.01$). The authors concluded that linaclotide significantly reduced bowel and abdominal symptoms of constipation, but long-term risk and benefits need to be assessed (59). Currently, linaclotide is approved in the United States for the treatment of irritable bowel syndrome with constipation and chronic idiopathic constipation.

Alvimopan, is a peripherally acting Mμ-opioid receptor antagonist that does not cross the blood-brain barrier and, therefore, does not inhibit the analgesic effect of opioids. Alvimopan can increase motility in opioid-induced colonic constipation without compromising analgesia; however, this does not seems to extend to patients with idiopathic constipation transit in healthy subjects (60,61). This drug has been shown to be effective in the treatment of acute postoperative ileus (62).

Other agents such as elobixibat (63,64), and procalopride (65), are currently under investigation and not formally approved by the U.S. Food and Drug Administration for the treatment of chronic idiopathic constipation. However, Plecanatide (66), which functions as a guanylate cyclase-C (GC-C) agonist and is taken orally once daily, acts locally on the luminal surface of the intestinal epithelium resulting in increased intestinal fluid and accelerated transit has been recently approved.

## BIOFEEDBACK THERAPY

As described previously, a subtype of constipation identified as pelvic constipation may be the result of pelvic floor dyssynergia also known as *anismus*. It is characterized by a failure of the abdominal, rectal, and pelvic floor and anal sphincter muscles to coordinate and complete the act of defecation resulting in an impaired propulsion of stool from the rectum, paradoxical anal contraction, inadequate anal relaxation, or a combination of these (67). This represents about one-third of patients with chronic constipation seen in tertiary care centers (68).

Biofeedback therapy plays an important role in patients with constipation due to pelvic floor dyssynergia, especially after failure of conservative management (69). Biofeedback therapy is based on operant conditioning to reinforce positive behavior; it uses electronically amplified recordings of pelvic floor muscle contractions (electromyography [EMG]) or anorectal pressure tracings to teach patients how to relax pelvic floor muscles and to strain more effectively when they defecate (2). Visual or auditory feedback is used to provide

patients with input regarding their performance during attempted defecation maneuvers.

The use of biofeedback therapy for the treatment of pelvic floor dyssynergia has been well documented (70,71). These studies report success rates ranging from 30% to 100% with over two-thirds of patients benefiting from biofeedback training. In a prospective randomized controlled trial, Rao et al. investigated the efficacy of biofeedback with either sham feedback therapy or standard therapy (diet, exercise, and laxatives) in 77 subjects with chronic constipation and dyssynergic defecation (68) at baseline and after 3 months of treatment. Physiologic changes were assessed by anorectal manometry, balloon expulsion, colonic transit study, and symptomatic changes. Subjects in the biofeedback group were more likely to correct their dyssynergia, improve defecation indexes, and decrease balloon expulsion time.

In regard to patients with outlet obstruction with associated pelvic floor dyssynergia, a 2006 randomized, controlled trial compared patients with pelvic floor dyssynergia treated with biofeedback versus laxative therapy with polyethylene glycol and education. The results favored the biofeedback-treated group, and benefits continued to be seen after 2 years of initial treatment. The authors conclude that biofeedback therapy should be the treatment of choice for this type of constipation (72).

Biofeedback therapy may rely on EMG monitoring of muscle tone or anorectal pressures for patient training. A 2003 meta-analysis compared both methods and concluded that patients with pressure biofeedback protocols showed significantly better outcomes (mean success rate of 78%) versus EMG biofeedback (mean success rate of 70%). Further analysis compared intraanal to perianal EMG biofeedback, and the results showed no significant difference between the two subgroups (69% versus 72%, respectively). The overall data showed a success rate ranging from 69% to 78%, regardless of which protocol or what instrumentation was used (69).

The treatment sessions are typically performed by nurses or physical therapists with advanced training and interest in pelvic floor disorders. Outcomes depend on the affect and patience of the therapist and patient acceptance to the therapist's technique. Other factors influencing the outcome of biofeedback therapy have been studied. In a recent review, additional predictors of successful outcome include the number of sessions attended (five or more) and whether the completion of therapy was determined by the therapist (63% success rate) as opposed to the patient terminating treatment prematurely (25% success rate) (73). Unfortunately, to date, no physiologic (manometry and balloon expulsion test), anatomic (rectocele, intussusception, or abnormal perineal descent), or demographic (age, gender, or duration of symptoms) variable has been able to be identified that would influence treatment outcome. Nevertheless, many researchers suggest that psychopathology may play an important role (2).

Despite the lack of a reproducible standardized technique, biofeedback therapy is a relatively inexpensive treatment option that has no related risk of side effects. Of note, the presence or absence of irritable bowel syndrome does not appear to impact the success rates of biofeedback for constipation (74).

There is insufficient data supporting the use of biofeedback therapy for the treatment of slow-transit constipation (75,76).

Failure of biofeedback therapy poses a significant treatment problem. Botulinum toxin injection has been proposed as an alternative therapeutic modality for patients with refractory pelvic floor dyssynergia. Injection is directed into the puborectalis muscle and external anal sphincter. Symptom improvement is reported to be short lived (1–3 months) with incontinence reported in 25% of patients. Because of these results and expense of the drug, this treatment modality should be reserved for those patients with severe symptomatic pelvic dyssynergia who have failed all other therapies (77).

## SURGICAL OPTIONS

The role of surgical intervention for patients who present with constipation should only be considered when the classification has been accurately identified as result of a thorough constipation workup, including colon transit studies and pelvic floor physiology testing. In addition, symptoms should be severe and incapacitating and are not responsive to nutritional or pharmacological therapy. Lahr evaluated over 2,000 patients who presented with severe constipation and found only 9.9% met criteria for surgical treatment (78). As with any operative procedure, patient selection is critical for success. A decision for surgery requires a detailed discussion regarding standard operative risk and postoperative complications as well as appropriate expectations as they relate to improvement in bowel frequency and the resolution of symptoms including abdominal pain and bloating, which are often associated in these patients and can persist after surgical intervention (79).

For patients who have documented slow-transit constipation and normal pelvic floor physiology, total abdominal colectomy with ileorectal anastomosis is generally considered to be the procedure of choice. Other options include subtotal colectomy with ileosigmoid anastomosis, subtotal colectomy with cecorectal anastomosis, and segmental colectomy.

Abdominal colectomy was first reported by the British surgeon Arbuthnot-Lane in 1908 for patients with constipation (80). Overall success of total abdominal colectomy with ileorectal anastomosis is exceedingly high with good rates of clinical improvement and patient satisfaction ranging from 50% to 100% (81–86) (Table 39.5). One summarizes many of the results of total abdominal colectomy with ileorectal anastomosis (87–92). Morbidity after total abdominal colectomy with ileorectal anastomosis can be significant, including anastomotic leak seen in up to 10% of patients, small bowel obstruction with a reported incidence up to 30%, and postoperative ileus seen in up to 25% of patients (83,85). Minimally invasive approaches have been successfully applied to this procedure with good results and are

Table 39.5 Results of total abdominal colectomy with ileorectal anastomosis

| Study | Number of patients | Success (%) | Follow-up (Mo) |
|---|---|---|---|
| Beck | 14 | 100 | 14 |
| Nylund | 40 | 72.50 | 132 |
| FitzHarris | 75 | 80 | — |
| Fan | 24 | 82 | 23 |
| Hassan | 104 | 85 | 104 |
| Webster | 55 | 89 | 12 |
| Zutshi | 64 | 92 | 128 |
| Pikarsky | 50 | 100 | 106 |
| Wexner | 16 | 94 | 15 |
| Pinedo | 20 | 95 | 25 |
| Glia | 14 | 86 | 60 |
| Riss | 12 | 50 | 84 |
| Sohn | 37 | 81.8 | 41 |
| Sheng | 68 | 94 | 40.7 |

Source: Pinedo G et al. Surg Endosc. 2009;23:62–5; Pinedo G et al. Surg Endosc. 2009;23:62–5; Sohn G et al. J Korean Soc Coloproctol. 2011;27(4):180–7; Fan CW, Wang JY. Int Surg. 2000;85:309–12; Hasson I et al. J Gastroinest Surg. 2006;10:1330–7; Riss S et al. Colorectal Dis. 2009;11(3): 302–7.

commonly performed (93,94). A report by Xu comparing laparoscopic versus open colectomy for slow-transit constipation confirms the established benefits of the minimally invasive techniques in colon surgery, including less blood loss, earlier return of bowel function, better cosmesis, and shorter hospital stays (95).

Variations of the procedure have been developed, including preservation of the cecum with cecorectal anastomosis or a portion of the sigmoid colon with ileosigmoid anastomosis. The intent is to reduce the side effects of diarrhea and electrolyte abnormalities that can be associated with total abdominal colectomy. Sarli reported an antiperistaltic anastomosis between the cecum and the rectum without mesenteric rotation with good results, with only one case of recurrent constipation (96). Marchese reported 22 patients who underwent cecorectal anastomosis for slow-transit constipation. Over 88% of the patients were pleased with the results and expressed a willingness to repeat the procedure given the same preoperative conditions. They initially concluded that cecorectal anastomosis did not appear to be inferior to subtotal colectomy with ileorectal anastomosis in terms of therapeutic effectiveness, postoperative morbidity, and overall impact on quality of life (97). However, a subsequent review by the same author reported three delayed surgical complications from cecorectal anastomosis relating to a dysfunctional or mobile cecal stump requiring surgical revision. Additional reports support the concept that maintenance of the cecal reservoir can result in dilatation and recurrence of constipation symptoms (98). In an attempt to improve functional results with this technique, Wei concluded that postoperative outcomes can be optimized by shortening the length of the ascending colon reservoir above the ileocecal junction to 2–3 cm as opposed to 10–15 cm (99).

Sigmoid preservation does not have any major advantage compared with other procedures and can predispose to postoperative constipation. Pemberton reported a 50% conversion rate from ileosigmoid anastomosis to ileorectal anastomosis (100). A retrospective comparison of cecorectal anastomosis versus ileosigmoid anastomosis demonstrated that the cecorectal anastomosis was more often associated with persistent constipation and lower patient satisfaction (73% versus 93%) (101). Despite the theoretical advantages of these procedures, preservation of the cecal reservoir and sigmoid colon can result in the recurrence of constipation symptoms.

Segmental colectomy has been advocated by some for the treatment of slow-transit constipation with the theoretical advantages being a reduction in the incidence of diarrhea that can be seen with total abdominal colectomy (102,103). Modifications of colon transit studies have been used to determine segmental colon transit impairment, which would subsequently influence a decision to perform a segmental resection, although the reliability of these studies has been questioned (103,104). You et al. reported a series of patients who underwent different types of colectomies including left and right colectomy according to the distribution or accumulation of markers in the colon. Follow-up in 2 years revealed that all but three patients had satisfactory bowel movements without worsening constipation. Three patients eventually went on to have subtotal colectomy with ileorectal anastomosis (105). In addition, Lundin reported on 28 patients who underwent segmental resections based on impaired transit in one segment by radiographic imaging. While 23 patients were satisfied with the outcome, 5 subsequently required additional surgery (106). It must be emphasized that interpretation of radial opaque marker studies has limitations, and the decision to proceed with segmental resection should be approached with caution since controlled data are lacking, and failure rates can be high (106).

The role of proctocolectomy as well as completion proctectomy after total abdominal colectomy and ileorectal anastomosis with ileo pouch anal anastomosis has been described for slow-transit constipation. Although the data are limited, Hosie reported on 13 patients with functional bowel disorders including 8 who had recurrent constipation after colectomy for slow-transit constipation and 5 who had constipation associated with megarectum and megacolon. Mean frequency of defecation was improved, and 85% of the patients surveyed felt the operation had been worthwhile with an improvement in their quality of life. Two patients had the pouch converted to an ileostomy due to persistent complications and a poor functional result (107). Keighley reported his series of patients who had previously undergone total colectomy with ileorectal anastomosis who had recurrent difficulty with evacuation of stool. Four of these patients subsequently underwent

excision of the pouches because of poor functional results (108). Proctocolectomy with ileoanal pouch creation should be chosen carefully as a surgical option for patients with refractory constipation, regardless of the circumstance, and should be considered only when a stoma is the only remaining option. The available literature does not justify the risk of complications from this procedure for this indication, and patients should be extensively counseled regarding functional expectations (109).

There is a subset of patients who may benefit from fecal diversion, albeit an extreme measure, as a reasonable alternative for the management of constipation and should be reserved for those who have failed other available treatments. In addition, this procedure can be considered in symptomatic patients who may have global intestinal motility disorder, combined slow-transit constipation, as well as a pelvic outlet problem, in which case it is uncertain as to whether the patient will benefit from colonic resection, fecal incontinence, or who may not tolerate a colon resection. Ileostomy is generally the preferred stoma, and relief of symptoms must be weighed against potential complications associated with an ileostomy, including electrolyte abnormalities, dehydration, and other stomal problems including hernia and retraction. Scarpa reviewed outcomes in 24 patients who underwent ileostomy for constipation with a 96% success rate in alleviating symptoms. Four patients subsequently underwent ileostomy closure, and 50% of them developed recurrent constipation (110).

Another less invasive option in the treatment of constipation is the use of antegrade colonic enema (ACE), which was initially described by Malone for the treatment of fecal incontinence in children, utilizing enemas delivered to the cecum to wash out the colon (111). The technique has also been described in adults with neurogenic constipation secondary to spinal cord injury, as well as slow-transit constipation or obstructive defecation (112–116). Over time, there have been modifications to the original technique with the creation of catheterizable conduit most commonly using the appendix left in situ to administer the enema, although a tube cecostomy and ileostomy have been described (117). The benefits of this approach are the avoidance of a colectomy and functioning stoma. The main disadvantage is a high incidence of surgical complications, including stenosis of the conduit occurring in up 23%–100% of patients and leakage (112,117). The placement of an indwelling catheter has been shown to decrease the incidence of stenosis, although wound infection and catheter dislodgement are frequent (118). Two series of just over 100 patients reported the use of the ACE procedure for constipation and reported satisfactory function in 42%–47% of patients (112). Success is generally reported as technical success, with less reliable data on the improvement of constipation symptoms and no comparison with other therapies for constipation. Hirst reported that 65% of patients experienced subjective improvement in defecation, but many patients were lost to follow-up (113). Patient compliance is an important factor in judging the success of this approach, and most series report only 50% of patients use the conduit for irrigations in the long term (112,113,119). Selection of this procedure should be reserved for highly motivated patients whose constipation is secondary to neurogenic causes and who understand the daily long-term commitment necessary to achieve success.

## SURGERY FOR COMBINED DISORDERS

In patients with mixed disorders of slow-transit constipation and obstructed defecation, treatment is complex and requires a multidisciplinary approach. The role of total abdominal colectomy with ileorectal anastomosis remains somewhat controversial, since a favorable outcome is less predictable than for patients with pure slow-transit constipation (82). Ragg evaluated 541 patients with chronic constipation and identified a 29% incidence of outlet obstruction in conjunction with colonic inertia (120). Hedrick created a classification scheme in patients with obstructed defecation based on functional and mechanical etiologies. Functional causes include short segment Hirschsprung disease, pelvic floor dyssynergia, and neuropathy which would include spinal cord lesions and neurologic disease such as multiple sclerosis. Mechanical causes include internal intussusception, enterocele, sigmoidocele, rectocele, and rectal prolapse (121). A comprehensive workup is critical in the assessment of these patients so that an appropriate treatment strategy can be formulated.

In general, patients with slow-transit constipation and pelvic floor dyssynergia should be treated with biofeedback before colectomy, because total abdominal colectomy with ileorectal anastomosis in this group of patients is associated with higher rates of recurrent constipation and lower rates of patient satisfaction (82). Biofeedback has been shown to help patients with constipation and obstructed defecation. A prospective randomized trial investigating the efficacy of biofeedback concluded that the use of biofeedback improved defecation indexes and decreased balloon expulsion time, resulting in an improvement in physiologic bowel function in patients with obstructed defecation (122). The timing of biofeedback therapy remains controversial with some authors advocating its use in the preoperative period, while others have reported efficacy in the postoperative period (123,124).

If the slow-transit constipation is associated with rectal intussusception or a nonemptying rectocele/enterocele on defecography, repair of the outlet obstruction is recommended before or concomitant with total abdominal colectomy with ileorectal anastomosis (109,125).

Rectocele repair has been described using transvaginal, transrectal, or transperineal approaches with and without mesh with good results in patients with symptoms of outlet obstruction. Indications for surgery include manual manipulation of the vaginal wall or rectum to evacuate, findings of an abnormal defecography with lack of emptying of contrast

from a rectocele, and size of a rectocele being greater than 4 cm (126). The basic premise of the operation is to recreate the rectovaginal septum to eliminate the bulge into the posterior wall of the vagina.

Theoretical benefits of the transvaginal repair include better visualization and access of the endopelvic fascia and the levator muscles as well as maintenance of the rectal mucosa integrity that may reduce infection and fistula complications (109). Transrectal repair has a theoretical advantage of less sexual and defecatory dysfunction as well as addresses any other anorectal pathology. A transperineal approach is appealing for patients with both a symptomatic rectocele and fecal incontinence as a result of a sphincter defect, which would allow for a concomitant sphincteroplasty to be performed.

There have only been a few prospective studies done to assess the efficacy of these different approaches. Arnold compared transrectal versus transvaginal approaches, which demonstrated an equal complication rate in both groups. Over 50% of the patients had postoperative constipation, and up to 30% had some component of gas or liquid stool incontinence (127). Nieminen examined transvaginal versus transrectal repair in 30 patients and demonstrated improvement of the outlet obstructive symptoms in over 70% of patients, with less recurrence in the transvaginal group 12 months after surgery (128).

Surgical repair of rectal intussusception can be considered in patients with severe symptoms of obstructive defecation only after failing nonoperative treatments, since in almost half of the cases, functional improvement can be achieved without the use of surgery (129). Several approaches have been described, including different rectopexy techniques, stapled transanal resection, and the Delorme procedure. Although these procedures may resolve anatomic issues like rectal ulcers and document improvement on repeat defecography, caution still needs to be applied, because they may not improve and can potentially worsen functional outcomes for patients (130,131).

Ventral mesh rectopexy is a relatively new and promising technique to correct rectal intussusception. A theoretical advantage of this approach is that it avoids posterior lateral rectal mobilization and thereby minimizes the risk of postoperative constipation. Several studies have shown improvement in constipation in 80%–95% of patients with minimal new-onset constipation (132,133). Portier reported a series of 40 patients who underwent ventral mesh rectopexy without sigmoid resection for rectal intussusception and found that 65% of patients on self-assessment responded as being cured, with another 33% showing improvement (133). Laparoscopic and robotic-assisted ventral mesh rectopexy is now being performed with acceptable recurrence rates, good functional results, and low mesh-related morbidity (134,135).

Stapled transanal rectal resection, initially reported by Longo (136), has been performed for the treatment of obstructed defecation resulting from rectocele and intussusception. The procedure utilizes a stapler for endorectal resection to remove the redundancy of the distal rectum, allowing for a less obstructed pathway to defecation. The literature is difficult to interpret because of the diverse patient population as well as a lack of prospective randomized studies. In addition, there has been inconsistent assessment of long-term outcomes. Despite this, several studies have attested to the successful results of this procedure in treating obstructed defecation with satisfaction rates ranging from 64% to 86% (137–139). In a review of 344 patients, 81% of the patients were highly satisfied, and rectal urgency was resolved in all patients at a median follow-up of 81 months (140). Concerns about long-term outcomes and serious postoperative complications including pain, urgency, incontinence, constipation, rectal diverticulum, retroperitoneal emphysema, bleeding, the development of rectovaginal fistula, and long-term proctalgia associated with inflammation from retained staplers have deterred rapid acceptance of this procedure in the United States (141,142). Careful patient selection, detailed informed consent outlining both benefits and potential risks, and surgeon experience in performing this procedure are vital to maximize the benefits and minimize potential complications.

The optimal surgical treatment for slow-transit constipation associated with concomitant obstructive defecation remains controversial. Based on the pathophysiologic changes of mixed constipation, a novel surgery entitled the Jinling procedure aims to solve the coexistence of obstructed defecation and delayed colon transit in one operation. This procedure adds a new side-to-side anastomosis to the low colorectal posterior anastomosis after subtotal colectomy, which fixates the right colon mesentery with the rectal stump acting as a rectopexy resulting in elevation of the pelvic floor musculature and relieving the symptoms of obstructed defecation (143). In a review of 117 patients who underwent this procedure, there was a reduction in validated constipation scores that was maintained for over 4 years, as well as improvement in the postoperative GI quality of life with high patient satisfaction rates (110). In addition, Reshef studied the outcomes for patients with pure slow-transit constipation (102) compared to those with slow transit and features of obstructed defecation (41) who underwent total abdominal colectomy with ileorectal anastomosis. They concluded that total abdominal colectomy can be offered to a highly select group of patients with a combined disorder, with the expectation of achieving equivalent long-term results and high patient satisfaction rates (144).

Sacral nerve stimulation (SNS) has been used successfully for pelvic floor disorders including urinary incontinence, overactive bladder, and fecal incontinence. The mechanism of action is poorly understood, but it is thought to alter pelvic afferent pathways and central mechanisms (145). Neurostimulation has now emerged as a potential treatment for chronic constipation from slow-transit or outlet dysfunction, primarily in institutions outside of the United States (145–150). A recent European consensus statement was in agreement that SNS could be considered for patients who have constipation symptoms for greater than

a year and have failed medical therapy (148). It is currently not approved by the U.S. Food and Drug Administration for this condition in the United States.

The reported success rates range from 42% to greater than 90%, and several prospective studies have shown improvement in the Cleveland Clinic constipation score (145,151,152). Thomas reviewed 13 studies demonstrating the use of SNS for the treatment of constipation. In patients who proceeded to permanent SNS, up to 87% showed improvement in symptoms based on quality of life and patient satisfaction scores at a medium follow-up of 28 months (146). Some studies do not report efficacy separating patients with slow-transit versus outlet obstruction, but Ratto reported that improvement was better in patients with obstructed defecation (147).

Dinning completed a randomized, double-blind placebo-controlled two-phase crossover study for SNS in slow-transit constipation. The short-term trial compared sham stimulation with SNS with the primary outcome being days per week with the feeling of complete evacuation. There was no significant difference in the response rate between the SNS group (30%) versus the sham stimulation group (21%) (153). A longer follow-up at 2 years concluded that SNS was not effective treatment for slow-transit constipation. One reason for such a low success rate in this study was that all patients proceeded to permanent implantation regardless of their response to peripheral nerve evaluation (PNE) (154).

A recent Cochrane Review for SNS for constipation in adults concluded that SNS did not seem to improve symptoms in people with constipation, but there were only two randomized trials providing evidence, of which one trial had only two participants (155).

While there is prospective case series data available supporting the beneficial effects SNS for chronic constipation, the majority of reports were uncontrolled and had no comparison with any other treatment modalities. In addition, there was no consistent definition of constipation or uniform methods to measure response and improvement in these studies. Additional studies are necessary to assess the potential efficacy of this treatment option and provide evidence to determine selection criteria for its use.

## COMPLICATIONS

The success rate for total colectomy with an ileorectal anastomosis for slow-transit constipation has been shown to be around 90% overall; however, morbidity is high, which can be attributed to those risks directly related to any colon resection as well as long-term functional problems. Short-term complications that can occur after any bowel operation include bleeding, urinary tract infections, thromboembolic events, adverse reaction to anesthesia, and surgical site infections, which can be superficial or intraabdominal secondary to an anastomotic leak, which has been reported up to 11% of patients (85). Postoperative ileus and small bowel obstruction are the most frequent complications seen after total abdominal colectomy for constipation. Long-term postoperative functional complaints include chronic abdominal pain, bloating, diarrhea, and incontinence.

In a review of 144 patients who underwent total colectomy for slow-transit constipation, postoperative ileus was the most common complication. And 10% of patients underwent reoperation in the immediate postoperative period, including 9 for anastomotic leak, 5 for postoperative bleeding, and 1 for a missed enterotomy. Wound infection was seen in 14% of patients, and urinary tract infection was seen in 12% (144).

Knowles reviewed 32 series looking at the outcome of colectomy for slow-transit constipation from 1991 to 1998. The mortality rate varied from 0% to 6%. The most common postoperative complication was small bowel obstruction, which generally occurs from adhesions created at the time of colectomy, although others have reported small bowel pseudo-obstruction secondary to a neuropathic disorder of the myenteric plexus limiting bowel motility (156). In his review, the median incidence was 18% with a reoperation rate of 14% (82). Others have reported an incidence of small bowel obstruction in up to 25% of patients with more than half requiring surgical intervention for lysis of adhesions (83,85,157). Other significant complications include diarrhea, which is generally a short-term complication resulting from the absence of the ability of the colon to absorb water, which has been reported in 14%–46% of patients. Medical treatment including fiber supplements, antimotility agents, and binders, as well as time to allow for intestinal adaptation may reduce bowel frequency and improve the consistency of stool. Some degree of incontinence has been reported in up to 50% of patients with a median 14% (79,82). Chronic abdominal pain can be a frequent complaint in this group of patients, with an incidence in up to 41% of patients. The need for permanent ileostomy as a result of these complications can be seen in up to 5% of patients (79,82,85).

FitzHarris noted that despite the statistically significant negative impact the long-term consequences of chronic abdominal pain, diarrhea, and incontinence had on gastrointestinal quality of life index scores, the vast majority of patients (over 90%) stated they would undergo subtotal colectomy again if given a second chance (79).

The unrecognized presence of gastrointestinal dysmotility may explain the high rate of ileus and postoperative small bowel obstruction. Glia looked at outcomes of colectomy for slow-transit constipation in relation to the presence of small bowel dysmotility evidenced by abnormal antral duodenal manometry. They found a trend toward better long-term results after surgery for slow-transit constipation in patients with normal manometry before the operation, specifically in the incidence of constipation, diarrhea, chronic abdominal pain, and abdominal bloating (158).

In addition, the indication for colectomy has been shown to influence postoperative morbidity. In comparing total abdominal colectomy with ileorectal anastomosis in patients undergoing surgery for colonic inertia versus other noninflammatory reasons, Reshef noted a significantly greater overall morbidity in the colonic inertia group. There were higher rates of postoperative abscess, more urinary tract infections, higher rates of wound infection, and higher rates of postoperative ileus and increased length of stay. In addition, the 30-day readmission rate was also significantly higher (159).

In an effort to improve outcomes specifically aimed at decreasing ileus rates and lowering the incidence and surgical treatment of small bowel obstruction, the implementation of enhanced recovery after surgery protocols and minimally invasive colorectal techniques has demonstrated a reduction in morbidity, decrease in overall length of hospital stay, earlier return of bowel function, as well as a low readmission rate in colectomy patients (160–164). In addition, the placement of an antiadhesive agent at the time of surgery has been shown to reduce the incidence of adhesions that can cause small bowel obstruction (165). In comparing laparoscopic versus open procedures in colorectal surgery, the need for operative intervention for small bowel obstruction has been shown to significantly lower after laparoscopic operations as compared to open procedures (166). Utilizing these protocols and surgical approaches achieves the goals of improving the quality of patient care and satisfaction, while reducing health care–related cost.

## RECURRENCE OF CONSTIPATION/ OUTCOMES

Total abdominal colectomy with ileorectal anastomosis is an effective method of treatment for medically resistant colonic inertia. After an appropriate preoperative workup including colon transit and pelvic floor studies, successful outcomes have been reported to be greater than 90%.

In 26 studies involving 1,047 patients with a mean follow-up of 44.8 months, the rate of bowel movements reported by the patients was 2.8 times per day, whereas recurrent constipation was reported in up to one-third of patients with a mean of 9% (0%–33%) of 683 patients in 17 series (167).

It must be noted that definitive conclusions regarding the effectiveness of surgery cannot be universally decided. The methods used to assess the outcome of surgery and patient satisfaction vary greatly. Some studies use patient satisfaction as a criterion for success, which can be very subjective and inaccurate. The ideal way to measure success should include standardized outcome measures such as questionnaire-based protocols that assess quality of life, postoperative complications, and functional outcome as it relates specifically to bowel function. The process of distributing and collecting questionnaires as well as patient compliance rates remains an obstacle and presents a challenge in accumulating outcome data when assessing the results of surgery for constipation. However, the overall rate of success or satisfaction documented in 39 studies involving 1,423 patients was 86% (39%–100%) (167).

Psychiatric history and mental well-being are also important factors to consider in the selection of patients for surgery and evaluating outcomes. Pluta et al. found superior results in patients with no psychiatric history compared to those with a psychiatric history, while others noted poor outcomes with higher permanent stoma rates in patients with psychologic conditions (168). In contrast, additional series reported by Nylund and Reshef did not find psychiatric history to be a predictor of poor outcomes (166,169). In a more detailed study by Heyman et al. utilizing the Minnesota Multiphasic Personality Inventory in a series of patients with severe constipation, it was noted that the incidences of hypochondriasis, depression, and hysteria were significantly increased (170). Furthermore, O'Brien et al. noted that a history of sexual abuse and not psychiatric history was associated with persistent abdominal symptoms after total abdominal colectomy (171).

Considerations for the recurrence or persistence of constipation after colectomy include the unrecognized presence of pelvic floor dysfunction and the presence of a neuropathic disorder that may extend proximally into the small bowel or even the entire gastrointestinal tract, resulting in a global gastrointestinal motility disorder or the direct result of incomplete colonic resection (2).

Evaluation of these patients requires an initial assessment for concomitant outlet obstruction with pelvic floor physiology testing, since the presence of pelvic floor dysfunction has been shown to significantly decrease successful outcomes after surgery. If pelvic dyssynergy is identified, then biofeedback therapy can be considered to improve symptoms and outcome (84).

Radiographic imaging with contrast enemas and endoscopic visualization to identify anatomical abnormalities related to prior surgery and the remaining rectum is essential to determine if recurrence of constipation is the direct result of a dysfunctional or mobile cecal stump from a cecorectal anastomosis or a dysmotile portion of colon as a result of a segmental resection or ileosigmoid anastomosis. All of these technical variants have been shown to be associated with a higher incidence of constipation recurrence, and reoperation with completion colectomy and conversion to ileorectal anastomosis may be necessary to correct these types of surgical failure (97,98,100).

If the above testing is inconclusive and does not provide sufficient evidence to proceed with either biofeedback or reoperative surgery, then further testing to assess whole gastrointestinal transit should be performed to identify patients with a neuropathic disorder causing pseudo-obstruction who may benefit from ileostomy.

## SUMMARY

Chronic constipation is a common disease that is multifactorial in origin. In most cases, it can be successfully managed by diet modification, medication, or rehabilitative treatment. Of all the patients who present with chronic constipation, only a small percentage will be refractory to medical management. Patients who do not respond to these forms of treatment may be candidates for surgical intervention. The goals of surgical management for constipation are to increase the number of bowel movements and improve the quality of life for patients. A precise and thorough evaluation of the morphology and function of the bowel and pelvic floor is essential to accurately categorize the classifications of chronic constipation, which include slow-transit constipation, obstructed defecation, and combined disorders. This fundamental principle will guide clinicians in their decisions to select the appropriate therapy necessary to achieve a successful outcome, satisfy expectations associated with treatment, and minimize the recurrence of symptoms.

Future developments in the field of neurostimulation and understanding its effect on the properties of nerves in the gastrointestinal tract may provide a less invasive treatment with better outcomes in the management of patients with chronic constipation.

## REFERENCES

1. Brandt LJ et al. *Am J Gastroenterol.* 2005;100(Suppl. 1):S5–21.
2. Papaconstantinou HT. Operative and nonoperative therapy for chronic constipation. In Whitlow CB et al. (eds). Improved Outcomes in Colon and Rectal Surgery. London: Informa, 2010, pp. 361–374.
3. Sandler RS et al. *Am J Public Health.* 1990;80:185–9.
4. Ribas Y et al. *Dis Colon Rectum.* 2011;54:1560–9.
5. Knowles CH et al. *Dis Colon Rectum.* 2003;46:1716–17.
6. Wexner SD et al. *Dis Colon Rectum.* 1991;34:851–6.
7. Tobon F et al. *N Engl J Med.* 1968;278:188–93.
8. Rao SS et al. *Am J Gastroenterol.* 2005;100:1605–15.
9. Ternent CA et al. *Dis Colon Rectum.* 2007;50:2013–22.
10. Beck DE. *Ochsner J.* 2008;8:25–31.
11. Hinton JM et al. *Gut.* 1969;10:842–7.
12. Nam YS et al. *Dis Colon Rectum.* 2001;44:86–92.
13. Videlock EJ et al. *Neurogastroenterol Motil.* 2013;25:509–20.
14. Metcalf AM et al. *Gastroenterology.* 1987;92:40–7.
15. Cowlam S et al. *Colorectal Dis.* 2008;10:818–22.
16. Felt-Bersma RJ et al. *Dis Colon Rectum.* 1990;33:277–84.
17. Karlbom U et al. *Int J Colorectal Dis.* 1998;13:141–7.
18. Jones PN et al. *Dis Colon Rectum.* 1987;30:667–70.
19. Bremmer S et al. *Dis Colon Rectum.* 1995;38:969–73.
20. Murad-Regadas SM et al. *Surg Endosc.* 2008;22:974–9.
21. Murad-Regadas SM et al. *Dis Colon Rectum.* 2014;57:228–36.

22. Vitton V et al. *Dis Colon Rectum.* 2011;54:1398–404.
23. Bozkurt MA et al. *Ulus Cerrahi Derg.* 2014;30:183–5.
24. Wieczorek AP et al. *World J Urol.* 2011;29:615–23.
25. Varma MG et al. *Dis Colon Rectum.* 2008;51:162–72.
26. Jones MP et al. *Dig Dis Sci.* 2002;47:2222–30.
27. Ramkumar D, Rao SS. *Am J Gastroenterol.* 2005;100: 936–71.
28. Siegel JD, Di Palma JA. *Clin Colon Rectal Surg.* 2005; 18:76–80.
29. Meshkinpour H et al. *Dig Dis Sci.* 1998;43:2379–83.
30. Young RJ et al. *Gastroenterol Nurs.* 1998;21:156–61.
31. Whitehead WE et al. *J Am Geriatr Soc.* 1989;37: 423–9.
32. Anti M et al. *Hepatogastroenterology.* 1998;45: 727–32.
33. Ashraf W et al. *Aliment Pharmacol Ther.* 1995;9: 639–47.
34. Rodrigues-Fisher L et al. *Clin Nurs Res.* 1993;2: 464–77.
35. Voderholzer WA et al. *Am J Gastroenterol.* 1997;92: 95–8.
36. Sturtzel B et al. *J Nutr Health Aging.* 2009;13:136–9.
37. Burkitt DP et al. *Lancet.* 1972;2:1408–12.
38. Schiller LR. *Aliment Pharmacol Ther.* 2001;15:749–63.
39. Madoff RD, Fleshman JW. *Gastroenterology.* 2003; 124:235–45.
40. Lembo A, Camilleri M. *N Engl J Med.* 2003;349: 1360–8.
41. DiPalma JA. *Rev Gastroenterol Disord.* 2004; 4(Suppl. 2):S34–42.
42. Bass P, Dennis S. *J Clin Gastroenterol.* 1981;3(Suppl.): 23–8.
43. Lederle FA et al. *Am J Med.* 1990;89:597–601.
44. Schiller LR et al. *Gastroenterology.* 1988;94:933–41.
45. Toledo TK, Di Palma JA. *Aliment Pharmacol Ther.* 2001;15:605–11.
46. Lee-Robichaud H et al. *Cochrane Database Syst Rev.* 2010;(7):CD007570.
47. Di Palma JA et al. *Am J Gastroenterol.* 2002;97: 1776–9.
48. DiPalma JA et al. *Am J Gastroenterol.* 2000;95: 446–50.
49. Corazziari E et al. *Gut.* 2000;46:522–6.
50. Kamm MA et al. *Clin Gastroenterol Hepatol.* 2011; 9:577–83.
51. Passmore AP et al. *Pharmacology.* 1993;47(Suppl. 1): 249–52.
52. Oster JR et al. *Am J Gastroenterol.* 1980;74:451–8.
53. Urso FP et al. *Radiology.* 1975;116:557–9.
54. Cupoletti J et al. *Am J Physiol Cell Physiol.* 2004;297: C1173–83.
55. Johanson JF, Ueno R. *Aliment Pharmacol Ther.* 2007; 25:1351–61.
56. Camilleri M et al. *Am J Physiol Gastrointes Liver Physiol.* 2006;290:G942–7.
57. Johanson JF et al. *Am J Gastroenterol.* 2008;103: 170–7.
58. Gras-Miralles B, Cremonini F. *Clin Interv Aging.* 2013; 8:191–200.
59. Lembo AJ et al. *N Engl J Med.* 2011;365:527–36.
60. Gonenne J et al. *Clin Gastroenterol Hepatol.* 2005; 3:784–91.
61. Webster L et al. *Pain.* 2008;137:428–40.
62. Camilleri M. *Neurogastroenterol Motil.* 2005;17: 157–65.
63. Acosta A, Camilleri M. *Therap Adv Gastroenterol.* 2014;7:167–75.
64. Wong BS, Camilleri M. *Expert Opn Investig Drugs.* 2013;22:277–84.
65. Woodward S. *Br J Nurs.* 2012;21:982, 984–6.
66. Shailubhai K et al. *Dig Dis Sci.* 2013;58:2580–6.
67. Rao SS et al. *Am J Gastroenterol.* 1998;93:1042–50.
68. Rao SS et al. *Clin Gastroenterol Hepatol.* 2007;5: 331–8.
69. Heymen S et al. *Dis Colon Rectum.* 2003;46:1208–17.
70. Enck P. *Dig Dis Sci.* 1993;38:1953–60.
71. Rao SS et al. *Dig Dis Sci.* 1997;15(Suppl. 1):78–92.
72. Chiarioni G et al. *Gastroenterology.* 2006;130: 657–64.
73. Gilliland R et al. *Br J Surg.* 1997;84:1123–6.
74. Ahadi T et al. *J Res Med Sci.* 2014;19:950–5.
75. Brown SR et al. *Dis Colon Rectum.* 2001;44:737–9.
76. Chiarioni G et al. *Gastroenterology.* 2005;129:86–97.
77. Maria G et al. *Dis Colon Rectum.* 2000;43:376–80.
78. Lahr SJ. *Am Surg.* 1999;65:1117–23.
79. FitzHarris GP et al. *Dis Colon Rectm.* 2003;46: 433–40.
80. Lane WA. *Br Med J.* 1908;1:126–30.
81. Wexner SD et al. *Dis Colon Rectum.* 1991;43:851–6.
82. Knowles CH et al. *Ann Surg.* 1999;230:627–38.
83. Webster C, Dayton M. *Am J Surg.* 2001;182:639–44.
84. Redmond JM et al. *Am J Gastroenterol.* 1995;90: 748–53.
85. Pikarsky A et al. *Dis Colon Rectum.* 2001;44:1898–9.
86. Ripetti V et al. *Surgery.* 2006;140:435–40.
87. Pinedo G et al. *Surg Endosc.* 2009;23:62–5.
88. Sheng QS et al. *J Dig Dis.* 2014;15:419–24.
89. Sohn G et al. *J Korean Soc Coloproctol.* 2011;27(4): 180–7.
90. Fan CW, Wang JY. *Int Surg.* 2000;85:309–12.
91. Hasson I et al. *J Gastroinest Surg.* 2006;10:1330–7.
92. Riss S et al. *Colorectal Dis.* 2009;11(3):302–7.
93. Hsiao KC et al. *Int J Colorectal Dis.* 2008;23:419–24.
94. Athanasakis H et al. *Surg Endosc.* 2001;15(10): 1090–2.
95. Xu LS, Liu WS. *Am Surgeon.* 2012;78:495–6.
96. Sarli L et al. *Dis Colon Rectum.* 2001;44(10):1514–9.
97. Marchesi F et al. *World J Surg.* 2007;31:1658–64.
98. Fasth S et al. *Acta Chir Scand.* 1983;149:623–7.
99. Wei D et al. *BMC Gastroenterol.* 2015;15:30.
100. Pemberton JH et al. *Ann Surg.* 1991;214:403–11.
101. Feng Y, Jianjiang L. *Am J Surg.* 2008;195:73–7.
102. Kamm MA et al. *Int J Colorectal Dis.* 1991;6(1):49–51.
103. De Graff EJ et al. *Br J Srg.* 1996;83(5):648–51.

104. Ehrenpreis ED et al. *Gastroenterology*. 1997;110A: 728.
105. You YT et al. *Am Surg*. 1998;64(8):775–7.
106. Lundin E et al. *Br J Surg*. 2002;89(10):1270–4.
107. Hosie KB et al. *Br J Surg*. 1990;77:801–2.
108. Keighley MR et al. *Gut*. 1993;34(5):680–4.
109. Paquete IM et al. *Dis Colon Rectum*. 2016;59: 479–92.
110. Scarpa M et al. *Colorectal Dis*. 2005;7(3):224–7.
111. Malone PS et al. *Lancet*. 1990;336(8725):1217–8.
112. Lees NP et al. *Colorectal Dis*. 2004;6:362–8.
113. Hirst GR et al. *Tech Coloproctol*. 2005;9:217–21.
114. Poirier M et al. *Dis Colon Rectum*. 2007;50:22–8.
115. Buntzen S, Laurberg S. *Dis Colon Rectum*. 2008;51: 1523–8.
116. Meurette G et al. *Gastroenterol Clin Biol*. 2010;34(3): 209–12.
117. Biyani D et al. *Colorectal Dis*. 2007;9:373–6.
118. Patton V, Lubowski DZ. *Dis Colon Rectum*. 2015;58: 457–65.
119. Worsøe J et al. *Dis Colon Rectum*. 2008;51:1523–8.
120. Raag J et al. *Colorectal Dis* 2011;13:1299–302.
121. Hedrick TL, Friel CM. *Gastroenterol Clin N Am*. 2013; 42:863–76.
122. Talley NJ et al. *Am J Gastroenterol*. 1996;91:19–25.
123. Nyam DC et al. *Dis Colon Rectum*. 1997;40(3):273–9.
124. Bernini A et al. *Dis Colon Rectum*. 1998;41(11): 1363–6.
125. Zenilman ME et al. *Arch Surg*. 1989;124:947–51.
126. Mellgren A et al. *Dis Colon Rectum*. 1995;38:7–13.
127. Arnold MW et al. *Dis Colon Rectum*. 1990;33:684–7.
128. Nieminen K et al. *Dis Colon Rectum*. 2004;47: 1636–42.
129. Murad-Regadas SM et al. *Arq Gastroenterol*. 2012;49: 135–42.
130. Van Tets WF, Kuijpers JH. *Dis Colon Rectum*. 1995;38: 1080–3.
131. Christiansen J et al. *Dis Colon Rectum*. 1992;35: 1026–8.
132. Slawik S et al. *Colorectal Dis*. 2008;10:138–43.
133. Portier G et al. *Colorectal Dis*. 2011;13:914–7.
134. Owais AE et al. *Colorectal Dis*. 2014;16:995–1000.
135. Van Iersel JJ et al. *World J Gastroenterol*. 2016; 22(21):4977–87.
136. Longo A. *Annual Cleveland Clinic Florida Colorectal Disease Symposium*. 2004.
137. Reboa G et al. *Dis Colon Rectum*. 2009;52: 1598–604.
138. Stuto A et al. *Surg Innov*. 2011;18:248–53.
139. Schwandner O, Fürst A, German StaRR Registry study Group. *Langenbecks Arch Surg*. 2010;395: 505–13.
140. Goede AC et al. *Colorectal Dis*. 2011;13:1052–7.
141. De Nardi P et al. *Tech Coloproctol*. 2007;11:353–6.
142. Pescatori M et al. *Int J Colorectal Dis*. 2005;20:83–5.
143. Ding W et al. *Dis Colon Rectum*. 2015;58:91–6.
144. Reshef A et al. *Int J Colorectal Dis*. 2013;28:841–7.
145. Carrington EV et al. *Neurogastroenterol Motil*. 2014; 26:1222–37.
146. Thomas GP et al. *Br J Surg*. 2013;100:174–81.
147. Ratto C et al. *Colorectal Dis*. 2015;17:320–8.
148. Maeda Y et al. *Colorectal Dis*. 2015;17:o74–87.
149. Graf W et al. *Neurogastroenterol Motil*. May 2015; 27(5):734–9.
150. Ortiz H et al. *Dis Colon Rectum*. 2012;55:876–80.
151. Pinto RA, Sands DR. *Gastrointest Endoscopy Clin N Am*. 2009;19:83–116.
152. Kamm ma et al. *Gut*. 2010;59:333–40.
153. Dinning PG et al. *Am J Gastroenterol*. 2015;110: 733–40.
154. Patton V et al. *Dis Colon Rectum*. 2016;59:878–85.
155. Thaha MA et al. *Sacral Nerve Stimulation for Fecal Incontinence and Constipation in Adults (Review)*. Cochrane Database of Systematic Reviews 2015, Issue 8. Art. No.: CD004464. DOI: 10.1002/14651858. CD004464.pub3.
156. Krishnamurthy S et al. *Gastroenterology*. 1985;88: 26–34.
157. Zutshi M et al. *Int J Colorectal Dis*. 2007;22:265–9.
158. Glia A et al. *Dis Colon Rectum*. 2004;47:96–102.
159. Reshef A et al. *Colorectal Dis*. 2012;15:481–6.
160. Senagore AJ et al. *Dis Colon Rectum*. 2009;52(2): 183–6.
161. Delaney CP et al. *Ann Surg*. 2008;247(5):819–24.
162. Bona S et al. *World J Gastroenterol*. 2014;20(46): 17578–87.
163. Feldman LS, Delaney CP. *Surg Endosc*. 2014;28(5): 1403–6.
164. Sample C et al. *J Gastrointest Surg*. 2005;9:803–8.
165. Becker JM et al. *J Am Coll Surg*. 1996;183:297–306.
166. Reshef A et al. *Surg Endosc*. 2013;27:1717–20.
167. Bove A et al. *World J Gastroenterol*. 2012;18(36): 4994–5013.
168. Pluta H et al. *Dis Colon Rectum*. 1996;39(2):160–6.
169. Nylund G et al. *Colorectal Dis*. 2001;3(4):253–8.
170. Heyman S et al. *Dis Colon Rectum*. 1993;36:593–6.
171. O'Brien S et al. *Dis Colon Rectum*. 2009;52(11): 1844–7.

# 40

# Colorectal trauma

ALISON ALTHANS AND SCOTT R. STEELE

## CHALLENGING CASE

A 19-year-old male was involved in a blast injury with multiple shrapnel wounds to the abdomen. He was initially alert and talking on presentation and slightly tachycardic (HR 118) and mildly hypotensive (systolic blood pressure 95 mm HG), but he responded to fluid resuscitation. Chest x-ray demonstrated a small left-sided pneumothorax and abdominal plain film showed multiple metallic fragments. Physical examination was significant for peritonitis on abdominal examination. After he was given cefazolin and metronidazole, he was taken to the operating room. He was found to have multiple small bowel, descending and sigmoid colon through-and-through injuries (Figure 40.1) and a moderate amount of intraabdominal contamination of stool.

## CASE MANAGEMENT

After initially packing the abdomen and continuing resuscitation, hemostasis was achieved on two small bowel mesenteric bleeding vessels. Further stool contamination was controlled by stapling off and resecting the bowel with significant injury and loss of wall integrity and oversewing smaller areas. The colon injuries were resected due to the >50% loss of colon wall. After washing the abdomen out with several liters of warm normal saline, the patient remained mildly hypotensive despite appropriate aggressive resuscitation. The bowel was left in discontinuity, the abdomen was packed and left open utilizing a sterile negative therapy wound device, and the patient was taken to the intensive care unit for continued resuscitation. The following day after his hemodynamics and laboratory values were normalized and he was normothermic, he was taken back to the operating room for a second

look. His bowel appeared healthy and in-continuity restoration was performed for both the small and large bowel. Following a negative air-leak test on the colon, he was closed, extubated, and recovered uneventfully.

## INTRODUCTION

Since the experience of military surgeons in managing colon and rectal traumas has been crucial in shaping the way civilian colorectal injuries are now managed, it is important to consider these traumas in the context of wartime history. During the American Civil War, the risk of infection and sepsis secondary to any surgical intervention for abdominal trauma made expectant management the mainstay (1). At the beginning of World War I, most abdominal wounds were managed nonoperatively. However, as the war continued on, Cuthbert Wallace and other defiant British surgeons insisted on laparotomy, arguing that hemorrhage was the chief cause of early mortalities (2,3). With the implementation of expedited evacuation of the injured from the battlefield and subsequent operation, mortality from abdominal wounds began to fall (4). Throughout World War II and the first half of the twentieth century, the procedure of choice was largely exteriorization of the affected bowel—taking the portion of the bowel wall that was injured and bringing it to the skin as a stoma. The most important work shaping these guidelines was Ogilvie's "Abdominal Wounds in the Western Desert," in which he advocated for exteriorization or proximal colostomy—even though his data did not clearly support this recommendation (5,6). Despite the fact that mortality rates were similar between primary repair and diversion/exteriorization groups in Ogilvie's series, the U.S. Office of the Surgeon General mandated against primary repair (6,7). Management of rectal injuries also improved during this time as presacral drainage and distal rectal irrigation were implemented (8). Along the way, mortality rates following colon and rectal traumas had dropped from the nearly 90% initially seen in the Civil War era to less than 40% (9).

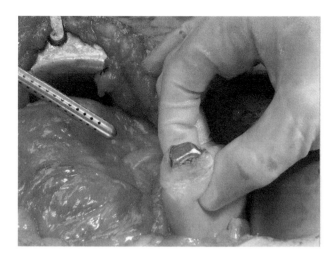

Figure 40.1 **(See color insert.)** Shrapnel injury to the small bowel with a hex nut. Similar injuries were present to the small and large bowel.

The transition to surgical management was also accompanied by simultaneous advances in antibiotic therapy, fluid resuscitation, blood banking, surgical techniques, and equipment. Continued experience with diversion and exteriorization procedures used during the Korean and Vietnam Wars, in alignment with the previously established doctrine against primary anastomosis, led to improved outcomes and dropped the mortality rate even further to ~10% (10). Although there was some experimentation with primary repair in some right-sided colon injuries during this time (11), colostomy remained standard practice until the 1970s. Civilian practices largely paralleled those of the combat setting, until the late 1970s at which point surgeons questioned the differences in militant and civilian traumas, the possible compounding factors that may have contributed to the success of diversion in military trauma, and the potential benefit of primary anastomosis in carefully selected and optimized cases (12,13). These questions were addressed by Stone and Fabian's randomized study that demonstrated better outcomes for repair rather than diversion, although they did exclude patients with extensive blood loss, organ damage, fecal contamination, or delay to operation (13). This study and the subsequent prospective randomized studies that supported these data led to increasing support for a single-staged procedure with primary anastomosis that continues today (14,15). Especially in the context of the recent military conflicts in Iraq and Afghanistan, however, management of colorectal trauma is still heavily debated and warrants continued appraisal and application of case-by-case decision-making (16). In this chapter, we focus on the management and controversies of the care of the patient with colorectal trauma.

## ETIOLOGY

The incidence, mechanism, and type of colorectal injury vary between civilian and combat settings. These traumas

have an incidence of somewhere between 1% and 3% in civilian trauma centers, and 5%–10% of those injured in combat (17). In both cohorts, penetrating injuries are most common (18,19). However, in war injuries, there is much greater concern for high-energy and blast mechanisms. These are far more important to consider, as they are often associated with concomitant damage to adjacent organs. In addition, the thermal injury that occurs with this type of mechanism often leads to a delay in the injury presentation, as it may evolve over time. What initially appears to be a normal appearing section of bowel adjacent to the wound may progress to more severe injury that warrants resection. Failure to recognize this injury pattern may contribute to subsequent complications. A recent series describing the epidemiology of colorectal trauma in Operation Iraqi Freedom and Operation Enduring Freedom found that 35% of colorectal injuries among combatants could be attributed to explosions or blasts, consistent with the widespread use of improvised explosive devices (16). While this mechanism of injury may also be seen in the civilian setting, especially in light of the more recent world events, the vast majority in the civilian sector are due to gunshot and stab wounds (15). Blunt trauma usually occurs in the context of motor vehicle crashes, and incidences are as infrequent as 0.02% in the civilian setting and 5% in war (20,21). Rectal injuries may also include accidental or intentional impalement, iatrogenic injury, secondary damage from bony fragments in a pelvic fracture, and insertion of foreign bodies, or with extensive perineal trauma (22) (Figure 40.2).

## PREOPERATIVE ASSESSMENT

As with all trauma patients, those with colorectal trauma are first evaluated for airway, breathing, and circulation issues, and assessed according to the Advanced Trauma Life Support primary and secondary surveys. Fluids and blood products are administered as needed. Additionally, patients with

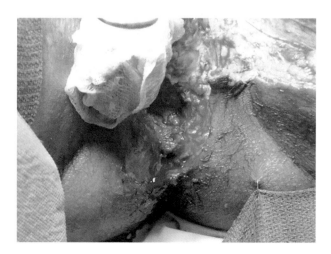

Figure 40.2 **(See color insert.)** Perineal injury.

life-threatening injuries (especially those with features of the "lethal triad" of acidosis, hypothermia, and coagulopathy) may be considered for urgent damage control laparotomy (DCL). Under this protocol, the patient undergoes a staged process of abbreviated laparotomy with control of hemostasis and fecal soilage, temporary closure, aggressive resuscitation in the intensive care unit, and a later operation for definitive repair or diversion after the patient has been stabilized (23). In the context of colorectal surgery, this approach has been particularly useful in patients with presacral bleeding and colorectal perforations (24), even in the setting of elective surgery. Patients not necessitating urgent laparotomy may undergo any of several diagnostic methods described in the following sections and summarized in Table 40.1.

## DIAGNOSIS OF COLON INJURIES

## PHYSICAL EXAMINATION

Depending on the severity and context of the injury at hand, conducting a physical examination may be impractical or have limited utility in establishing a definitive diagnosis, especially in those with blunt trauma (25). Examination is especially difficult in patients who are intoxicated, have neurological impairments, or have multisystem trauma. Potential pertinent positives may include evidence of penetrating wounds, peritoneal signs associated with hollow viscous perforation, "seat belt sign" ecchymosis in blunt injuries, signs of chance fracture, and gross blood on digital rectal exam (DRE) (7,26). While physical examination and thorough history when possible remain important first

steps in diagnosis, most colorectal injuries are identified intraoperatively or by other diagnostic techniques (27).

## DIAGNOSTIC PERITONEAL LAVAGE

Diagnostic peritoneal lavage (DPL) was first introduced by Root and colleagues in 1965 and is particularly applicable for the evaluation of hemodynamically unstable patients that are suspected to have blunt intraperitoneal colorectal trauma. While not performed as commonly as in the past, it still is a useful adjunct to obtain urgent information and stratify patients. Before proceeding with DPL, an attempt is made to aspirate free intraperitoneal fluid (the diagnostic peritoneal aspirate). If 10 mL or more of gross blood is aspirated, no further steps are taken because an injury is likely and exploration is often warranted. If not, the peritoneal cavity is lavaged with 1 L of either normal saline or lactated Ringer solution, and then the effluent fluid is evaluated. The lavage is considered positive if more than 100,000 red blood cells/mm$^3$ or 500 white blood cells/mm$^3$, bile, amylase, bacteria, or particulate matter are present on microscopic analysis. These patients necessitate laparotomy.

DPL is more sensitive than physical examination and is also rapid and inexpensive (27,28). The extremely high sensitivity, however, comes at the cost of false-positive results that may occur in the context of solid organ lacerations, retroperitoneal hematoma, or iatrogenic injury that results in nontherapeutic laparotomy (29). Additionally, because DPL is an invasive procedure, it may result in complications, such as intraabdominal organ or neurovascular damage (30). DPL is often contraindicated when the patient is pregnant. Care should be taken in the morbidly obese patient and in those with a prior laparotomy.

Table 40.1 Comparison of diagnostic techniques for colorectal injury

|  | Accuracy | Sensitivity | Specificity | Advantages | Disadvantages |
|---|---|---|---|---|---|
| DPL | 92%–98% | 87%–100% | 84%–98% | Inexpensive<br>Rapid<br>Mobile<br>Very sensitive<br>No radiation | Invasive<br>Misses retroperitoneal injury<br>Relatively low specificity |
| Abdominal CT | 82%–99% | 92%–98% | 97%–99% | Noninvasive<br>Very sensitive and specific<br>Identification of specific injury<br>Identification of concurrent extraabdominal injury<br>Not operator dependent | Expensive<br>Timely<br>Radiation exposure<br>Requires transport |
| FAST | 96%–98% | 73%–88% | 98%–100% | Inexpensive<br>Rapid<br>Mobile<br>Noninvasive<br>Highly specific<br>Allows for concurrent resuscitation<br>Can be repeated<br>No radiation | Interobserver variability<br>Can be hampered by obstruction of view (e.g., obesity, fractures, intraabdominal air)<br>Relatively low sensitivity |

## FOCUSED ABDOMINAL SONOGRAPHY FOR TRAUMA

As an alternative to DPL, a focused assessment with sonography for trauma (FAST) may be utilized for initial evaluation of a hemodynamically unstable blunt trauma patient. This technique may also be used for stable patients with both blunt and penetrating injuries, and involves ultrasound views of Morison's pouch (hepatorenal recess), the pouch of Douglas (retrovesical intraperitoneal cavity), the splenorenal space, and the pericardium. If an extended examination (E-FAST) is performed, bilateral hemithoracic and upper anterior chest wall views are also obtained. The ultrasound is positive if hemoperitoneum is observed. Similar to DPL, a positive FAST often requires laparotomy in the unstable patient. In the stable patient, the free fluid can be followed with other diagnostic imaging such as a computed tomography (CT) scan to look for solid organ injury that may not require a laparotomy.

FAST is easily accessible, can be performed while resuscitation is ongoing, is noninvasive, and is specific (27,31,32). It is safe for pregnant patients and children and may be repeated in serial investigations to potentially avoid DPL, CT, and/or laparotomy. However, because a positive exam relies on the presence of intraperitoneal fluid (for most operators, about 200 mL), sensitivity is decreased, and a CT scan should be obtained before a course of nonoperative management is begun (33,34). Finally, care should be taken for the patient with retroperitoneal fluid that may not be picked up as readily on FAST examination.

## COMPUTERIZED TOMOGRAPHY

CT is the imaging modality of choice for colorectal injury, typically used in the evaluation of hemodynamically stable patients who either had a positive FAST examination or went straight to CT. Views of the head, chest, abdomen, and pelvis with IV contrast are typically obtained in order to scan for multiple injuries.

The high levels of sensitivity, specificity, and accuracy in abdominal CT for blunt abdominal trauma have been well established in the literature (35–37). These values are somewhat decreased in the context of mesenteric injury and potentially in hollow viscous, where DPL may be more appropriate (27). Though CT requires more time and patient transport than FAST and DPL, it has the unique ability to detect occult injury and identify the specific lesion. Improvements in radiologic technology over time have decreased scan time and allowed for detection of more subtle signs of bowel injury. Findings that may indicate injury include thickening of the bowel wall, tearing of the bowel wall, abdominal free fluid or air, and mesenteric fat stranding (38). In addition, due to the availability of rapid thin-slice CT imaging, trajectory of projectile fragments or bullets can often be identified on CT (Figure 40.3).

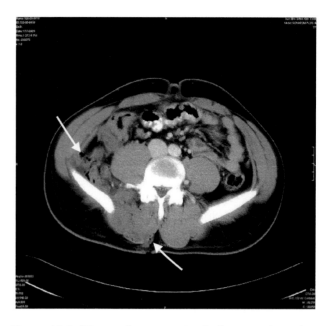

Figure 40.3 CT scan demonstrating bullet tract through the retroperitoneum (white arrows).

## DIAGNOSTIC LAPAROSCOPY

Laparoscopy is unique in that it may be used in both the diagnosis and minimally invasive treatment of colorectal traumas (Figure 40.4). Laparoscopic exploration following penetrating abdominal wounds is especially useful in detecting injuries missed by standard imaging (especially diaphragmatic), and also in minimizing rates of nontherapeutic laparotomy (39). A prospective study conducted by Lin et al. in 2010 found that the implementation of diagnostic laparoscopy decreased the nontherapeutic laparotomy rate from 58% to 0% in hemodynamically stable patients with abdominal stab wounds, with an accuracy of 100% (40). Similarly, a 2014 retrospective study by Lee et al. showed that 16% of their blunt abdominal trauma patients avoided unnecessary laparotomy when initially evaluated with laparoscopy (41). In select cases, surgeons who are experienced in advanced laparoscopic techniques may take the opportunity to address the injuries identified on diagnostic laparoscopy in a minimally invasive manner. Laparoscopy does

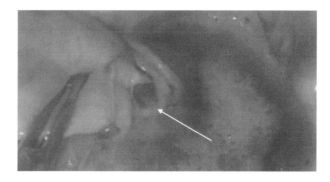

Figure 40.4 **(See color insert.)** Rectal injury identified on laparoscopy (white arrow).

come with the small risk for inducing tension pneumothorax, hypotension, or gas embolism (42). The role of laparoscopy in the diagnosis and treatment of colorectal trauma will likely evolve as the technology progresses and more surgeons gain expertise in the involved techniques.

## Diagnosis of rectal injuries

Diagnosis of rectal injuries is particularly complicated by the fact that they may occur in the context of trauma to the pelvic bone, which may need to be concomitantly addressed. DRE has classically been used in secondary survey to assess for sphincter tone, bleeding, or palpable injury to the rectal wall, but its use has become somewhat controversial as it has varying rates of sensitivity in detecting rectal injury (43,44). More accurately, the finding of gross blood, bone segments, or a palpable defect should indicate the need for other tests to definitively diagnose the injury. A negative DRE in the setting of other information that is potentially compatible with a rectal injury warrants further investigation. Comparing DRE to rigid sigmoidoscopy, sigmoidoscopy has been demonstrated to be more specific, especially in the context of extraperitoneal rectal lesions (45). Proctosigmoidoscopy, however, may have limited utility without a bowel preparation. Because there is little downside to DRE, the authors would still recommend DRE when possible for identification and treatment of injuries that may not be detected on imaging. Finally, because up to one-third of rectal injuries are accompanied by a genitourinary injury, a CT scan with both rectal and bladder contrast is often recommended in hemodynamically stable patients (21,46).

## Injury scales

As a means of standardizing the assessment of traumatic colorectal injury, several injury scales have been developed. The first was established by Flint and associates in 1981 and was used to classify which levels of injury could safely undergo primary repair versus colostomy (47). The Penetrating Abdominal Trauma Index (PATI) was developed the same year by Moore et al., and takes into account all injured intraabdominal organs and the severity of each injury (48). Most recently, the American Association for the Surgery of Trauma (AAST) developed a similar scale for all abdominal organs with the goal of further standardizing assessment for unifying research and management efforts (49). The AAST scales for colon and rectal injury can be seen in Table 40.2.

## MANAGEMENT OF COLON INJURY

## THE CONTROVERSY OF PRIMARY REPAIR

We have come a long way since the time of Ogilvie when exteriorization was standard and primary repair was mandated against, and primary repair is now the procedure of

Table 40.2 AAST colon and rectal injury scales

| Grade | Injury description |
|---|---|
| **Colon** | |
| I | (a) Contusion or hematoma without devascularization |
| | (b) Partial-thickness laceration |
| II | Laceration ≤50% of circumference |
| III | Laceration >50% of circumference |
| IV | Transection of the colon |
| V | Transection of the colon with segmental tissue loss |
| **Rectum** | |
| I | (a) Contusion or hematoma without devascularization |
| | (b) Partial-thickness laceration |
| II | Laceration ≤50% of circumference |
| III | Laceration >50% of circumference |
| IV | Full-thickness laceration with extension into the perineum |
| V | Devascularized segment |

choice for the majority of colon injuries. This was set into motion by the aforementioned Stone and Fabian's classic randomized trial that resulted in equivalent mortality between the primary repair and colostomy groups (1.5% versus 1.4%, $p > 0.05$), as well as increased morbidity and length of stay for patients in the colostomy group (13). Several prospective series since this study have demonstrated the favorable use of primary repair, resulting in safe and successful treatment of ~73%–85% of civilian injuries and a more uncertain range in the military setting (50–54). These studies have proven primary repair to have equivalent if not superior outcomes to diversion in most clinical scenarios.

Stone and Fabian's study, however, required mandatory colostomy for patients with extensive blood loss, organ damage, fecal contamination, or delay to operation in approximately half their cohort—thus eliminating the sickest of patients and preventing assessment of how these patients fare with primary repair. This issue was addressed by Chappuis et al., who only excluded patients who had a rectal injury rather than a colonic one. They found that complication rates were similar between the two groups, and concluded that primary repair could safely be performed in all civilian penetrating colon traumas; however, they did not report any statistics on their sample size of only 56 patients (55).

Since Chappuis and colleagues' study, there have been three major prospective randomized trials comparing primary repair and diversion while only excluding rectal injuries (56–58). Gonzalez et al. also published the results of the first 109 patients in their study 4 years prior but continued the study in an attempt to assess outcomes of repair of destructive injuries (57,59). The results of the subsequent

Table 40.3 Prospective randomized trials comparing primary repair and diversion for colon injury without exclusion based on risk factors

| Author (year) | Number of patients | Morbidity of primary repair, % | Morbidity of diversion, % | Other conclusions | Study weaknesses |
|---|---|---|---|---|---|
| Sasaki (1995) (56) | 71 | 19 | 36 | Broke primary repair group into resection and nonresection groups and found no differences | Small study sample; only 28 patients diverted |
| Gonzalez (2000) (57) | 176 | 18 | 21 | Patients with PATI score >25 have similar complication rates regardless of treatment modality | Only 9% of injuries were destructive |
| Kamwendo (2002) (58) | 240 | 26 | 18 | Delay from time of penetrating colon injury is not a contraindication to primary repair; primary repair is associated with shorter operation time and length of stay | Majority of injuries (80%) were due to low-energy gunshot |

study published in 2000 and the other two major randomized trials are summarized and compared in Table 40.3. Each of these studies showed similar complication rates between the two groups, with Sasaki and Gonzalez demonstrating lower rates in the primary repair group, and Kamwendo showing a statistically insignificant ($p = 0.21$) higher rate in the primary repair group. All three studies concluded in support of primary repair as the standard of care for penetrating colon injury.

Despite these data, uncertainty regarding the safety of a single-staged operation with primary anastomosis persisted. In 2003, a Cochrane meta-analysis of the previously mentioned randomized studies (plus a 1992 study by Falcone et al. that had stringent exclusion criteria similar to Stone and Fabian) was compiled to conduct a review of 361 patients in the primary repair group and 344 in the diversion group (60,61). This analysis found no difference in mortality, total infectious complications (odds ratio [OR] = 0.44; 95% confidence interval [CI], 0.17–1.1), abdominal infections including dehiscence (OR = 0.67; 95% CI, 0.35–1.3), or abdominal infections excluding dehiscence (OR = 0.69; 95% CI, 0.34–0.9) between primary repair versus diversion (61). Total complications (OR = 0.54; 95% CI, 0.39–0.76), and wound complications excluding dehiscence (OR = 0.43; 95% CI, 0.24–0.77) all significantly favored primary repair (61). Another meta-analysis conducted the year before the Cochrane Review that did not include the Kamwendo study, which was found to contribute heterogeneity to the Cochrane review, yielded ORs in favor of primary repair for each condition (62).

## THE ROLE OF RESECTION WITH ANASTOMOSIS OR DIVERSION

All of the randomized trials describe thus far classified all surgeries that occurred in one operation with anastomosis

as a "primary repair," without distinguishing a direct anastomosis from one requiring resection before restoring continuity. The Sasaki et al. study did conduct a subanalysis where the primary repair group was separated by resection versus no resection, and found no differences between the two groups (56). However, there were only 29 patients in the resection group and 24 patients in the nonresection group. As suggested by the development of injury scales, stratifying colon injuries by the extent of damage may be helpful in determining whether primary repair with no resection, resection with primary anastomosis, or resection with diversion is the most suitable management for the patient at hand (see Colon Algorithm, Figure 40.5).

First, it is helpful to distinguish whether the colon injury is nondestructive or destructive. A nondestructive injury is one that would be classified as grades I–III on the AAST colon injury scale (63). Based on the findings of the randomized trials and reviews of these studies conducted throughout the years, ample evidence supports the safety and efficacy of primary repair without resection or diversion for nondestructive trauma to the colon. This was further supported by a 2003 Maxwell and Fabian review of prospective and retrospective studies of civilian colon injury that separately analyzed nondestructive and destructive wounds, showing that primary repair with minimal amounts of debridement was clearly the treatment of choice for nondestructive injuries (64). For these patients, the overall complication rate was 14% in the primary repair group and 30% in the colostomy group, and intraabdominal abscess rates were 4.9% and 12%, respectively (64).

Destructive wounds, on the other hand, typically require some degree of resection, as a result of transection of the bowel or devascularization due to mesenteric injury. Because most of the prospective studies conducted through the early 2000s did not include a substantial amount of destructive

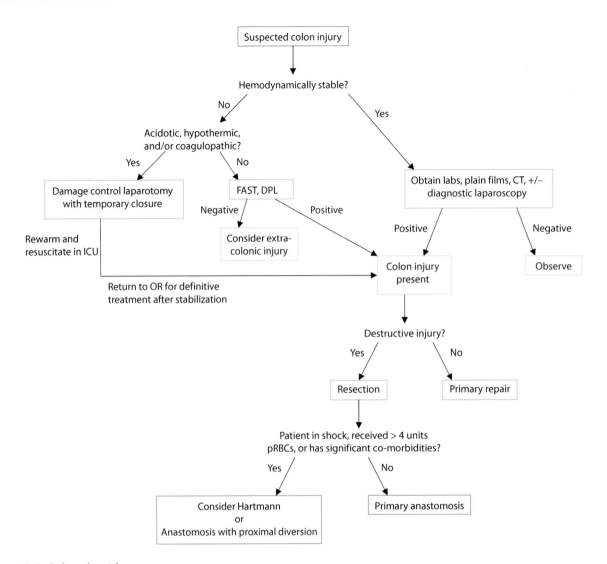

Figure 40.5 Colon algorithm.

injuries, it was less clear if primary repair was just as safe and effective for these patients as for those with nondestructive injuries. In 2001, Demetriades and colleagues published a landmark study that, though not randomized, prospectively evaluated the outcomes of resection with primary anastomosis versus diversion for 297 patients with destructive colon injuries (15). Treatment was determined at the surgeon's discretion, resulting in two-thirds of patients treated with primary anastomosis and one-third with diversion. There was lower colon-related mortality in the primary anastomosis group (0% versus 4%, $p = 0.012$), and similar rates of abdominal complications (22% versus 27%, $p = 0.373$). Univariate analysis demonstrated that severe fecal contamination, transfusion requiring greater than 4 units of packed red blood cells within the first 24 hours, and single-agent antibiotic prophylaxis were all independently associated with increased complications. However, when controlling for these risk factors on multivariate analysis comparing primary anastomosis with diversion, there was no significant difference in risk for complications. They also found no differences between the two treatment arms when

controlling for the traditional risk factors described in the literature, such as shock, transfusion >6 units of packed red blood cells, PATI score >25, and delay to operation >6 hours. Thirteen patients in the primary repair cohort experienced an anastomotic leak, and one patient in the diversion group had a leak from the Hartmann pouch. No patients died from leak, and no risk factors were identified for leak. The authors of this study concluded that all destructive colon injuries requiring resection should be managed with primary repair regardless of risk factors present.

There remain adamant supporters on either side of the argument for primary anastomosis versus either proximal diversion or Hartmann, especially for destructive colon injuries in patients with the traditional risk factors. Rather than universally implementing primary repair regardless of risk factors, some have attempted to standardize a clinical algorithm based on the presence of potential risk factors for anastomotic leak and/or mortality related to suture line failure. Stewart et al. found that patients with destructive wounds that also received >6 units of packed red blood cells and/or had significant comorbid conditions were had a 42%

risk for leak, while their healthy counterparts who did not require massive transfusion had a leak rate of just 3% (65). Furthermore, one-third of patients suffering a leak died. Considering these concerning data, this institution implemented a clinical pathway, whereby patients with destructive injuries and either significant comorbid conditions or >6 unit transfusion were treated with end colostomy and those with destructive injury but without either of these conditions were treated with resection and primary repair (50). By following this algorithm, the authors were able to reduce their overall leak rate from 14% to 3%, as well as decrease their abscess and mortality rates. Despite the clear improvements made by this series, conflicting data continue to emerge that still support routine primary repair regardless of any patient risk factors (66). The authors believe that diversion is still useful in select cases, and that the judgement of an experienced surgeon is required on a case-by-case basis to choose between primary repair and diversion. The risk factors shown in some of the literature, technical issues encountered during the case, and circumstances unique to each patient must be considered when weighing treatment options.

Of note, there are important differences between civilian and military colon traumas, but primary repair is still applicable to combat injuries. As stated, these patients are more likely to have trauma involving high-energy mechanisms, have multiple associated injuries, and have burns, and care should be taken to consider the evolution of the injury over time. The limitations of treatment in some combat settings also pose challenges as compared to civilian trauma centers, with limited supplies and prolonged transport time often required. Considering these factors, primary anastomosis has thus far been utilized less frequently in the military setting than in civilian traumas and has been encouraged to be approached with increased caution (67,68). However, when implemented appropriately, similar results may be obtained to those in the civilian literature. A 2007 study of Operation Iraqi Freedom colorectal trauma patients from 2003 to 2004 showed that diversion was associated with lower leak rates compared to primary anastomosis, but rates of sepsis and mortality did not differ between the two groups (54).

## DAMAGE CONTROL

The concept of damage control has been useful in preventing the rapid decline of patients that are acidotic, hypothermic, and coagulopathic in order to avoid the lethal triad. After an abbreviated procedure for control of hemorrhage and prevention of further intraabdominal contamination, the patient is taken to the ICU for stabilization, re-warming, and resuscitation. Not only does this save the patient from deteriorating, but it also permits time for the surgeon to decide if an anastomosis or diversion will be performed in the subsequent operation. This protocol was first elaborated by Rotondo et al. in 1993, based on the experience of the Navy with damaged ships, and proved to be a promising methodology to improve morbidity and mortality in an initially unstable state (69).

The literature describing long-term outcomes of patients undergoing repair of colon injury after damage control surgery is sparse, lacking randomized studies. The current set of reviews of DCL patients yields conflicting data, with some studies suggesting that restoration of continuity is unsafe after DCL, and others that repair after DCL is equivalent to a single operation. It is important to note that patients undergoing DCL have been shown to have higher leak rates, increased risk of ventral hernia, and more colon-related complications than those who undergo repair by a single laparotomy (both primary repair or resection with anastomosis or diversion) (70,71). Another study also showed higher leak rates in the DCL group, but still concluded that it was a safe option (72). Miller and associates found no leaks in the DCL group and one in the primary repair group, and no differences in abscess rates and overall survival between the patients who underwent anastomosis versus diversion after DCL (73). A more recent study concluded that anastomosis in DCL patients is feasible if completed during the first operation post-DCL, but anastomoses performed beyond this point are associated with an eight times greater risk of leak compared to those in single laparotomy and first operation post-DCL patients (74).

There are even fewer studies detailing DCL in the military setting, but it has been shown to minimize complication rates for severely injured patients (19). Despite the varying data that exist, damage control laparotomy remains a useful strategy for improving outcomes of rapidly deteriorating patients and delaying decision-making regarding definitive repair of the colon. This may be particularly relevant for treating some of the high-energy and blast injuries encountered especially in the battlefield (Figure 40.6).

## COLOSTOMY CLOSURE

It has classically been thought that diversion is a "safer" option as compared to primary anastomosis, especially in hemodynamically unstable patients with increased comorbidities. However, colostomy creation and takedown are

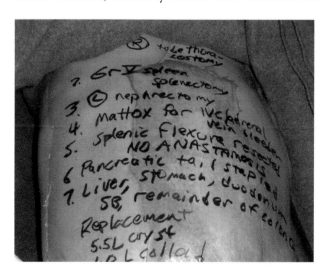

Figure 40.6 (See color insert.) Damage control laparotomy in a combat environment.

procedures that are not without risks of their own. In a 2000 review of 311 patients admitted for penetrating trauma to the colon at a level I urban trauma center, ostomy creation was found to be one of the most significant risk factors for postoperative complications on both univariate ($p < 0.0001$) and multivariate ($p = 0.004$) analysis (75).

Patients who have a complicated initial procedure have been shown to also be more likely to experience complications after colostomy closure, especially if performed within 3 months of the trauma (76). The rates of complications associated with colostomy closure reported in the literature vary greatly, anywhere from 5% to 55% but most somewhere around 20%–30% and some studies showing lower complication rates with loop compared to end colostomies (77–80). Pertinent complications include enterotomy, wound infection and dehiscence, anastomotic leakage and stricture, enterocutaneous fistula, ileus, and ventral hernia. The fact that an additional operation and hospital stay are required for reversal also increases costs associated with colostomy. Although the timing of reversal remains controversial, same-admission reversals may be an effective strategy to reduce costs while also minimizing complications (81). In summary, while there is certainly a role for diversion, the morbidity associated with not only colostomy creation but also takedown must also be considered when deciding against primary anastomosis.

## SUMMARY: COLON INJURIES

Patients with traumatic colon injuries can often be managed by in-continuity methods (i.e., primary resection, resection with primary anastomosis). Patients should first be evaluated for hemodynamic stability, and if needed, undergo a damage control laparotomy followed by resuscitation and secondary laparotomy when stabilized. Complications may still occur, but sound technique and good surgical judgment are required when confronted with colon injuries.

## MANAGEMENT OF RECTAL INJURY

## COMPARING TO COLON INJURY

In general, the diagnosis and management of rectal injury are more complex than that of colon injury for several reasons. Because the rectum is largely protected by the pelvic bones and surrounding soft tissue, it is less likely to sustain injury; when injury does occur, however, these barriers make exposure and treatment of the affected area much more difficult. Additionally, the rectum has both intraperitoneal and extraperitoneal portions. In general, the same principles for management of colon injuries discussed previously can be applied to intraperitoneal rectal injuries, but lower rectal injuries have different diagnostic and management implications. Finally, the close proximity of the rectum to the genitourinary system requires a high index of suspicion for concurrent injuries to these organs and to the surrounding bony pelvis and major vasculature as well. This makes the principles of damage control laparotomy especially pertinent to rectal injury (82).

## THE FOUR D'S

While the management of rectal injuries has evolved on a timeline similar to colon injuries, the adoption of primary repair has been somewhat slowed and wary due to the paucity of class I data evaluating the outcomes of management of rectal trauma. Classically, the surgical treatment of rectal injury has been based on "the four D's": diversion, drainage, distal washout, and direct repair when feasible. The use of these four pillars was supported by reduced mortality in a study of rectal injuries during the Vietnam War, but the study included just 29 patients considering the rare nature of the injury (83). Each of these components, which have been considered central dogma for the treatment of rectal trauma, has been challenged in the subsequent literature, but small sample sizes, lack of randomized control trials, and conflicting results have made coming to a uniform consensus quite difficult. A summary of the data reviewed for the 2016 Eastern Association for the Surgery of Trauma (EAST) guidelines on the management of penetrating extraperitoneal rectal injury can be found in Table 40.4.

### Diversion

Similar to decision-making for the approach to colon management, considering the extent and location of the rectal damage as well as the overall stability of the patient can be used to determine when diversion versus primary anastomosis is most appropriate (see Rectal Algorithm, Figure 40.7). As with colon injury, primary repair should be considered for nondestructive intraperitoneal rectal injury, but resection is necessary with destructive injury. Primary anastomosis is an option for the otherwise healthy and hemodynamically stable patient, but those with comorbidities or hemodynamic instability should be diverted (84,85).

In general, at least some form of diversion is considered necessary in the context of the majority of extraperitoneal rectal injuries in both civilian and military cases. This is largely because diversion has been confirmed to be safe and effective for rectal injury, while studies describing repair without any diversion are few, and conclusions are based mainly on class III data. A 2006 prospective study conducted by Gonzalez et al. managed 14 patients with nondestructive extraperitoneal rectal injuries without fecal stream diversion, with no infectious complications related to the rectal defect (86). This management style is yet to become common practice as these results have not been replicated in any substantial sample size or in a randomized study, while several larger studies have demonstrated consistent sepsis rates <33% and mortality rates <7% in the context of stoma placement (67,87–91). Colostomy creation may be even more

Table 40.4 Data reviewed in the 2016 EAST guidelines for penetrating extraperitoneal rectal injury

|  | Number of studies | Number of patients | Mortality, % | Infectious complications, % |  |
|---|---|---|---|---|---|
| Diversion versus repair | 14 | 549 |  |  | Proximal diversion |
|   Diversion |  | 523 | 1.7 | 8.8 |  |
|   Primary repair + no diversion |  | 26 | 0 | 18.2 |  |
| Drainage versus no drainage | 17 | 653 |  |  | No drainage |
|   Drainage |  | 388 | 1.8 | 9.3 |  |
|   No drainage |  | 265 | 0.75 | 6.1 |  |
| Washout versus no washout | 13 | 487 |  |  | No washout |
| Washout |  | 200 | 1 | 11 |  |
| No washout |  | 287 | 1.4 | 11.5 |  |

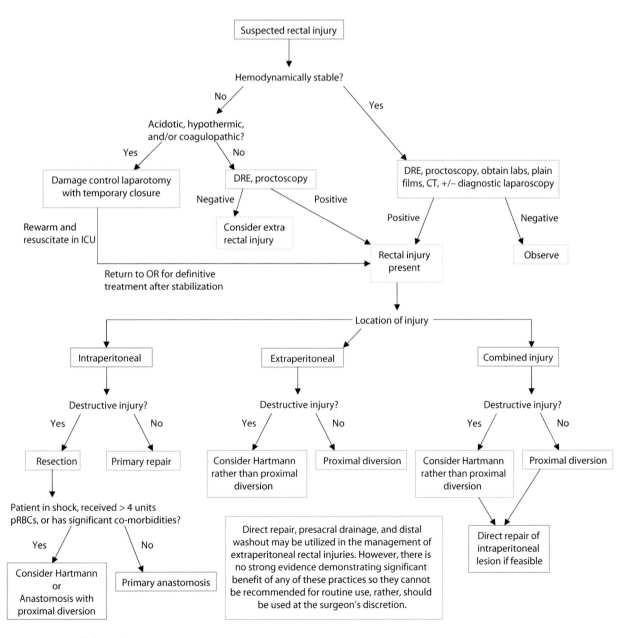

Figure 40.7 Rectal algorithm.

crucial in the military setting, where injury severity is often escalated, and multiple traumas are sustained simultaneously (16,67).

The type of diversion performed is dependent on both the extent of the injury, the skill and experience of the surgeon, and whether or not the stoma is to be reversed in the future. Considering the increased morbidity and mortality associated with reversal of colostomy after a Hartmann procedure, loop ostomy diversion is preferable when feasible (92–94). However, if there is significant damage to the sigmoid and/or rectum, a Hartmann procedure is often necessitated (89).

## Direct repair

It is generally accepted that rectal wounds that are intraperitoneal should be repaired, because they can easily be accessed without major dissection. Furthermore, intraperitoneal wounds can be treated similar to colon injuries as previously discussed. Extraperitoneal lesions, however, are less amenable to repair and require significant operative time. Therefore, the potential benefits of repair are often outweighed by the risks, and it is generally accepted that extraperitoneal injury repair should not be attempted unless the wound is easily visualized and requires minimal dissection (95–97).

Whether or not a diversion is performed may also dictate whether or not direct repair of the rectal wound is necessary. When the fecal stream is diverted away from the rectum, the risk of infectious complications is minimized, and foregoing direct repair has been shown to have no correlation with infection (88,97). This was demonstrated in a study by Weinberg et al. that followed an algorithm by which intraperitoneal rectal injuries treated with primary repair, extraperitoneal injury to the proximal two-thirds or accessible distal segments of the rectum were managed with direct repair and diversion, and inaccessible injuries to the distal one-third were managed with proximal diversion and presacral drainage without direct repair (85). Following this clinical pathway, they were able to reduce the incidence of infectious complications by 50%. Others have attempted primary repair of an accessible rectal injury without proximal diversion, demonstrating no associated morbidity but only in very small sample sizes (96).

## Drainage

Presacral drainage is one of the other classic pillars of extraperitoneal rectal injury management, but this practice has also been supported by only weak evidence and has been proven futile in other studies. Drains allow for extraction of contaminated fluid or blood but also involve the invasive nature of drain placement. While older studies of combat trauma demonstrated decreased rates of pelvic infection with drain placement, more recent studies have concluded that drainage does not significantly reduce infection rates and is not as imperative as once thought (98). Similar to the train of thought for the role of direct repair, drainage is even less useful in the context of a stoma.

The largest retrospective study conducted thus far reviewed 92 patients with rectal injuries, 86 of which received a proximal colostomy. None of these patients had a drain placed, the infection rate was just 10%, and there was no incidence of sepsis (99). Similar results have been obtained by other reviews (100,101). Additionally, a randomized control trial was conducted by Gonzalez et al. in which all 48 patients were diverted but 23 received a drain and 25 did not. Infectious complications occurred in just 4% of the no-drain group and 8% of the drain group, leading the authors to conclude in favor of omission of presacral drainage in most cases (102). This practice may still be useful in the setting of large destructive wounds with increased serosanguinous fluid drainage into the pelvis.

## Distal washout

Distal washout involves either a washout from below or on-table lavage through a separate injury, colotomy, or appendectomy opening (Figure 40.8). Although distal rectal irrigation was initially implemented for fear of leaving remaining stool to act as a substrate for sepsis, opponents of this practice argue that forcing fluid into the rectum may actually facilitate spread of feces and bacteria into previously uncontaminated planes. With little benefit attributable to washout, most surgeons have abandoned this component of management. The majority of data evaluating the outcomes of washout are retrospective in nature, but most studies in the last two decades have shown no significant decrease in morbidity associated with distal washout, and EAST similarly recommends against it (91,97,103).

## SUMMARY: RECTAL INJURY

Rectal injuries need to be stratified by the location—intra- versus extraperitoneal. Intraperitoneal injuries can often be treated as colon injuries, with the same issues of need for primary repair, resection, or diversion, along with the DCL. Extraperitoneal injuries often still require diversion. Drainage, direct repair, and distal washout are more controversial. The senior author prefers to avoid washout from above and simply remove the gross stool where possible; direct repair only when easy and directly amenable (foregoing extensive dissection to get at the site of injury), and drainage only when the area is open (avoiding making new planes to place drains).

## OTHER STRATEGIES TO MINIMIZE INFECTION IN COLORECTAL TRAUMA

Patients with penetrating abdominal trauma, especially when the colon and rectum are affected, are almost the perfect hosts for infection. Discontinuity of the gastrointestinal tract allows for microbial translocation, ischemic tissue and retained fragments allow for seeding and growth of

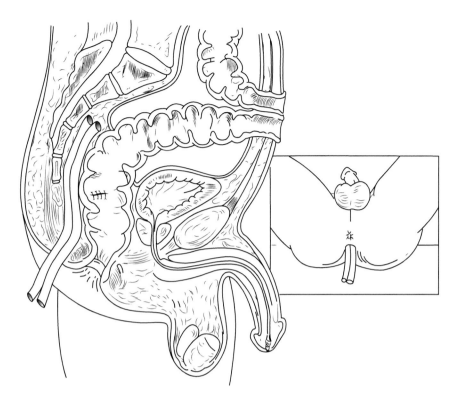

Figure 40.8 Rectal washout.

organisms, and a patient with sustained blood loss in shock will have an impaired immune response (104). Therefore, extra precaution must be taken to prevent infectious complications in these trauma patients. There are several strategies that are commonly described in the literature and are typically recommended in these cases.

Aggressive wound debridement should be undertaken at the time of surgery. The goal is to remove all of the necrotic and nonviable tissue, and then clean the wound with irrigation using normal saline or sterile water (105). At this point in time, any retained fragments from the penetrating weapon that are visualized should also be carefully removed. These foreign objects may serve as a foundation for abscess formation, thus increasing the risk for sepsis if left in the abdominal cavity (106). After these procedures, the abdominal skin wound is usually left open to heal by secondary intent in order to prevent surgical site infection (107).

The use of prophylactic antibiotics in this setting has been well described and supported by sufficient class I and class II data. The cornerstone for antibiotic therapy in colorectal trauma is preoperative administration of broad-spectrum IV antibiotics with anaerobic coverage continued for up to 24 hours. The accumulation of high-quality data supporting this tenant has led to recommendations in both the civilian and military sectors that are widely accepted (105,108). Following these guidelines can minimize the rate of postoperative infection to just 11% (109). A single-drug regimen is typically adequate for nondestructive injuries, but more extensive wounds may benefit from combination therapy (15,110). The administration of antibiotics for longer than 24 hours has not been shown to add any benefit, even in the context of DCL or high-risk patients (111–113). It is important to not prolong antibiotic use so as to avoid promotion of antibiotic-resistant strains (114).

## ANORECTAL FOREIGN BODIES

In this section, we cover anorectal foreign bodies. The reader is encouraged to review other extensive reviews on this topic by the senior author including an UpToDate discussion on management (available at www.UpToDate.com). Retained foreign bodies in the rectum are encountered relatively infrequently, but diagnosis and management are complicated by the vast array of objects that may be found and the potential damage that each object can cause. Examples of items recovered are drugs, torches, broomsticks, aerosol cans, pipes, vibrators, a variety of foods, light bulbs, knives, enema tips, and more. Most of the literature represents single-center case studies, but a recent Nationwide Inpatient Sample (NIS) database review identified 3,359 cases with a primary diagnosis of rectal foreign body between 2009 and 2011 (115). The majority of patients presenting in these cases are men, with published studies showing between 65% and 100% of their sample to be men (116). Most patients are between ages 30 and 40, but patients as old as 90 have been reported (117–119).

Placement of the foreign object is typically classified as voluntary versus involuntary, and/or sexual versus nonsexual. Examples of scenarios and objects typical for each category can be found in Table 40.5. A 2010 systematic review of colorectal foreign bodies in 193 patients found that sexual activity was implicated in 49% of cases, iatrogenic injury following self-treatment for anorectal pathology in 25% of cases, self-insertion in the mentally ill in 5%, and accidents or assaults in the remaining 21% of cases (120). The injury may also be classified by the AAST rectal injury scale (Table 40.2), but the majority of foreign body–related injuries are grade I or less commonly grade II (116,118).

Obtaining an accurate history is often challenging in these instances, as it is not uncommon for patients to feel embarrassed and reluctant to disclose all relevant information. The physician must also be prepared for the possibility of providing emotional support and a safe environment for rape and assault victims. Most patients will present on the day of or several days after insertion of the object, but some will wait months, making careful examination and removal even more imperative (120). Patients may report constipation, anorectal or abdominal pain, bright red blood per rectum, or anal mucous discharge. Physical examination findings will vary depending on the location of the object and the degree of injury caused. The item may be palpated in the lower quadrants of the abdomen if located more proximally, or may be visualized or palpable upon DRE if more distal. Gross blood may be found, and in cases of sphincter injury, tone will be decreased on DRE. If the rectum has been perforated above the peritoneal reflection, there may be peritoneal signs. When foreign-body placement is suspected but has not been disclosed by the patient, the physician should directly inquire about this possibility in a nonconfrontational and nonjudgmental manner—emphasizing the importance of obtaining details regarding the object, timing, and circumstances of the insertion in order to best proceed with management.

Diagnosis is typically established using plain film radiographs to identify the object and rule out pneumoperitoneum. Pneumoperitoneum, hypotension, fever, tachycardia, and peritoneal signs indicate perforation. In this case, the patient should be immediately resuscitated and broad-spectrum antibiotics should be administered. If the patient is stable enough for CT, this may be useful in locating the site of rectal perforation. Patients with an intraperitoneal perforation of the rectum or distal colon require laparotomy, and the approach to repair follows the same guidelines as the trauma management algorithms discussed previously (121). Extraperitoneal perforations may be managed more conservatively (122).

In most cases, the patient is stable without perforation and may be managed nonoperatively. The majority of foreign bodies can be removed transanally at the bedside (120,121). Patient relaxation can be encouraged with the use of a perianal nerve block or conscious sedation. Additionally, Foley catheter inflation, clamps, obstetric vacuum extractors, and endoscopy may be utilized to help retrieve the object if manual manipulation is not successful. If this becomes challenging, the patient may be asked to perform a Valsalva maneuver or can be admitted and observed to allow the object to descend distally. When none of these techniques facilitate removal of the object, then transfer to the operating room and use of general anesthesia or spinal anesthetic may be required. The goal is to milk the object distally so that it may be accessed transanally. Some surgeons have utilized laparoscopy to achieve this (123,124). Finally, if none of these approaches are successful, then colotomy must be performed to remove the object.

In general, patients with anorectal foreign bodies recover without major complications. However, there have been cases of sepsis and even death reported in severe cases with perforation (125). Patients with perforation may require diversion, which facilitates subsequent operation for reversal. Finally, injury to the sphincters can result in long-term fecal incontinence or require sphincterotomy (126–128).

Table 40.5 Classification of anorectal foreign bodies and common presentations of each

| | Common patient profile/objects |
| --- | --- |
| Sexual + voluntary | Vibrators and dildos most commonly, but many other objects have been implicated in these scenarios |
| Sexual + involuntary | Rape or assault victims, sodomy with a variety of objects |
| Nonsexual + voluntary | Body packing with illicit drugs or illegal paraphernalia |
| Nonsexual + involuntary | Children following ingestion of plastic objects or utensils. Ingestion of bones from food. Mentally ill patients. Iatrogenic injury, retained thermometers or enema tips |

## ANAL SPHINCTER AND PERINEAL INJURY

Anal sphincter injury occurs most commonly in the setting of obstetric trauma but may also result from anorectal foreign-body placement or iatrogenic during anorectal operations (129). The extent of the injury determines management strategy, as described by Hellinger (130). Superficial injuries may be debrided, and if the extent of injury is limited to minimal damage to the internal sphincter, it may be left unrepaired. Destructive injuries often mandate proximal diversion and repair of the sphincter damage. This was classically achieved with end-to-end direct apposition of the anal sphincters, but more recently the practice of overlapping sphincteroplasty has been introduced (129). Surgeon preferences and data literature on method of repair vary, but end-to-end apposition may be more effective in acute scenarios, while overlap may be suitable for delayed repairs (131). More advanced techniques include sphincter reconstruction with the gluteal and gracilis muscles, as well as construction of artificial sphincter systems (132–134). These methods are complex and have variable success and fecal incontinence rates, and they should only be attempted by surgeons in a delayed setting with extensive training and experience with these procedures. Ultimately, up to 10% of sphincter repairs may degenerate in the long term, and fecal incontinence rates vary from study to study and may be underestimated, as this is a difficult endpoint to ascertain from patient interviews (135,136). The timing of this procedure is variable and somewhat controversial. Often the injury and surrounding tissues are not amenable to repair at the time of the surgery and are best left alone to attempt definitive repair at a later date. To divert at the time of the initial injury also is variable, but discussion with the patient should be performed ahead of time when possible.

Complex perineal injuries may be associated with more life-threatening conditions such as hemorrhage and pelvic fracture. Management of these issues takes priority over repair of any sphincter damage, and the principles of Advanced Trauma Life Support as well as damage control surgery apply when needed. A review of these rare, complex clinical scenarios was published by Kudsk and Hannah in 2003, demonstrating an overall mortality rate of 32%, and 21% pelvic sepsis rate (137). The initial surgical goals should be pelvic fixation and control of hemorrhage, and fecal diversion with wound debridement and irrigation can be addressed during later return to the operating room after stabilization. Wound coverage and restoration of sphincter function are long-term goals.

# REFERENCES

1. Welling DR, Duncan JE. *Clin Colon Rectal Surg.* 2008; 21(1):45–52.
2. Bennett J. *J R Soc Med.* 1991;84:554–7.
3. Wallace C. *Lancet.* 1917;(ii):561–8.
4. Bowlby A. *Br Med J.* 1917;I:705–21.
5. Perry WB et al. *Semin Colon Rectal Surg.* 2005;15(2):70–9.
6. Ogilvie W. *Surg Gyn Obs.* 1944;78(2):225–38.
7. Steele SR et al. *Dis Colon Rectum.* 2011;54(9):1184–201.
8. Hughes L. *Br J Surg.* 1969;56(3):169–72.
9. MacFarlane C et al. *J R Army Med Corps.* 2002;148(1):27–31.
10. Ganchrow MI et al. *Arch Surg.* 1970;100(4):515–20.
11. Aldrete JS et al. *Ann Surg.* 1970;172(6):1007–14.
12. LoCicero J et al. *J Trauma.* 1975;15(7):575–9.
13. Stone HH, Fabian TC. *Ann Surg.* 1979;190(4):430–6.
14. Morken JJ et al. *Surgery.* 1999;126(4):693–700.
15. Demetriades D et al. *J Trauma.* 2001;50(5):765–75.
16. Glasgow SC et al. *J Trauma Acute Care Surg.* 2012;73(6 Suppl 5):S503–8.
17. Johnson EK, Steele SR. *J Gastrointest Surg.* 2013;17(9):1712–9.
18. Hatch Q et al. *Surgery.* 2013;154(2):397–403.
19. Cho SD et al. *Dis Colon Rectum.* 2010;53(5): 728–34.
20. Causey M et al. *Clin Colon Rectal Surg.* 2012;25(4): 189–99.
21. Perry WB. Trauma of the colon, rectum, and anus. In: Steele SR, Hull TL, Read TE, Saclarides TJ, Senagore AJ, Whitlow CB (eds.) *The ASCRS Textbook of Colon and Rectal Surgery.* Cham, Switzerland: Springer International, 2016, pp. 735–47.
22. Herzig D. *Clin Colon Rectal Surg.* 2012;25(4):210–3.
23. Shapiro MB et al. *J Trauma.* 2000;49(5):969–78.
24. McPartland KJ, Hyman NH. *Dis Colon Rectum.* 2003; 46(7):981–6.
25. Schurink GW et al. *Injury.* 1997;28(4):261–5.
26. Chandler CF et al. *Am Surg.* 1997;63(10):885–8.
27. Hoff WS et al. *J Trauma.* 2002;53(3):602–15.
28. Blow O et al. *J Trauma Acute Care Surg.* 1998;44(2): 287–90.
29. Liu M et al. *J Trauma.* 1993;35(2):267–70.
30. Davis JW et al. *J Trauma.* 1990;30(12):1506–9.
31. Smith IM et al. *Ann Surg.* 2015;262(2):389–96.
32. Rozycki GS et al. *J Trauma.* 1995;39(3):492–500.
33. Branney SW et al. *J Trauma.* 1995;39(2):375–80.
34. Udobi KF et al. *J Trauma.* 2001;50(3):475–9.
35. Malhotra A et al. *J Trauma.* 2000;48(6):991–1000.
36. Butela ST et al. *Am J Roentgenol.* 2001;176(1): 129–35.
37. Shanmuganathan K et al. *Am J Roentgenol.* 2001; 177(6):1247–56.
38. Killeen KL et al. *J Trauma.* 2001;51(1):26–36.
39. Powell BS et al. *Injury.* 2008;39(5):530–4.
40. Lin HF et al. *World J Surg.* 2010;34(7):1653–62.
41. Lee PC et al. *Surg Innov.* 2014;21(2):155–65.
42. Villavicencio RT, Aucar JA. *J Am Coll Surg.* 1999; 189(1):11–20.
43. Shlamovitz GZ et al. *Ann Emerg Med.* 2007;50(1): 25–33.
44. Esposito T et al. *Int Braz J Urol.* 2006;32(1):107–9.
45. Hargraves MB et al. *Am Surg.* 2009;75(11):1069–72.
46. Anderson SW, Soto JA. *Semin Ultrasound, CT MRI.* 2008;29(6):472–82.
47. Flint LM et al. *Ann Surg.* 1981;193(5):619–23.
48. Moore E et al. *J Trauma.* 1981;21(6):439–45.
49. Moore EE et al. *J Trauma.* 1990;30(11):1427–9.
50. Miller PR et al. *Ann Surg.* 2002;235(6):775–81.
51. Baako BN. *West Afr J Med.* 1998;17(2):109–12.
52. Hudolin T, Hudolin I. *Br J Surg.* 2005;92(5):643–7.
53. Uravic M et al. *Mil Med.* 2000;165(3):186–8.
54. Steele SR et al. *Dis Colon Rectum.* 2007;50(6):870–7.
55. Chappuis CW et al. *Ann Surg.* 1991;213(5):492–8.
56. Sasaki LS et al. *J Trauma.* 1995;39(5):895–901.
57. Gonzalez RP et al. *Am Surg.* 2000;66(4):342–7.
58. Kamwendo NY et al. *Br J Surg.* 2002;89(8):993–8.
59. Gonzalez RP et al. *J Trauma.* 1996;41(2):271–5.
60. Falcone RE et al. *Dis Colon Rectum.* 1992;35(10):957–63.

61. Nelson RL, Singer M. *Cochrane Database Syst Rev.* 2003;(3):CD002247.

62. Singer MA, Nelson RL. *Dis Colon Rectum.* 2002;45(12): 1579–87.

63. Choi WJ. *J Korean Soc Coloproctol.* 2011;27(4): 166–72.

64. Maxwell RA, Fabian TC. *World J Surg.* 2003;27(6): 632–9.

65. Stewart RM et al. *Am J Surg.* 1994;168(4):316–9.

66. Dubose J. *J Gastrointest Surg.* 2009;13(3):403–4.

67. Duncan JE et al. *J Trauma.* 2008;64(4):1043–7.

68. Sambasivan CN et al. *Am Surg.* 2011;77(12):1685–91.

69. Rotondo MF et al. *J Trauma.* 1993;35(3):375–83.

70. Weinberg J et al. *J Trauma.* 2009;67(5):929–35.

71. Brenner M et al. *Arch Surg.* 2011;146(4):395–9.

72. Kashuk JL et al. *Surgery.* 2009;146(4):663–70.

73. Miller PR et al. *Am Surg.* 2007;73(6):606–9.

74. Anjaria DJ et al. *J Trauma Acute Care Surg.* 2014; 76(3):594–600.

75. Dente CJ et al. *J Trauma.* 2000;49(4):628–37.

76. Sola JE et al. *Injury.* 1993;24(7):438–40.

77. Parks SE, Hastings PR. *Am J Surg.* 1985;149(5):672–5.

78. Pachter HL et al. *J Trauma.* 1990;30(12):1510–3.

79. Berne JD et al. *Surgery.* 1998;123(2):157–64.

80. Pokorny H et al. *Arch Surg.* 2005;140(10):956–60.

81. Khalid MS et al. *Surgeon.* 2005;3(1):11–4.

82. Arthurs Z et al. *Am J Surg.* 2006;191(5):604–9.

83. Lavenson GS, Cohen A. *Am J Surg.* 1971;122(2): 226–30.

84. Herr MW, Gagliano RA. *Curr Surg.* 2005;62(2):187–92.

85. Weinberg J et al. *J Trauma.* 2006;60(3):508–14.

86. Gonzalez RP et al. *J Trauma.* 2006;61(4):815–9.

87. Ivatury RR et al. *Am Surg.* 1991;57(1):50–5.

88. Velmahos GC et al. *World J Surg.* 2000;24(1):114–8.

89. Merlino JI, Reynolds HL. *Semin Colon Rectal Surg.* 2005;15(2):95–104.

90. Bostick PJ et al. *J Natl Med Assoc.* 1993;85(6):460–3.

91. Burch JM et al. *Ann Surg.* 1989;209(5):600–11.

92. Sharma A et al. *Color Dis.* 2013;15(4):458–62.

93. Ince M et al. *Color Dis.* 2012;14(8):492–8.

94. Mosdell DM, Doberneck RC. *Am J Surg.* 1991;162(6): 633–7.

95. Tuggle D, Huber PJ. *Am J Surg.* 1984;148(6):806–8.

96. Levine JH et al. *Am J Surg.* 1996;172(5):575–9.

97. Mcgrath V et al. *Am Surg.* 1998;64(12):1136–41.

98. Armstrong R et al. *Surgery.* 1973;74:570–4.

99. Navsaria PH et al. *World J Surg.* 2007;31(6):1345–51.

100. Levy R et al. *J Trauma.* 1995;38:273–7.

101. Steinig JP, Boyd CR. *Am Surg.* 1996;62(9):765–7.

102. Gonzalez RP et al. *J Trauma.* 1998;45(4):656–61.

103. Shannon F et al. *J Trauma.* 1988;28(7):989–94.

104. Fabian TC. *Am J Surg.* 1993;165(2A Suppl.):14S–9S.

105. Hospenthal DR et al. *J Trauma.* 2008;64(3 Suppl): S211–20.

106. Poret HA3rd et al. *J Trauma.* 1991;31(8):1085–8.

107. Velmahos GC et al. *Am Surg.* 2002;68(9):795–801.

108. Goldberg SR et al. *J Trauma Acute Care Surg.* 2012; 73(5 Suppl 4):S321–5.

109. Fullen W et al. *J Trauma.* 1972;12(282):289.

110. Greer CLT et al. *Am Surg.* 2013;79(2):119–27.

111. Fabian TC et al. *Surgery.* 1992;112(4):788–95.

112. Cornwell EE et al. *J Gastrointest Surg.* 1999;3(6):648.

113. Kirton OC et al. *J Trauma.* 2000;49(5):822–32.

114. Velmahos GC et al. *Arch Surg.* 2002;137(5):537–42.

115. Pathak R et al. *N Am J Med Sci.* 2016;8(4):191.

116. Goldberg JE, Steele SR. *Surg Clin North Am.* 2010; 90(1):173–84.

117. Ooi BS et al. *Aust N Z J Surg.* 1998;68(12):852–5.

118. Rodríguez-hermosa JI et al. *Color Dis.* 2007;9(6): 543–8.

119. Clarke D et al. *Color Dis.* 2010;7(1):98–103.

120. Kurer MA et al. *Color Dis.* 2010;12(9):851–61.

121. Lake JP et al. *Dis Colon Rectum.* 2004;47(10):1694–8.

122. Fry RD et al. *Dis Colon Rectum.* 1989;32(9):759–64.

123. Rispoli G et al. *Dis Colon Rectum.* 2000;43(11): 1632–4.

124. Berghoff KR, Franklin ME. *Dis Colon Rectum.* 2005; 48(10):1975–7.

125. Waraich NG et al. *N Z Med J.* 2007;120(1260):U2685.

126. Madiba TE, Moodley MM. *East Afr Med J.* 2003; 80(11):585–8.

127. Fernando R et al. *Cochrane Database Syst Rev.* 2006; 3(12):CD002866.

128. Fitzpatrick M et al. *Am J Obstet Gynecol.* 2000;183: 1220–4.

129. Brill SA, Margolin DA. *Semin Colon Rectal Surg.* 2005; 15(2):90–4.

130. Hellinger MD. *Surg Clin North Am.* 2002;82(6): 1253–60.

131. Cherry D, Greenwald M. Anal incontinence. In: Beck D, Wexner S. (eds.) *Fundamentals of Anorectal Surgery.* New York, NY: McGraw-Hill, 1992, pp. 104–30.

132. Wexner SD et al. *Dis Colon Rectum.* 2002;45(6): 809–18.

133. Madoff RD et al. *Gastroenterology.* 1999;116:549–56.

134. Wong WD et al. *Dis Colon Rectum.* 2002;45(9): 1139–53.

135. Halverson AL, Hull TL. *Dis Colon Rectum.* 2002;45(3): 345–8.

136. Jorge JM, Wexner SD. *Dis Colon Rectum.* 1993;36(1): 77–97.

137. Kudsk KA, Hanna MK. *World J Surg.* 2003;27(8): 895–900.

# 41

# Prevention and management of urologic complications after colorectal surgery

JACOB A. McCOY, J. CHRISTIAN WINTERS, AND SCOTT E. DELACROIX JR.

## CHALLENGING CASE

An elderly man presents with gross hematuria. Cystoscopic examination reveals a mass invading the left lateral bladder wall. Computed tomography (CT) scan of the abdomen and pelvis demonstrates a 6.6 cm pelvic mass originating from the sigmoid colon with bladder invasion and moderate left hydroureteronephrosis; colonoscopy with biopsy confirms sigmoid colon adenocarcinoma.

## CASE MANAGEMENT

The patient undergoes en bloc resection of the tumor via open sigmoid colectomy with distal ureterectomy and partial cystectomy. Four centimeters of left ureter is removed along with the left lateral bladder wall. Reconstruction of the left ureter and bladder is accomplished with a Boari flap, psoas hitch, and ureteral reimplantation over a JJ stent. A drain is placed in the region of the ureteroneocystotomy.

The patient progresses well postoperatively with low drain output and is removed prior to discharge. A cystogram performed 10 days postoperatively shows no evidence of leak from the bladder repair; his Foley catheter is removed at this time, and 3 weeks later the JJ stent is removed. Six months postoperatively, a renal ultrasound shows no evidence of hydronephrosis, and his creatinine is at his preoperative baseline.

## URETHRAL INJURIES

The most common urologic injury in surgery is the traumatic Foley catheter placement, often caused by premature inflation of the retention balloon within the prostatic urethra. A standard 16-French Foley catheter is an appropriate choice for the initial attempt for most patients. It is not necessary to "test" inflate the balloon prior to attempted placement, as this will increase the size and decrease the rigidity of the distal aspect of the catheter. In men with a known history of benign prostatic hyperplasia, a 16- or 18-French coude-tipped catheter may be helpful as an initial intervention.

It is essential to adequately lubricate the catheter and insert the catheter past the point at which urine is returned into catheter tubing prior to inflating the balloon. In men, it is recommended to grasp the penis firmly, hold it on stretch (toward the ceiling), and advance the Foley to the point at which the balloon inflation port projects off the side of the catheter ("hubbed"). This ensures that the balloon of the catheter has passed the prostatic urethra and entered the bladder prior to balloon inflation. Men with a tightly phimotic foreskin not allowing visualization of the glans may require gentle dilation of the phimotic band with a hemostat, or urologic consultation. It may be difficult to locate the urethral meatus of the obese female or in a woman with a posteriorly located meatus (postradiation for anal squamous cell carcinoma [SCC]). An often-employed method of dealing with difficult female anatomy is to block the anterior vaginal introitus with a finger, guiding the catheter ventrally toward the meatus. Intravesical placement of the catheter is confirmed with return of urine; if necessary, a Crede maneuver (manual pressure on the lower abdomen) can be performed. Patient dehydration secondary to nothing-by-mouth status or bowel preparation can make it difficult to determine proper placement if one only looks for urine return. If the entire catheter has been inserted and no urine has been returned, gentle irrigation of the catheter with a 60 cc catheter-tipped syringe prior to balloon inflation is recommended. If the catheter is in appropriate position, the catheter should easily irrigate and return fluid with aspiration. If irrigant goes in easily but does not return, a second syringe of saline may be injected and aspirated, as the bladder may be inadequately distended to allow for aspiration. If aspiration is not easily accomplished after 120 cc has been injected, the balloon should not be inflated. Intraoperative urologic consultation for evaluation and Foley catheter placement can be performed if the above measures fail.

A common algorithm employed by urologists for difficult Foley catheter placement includes first attempting a standard 16-French Foley. If the patient is male and there is suspicion for prostatic hypertrophy, an 18-French coude-tipped catheter is often employed next. For nonurologists, this may seem to be counterintuitive. The larger catheter provides more rigidity to pass the enlarged prostate. Cystoscopy can aid in catheter placement over a wire or urethral dilation, if necessary. If cystoscopy is unsuccessful, a suprapubic tube may be necessary and can be accomplished open or percutaneously.

Artificial urinary sphincters (AUSs) must be deactivated prior to insertion of a Foley catheter. Deactivation is a different mechanism than the normal operating "on" and "off" cycling. It is the author's experience that most patients do not know how to deactivate their AUS beyond the normal cycling mode. This deactivation must be performed prior to placement of a Foley catheter. Either a device representative or a urologist can deactivate the sphincter preoperatively as an outpatient or on the day of surgery. A 12-French Foley catheter can then be placed with lubrication and care to ensure placement in the bladder prior to inflation of the balloon. Failure to deactivate the AUS can result in erosion of the urinary sphincter by means of pressure necrosis between the Foley catheter and the sphincter device. Removal of the catheter should be done in standard fashion postoperatively. The patient should be able to reactivate their AUS by cycling it as they normally would. If unable to obtain urologic consultation prior to or intraoperatively, a suprapubic catheter can be placed either by open or percutaneous methods (preferably under ultrasound guidance to avoid components of AUS). Care must be taken to avoid intraabdominal components, which are normally placed in the retropubic space. An inflatable penile prosthesis (IPP) should not pose any additional difficulty in placing a urethral catheter if lubrication and the aforementioned guidelines are adhered to.

Urethral injuries are associated with extensive rectal neoplasm or any inflammatory processes that alter surgical planes, including pelvic radiation. Urethral injuries are usually identified at the time of surgery secondary to identification of the indwelling Foley catheter. Repair of a small urethral laceration can be performed with absorbable 3-0 or 4-0 synthetic absorbable suture (SAS) on a tapered needle and delayed Foley catheter removal. If the patient has had prior radiation or there is poor tissue composition, placement of either an omental flap or local tissue flap to support coverage of the repair is recommended. Injuries not identified at surgery can present postoperatively as urine drainage per rectum, pneumaturia, or fecaluria if fistula is present.

Sequelae from treatment and/or intraoperative injury can include delayed urethral stricture with difficult voiding and bladder outlet obstruction. A retrograde urethrogram will confirm the presence of a urethral stricture but must be done in the bilateral oblique as well as anterior-posterior views. A retrograde urethrogram (RUG) can be performed by affixing a 14-gauge angiocatheter to a 60 cc syringe filled with standard water-soluble contrast. A RUG should be performed around an indwelling catheter if already in place. If a radiographic enema is performed, water-soluble contrast is preferred, as it does not form concretions in the bladder. Spontaneous closure of a urinary fistula is rare, but a trial of conservative urinary diversion (Foley catheter) for 4–6 weeks for low-grade fistulas is recommended.

Urinary fistulas are staged according to location, size, and patient's history (1):

- *Stage 1*: Low (less than 4 cm from the anal verge and nonirradiated)
- *Stage 2*: High (greater than 4 cm for the anal verge and nonirradiated)
- *Stage 3*: Small (less than 2 cm irradiated fistula)
- *Stage 4*: Large (more than 2 cm irradiated fistula)
- *Stage 5*: Large (ischial decubitus fistula)

Enteric diversion by means of a diverting colostomy or ileostomy is recommended for stages 3–5. The choices for repair are diverse and depend on local tissue integrity and staging. A suprapubic catheter can be placed at the time of repair in addition to a Foley catheter for maximal drainage (2). Transanal rectal flap advancement can be used for stage 1 fistulae or in combination with other techniques for higher-stage fistulae (3). Other techniques described include:

- Transanal-transsphincteric approach (dorsal lithotomy anterior sphincterotomy) (4)
- York Mason/transsphincteric with rectal advancement flap (2,5,6) (jackknife posterior sphincterotomy)
- Perineal approach (jackknife or dorsal lithotomy) (7,8)
- Gracilis and rectus abdominus flaps (9,10)

Surgical selection is based on fistula stage and the experience of the reconstructive surgeon. Higher-stage fistulas and recurrences normally require regional flaps and possibly even urinary diversion (11). Outcomes for surgically repaired rectourethral fistulas are overall favorable, with recurrences mostly dependent on stage and appropriate choice in initial surgical treatment. Success rates vary from greater than 90% for low-grade fistulas to 70% for higher-grade fistulas (1–11). A retrograde urethrogram around a Foley catheter ("pericatheter RUG") at 4–6 weeks postoperatively can be performed prior to urethral catheter removal. Alternatively, a voiding cystourethrogram can be performed through a suprapubic tube after Foley catheter removal.

## BLADDER INJURIES

The location of the bladder within the pelvis and its close proximity to the sigmoid colon and rectum predisposes the bladder to injury during surgery of the colon and rectum. Iatrogenic injuries to the bladder can be staged as follows (12,14):

*Grade 1:* Contusion, intramural hematoma, or partial-thickness laceration
*Grade 2:* Extraperitoneal bladder wall laceration <2 cm
*Grade 3:* Extraperitoneal >2 cm or intraperitoneal <2 cm bladder laceration
*Grade 4:* Intraperitoneal bladder wall laceration >2 cm
*Grade 5:* Intra- or extraperitoneal bladder wall laceration extending into the bladder neck or trigone (near ureteral orifice)

Risk factors for bladder injury include any process that distorts tissue planes and reduces surgical exposure. This includes adhesions or scarring from prior surgery, radiation, malignant infiltration, chronic inflammation, or infection. Injuries can be apparent intraoperatively or present in a delayed fashion. Intraoperative identification of the injury allows for immediate cystorrhaphy usually in a two-layer fashion (13). In open or robotic surgery, the mucosa is closed in a running fashion using a 3-0 SAS followed by a seromuscular running 2-0 SAS. The bladder can then be irrigated to ensure a watertight closure. In the laparoscopic setting, a running one-layer closure is performed using a 2-0 SAS to close all three layers of the bladder. Care must be taken to ensure closure of the mucosal layer in the laparoscopic one-layer technique. Again, the bladder should be irrigated to ensure a watertight closure.

Repair can also differ depending on the location of the injury. Anterior and dome injuries can be repaired primarily as above. Posterior injuries involving the trigone or those near the ureteral orifices (possible grade 5) dictate a more thorough inspection of the bladder and an assurance of ureteral integrity prior to closure. This is done through an anterior cystotomy in the sagittal plane extending down toward the pubic symphysis. This will allow placement of a Balfour or Bookwalter self-retaining retractor and placement of bilateral ureteral open-ended catheters. Giving the patient indigo carmine or methylene blue with Lasix can aid in identification of the ureteral orifices by visualization of blue efflux. Closure of the posterior bladder injury can then be done from the bladder lumen, closing the muscular layer first using 2-0 SAS followed by closure of the mucosal layer using 3-0 SAS. The anterior cystotomy is then closed as described previously. In cases where neoadjuvant radiotherapy has been used, an interposition of omentum or perivesical fascia/peritoneal flap is prudent to decrease the risk of fistula formation.

A bladder injury will usually manifest in the early postoperative period, especially after removal of Foley catheter.

The injury can present as drainage from surgical incision, increased output from surgical drain, vaginal leakage, ileus, apparent oliguria, urinary ascites (with increasing potassium, blood urea nitrogen, and serum creatinine secondary to reabsorption of urine through parietal peritoneum in the case of an unrecognized intraperitoneal injury), pneumaturia, or fecaluria in the cases of an enterovesical or colovesical fistula. Delayed urine leaks can be diagnosed radiographically by fluoroscopic cystogram or the CT cystogram (15). Traditional cystogram is performed by obtaining a prefilling film, placing a catheter, and distending the bladder with 200–300 cc of contrast, obtaining anterior-posterior and lateral films with the bladder distended, and obtaining a postdrainage film. A CT cystogram should similarly be performed with *active retrograde filling* of the bladder and adequate distention of the bladder. Passive opacification from IV contrast or inadequate retrograde distention of the bladder is usually inadequate to identify smaller bladder injuries.

The development of a colovesical or enterovesical fistula is a delayed complication of cystotomy and/or pelvic radiation and/or inflammatory bowel disease (16,17). Abdominal-pelvic CT scan with oral and/or rectal water-soluble contrast has a greater sensitivity than cystoscopy in diagnosing an enterovesical fistula (Figure 41.1). The most sensitive test to diagnose an enterovesical or colovesical fistula is the poppy seed test (17). A 1.25-ounce container of poppy seed is mixed into a 12-ounce beverage or a 6-ounce serving of yogurt and orally ingested by the patient. Urine is visually inspected for 48 hours, during which time identification of poppy seeds in the urine is a positive confirmatory test for gastrointestinal fistula to the urinary tract. The sensitivity and specificity in prior studies were 100% (17). This test does not provide anatomical information as in the case of the abdominal-pelvic CT scan, but it is a much more cost-effective screening test in patients with equivocal symptoms

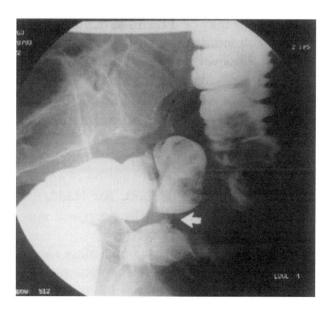

Figure 41.1 Enterovesical fistula (arrow).

($5 versus more than $600) (17). When using barium contrast, it is the authors' recommendation to empty the bladder after a fistula is diagnosed, as there have been reports of barium concretions within the bladder.

## URETERAL INJURIES

Injury to the ureter is one of the most common intraoperative urologic injuries in colorectal surgery. The incidence of iatrogenic injury to the ureter is reportedly from 1% to 10% (18–22). Iatrogenic ureteral injuries are of four types: laceration, ligation, devascularization, and thermal or energy related. Optimal treatment is early recognition and repair of any ureteral injury.

## ANATOMY

Iatrogenic ureteral injuries in colorectal surgery usually occur in three distinct locations: at the takeoff of the inferior mesenteric artery, where the infundibulopelvic ligament/uterine vessels cross the pelvic brim, and between the lateral rectal ligaments (Figure 41.2) (23). The course of the ureter begins posterior to the renal artery around the vertebral level L3 and continues along the anterior edge of the psoas muscle. The gonadal vessels cross the ureter from lateral to medial in this region. The ureter next passes over the iliac vessels, generally marking the bifurcation of the common iliac into internal and external iliac arteries

(24). Of greatest importance to the surgeon is that arterial branches to the abdominal ureter approach from the medial direction, whereas arterial branches to the pelvic ureter approach from the lateral direction (24). For the abdominal ureter, these branches originate from the renal artery, gonadal artery, abdominal aorta, and common iliac artery. After entering the pelvis, additional small arterial branches may arise from the internal iliac artery or its branches, and also from the middle rectal and vaginal arteries (24).

The ureter will tend to adhere to the peritoneum during its reflection rather than staying adherent to the psoas muscle and underlying tissue. The ureter can be identified by visualization and by its peristaltic activity. Gentle pressure applied to the ureter will frequently cause peristalsis—termed the Kelly sign. The right ureter is adjacent to the cecum, terminal ileum, and appendix. The left ureter is related to the descending and sigmoid colon and their mesenteries.

## PREVENTION

Ureteral catheterization is used to aid in identification of the ureters and to help identify ureteral injury, but catheters do not prevent ureteral injury. The clinical value of prophylactic ureteral catheter placement prior to 162 laparoscopic segmental left and right colectomies was assessed by Nam et al. There were no complications from placement of ureteral catheters (18). Postoperative urinary tract infection was not increased. Total operative time was increased by 11.3 minutes. The ureteral catheter group included more difficult

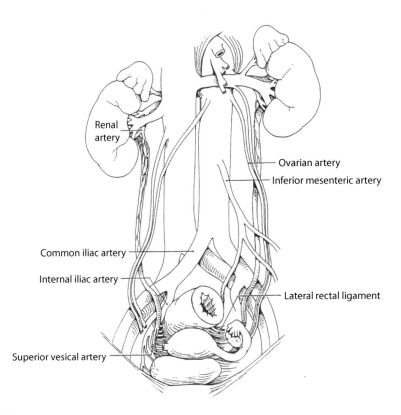

Figure 41.2 Anatomy of the ureter.

cases, including patients with Crohn disease and diverticulitis. There were no ureteral injuries in any of the 162 patients (18). An earlier study deemed ureteral catheterization necessary in 27.5% of patients when assessed in a standardized retrospective fashion (22). There were four complications, presumably due to ureteral catheterization, which included renal colic, oliguria, and one case of anuria attributed to ureteral edema after removal of the ureteral catheters (20,25). Chahin et al. studied lighted ureteral stents/catheters placed prior to laparoscopic colectomy in 66 patients (20). The most common complication was self-limiting hematuria in 98.4% of patients with an average duration of 2.5 days for unilateral stenting and 3.3 days with bilateral stenting.

It is the authors' opinion that the choice for ureteral stenting is a surgeon preference and depends on multiple variables, including complexity of case, anatomy, and experience—especially with the laparoscopic approach in a hostile abdomen. With greater operative experience, iatrogenic ureteral injury decreases. In a study by Larach et al., the incidence of conversions due to iatrogenic injuries showed a decline from 7.3% in the early group to 1.4% in the later experience group (26). Once again, ureteral catheters have not been shown to decrease ureteral injuries but do aid in identification of the ureters, and most importantly, of an iatrogenic ureteral injury. Ureteral catheters can be used to aid in diagnosis of ureteral injury by retrograde injection of methylene blue through the ureteral catheter or visualization of the catheter itself. They can also be used to place a retrograde wire under fluoroscopic guidance for placement of an indwelling ureteral double-J stent after identification of an injury.

## TYPES OF INJURY

### Laceration/transection

A laceration or transection of the proximal or mid-ureter can usually be repaired with primary anastomosis (ureteroureterostomy with spatulated ends), ureteral stent, and placement of a closed suction drain in the area of the repair (Figure 41.3).

### Ligation

If a ligation injury is apparent intraoperatively, the clamp or tie can be removed followed by ureteral stent placement for up to 1 month. The patient should undergo repeat renal imaging at 3 months to assess for hydronephrosis to ensure a ureteral stricture has not developed. If the injury is not identified until postoperatively, a retrograde ureterogram and stent placement or percutaneous nephrostomy tube placement may be needed prior to surgical correction.

### Devascularization

A devascularization injury will not be evident intraoperatively and results from the sacrifice of the segmental ureteral blood supply. Intraoperatively a devascularized ureter

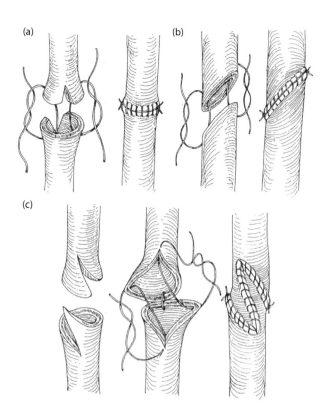

Figure 41.3 Ureteroureterostomy. **(a)** Spatulation of ureteral margins and placement of running locked sutures. Preferred technique. **(b)** Oblique anastomosis. **(c)** Spiral anastomosis.

may appear discolored, lack peristalsis, and may not bleed at a transected site. The irradiated ureter is especially susceptible to this type of injury, as the normal healthy ureter has numerous collaterals and is very resistant to devascularization, even with extensive dissection. The anatomy of the blood supply to the ureter (as previously described) should be known as the surgeon is carrying his or her dissection over the pelvic brim. Postradiation, many delayed ureteral strictures are not necessarily due to an iatrogenic injury but rather due to "treatment effect" in the surgical field.

### Thermal

Thermal injuries will usually present in the early postoperative period with either fistula or stricture formation. These injuries are repaired in the same fashion as above depending on the location of the injury. Many laparoscopic surgeons use alternatives to monopolar dissectors because of the risk of thermal injury and delayed presentation of injuries. Even with these newer technologies, collateral tissue damage can be produced depending on the energy level and duration of exposure. In animal models, use of the ultrasonic dissector (Ethicon or USSC) at a level of 3 for less than 10 seconds per burst resulted in little to no collateral tissue damage (27). When using an ultrasonic dissector at levels of 4 or 5, energy time should be reduced to less than 5 seconds to prevent collateral damage due to spread of thermal energy (27).

## Location-dependent repair of the iatrogenic ureteral injury

Repair of the injured ureter does not necessitate open conversion if a urologist is available with advanced laparoscopic skills. The basic principles of a ureteral anastomosis are as follows: a tension-free anastomosis; well-vascularized spatulated ends anastomosed over an indwelling ureteral stent; use of an absorbable suture material 4-0 or 5-0; and placement of a closed drain near the area of the repair. Do not use nonabsorbable suture, as stone formation is inherent with these nonabsorbable materials.

### Proximal one-third

The boundaries of the proximal one-third ureter are the ureteropelvic junction (level of the kidney) and the pelvic brim (sacroiliac joint on pelvic X-ray). Repairs of injuries to the proximal ureter depend on the length of the damaged segment. Simple spatulated ureteroureterostomy ("U-U") with ureteral stent placement is the preferred method of repair if there is significant length of the uninjured ureter to allow for a tension-free anastomosis. A nephropexy can be performed to bring the kidney caudad to decrease tension, if needed. In cases with long segments of damaged ureters, a bowel interposition with tapered ileum or an appendiceal interposition can be used (Figure 41.4). At specialized centers, autotransplantation with reanastamosis to the iliac vessels and native more distal ureter can be performed.

### Middle one-third

The preferred technique for midureteral repair is ureteroureterostomy, either laparoscopically or through the open technique. Care must be taken to maintain a tension-free anastomosis. This can usually be accomplished with a psoas hitch (Figure 41.5). The bladder is mobilized by ligating the superior vesical pedicle on the contralateral side of the injury. It is prudent to locate the contralateral ureter and ensure its integrity prior to this maneuver. The bladder can then be opened through an anterior cystotomy and then secured to the psoas muscle and tendon using several 0-0 SAS sutures through the seromuscular layer of the bladder. Care must be taken not to include the genitofemoral nerve, which is located within the belly of the psoas muscle. Suture should be placed in a linear fashion in line with the fascicles of the muscle. The ureter can then be tunneled by passing a clamp from the lumen of the bladder through all layers of the bladder and then withdrawn with the distal aspect of the proximal salvaged ureter. The ureter should then be widely spatulated, and interrupted mucosal stitches (4-0 SAS) should be used circumferentially to create the neo-orifice. A ureteral stent can also be placed. The anterior cystotomy is then closed as previously described. A closed suction drain and Foley catheter are then left in place.

The Boari flap is another effective yet more complex method for replacing an extensive loss of the distal and

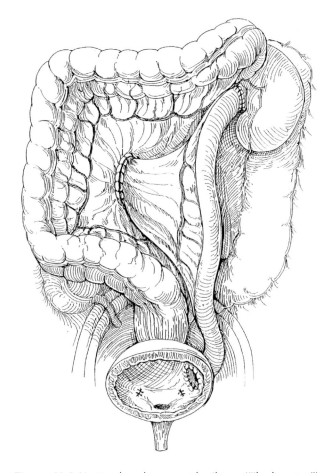

Figure 41.4 Ureteral replacement by ileum ("ileal ureter"). Left colon retracted medially. Ileum brought through a hiatus in the colonic mesentery. Ileal ureter is in retroperitoneal position.

midureter. A flap of the anterior bladder wall is raised in a rectangular fashion and affixed to the psoas muscle in the same fashion as a psoas hitch. The ureter is tunneled through the most proximal portion of the flap, and a neo-orifice is created as previously described. The bladder flap is then tubularized and closed in a two-layer fashion using running 3-0 SAS to close the mucosa, followed by closure of the seromuscular layer using 2-0 SAS (Figure 41.6). Prolonged bladder drainage with a Foley catheter for 7–14 days is warranted.

The final option is the transureteroureterostomy. The surgeon tunnels the injured ureter under the posterior peritoneum overlying the great vessels. This allows a spatulated end-to-side anastomosis of the injured ureter to the patient's contralateral native uninjured ureter (Figure 41.7). Contraindications include distal ureteral obstruction in the uninjured ureter or a history of nephrolithiasis (relative contraindication) (48).

### Distal one-third

The procedure of choice for the lower one-third ureteral injury is the ureteroneocystotomy (ureteral reimplant). This may be accomplished primarily for very distal ureteral injuries or may require a psoas hitch or Boari flap for patients with small capacity bladders and injuries near the iliac vessels (24).

## Delayed recognition

Ureteral injury may not be recognized at the time of surgery, especially if ureteral catheters were not placed. Urine leaks often present as urinoma, azotemia, ileus, sepsis, high drain output, or flank pain. Cross-sectional imaging, especially with a delayed contrast phase, may be helpful in identifying a urine leak or ureteral obstruction. If a urine leak is suspected due to high drain output, the drain fluid may be sent for a creatinine level; results two to five times that of serum (or higher) are indicative of the presence of urine. Cystoscopy with retrograde urography is the most sensitive method of identifying a ureteral injury and demonstrates the exact location of a ureteral injury and also allows attempted retrograde stent placement. If a stent cannot successfully be placed retrograde, either due to stricture/ligation or a significant ureteral disruption, a percutaneous nephrostomy tube can be placed. Repair of an injury may be performed at any point once the patient is stable for a return to the operating room.

## RENAL INJURIES

Direct renal injury is a rare occurrence in colorectal surgery. McAnich et al. have reported that 90% of renal injuries can be managed without nephrectomy (28). Though this work does not address iatrogenic injuries, the principle of renal salvage should be adhered to. Every attempt to evaluate the

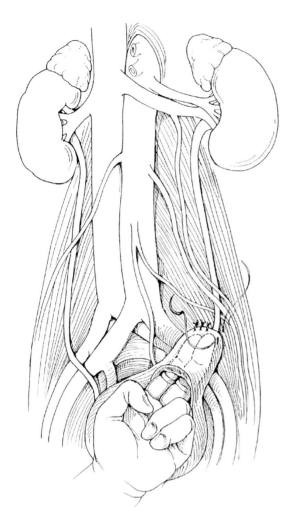

Figure 41.5 Psoas bladder hitch. Mobilized bladder being anchored to psoas muscle, and the ureter is reimplanted.

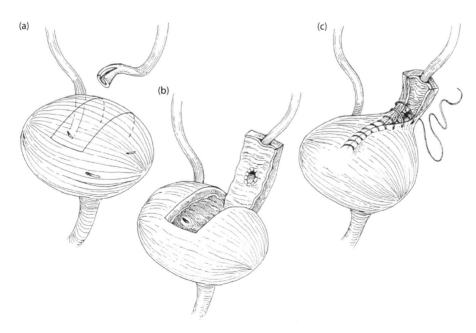

Figure 41.6 Boari or bladder flap procedure. **(a)** Creation of tapered bladder flap, based posteriorly. **(b)** Submucosal ureteral reimplantation. **(c)** Closure of bladder flap.

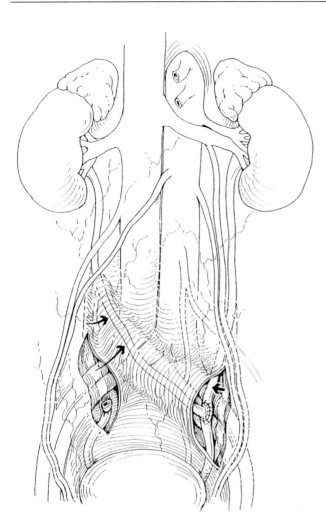

Figure 41.7 Transureteroureterostomy. Right-to-left, showing retroperitoneal tunnel anterior to the great vessels.

extent of the injury as well as assess the entire genitourinary tract should be done prior to undertaking repair. A one-shot intravenous pyelogram (IVP) can confirm contralateral renal function. This can be done by giving the patient 2 mL of contrast per kg IV up to a maximum of 150 mL. An on-the-table KUB is then done 10 minutes later. Simple palpation of the contralateral kidney does not ensure function. The literature is full of anomalous solitary kidneys that were removed, necessitating dialysis or transplantation (29,30). Pelvic kidneys have an anomalous blood supply generally arising from multiple arteries along the aorta and iliac vessels. Ten percent are solitary and may easily be taken for a pelvic mass, as they are not reniform and have a discoid shape (23). If calyceal or renal pelvis injury is suspected, a retrograde pyelogram can be performed.

Once the injury is well defined, repair can be decided. Minor renal lacerations or penetrating injuries may be repaired primarily with absorbable sutures and re-retroperitonealized with perinephric fat, omentum, or hemostatic materials. Hilar control is paramount if an attempt at repair is to be performed. If the injury is to the collecting system or renal parenchyma

and the ensuing blood loss is able to be managed by pressure and hemostatic agents alone, a ureteral stent and Foley catheter can be placed from below and the area drained with a closed suction to prevent urinoma formation. Conservative management is optimal as renorrhaphy, and exploration can lead to unnecessary nephrectomy.

The left renal vessels are located posterior to the mesentery between the inferior mesenteric vein and aorta. If a major vascular injury occurs and the patient's intraoperative condition permits, every attempt should be made to reestablish vascular integrity.

## BLADDER DYSFUNCTION

The reported incidence of difficulty in reestablishing micturition ranges from 15% to 25% after low anterior resection and up to 50% after abdominoperineal resection (31). A thorough understanding of the neuroanatomy of the pelvis and the technique of total mesorectal excision (TME) and autonomic nerve preservation (ANP) can enable both local tumor control and preservation of autonomic nerve structures, thus reducing the risk of urogenital dysfunction (34,35). Favorable oncologic outcomes have been reported for these nerve-sparing techniques (35–39). APR, when performed in accordance with the principles of TME and ANP, ensures the greatest likelihood of resecting all regional disease while preserving both urinary and sexual function (39). Locally advanced tumors and preoperative chemotherapy and radiation can make identification of the autonomic nerves and plexus more difficult and sometimes impossible (34). The most common sequela from autonomic nerve damage during surgery of the colon and rectum is detrusor denervation and areflexia. This normally requires clean intermittent catheterization, Foley catheter placement, or suprapubic tube placement depending on the overall dexterity and functional status of the patient. Damage to the pudendal nerve or its branches from Alcock canal can result in weakening of the striated urinary sphincter with resultant stress urinary incontinence and intrinsic sphincter deficiency (rare).

Detrusor function (bladder contractility) is predominantly mediated by the parasympathetic nervous system, namely, the pelvic nerve (33). These parasympathetic fibers originate from the spinal cord at the S2-S4 level. Pelvic nerve branches are redundant within the pelvis. The main trunks to the bladder and proximal urethra course in the visceral pelvic fascia, also called the posterior endopelvic fascia (33). These preganglionic autonomic fibers course alongside the superior vesical vasculature to synapse with postganglionic autonomic fibers within the bladder wall. Multiple pelvic preganglionic nerves pass laterally from the pelvic floor over the rectal fascia investments en route medially to the bladder (Figure 41.8) (33).

Sympathetic innervation to the bladder arises at the level of L2-L4 with a presynaptic fiber to the sympathetic

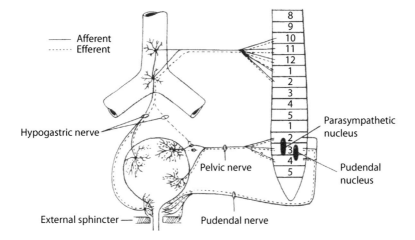

Figure 41.8 Innervation of lower urinary tract.

ganglion adjacent to the spinal cord. Synapse occurs in the ganglion, and a long postganglionic fiber travels through the pelvis to innervate the bladder. Through different end receptors located within the bladder, the sympathetic component of the autonomic nervous system helps to cause relaxation of the bladder body (compliance for storage) and contraction of the trigone and bladder neck at resting/storage states.

Somatic motor innervation to the striated pelvic floor musculature and sphincter arises from the S2-S4 level and travels via the pudendal nerve through Alcock canal. The perineal branches of the pudendal nerve follow the perineal artery into the superficial pouch to supply the ischiocavernosus, bulbospongiosus, and transverse perinei muscles. Some branches continue anteriorly to supply sensation to the posterior scrotum and perineum. Additional perineal branches pass deep to the perineal membrane to supply the levator ani and striated urethral sphincter (40).

In the study by Junginger on TME, identification of the pelvic autonomic nerves was complete in 72%, partial identification in 10.7%, and not at all in 17.3% of patients (34). Univariate analysis showed that the case number (experience), gender (males greater than females), and T-stage (T1-2 versus T3-4) exerted an independent influence on the achievement of complete pelvic nerve identification. In this series of 150 patients with adenocarcinoma of the rectum, identification and preservation of the autonomic nerves were achieved in a majority of patients and led to the prevention of urinary dysfunction (4.5% versus 38.5%, $p < 0.001$) (34).

A Swiss group investigated the incidence and risk factors for postoperative urinary retention in 513 consecutive patients undergoing colorectal surgery with early Foley removal due to an enhanced recovery pathway (49). Fourteen percent of these patients experienced urinary retention postoperatively; male gender and postoperative thoracic epidural anesthesia were independent risk factors for retention. Complications of urinary retention included decreased mobilization, increased pain, and longer duration of IV hydration.

Management of the postoperative patient with urinary retention varies widely between urologists. Of paramount importance in treating urinary retention is accurate documentation of voided volumes and postvoid residuals, determined either by ultrasound (bladder scan) or initial urine return after catheterization. A lack of voiding may be due to oliguria rather than retention. After a patient's Foley catheter is removed, a period of 6–8 hours is usually given to the patient to allow for spontaneous voiding. A bladder scan may be performed if the patient has not urinated after this trial, or sooner if the patient feels an urge to void and is unable to. It is the authors' practice to leave a Foley catheter indwelling for a period of 48–72 hours after a failed voiding trial with a volume greater than 400 mL to allow the bladder to decompress and recover from distention. A voiding trial may again be attempted in the same fashion afterward.

Repeated voiding trial failure may be an indication of bladder dysfunction. Management includes teaching clean intermittent catheterization (CIC) or leaving an indwelling Foley and having the patient return for full urodynamic evaluation around 2–3 months postoperatively. Urodynamics can be a combination of pressure/flow studies with electromyography tracings under fluoroscopic observation and, sometimes, urethral pressure profiling. It may take up to 6 months for bladder function to return to its new baseline, and CIC may be a lifelong therapy. CIC is performed with a 12- to 14-French low-friction catheter every 4–6 hours, and the duration can be adjusted based on the storage pressures and bladder capacity at the time of urodynamic evaluation. There are no drugs (including Bethanechol) with acceptable pharmacokinetics and side-effect profiles that have been shown to clinically increase/improve contractility in the bladder.

In a meta-analysis, Branagan et al. reviewed the colorectal surgery literature on suprapubic catheter placement followed by voiding trial versus urethral catheter placement and standard trial of voiding postoperatively (31). They found favorable results for the suprapubic catheter in terms of incidence of urinary tract infection, and a shorter magnitude and duration of pain and discomfort. The ability to simply clamp and unclamp the suprapubic catheter makes management and voiding trials relatively simple, especially in patients unable to perform CIC or those at especially high risk for postoperative bladder dysfunction. Suprapubic catheters are particularly useful if autonomic nerves have to be removed during radical pelvic surgery, because normal voiding may be difficult to reestablish and may take several months to recover. In the select patient with voiding dysfunction and delayed recovery, suprapubic catheter placement results in less morbidity and patient discomfort than urethral catheterization (32).

## SEXUAL DYSFUNCTION

In the urologic community, an emphasis on postoperative sexual function has arisen from studies by Walsh on the anatomic retropubic prostatectomy with preservation of the neurovascular bundles that contribute to erectile function (41). Most recently, postoperative penile rehabilitation is being performed in multiple settings with a theoretical benefit of reducing the time of neuropraxia to the penis and prevention of apoptosis-induced atrophy. Although no standardization exists with these rehabilitation programs, patients are very interested, and at the authors' institution this is discussed preoperatively. Sexual dysfunction has long been associated with rectal surgery in both male and female patients. In male patients, erectile dysfunction is reported in 5%–65% of patients, and ejaculatory dysfunction is reported in 14%–69% (43). Damage to the sacral splanchnic nerve (parasympathetic) or the hypogastric nerve (sympathetic) during surgery is the proposed mechanism of injury (43).

Sexual dysfunction is a broad term that encompasses failure of arousal, erection, orgasm, ejaculation, and emission. Complaints from patients after radical pelvic surgery are usually mixed. Erection is parasympathetically mediated and is governed by impulses traveling along the nervi ergentes (S2-S4) (41). The pelvic plexus is located retroperitoneally on the lateral surface of the rectum 5–11 cm from the anal verge with its midpoint located at the tip of the seminal vesicles. The preganglionic fibers from the nervi ergentes coalesce on the pelvic wall with contributions from the sympathetic fibers from the hypogastric plexus (T10-L4). Damage to the sympathetic plexus will result in problems with ejaculation, including retrograde ejaculation or anejaculation.

In a study by Henderson et al., 81 women and 99 men who had undergone curative rectal cancer surgery were given a validated sexual function questionnaire (42). Thirty-two percent of women and 50% of men were sexually active compared with 61% and 91% preoperatively. Twenty-nine percent of women and 49% of men reported that "surgery made their sexual lives worse." Specific sexual problems in women were libido 41%, arousal 29%, lubrication 56%, orgasm 35%, and dyspareunia 46%. In men complaints were impotence/erectile dysfunction 84%, libido 47%, orgasm difficulty 41%, and ejaculation difficulties 43%. Patients seldom remembered discussing sexual risks preoperatively

and were seldom referred or treated for symptoms postoperatively. Sexual dysfunction should be discussed with rectal cancer patients, and when appropriate, efforts to prevent and treat sexual dysfunction should be instituted (42).

In a study by Nam et al. of patients undergoing TME and ANP for rectal carcinoma, factors that most affected postoperative sexual dysfunction were age older than 60 (sexual desire, $p = 0.019$), time period within 6 months of surgery (erectile function, $p = 0.04$), and lower rectal cancer (erectile function $p = 0.02$) (43). In the urologic literature, penile "rehabilitation" is started at approximately 1 month postoperatively with evidence suggesting that lack of natural erections during this period of time produces cavernosal hypoxia (44). Prolonged periods of cavernosal hypoxia induce fibrosis, which later increases the incidence of venous leak and thus potentiates long-term or permanent erectile dysfunction.

In consultation with a urologist, sexual dysfunction in the man can be treated with many different modalities. For erectile dysfunction, oral phosphodiesterase inhibitors, intraurethral vasoactive suppositories, intracavernosal injections, vacuum erection devices, and implantable devices are all options. For ejaculatory dysfunction in a patient desiring pregnancy, semen may be collected from the bladder in the case of retrograde ejaculation. Sympathomimetic agents may also be used. For refractory cases, electrovibratory ejaculation can be performed at specialized centers. It is important to discuss sexual function with the patient both pre- and postoperatively, as there are many therapeutic options that have been shown to be very satisfactory for both partners.

## ARTIFICIAL DEVICES

Thousands of AUS and IPP have been implanted worldwide for the treatment of stress urinary incontinence and erectile dysfunction, respectively (Figure 41.9). The IPP has one to three components, while the AUS has three components. The three-component systems will have a reservoir, pump, and cuff or prosthesis that is interconnected with reinforced tubing. These devices are silicone but develop a capsule around them after implantation. The reservoir is typically found suprapubically in the space of Retzius. One should make every attempt to refrain from entering this capsule and to prevent contamination of these silicone devices. If contamination occurs, either device removal or salvage therapy with copious antibiotic irrigation is recommended. A urologist should be consulted if available. The risk of device contamination, postoperative infection, and damage to the tubing necessitating device removal or reoperation should be discussed with the patient preoperatively. It is the authors' practice to be very conservative in patients with AUS, and we recommend all patients have their device deactivated by a urologist familiar with the AUS prior to placement of a urethral catheter. There are numerous reports of

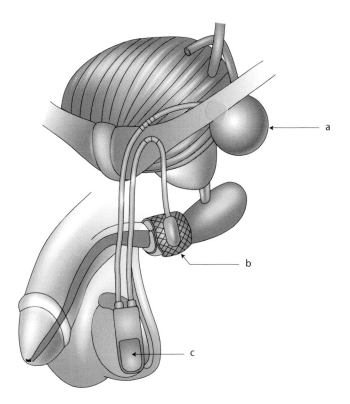

Figure 41.9 Artificial urinary sphincter (AVS-800);
American Medical Systems Inc, Minnetonka, Minnesota.
**(a)** Reservoir. **(b)** Cuff. **(c)** Pump.

patients "turning off" their own AUS, when in reality, they only cycle them followed by urethral catheterization at the time of surgery and resulting device erosion. This is a medicolegal issue that usually can be averted with a preoperative consultation with a urologist.

The U.S. Food and Drug Administration approved sacral neuromodulator is the Interstim device manufactured by Medtronic Corp. (45). It is approved for use in patients with refractory urgency and frequency or nonobstructive, nonneurogenic urinary retention. A tined lead is placed through the S3 foramen, and an implanted generator is placed in a pocket created in the gluteal area/upper hip. The manufacturer recommends against using electrocautery near the generator and not performing magnetic resonance imaging (MRI) on any patients with the Interstim device. It is the authors' practice to turn off the device with a Medtronic supplied magnet prior to any radical pelvic operation. In thin patients, appropriate padding must be applied to the area of the implanted generator. MRI is contraindicated, although there has been at least one study to show deactivation of the device prior to MRI to be safe (46,47).

## REFERENCES

1. Rivera R et al. *J Urol* 2007;177:586–8.
2. Fengler SA, Abcarian H. *Am J Surg* 1997;173:213–7.
3. Dreznik Z et al. *Colorectal Dis* 2003;5:53–5.
4. Culkin DJ, Ramsey CE. *J Urol* 2003;169:2181–3.
5. Mason AY. *Proc R Soc Med* 1970;63(suppl.):91–4.
6. Crippa A et al. *Clinics* 2007;62:699–704.
7. Yousseff AH et al. *J Urol* 1999;161:1498–500.
8. Visser BC et al. *JACS* 2006;195:138–43.
9. Zmora O et al. *Dis Colon Rectum.* 2006;49(9):1316–21.
10. Bruce RG et al. *J Urol* 2000;163:1212–5.
11. Elliott SP et al. *J Urol* 2006;176:2508–13.
12. Moore EE et al. *J Trauma* 1992;33:337–9.
13. Armenakas NA et al. *JACS* 2004;198:78–82.
14. Van Goor H. *Colorectal Dis* 2007;9(Suppl 2):25–34.
15. Deck AJ et al. *J Urol* 2000;164:43–6.
16. Jarrett TW, Vaughan Jr ED. *J Urol* 1995;153:44–6.
17. Kwon EO et al. *J Urol* 2008;179:1425–7.
18. Nam YS, Wexner SD. *J Korean Med Sci* 2002;17:633–5.
19. Larach SW, Gallagher JT. *Semin Surg Oncol* 2000;18:265–8.
20. Chahin F et al. *JSLS* 2002;6:49–52.
21. Scala A et al. *Colorectal Dis* 2007;9:701–5.
22. Fry et al. *Arch Surg.* 1983;118:454–7.
23. Perlmutter AD et al. Anomalies of the upper urinary tract. In Harrison JH, Gittees RF, Perlmutter AD et al. (eds.) *Campbell's Urology,* 4th Edition. Philadelphia, PA: WB Saunders, 1979, pp. 1309–98.
24. Anderson KJ et al. Surgical anatomy of the retroperitoneum, adrenals, kidneys, and ureters. In *Campbell-Walsh Urology,* 9th Edition. New York, NY: Elsevier, 2007, pp. 34–7.
25. Kyzer S, Gordon PH. *Am Surg* 1994;60:212–6.
26. Larach SW et al. *Dis Colon Rectum* 1997;40:592–6.
27. Emam TA, Cuschieri A. *Ann Surg* 2003;237:186–91.
28. McAninch JW et al. *J Urol* 1991;145:932–7.
29. Granat M et al. *Am J Obstet Gynecol* 1980;138:233–5.
30. Zusmer NR et al. *Rev Interam Radiol* 1980;5:95–6.
31. Branagan GW, Moran BJ. *Dis Colon Rectum* 2002;45:1104–8.
32. Chaudhri S et al. *Dis Colon Rectum* 2006;49:1066–70.
33. Hollabaugh Jr RS et al. *Dis Colon Rectum* 2000;43:1390–7.
34. Junginger T et al. *Dis Colon Rectum* 2003;46:621–8.
35. Shirouzu K et al. *Dis Colon Rectum* 2004;47:1442–7.
36. Saito N et al. *World J Surg* 1999;23:1062–8.
37. Yamakoshi H et al. *Dis Colon Rectum* 1997;40:1079–84.
38. Moriya Y et al. *World J Surg* 1997;21:728–32.
39. Enker WE et al. *World J Surg* 1997;21:715–20.
40. Brooks. *Anatomy for the Lower Urinary Tract and Male Genitalia.* 2;p69. *Campbell-Walsh Urology,* 9th Edition. New York, NY: Elsevier, 2007.
41. Walsh PC, Schlegel PN. *Ann Surg* 1988;208:391–400.
42. Hendren SK et al. *Ann Surg* 2005;242:212–23.
43. Kim NK et al. *Dis Colon Rectum* 2002;45:1178–85.
44. Raina R et al. *Int J Impot Res* 2008;20:121–6.
45. Interstim Device Trademarked by Medtronic Corp.
46. Holley et al. *Presentation at SESAUA Annual Meeting,* Orlando, Florida, USA, 2007.
47. Elkelini MS, Hassouna MM. *Eur Urol* 2006;50:311–6.
48. Delacroix SE, Winters JC. *Clin Colon Rectal Surg* 2010;23(2):104–12.
49. Grass F et al. *J Surg Res* 2017;207:70–6.

# Index

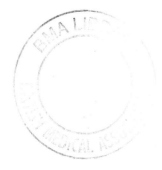